Y0-AET-119

HANDBOOK OF TREATMENT OF MENTAL DISORDERS IN CHILDHOOD AND ADOLESCENCE

HANDBOOK OF

BENJAMIN B. WOLMAN, *Editor*

JAMES EGAN, *Co-Editor*

ALAN O. ROSS, *Co-Editor*

TREATMENT OF MENTAL DISORDERS IN CHILDHOOD AND ADOLESCENCE

PRENTICE-HALL, INC., ENGLEWOOD CLIFFS, NEW JERSEY 07632

Library of Congress Cataloging in Publication Data

Main entry under title:
Handbook of treatment of mental disorders in childhood and adolescence.

Bibliography: p.
Includes index.
1. Child psychotherapy—Handbooks, manuals, etc.
2. Mentally ill children—Handbooks, manuals, etc.
3. Adolescent psychiatry—Handbooks, manuals, etc.
I. Wolman, Benjamin B. II. Ross, Alan O. III. Egan, James. [DNLM: 1. Mental disorders—In infancy and childhood—Handbooks. 2. Mental disorders—Therapy—Handbooks. WS350 H236]
RJ504.H364 1978 618.9'28'91 77-7928
ISBN 0-13-382234-6

HANDBOOK
OF TREATMENT OF MENTAL DISORDERS
IN CHILDHOOD AND ADOLESENCE

Benjamin B. Wolman, Editor
James Egan & Alan O. Ross, Co-Editors

Printed in the United States of America

10 9 8 7 6 5 4 3 2

PRENTICE-HALL INTERNATIONAL, INC., *London*
PRENTICE-HALL OF AUSTRALIA PTY. LIMITED, *Sydney*
PRENTICE-HALL OF CANADA, LTD., *Toronto*
PRENTICE-HALL OF INDIA PRIVATE LIMITED, *New Delhi*
PRENTICE-HALL OF JAPAN, INC., *Tokyo*
PRENTICE-HALL OF SOUTHEAST ASIA PTE. LTD., *Singapore*
WHITEHALL BOOKS LIMITED, *Wellington, New Zealand*

CONTENTS

21

CHILDHOOD PSYCHOSIS: PSYCHOTHERAPY, *354*

Clarice J. Kestenbaum

22

CHILDHOOD PSYCHOSIS: BEHAVIORAL TREATMENT, *385*

O. Ivar Lovaas, Douglas B. Young & Crighton D. Newsom

23

CHILDHOOD PSYCHOSIS: RESIDENTIAL TREATMENT AND ITS ALTERNATIVES, *421*

Mary B. Hagamen

24

CHILD ABUSE, *430*

Arthur H. Green

PREFACE

Treating mental disorders in childhood and adolescence serves a dual purpose. Its main aim is to alleviate the suffering of children and adolescents and help them to overcome their handicaps and shortcomings, thus enabling them to lead a normal life. The second task is of preventive nature, for an early treatment of mental disorder may prevent mental disorder in adulthood.

With these two broad objectives in mind, the Editors of the present volume invited 32 leading experts and assigned to them 24 chapters covering the entire field of child psychopathology, limiting the topics to treatment methods. The first part of this volume describes the main approaches, namely, psychopharmacology, behavior modification, psychoanalysis, institutional and family treatment, and community aspects of dealing with disturbed children and adolescents. The second part describes specific syndromes and disorders and the appropriate therapeutic techniques. The entire volume is geared to the needs of students of advanced standing in the above-mentioned areas and to practicing professionals.

The Editors of this collective volume are fully aware of the fact that they do not offer a homogeneous presentation, but then, an artificial homogeneity in this highly diversified field was precisely what the Editors avoided. They planned the volume as a comprehensive, objective, up-to-date presentation of all major treatment methods currently applied by clinical child psychologists, child psychiatrists, and other professionals concerned with mental health problems in childhood and adolescence and prevention of mental disorders in adult years.

The Editors and Authors represent diverse approaches and techniques, but all of them are united in a genuine desire to be of service to their colleagues who treat suffering children and adolescents, and to advanced programs of study which train the future professionals.

THE EDITORS

CONTRIBUTORS

Delia Battin (Chapter 5), M.S.W., Columbia University, is a Psychiatric Social Worker on the staff of the St. Luke's Hospital, Division of Child and Adolescent Psychiatry and the Therapeutic Nursery. She is on the faculty of Marymount Manhattan College. She is a psychoanalytic candidate at the New York Society of Freudian Psychologists. She is in private practice in New York City. From 1966 to 1976 she served as Psychiatric Social Worker on a federally funded project on Bereavement and also published many articles in journals, while others in the book, *Bereavement: It's Psychosocial Aspects*, Eds. Schoenberg, et al. Her main interests at present are treatment of children and their families, and the applications of psychoanalysis to literature.

Jules R. Bemporad (Chapter 11), M.D., University of Florida, is Director of Pediatric Psychiatry, Babies Hospital, Columbia-Presbyterian Medical Center and Associate Clinical Professor of Psychiatry, College of Physicians and Surgeons, Columbia University. He is also a training and supervising analyst in the Psychoanalytic Division of New York Medical College and an Assistant Editor of the *Journal of the American Academy of Psychoanalysis*. His major interests are the interrelationships of affective and cognitive development in children, aspects of attribution theory, and the psychodynamics of depression.

Magda Campbell (Chapter 2), M.D., University of Belgrade, Yugoslavia, is an associate professor of psychiatry at New York University School of Medicine, and Director of Children's Psychopharmacology Unit, New York University Medical Center. Dr. Campbell's special fields of research interest are children's psychopharmacology and psychoses of childhood, and she has published numerous articles in journals and contributed to various books.

Emory L. Cowen (Chapter 7), Ph.D, Syracuse University is Professor of Psychology and the Director of the Center for Community Study at the University of Rochester. He is a past President of the APA Division of Community Psychology and past Chairman of the New York State Board of Examiners of Psychologists. He has been an Associate Editor of the *American Journal of Community Psychology* and Advisory Editor of the *Journal of Consulting and Clinical Psychology*. He has authored or co-authored five books, a number of chapters and monographs, and more than 100 journal articles. His primary research interests are in the area of community psychology with special emphasis on early detection and prevention of school adjustment problems, and nonprofessional help-agents.

Melvyn A. Davine (Chapter 15), Ph.D., Queen's University at Kingston, Ontario, Canada, is a staff psychologist at the Community Clinic and Thistletown Regional Centre School, Thistletown Regional Centre for Children and Adolescents, Toronto. Dr. Davine's major interests are developmental psycholinguistics, learning and language disorders in children and behavioral management counselling with parents and teachers.

James Egan (Co-editor, Chapter 12), M.D., College of Physicians and Surgeons, Columbia University. Certificates in adult and child psychoanalysis from the Columbia Clinic for Psychoanalytic Training and Research. He is currently Chairman of the Department of Psychiatry at the Children's Hospital National Medical Center in Washington, D.C., Associate Professor of Psychiatry and the Behavioral Sciences, and Child Health and Development, and Director of Child and Adolescent Psychiatry at the George Washington University School of Medicine. His major fields of professional interest are in psychiatric education and psychotherapy.

Dean L. Fixsen (Chapter 18), Ph.D., University of Kansas, is co-director of the Teaching-Family Program at the Boys Town Center for the Study of Youth Development and adjunct Associate Professor in the Department of Human Development at the University of Kansas. He was codirector of the Achievement Place Research Project which developed the Teaching-Family Model. He serves as an Associate Editor of the *Journal of Applied Behavior Analysis*. His main interests are in developing a model for evaluating and disseminating social service programs for children and youth and he has published articles and books on program evaluation and staff training.

Donna M. Gelfand (Chapter 20), Ph.D., Stanford University, is Professor of psychology at the University of Utah. Her main areas of interest are in children's social development and in prevention and treatment of childhood behavior disorders. She currently serves on the editorial boards of *Child Development*, *Journal of Applied Behavior Analysis*, and *Annual Progress in Child Clinical Psychology*. She is a regular contributor to various professional journals, and has edited one book, *Social Learning in Childhood* (2nd edition, 1975); and written another, *Child Behavior Analysis and Therapy* (with D. P. Hartmann, 1975).

Ellis L. Gesten (Chapter 7), Ph.D., University of Rochester is research associate in psychology at the University of Rochester. Most of his work has been in the broad areas of community mental health and community psychology. Specific research interests relate to competence acquisition, preschool programs, and school mental health.

Anthony M. Graziano (Chapter 3), Ph.D., Purdue University, is Professor of Psychology at the State University of New York at Buffalo. He has published numerous articles and three books on child therapy (*Behavior Therapy With Children*, Vol. 1, 1971; Vol. 11, 1975; *Child Without Tomorrow*, 1974) and has written on a range of topics including psychological testing, mental health history and politics, and children's rights. He has served as consultant to children's agencies, initiated children's treatment programs, and worked with action groups of parents of exceptional children. Professor Graziano's current research and writing are in the areas of children's self-control and the "quality of life" for children.

Arthur H. Green (Chapter 24), M.D., is Clinical Associate Professor of Psychiatry, Downstate Medical Center and Director, Comprehensive Treatment Center for Abused Children and Their Families, Kings County Hospital Center. His main interest is the prevention and treatment of child abuse and neglect. Dr. Green has published numerous articles based upon his clinical observations and research in child maltreatment. He is currently a principal investigator of a research project on child abuse sponsored by the National Center for Child Abuse and Neglect. Dr. Green is a diplomate of the American Board of Psychiatry and Neurology in Psychiatry and Child Psychiatry, and a faculty member of The Psychoanalytic Clinic for Training and Research at Columbia University. He is also engaged in private practice in child and adult psychiatry and psychoanalysis.

Mary B. Hagamen (Chapter 23), M.D., Western Reserve University, is Director of Sagamore Children's Center, Melville, Long Island, New York. She is Associate Clinical Professor of Psychiatry at the Health Science Center of the State University of New York at Stony Brook. Her main interest has been the delivery of mental health services to severely emotionally disturbed children.

Clarice J. Kestenbaum (Chapter 21), M.D., U.C.L.A., is Director of the Division of Child and Adolescent Psychiatry, St. Luke's Hospital, New York City, and Associate Clinical Professor of Psychiatry, Columbia University. She is on the faculty of Columbia Psychoanalytic Institute for Training and Research. She served as consultant to the Therapeutic Nursery Group of the Hudson Guild Day Care Center between 1965 and 1970. She has produced a series of child development videotapes for the Education Textbook, Department of Educational Research, New York State Psychiatric Institute. Her chief research interest is a long term prospective study in children at risk for schizophrenia.

Ruth LaVietes (Chapter 14), M.D., Stanford University, is Professor of clinical psychiatry and director of child and adolescent psychiatry at New York Medical College. She is also director of child psychiatry at Westchester County Medical Center and director of psychiatry at the Mental Retardation Institute of New York Medical College. Her major interests are in therapeutic education and residency training.

O. Ivar Lovaas (chapter 22), Ph.D., University of Washington, Seattle, is Professor of psychology at the University of California, Los Angeles. He was clinic supervisor in the Institute of Child Development at the University of Washington from 1958 to 1961. He joined the faculty of the UCLA Psychology Department in 1961, where he supervises training of clinical psychology students, is a member of the developmental area, and is director of a treatment/research project funded by NIMH for young autistic children. He is well known for his work in behavior modification with psychotic children and has contributed to treatment of children with deviant gender identity problems and hyperactive children. His research interests, which have resulted in numerous publications, include the experimental analysis of psychotic behavior, research on deviant perception and motivation, and the control of self-destructive behavior. He is a co-editor of *Perspectives in Behavior Modification with Deviant Children* (with Bradley Bucher), author of a forthcoming book, *The Autistic Child: Language Development through Behavior Modification*, and director of two training films in behavior therapy, including "Behavior Modification: Teaching Language to Psychotic Children," distributed by Prentice-Hall. He is on the editorial board of numerous professional journals. He has been the recipient of an honorary doctorate and is a former Guggenheim fellow.

Eugene Mahon (Chapter 5), M.D., National University of Ireland, is director of St. Luke's Hospital Therapeutic Nursery. He is on the faculty of Columbia University in the Department of Psychiatry and candidate in the child and adult psychoanalytic programs at the Columbia University Psychoanalytic Clinic for Training and Research. He is a member of the American Academy of Child Psychiatry and serves on their Committee on Program. His main interests are therapeutic nursery education, psychoanalysis of children and adults, and the applications of psychoanalysis to literature. He has published articles on family therapy and childhood mourning.

Dennis M. Maloney (Chapter 18), Ph.D., University of Kansas, is co-director of the Teaching-Family Program at the Boys Town Center for the Study of Youth Development, and adjunct professor in the Department of Psychology at the University of Nebraska in Omaha. He was Director of Research and Evaluation for a regional network of group homes headquartered at Western Carolina Center in Morganton, North Carolina (1973–1975). His main research interests are staff training and program evaluation for youth services and he has contributed to professional journals and books.

Karen B. Maloney (Chapter 18), Ph.D., University of Kansas, is co-director of the Teaching-Family Program at the Boys Town Center for the Study of Youth Development, and adjunct professor in the Department of Psychology at the University of Nebraska in Omaha. Currently, she serves on the editorial board of the *Journal of Applied Behavior Analaysis*. She was Director of Training for a regional network of group homes headquartered at Western Carolina Center in Morganton, North Carolina and also was an assistant professor in the Department of Special Education at Appalachian State University (1973–1975). Her main research interests are staff training, program evaluation and dissemination of youth programs and she has contributed to books and professional journals.

Robert B. Millman (Chapter 16), M.D., is clinical associate professor of public health at Cornell University Medical College and adjunct assistant professor at The Rockefeller University, both in New York City. Trained in internal medicine and psychiatry, he is director of the Adolescent Development Program, a research and treatment program for adolescent drug abusers, operated under the aegis of these institutions. His major research interests include the pathogenesis of substance-abuse behavior, characterization of the disabilities incident to psychoactive drug taking, and the development of effective treatments for these behaviors. He is also interested in the delivery of medical and psychiatric care to inner-city populations.

Crighton D. Newsom (Chapter 22), Ph.D., University of California, Los Angeles, is a staff psychologist at Sagamore Children's Center, Melville, New York. He was the director of the Children's Learning Laboratory at Camarillo State Hospital, Camarillo, California from 1972 to 1976. His main areas of research interest are stimulus control, experimental child psychopathology, and behavior modification. Besides contributing to various professional journals, he has co-authored chapters in H. Leitenberg (Ed.), *Handbook of Behavior Modification* (with O. I. Lovaas, 1976) and R. S. Davidson (Ed.), *Experimental Analysis of Clinical Phenomena* (with E. G. Carr and O. I. Lovaas, in press).

George A. Rekers (Chapter 17), Ph.D., University of California at Los Angeles, is an Assistant Professor of Psychology at the Graduate School of Psychology, Fuller Theological Seminary, and an Adjunct Assistant Professor of psychology at UCLA. He has been a visiting scholar in the Center for the Behavioral Sciences at Harvard University. Dr. Rekers is a clinical child psychologist with special research interest in early identification, prevention, and treatment of gender disturbances, sexual deviance, and adolescent alcohol drinking problems. Professor Rekers has published numerous articles in professional journals, including *Journal of Experimental Child Psychology*, *Journal of Applied Behavior Analysis*, *Journal of Abnormal Child Psychology*, *Behaviour Research and Therapy*, *Journal of Behavior Therapy and Experimental Psychiatry*, and *Child Development*.

Alan O. Ross (Co-Editor), Ph.D., Yale University, is professor of psychology and director of the doctoral program in clinical psychology at State University of New York at Stony Brook, New York. He is a Diplomate in Clinical Psychology of the American Board of Professional Psychology and served for many years as chief psychologist in various community child guidance clinics before joining the Stony Brook faculty in 1967. His research and clinical interests are in child behavior therapy and learning disabilities. He serves on the editorial boards of *Behavior Therapy* and *Journal of Abnormal Child Psychology* and, in addition to numerous articles and contributed chapters, has written *The Practice of Clinical Child Psychology* (1959), *The Exceptional Child in the Family* (1964), *Psychological Disorders of Children* (1974), and *Psychological*

Aspects of Learning Disabilities and Reading Disorders (1976).

Clyde L. Rousey (Chapter 13), Ph.D., Northwestern University and graduate Topeka Institute for Psychoanalysis, is a psychologist, speech pathologist, and audiologist in private practice in Topeka. Prior to this, he was Director of the Speech and Hearing Clinic at the Menninger Clinic from 1961 to 1975. He presently serves as editorial consultant for the *Journal of Speech and Hearing Disorders* and abstractor for *Excerpta Medica*. His most recent book is *Psychiatric Assessment by Speech and Hearing Behavior* (1974). Further explanation and discussion of the theory utilized in the present chapter will appear in the forthcoming book *Basic Handbook of Child Psychiatry* edited by J. Noshpitz.

Melvin A. Scharfman (Chapter 4), M.D., New York Medical College, is a Professor of clinical psychiatry at State University of New York, Downstate Medical Center. He is the director of residency training in psychiatry at State University Hospital-Kings County Hospital Center. He is Chairman, Section on Child Analysis of the Division of Psychoanalytic Education of S.U.N.Y., Downstate Medical Center, where he is a training and supervising analyst in adult and child analysis. He has published in the field of child development and adolescence.

Jesse Schomer (Chapter 6), M.D., New York University is Clinical Associate Professor of Psychiatry at Cornell University and Director of the Outpatient Department at New York Hospital, Westchester Division. He was previously Director of the Child Psychiatry Clinic at Hillside Hospital in New York. One of his current teaching and research interests is the relationship between family and intrapsychic systems relevant to mental health.

Carolyn S. Schroeder (Chapter 15), Ph.D., University of Pittsburgh, is Head of the Psychology Section in the Division for Disorders of Development and Learning and associate professor of psychology in the Psychiatry Department at the University of North Carolina at Chapel Hill. She is also a research scientist in the Child Development Research Institute. Her main areas of interest are behavioral analysis of developmental and management problems with children, consultation techniques, and parent education programs. Dr. Schroeder has been Secretary-Treasurer (1974–1976) and President (1977) of the Society of Pediatric Psychology.

Stephen R. Schroeder (Chapter 15), Ph.D., University of Pittsburgh, is a research scientist in the Child Development Institute and clinical associate professor of psychology and psychiatry at the University of North Carolina at Chapel Hill. He also serves as director of research and development at Murdoch Center. Dr. Schroeder's main areas of interest are behavior analysis, abnormal development, and adaptation of laboratory experimental design and instrumentation to field settings.

Arthur M. Small (Chapter 2), M.D., State University of New York, Downstate Medical Center, is a clinical associate professor of psychiatry at New York University School of Medicine and an assistant attending psychiatrist at Bellevue and University Hospitals in New York City. He is a research child psychiatrist on the Children's Psychopharmacology Research Unit, N.Y.U. Medical Center, and the medical director of St. Agnes Home and School for Children in Sparkill, New York. His main research interest is the etiology and treatment of autism and childhood schizophrenia and has co-authored several chapters on this topic.

Gail E. Solomon (Chapter 8), M.D., Smith College, A.B.—1958, Albert Einstein College of Medicine, M.D.—1962, Clinical Associate Professor of Neurology and Pediatrics—Cornell University Medical College, Director of Electroencephalography—The New York Hospital, Associate Attending in Neurology and Pediatrics—The New York Hospital, Fellow-American Academy of Pediatrics, Fellow-American Academy of Neurology, certified in Neurology with Special Competence in Pediatric Neurology, Special Interest and Publications in Child Neurology especially relating to Convulsive Disorders, Minimal Cerebral Dysfunction, Cerebrovascular Disease in Children. Co-Author of recent book: *Clinical Management of Seizures: A Guide for the Physician* (W. B. Saunders, 1976).

John A. Sours (Chapter 10), M.D., Cornell University Medical College, is Clinical Assistant Professor of Psychiatry, College of Physicians and Surgeons, Columbia University and is training analyst and supervising adult and child analyst at the Columbia Psychoanalytic Clinic for Training and Research. After a medical internship at The New York Hospital—Cornell Medical Center he was a Fulbright Scholar (1958–1959) in Neurology and Psychiatry at London University (Maida Vale and National Hospitals and The Maudsley Hospital). From 1965 to 1967 he held a National Institute of Mental Health Career Teacher Award in Child Psychiatry at the Columbia—Presbyterian Medical Center and the N.Y.S. Psychiatric Institute. He has written on philosophy and psychoanalysis, neuropsychiatry, aviation and space medicine, narcolepsy and somnambulism, anorexia nervosa, and child development. With Jerome Goodman, M.D. he published *The Child Mental Status Examination*. His research interest is the theory and technique of child and adult treatment.

Thornton A. Vandersall (Chapter 9), M.D., Jefferson Medical College, is Associate Professor of psychiatry and assistant professor of pediatrics at Cornell University Medical College. A child psychiatrist, and former pediatrician, Dr. Vandersall received some of his early pediatric training with pediatric gastroenterologist, Dr. Murray Davidson. Dr. Vandersall currently serves as liaison child psychiatrist to the pediatric g.i. clinic of Dr. Mervin Silverberg. Dr. Vandersall is the Director of the Department of Psychiatry at North Shore University Hospital, a Cornell affiliated hospital.

Benjamin B. Wolman (Editor) Ph.D., 1935, University of Warsaw. Clinical Psychologist and Assistant Director, Centos Institute for Disturbed Children, 1932–33; Chief Psychologist and Director, Mental Health Clinic, Tel-Aviv, Israel, 1935–42; Director, Educational Services for Jewish Servicemen's Families in World War II, 1942–45; Lecturer in Psychology, Teachers College, Tel-Aviv, Israel, 1945–48; Visiting Lecturer, Columbia University, 1949–53; Visiting Associate Professor of Psychology, Yeshiva University, 1953–57; Clinical Lecturer in Psychiatry and Supervisor of Psychotherapy, Post Doctoral Program, Albert Einstein College of Medicine, 1958–62; Clinical Professor in Psychoanalysis and Psychotherapy, Post Doctoral Program, Adelphi University, 1963–65; Professor, Doctoral Program in Clinical Psychology, Long Island University, 1965 to the present; private practice of psychoanalysis and psychotherapy since 1939. Author of over 160 scientific papers and sixteen books in psychology and related fields.
Among the books, *Contemporary Theories and Systems in Psychology*, Harper & Row, 1960; *Vectoriasis Traecox or the Group of Schizophrenias*, Thomas, 1966; *The Unconscious Mind*, Prentice-Hall, 1967; *Children Without Childhood*, Grune and Stratton, 1970; *Call No Man Normal*, International Universities Press, 1973; *Victims of Success*, Quadrangle/New York Times, 1973; Editor-in-chief, *International Encyclopedia of Psychiatry, Psychology, Psychoanalysis, and Neurology*, Aesculapius, 1977; and others.

Douglas B. Young (Chapter 22), M.A., University of California, Los Angeles, is a graduate student working toward the doctorate at UCLA in the areas of child development and clinical psychology. He has been active in treatment and research with psychotic children. Additional fields of special interest include pediatrics and child psychiatry.

Louis Culberson Zang (Chapter 19), M.D., Baylor University, is Assistant Professor of psychiatry at Cornell University College of Medicine. He is the founder and director of the New York Hospitsl Children's Day Hospital for emotionally disabled children. Having practiced pediatric allergy for many years, he has an interest in the psychophysiological problems as well as the aggressive, antisocial problems of children. At present he is attempting to incorporate a psychoeducation training program into the in-service training given to day hospital staff.

I

METHODS OF TREATMENT

I

THE RATIONALE OF CHILD THERAPY

Benjamin B. Wolman

Treatment methods of mental disorders in childhood and adolescence must take into consideration the dual task of developmental years. On one hand, a child has the right to be a child and need not be prematurely forced to accept the social role and responsibility of adulthood. Children robbed of their childhood and burdened with worries and anxieties of their parents may seek escape in withdrawal from social contacts and regression to infantile modes of living where they expect to be able to survive undisturbed by their overdemanding parents. A study of schizophrenic children and their families called *Children Without Childhood: A Study of Childhood Schizophrenia* (Wolman, 1970) pointed to this morbid regression for survival.

Rational parents and parental substitutes allow the child to be a child and act in accordance with his age and his age-sex related social status and role. However, a child cannot and must not remain a child forever. Biological and sociocultural forces produce gradual changes in a child's personality and behavior. Some of these changes are determined by maturation and developmental processes, while other changes are brought about by social interaction and learning.

This dual social role of a child who *is* a child but *must not remain* a child, who can't act like an adult but must not be allowed forever to act like a child, requires a great deal of attention on the part of the child therapist. Children who come for treatment do not come voluntarily as adult patients do. Children are *brought* to our offices or clinics and, as a rule, they are brought by people who, in a majority of cases, are at least partially responsible for their abnormal behavior. The parent who comes with the child is usually the more active one and the one who exercises more influence in the child's life. As a rule, this is the parent who demands too much and too early or who overprotects and infantilizes or who outrightly rejects the child or relates toward the child in some other irrational manner.

The work of the child and adolescent therapist is much more complex than that of his colleague who treats adults. The diagnostic task is further complicated by a lack of clearly established nosological categories. The present classificatory system of the American Psychiatric Association, the Diagnostic and Statistical Manual of Mental Disorders, (DSM II) (1968) is neither consistent, nor popular among practitioners. Moreover, it is being currently revised and will be published in DSM III. The Group for Advancement of Psychiatry (1973) came up with a totally different classificatory system which is neither generally accepted nor easy to follow.

The scope of the difficulties encountered in the treatment of disturbed children can be best assessed by analyzing the therapeutic interaction from two poles, the patient and the therapist.

THE PATIENT

Every therapeutic relationship involves at least two partners, the one who needs help, the patient, and the other who supplies the needed help, the therapist (psychiatrist, clinical psychologist, or psychiatric social worker).

All living matter, with rare exceptions, resists destruction. Survival is the intrinsic, immanent goal of all living organisms, and almost all their actions are geared toward this universal goal. Survival-directed actions include intake of oxygen, water and food, assimilation, digestion and elimination, rest and sleep, and defense against destructive forces such as floods, hurricanes, germs, diseases, predators.

When one says, "I need food or rest or weapons," the term *need* represents a means which leads toward the satisfaction of the main goal which is survival.

The ability to satisfy needs is a term synonymous to one's chances for survival. Individuals capable of procuring whatever is needed for survival are *strong*; thus the ability to satisfy needs should be called *power*. Those who are unable to satisfy their needs are *weak*, and the degree to which one is capable of satisfying his needs is a measure of one's power or lack of it. The zero point of power is death, the maximum point of power is omnipotence and immortality (Wolman, 1974).

No human being is omnipotent, nor is he totally helpless. Moreover, human behavior is not determined by things as they are but as they are perceived.

K. Lewin observed that one's level of aspiration does not necessarily correspond to one's potentialities but to the estimate of one's own potentialities (Frank, 1941). In other words, human behavior is greatly influenced by how the individual sees himself, and human actions are more related to these perceptions than to what one really is.

Emotional Correlates

Apparently, many emotional responses are reactions to one's estimate of personal power. Pleasant emotions, such as joy, hope, reflect high estimates of one's ability to satisfy his needs. Elation usually corresponds to a high estimate of one's own power, and depression represents a low estimate. The feeling of courage is related to one's faith in being able to overcome obstacles and threats, while fear reflects one's doubts about successfully coping with hardships.

In the patient-therapist interaction the patient perceives himself as weak, that is, in need of help, and believes that the therapist is strong, that is, capable of giving the help. However, there are realistic limits to the weak versus strong interaction, for the patient is aware of the fact that therapeutic practice provides the therapist with livelihood. The patient himself, or the society in which the patient participates and to which he contributes as a taxpayer, pays for the treatment and thus satisfies the therapist's needs. Therefore the patient's position is not one of total weakness, nor is the therapist's position one of uncontestable strength.

The above reasoning does not apply to the role of a child as a patient. The child sees the therapist as a grownup who exercises more power than most other adults, for even the parents, who are the power symbols par excellence, need the therapist's help. Evidently, they are unable to cope with some not too clearly defined problems and accordingly renounce some part of their authority. "You must listen to the doctor," they say, implying that they themselves must listen too.

Fear of the Therapist

Whenever one faces someone who is perceived as being definitely stronger, one may experience fear or safety, depending on the intentions of the stronger individual. Most often, at home, children experience both fear and safety, for they feel that they are at the mercy of their not always rational and not always consistently merciful parents. In most cases the ratio of fear versus security is the single greatest determinant of mental health, as described by Freud, Horney, Sullivan, Erikson, Wolman, Bandura, and many others, irrespective of their particular theoretical orientation. Insecure, inconsistent, punitive, hostile, and outright rejecting parents play a highly significant role in the etiology of mental disorders in their offspring.

An emotionally disturbed child whose suffering is a result of parental attitudes may have great difficulty in relating to the therapist. These difficulties are not limited to psychotherapy, for the child who needs physical or chemical therapy probably had certain experiences with his parents who may or may have not offered support and comfort to him as an individual afflicted with an organic disorder. The child may suspect that the professional person whom they recommend for treating him might be as inconsiderate, critical, and/or hostile as the parents are.

Fear of disapproval, blame, and/or punishment is a typical child-therapist attitude. H. Colm (1966) has been critical even of the obviously permissive atmosphere in play-therapy. She writes:

> The play therapy approach of merely bringing "things in the open" with an accepting the other person fails in the face of the child's suspiciousness and defensiveness, for his self-condemnation makes him distrust the adult's interest. . . . He knows that the adult is to blame him. . . . Any discussion of his fear and control and distrust makes him withhold more: he feels that someone tries to break in and this must be prevented (Colm, 1966, p. 105).

Powerful allies are often suspected of imposing their will on their weak allies. Sometimes they do it in a paternalizing manner, "for your well-being." Sometimes they do it for their own gain. Power can be used and abused in more than one way, and the fact that the therapist seems to exercise tremendous power may encourage or discourage the child, depending on the way he perceives the therapist's intentions.

ACCEPTANCE

Power can be used to help or to hurt. Whenever it is used to help, it is friendly; when it hurts, it is hostile. Friendly means supportive and protecting one's life. Hostile means destructive, aiming at damaging and/or destroying one's life.

Interindividual relations are apparently a function of *power* and *acceptance*, power meaning the ability to satisfy needs, acceptance implying the willingness to do so.

In normal families, the child perceives his parents as strong and friendly, and his wholesome development greatly depends upon this perception. The child feels satisfied when he feels that his needs are taken care of by his parents and when he is sure that their caring attitude will be forthcoming. Such a belief creates a feeling that has been described as safety (Horney) or euphoria (Sullivan), and it is the foundation of the child's mental health (Wolman). The child who views his parents as *strong* and *friendly* develops the feeling of *awe*, which is a combination of love and fear. The child loves his parents but also fears losing their love. The development of superego (Freud) and of own identity (Erikson) is facilitated by the child's love for and fear of his parents or parental substitutes.

Every child is exposed to multiple social relations with other adults, grandparents, relatives, acquaintances. The child learns to distinguish the amount of power and degree of acceptance of those nonparental figures. "You have no right to punish me, you are not my mother," a child may say to anyone who tries to discipline him. In most European countries the parents vest a great deal of authority in the teachers. One of the major difficulties in the American educational system is linked with the decline of parental authority and exceedingly low teacher authority. Authority can be defined as recognition of and submission to another person's power.

A sick child is doubly weak: he is weak for being a child and weak for being sick. He may or may not trust his parents; he may perceive them as weak and friendly or weak and hostile or strong and hostile. In any one of these three cases he is poorly prepared to view the therapist as a strong and friendly person, but unless he perceives the therapist as strong and friendly, he will be not inclined to cooperate.

Thus the therapist who treats emotionally disturbed children may face more than what Freud described as unconscious resistance. In a great many cases, the child brought for treatment against his will, may be hostile toward the therapist whose intentions he doubts and often resents.

Transference

Transference is a reactivation of past emotional involvement and attachment (cathexis) of these emotions onto the therapist. Anna Freud originally (1926) rejected the idea that children develop transference neurosis. After almost 40 years of experience she wrote as follows:

> I have modified my former opinion that transference in childhood is restricted to simple "transference reactions" and does not develop to the complete status of a "transference neurosis." Nevertheless, I am still unconvinced that what is called transference neurosis in children equals the adult variety in every aspect (A. Freud, 1965).

Transference phenomena are not limited to the psychoanalytic process. They take place in everyday life. One's preference for certain colors that evoke pleasant memories, a vehement dislike for certain dishes which mildly resemble past infancy conflicts, and one's instant like or dislike for newly met human faces are examples of transference. Every therapeutic relationship necessarily creates transference, and the most detailed studies of transference phenomena have been conducted by psychoanalysts.

> The roots of the transference are embedded in the life history of the child during his development. He simultaneously forms a more or less realistic picture of his parents and a distorted picture based on his own wishes, needs, fantasies and emotions. . . . We are familiar with the child who views the analyst only as a beneficial protective figure (the partial introject of the "good mother") and with the child who treats the analyst as though any relationship with him will mean the loss of his parent . . . (in the "good mother" transference any negative thoughts or feelings that threaten the return of the split-off "bad mother"; and in the dangerous stranger transference, any positive expression threatens disintegration of the poorly integrated internal representation of the mother" (Lesser, 1972, p. 853).

The child can perceive the therapist as a "good doctor," friendly nursemaid, or a pain-inflicting, needle-giving monster, and so on. Rarely is chemotherapy the sole method of treatment with children. More often pharmacotherapy should be applied as part of a comprehensive therapeutic program. For instance, "The most important therapeutic function of psychoactive medication (of anxiety states) is to help the organic components of the ego become better organized so that a steadier, higher level of functioning is maintained. . . . The psychopharmacological agent may help the child to respond to psychotherapy directed toward resolving his conflicted thoughts, wishes, urges and fears" (Greenberg and Lourie, 1972, p. 1011).

Treatment of a child, whether by psychotherapeutic method, for example, psychoanalysis or behavior modification, or any of the physical or chemical methods *always* involves child-adult interaction. In this interaction the here and now elements are colored by the relationship between the child and other significant adults, especially his parents. Some of these influences originate in repressed past experiences of the child and may be defined as transference, and some are related to the here and now tripartite relationship between the child, his parents, and the therapist.

THE THERAPIST

One can distinguish three types of voluntary interaction, depending on the intentions of the participants. When one enters a social relationship with the aim of having his own needs satisfied, it is *instrumental*; the relationship is a means of meeting the individual's needs. All breadwinning activities and almost all business relationships are instrumental, for both the employer's and the employee's aims are selfish. When, however, people enter a relationship in order to give and to get, such as a friendship or a marriage, it is a *mutual* relationship. When people aim to give without expecting anything in return, it is a *vectorial* relationship (Wolman, 1970).

While the instrumental, breadwinning elements in the therapist's behavior are inevitable, they are common elements in everyone's life and, unless unduly fanned by some therapists' greediness, they do not interfere with the vectorial concern for the well-being of the patients (Wolman, 1976a).

Some therapists may, however, seek additional, noneconomic gains in their work which may seriously impair their therapeutic tasks. To be a "healer" and especially a "mind healer" may serve as a source of unearned conceit. Any therapy, whether physicochemical or psychological, is a service to those who need it and a job to be conscientiously performed. However, past experiences and emotions may activate in the therapist irrational ideas concerning himself and his role. These irrational ideas form the core of countertransference.

COUNTERTRANSFERENCE

Some irrational elements are typical for any therapeutic interaction and, probably, for all healing professions. In prehistorical times people ascribed magical powers to the individual who could heal sick bodies and sick souls. He was called priest, shaman, witch doctor, and so on, and in many instances he himself believed in his miraculous talents. Something of this megalomania survived through the millennia, and many a practitioner is tempted to believe in his superhuman abilities. Perhaps people who deal with emotional problems are more inclined to believe in their world-saving, divine powers than other professionals (Wolman, 1976b). However, the art of healing in general may be conducive to omnipotence fantasies which represent a gross distortion of reality and thus may adversely affect the judgment, caution, and professional responsibility of the therapist.

Both transference and countertransference are processes of investing (cathecting) emotional energy (Wolman, 1966). Uncontrolled countertransference conveyed in the form of overprotecting the child, identifying with the child, disliking him, and so on may cause a great deal of harm to the therapeutic interaction and, consequently, to the child. However, some elements of countertransference may or may not harm the therapist's proficiency depending on the extent to which he (or she) is aware of his regressive feelings and how good his self-control is.

The following two types of countertransference are most frequently encountered in child therapy:

1. Recollections from the therapist's childhood which may induce unconscious identification with the child and hostile feelings toward his parents.
2. Unconscious parental feelings toward the child with a tendency to overprotect/overindulge or overdiscipline/punish the child. The therapist may be guilty of substituting the parental caring role for his professional healing role.

Child therapists must be aware of the fact that children and adolescents are quite likely to evoke unconscious and irrational countertransference feelings. The therapist must be aware of these dangers in order to control them and retain an objective, professional attitude toward the patients.

THE PARENTS

Many years ago I was the director of a mental health institution for children overseas which conducted both out-patient and in-patient services. In the out-patient division we unconditionally adhered to the principle that no child was to be admitted unless both parents agreed simultaneously to undergo the appropriate psychotherapy. We were, however, only partially successful, for on many occasions parents did not come to the therapist's group sessions or discontinued their individual therapy. We avoided institutionalization and we admitted children to the in-patient services only when there was no one to take care of the child at home.

Some clinicians *prefer* to separate the child

from the apparently noxious parent-child interaction and to create for him instead an adequate protective and therapeutic home away from home (Bettelheim, 1950; Riese, 1962). But, whether the child is or is not physically separated from his parents, the parents and/or their images play a most significant role in child therapy.

In the vast majority of cases the child therapist deals with non-hospitalized children and adolescents, and parental cooperation is a prerequisite of successful treatment.

Siding with the child and an antagonistic attitude toward the parents is one of the frequent mistakes committed in child therapy. Many a parent resents being blamed, rightly or wrongly, for his child's ills.

The chances of successful treatment are greatly improved by parental cooperation. Frequent consultations with the parents, group or family therapy, simultaneous or (if advised) conjoint parent-child therepy are the standard devices which may contribute to successful psychotherapy with the child. Also in physical and chemical therapy a close cooperation with the parents may make the therapist's task easier and probably also more successful.

REFERENCES

BETTELHEIM, B. *Love is not enough.* Glencoe, Ill.: Free Press, 1950.

COLM, H. *The existential approach to psychotherapy.* New York: Grune and Stratton, 1966.

FRANK, J. D. Recent studies of the level of aspiration. *Psychological Bulletin*, 1941, *38*, 218–226.

FREUD, A. *Normality and pathology in childhood.* New York: International Universities Press, 1965.

GREENBERG, L. M. and LOURIE, R. S. Physicochemcial treatment methods. In B. B. Wolman (Ed.), *Manual of child psychopathology.* New York: McGraw-Hill, 1972, pp. 1010–1034.

GROUP FOR THE ADVANCEMENT OF PSYCHIATRY. *Psychopathological disorders in childhood: Theoretical considerations and a proposed classification.* 1966.

LESSER, S. R. Psychoanalysis with children. In B. B. Wolman (Ed.), *Manual of Child Psychopathology.* New York: McGraw-Hill, 1972, pp. 847–864.

LEWIN, K. *Field theory in social science.* New York: Harper, 1951.

RIESE, H. *Heal the hurt child.* Chicago: University of Chicago Press, 1962.

WOLMAN, B. B. Transference and countertransference as interindividual cathexis. *Psychoanalytic Review*, 1966, *53*, 225–265.

WOLMAN, B. B. *Children without childhood; a study of childhood schizophrenia.* New York: Grune and Stratton, 1970.

WOLMAN, B. B. (Ed). *Manual of child psychopathology.* New York: McGraw-Hill, 1972.

WOLMAN, B. B. (Ed.). *Handbook of child psychoanalysis.* New York: Van Nostrand-Reinhold, 1972.

WOLMAN, B. B. Power and acceptance as determinants of social relations. *International Journal of Group Tensions*, 1974, *4*, 151–183.

WOLMAN, B. B. The process of treatment. In B. B. Wolman (Ed.), *The Therapist's Handbook.* New York: Van Nostrand-Reinhold, 1976, pp. 3–17. (a)

WOLMAN, B. B. Success and failure in group psychotherapy. *Small Group Behavior*, 1976, *7*, 99–113. (b)

2

CHEMOTHERAPY[1]

Magda Campbell & Arthur M. Small

In medicine it is essential to know the following. First, how one treatment compares with another in a specific condition. Second, which treatment is most effective, and whether the efficacy of the best single treatment is enhanced by combining it with another therapeutic modality. Third, how do the immediate and long-term results differ in treated and untreated illness.

There is scientific evidence regarding the efficacy of drug therapy versus other treatment modalities and their relationships in adult psychiatric patients. The efficacy of neuroleptics and their superiority over psychosocial treatments in schizophrenics has been confirmed (Group for the Advancement of Psychiatry, GAP, 1975). Relatively good agreement on diagnostic criteria, the use of sophisticated methodology, and the availability of large numbers of subjects in collaborative studies have resulted in a vast body of knowledge. Acquisition of such information has been possible because treatments were compared in samples of patients as homogeneous as possible with regard to diagnosis, duration of illness, and other pertinent variables. We now know that pharmacotherapy not only decreases symptoms, but can also modify the course of schizophrenia (WHO, 1967).

In children and adolescents, such effect of drug treatment has not been demonstrated. There is a scarcity of well-controlled and designed studies comparing drug treatment to other treatments (psychotherapy, behavior therapy, etc.) in diagnostically homogeneous and sizable samples of patients, and of the effect of drug therapy in conjunction with such treatments (Christensen, 1973; Christensen & Sprague, 1973; Cytryn, Gilbert, & Eisenberg, 1960; Eisenberg, Gilbert, Cytryn, & Molling, 1961; Gittelman-Klein, 1975b). Anterospective studies comparing the natural history of illness with pharmacologic interventions are lacking.

Longitudinal studies of disturbed children have shown that with the exception of the neurotics, they do not outgrow their disorders but in most cases remain deviant, retarded, and/or psychotic adolescents and adults (Annell, 1963; Bender & Faretra, 1972; Eisenberg, 1956; Fish, Shapiro, Halpern, & Wile, 1966; Pichel, 1975; Robins, 1966, 1970; Rutter, 1970; Weiss, 1975). No type

[1]This work was supported in part by U.S. Public Health Service Grant MH-04665 from the National Institute of Mental Health.

of treatment, including lengthy and costly procedures, produces significant results. It would seem, therefore, that the use of psychoactive agents, a relatively inexpensive and quantifiable treatment with often immediate results, should have been adequately explored.

Although drugs are in wide use, the state of psychopharmacology is unsatisfactory in this age group. With the exception of the MBD (minimal brain dysfunction) child, the effect of drug treatment has been barely investigated in a systematic fashion; nor do we know enough about long-term adverse effects.

Therefore, in our present state of knowledge, the use of currently available therapeutic psychoactive drugs, when indicated, is not viewed as a long-term treatment modality but rather as a temporary, though often essential adjunct in the total treatment of the disturbed child and adolescent. Drugs should not be used if their risk and toxicity outweigh the possible therapeutic effects.

METHODOLOGY

The assessment of the efficacy of drugs in the treatment of behavioral disorders of children and adolescents is particularly difficult because of the unsatisfactory state of diagnostic classification, lack of appropriate and sensitive rating instruments for certain diagnostic categories (an exception is the MBD child), and such variables as chronological age, maturation, development, IQ, teacher's attitude, and parental influences. Various environmental manipulations can also obscure drug effects or interact with drugs. These environmental variables could be more powerful than drugs, particularly in the milder disturbances.

In the assessment of therapeutic efficacy and safety of a drug, a *single dose study* is the first step. The next stage of investigation is frequently an *open maintenance study*. The dosage based on single dose study is increased until therapeutic response or adverse effects are noted. A *controlled clinical trial* with carefully selected patients, adequate sample size, and good design is necessary to evaluate critically the therapeutic efficacy of a drug and to rule out placebo effect and investigator bias. Patients are randomly assigned to treatment or placebo groups. In chronic diseases, a *crossover design* is sometimes used, where each subject serves as his own control in every treatment condition. Controlled studies are usually carried out under *double-blind* conditions, where both patient and evaluating physician (or raters) are unaware of the nature of the treatment, and drug and placebo are identical in shape, size, and even taste. Placebo effects consist of those upon the patient, parents, teacher, and treating physician; they can be both positive and negative. Placebo effects are common and placebo responders were found even among the most severely impaired populations of children (Fish, Shapiro & Campbell, 1967).

Assessment of baseline behavior and changes with treatment in clinical studies is usually done by means of psychiatric rating scales or symptom lists developed for specific populations, by global evaluations, and by administering various performance tasks (Conners, 1970; Psychopharmacology Bulletin, 1973). In children, the use of independent, multiple raters is essential; in addition to the clinical assessment done by the psychiatrist, the parents', teachers', and/or nurses' reports are required.

Review articles on the subject of drug studies clearly show, again with the exception of those on MBD children (Conners, 1974; Gittelman-Klein, 1975b) that the above requirements for evaluating the efficacy of drug treatment were only infrequently met (Campbell, 1975; Conners, 1972a; Freeman, 1966, 1970; Sprague & Werry, 1971; Werry, 1972).

Methodology in children has been discussed by Conners (1973), Eisenberg and Conners (1971), Fish (1968), Lipman (1968) and Sprague and Werry (1971), and medical statistics by Bradford Hill (1971).

INDICATIONS AND CHOICE OF DRUG

Before instituting drug therapy, the relation of the patient and his symptoms to his family should be assessed. The patient's response to out-patient or institutional psychiatric treatment should be evaluated within two to four weeks before beginning medication. Such a baseline period of observation is not feasible in emergency situations.

Below are listed the disorders in which a trial of drug treatment is indicated.

In the category of *psychoneurotic disorders* (phobic type and depressive type), drug treatment should be instituted only if psychosocial therapies with patient and/or parents have failed. Imipramine was reported to be effective in the treatment of nonpsychotic children (6 to 14 years of age) with school phobia, in conjunction with other therapies (Gittelman-Klein and Klein, 1971, 1973a).

In adults, the effectiveness of imipramine-like drugs in retarded depression has been demonstrated. These states are poorly defined in children and adolescents (Anthony, 1967; Cytryn & McKnew, 1974; Weinberg, Rutman, Sullivan, Penick, & Dietz, 1973), and well-controlled and designed studies with clearly defined samples are lacking. The tricyclic antidepressants and monoamine-inhibitors have been used both in this country and abroad (Frommer, 1968, 1972; Lucas, Lockett, & Grimm, 1965; Stack, 1972; Weinberg et al., 1973), but their efficacy has not been critically evaluated. Until this has been done, these drugs should be restricted to investigational use in depressed children. Currently, a few controlled studies have been initiated. Although adequate studies are lacking, it seems that imipramine can be used with caution in adolescents with moderate to severe depressive states.

There is no evidence, based on well controlled studies, that drug treatment is more effective than any other type of therapy in the *psychotic disorders* (psychoses of infancy and early childhood, psychoses of later childhood and of adolescence). Nor has it been demonstrated that drugs are more effective when combined with other types of treatment in these populations.

Clinical experience, however, has shown that drugs can be a valuable addition or an essential modality in the total treatment of the psychotic child, particularly in the adolescent with acute onset of schizophrenia.

In general, the more severely disturbed and impaired (low IQ) patients require potent psychoactive agents such as the neuroleptics; they respond less favorably or even fail to respond to treatment with milder drugs, such as diphenhydramine. The less impaired psychotic children may show clinical improvement even on placebo or milieu treatment. In higher functioning school-age children, diphenhydramine, a safe drug and easy to regulate, can be tried first. If the child fails to respond, a neuroleptic should be prescribed, as would also be prescribed for severely disturbed and/or lower functioning children. Prepubertal children frequently respond even to low doses of sedative neuroleptics, such as chlorpromazine, with excessive sedation (Fish, 1960), and this interferes with learning. This may preclude drug treatment since psychosis in the child is frequently associated with retarded functioning and low IQ. Clinical experience shows that the more stimulating neuroleptics such as trifluoperazine, thiothixene, haloperidol, or molindone, are more therapeutic because they lack the sedative effect (for review, see Campbell, 1973, 1975).

There is some evidence that the degree of involvement of CNS functions underlying behavior may determine or influence the patient's response to drugs. Patients with perinatal complications, neurologic and neurophysiologic findings indicative of CNS dysfunction; that is, "organic" schizophrenics and autistics (Goldfarb, 1961, 1974; Kolvin, 1971; Quitkin, Rifkin, & Klein, 1976; Rutter & Lockyer, 1967), may respond differentially to psychoactive agents (Klein, 1967, 1968; Klein & Davis, 1969; Campbell, Fish, Korein, Shapiro, Collins, & Koh, 1972; Campbell, Small, Collins, Friedman, David & Genieser, 1976). On the other hand, it appears that a behaviorally therapeutic psychoactive agent may also produce positive changes in altered biochemical or neurophysiological parameters (Brambilla & Penati, 1971, 1974; Campbell et al., 1972; Campbell et al., 1976; Korein, Campbell, & Small, submitted for publication). These clinical findings, however, need further careful investigation.

Although many neuroleptics are in use today, it is sufficient to be familiar with one or two from each class or subclass. As a rule, the most familiar and seasoned drug should be tried first, that is, a *phenothiazine*. *Chlorpromazine* or *thioridazine* can be effective, particularly in cases of marked hyperactivity or agitation. When symptoms such as apathy and anergy predominate, a stimulating type of neuroleptic such as *trifluoperazine* is indicated. Although the superiority of one class of neuroleptics over another in the treatment of schizophrenia has not been demonstrated, the individual patient may respond more favorably to another class of neuroleptics than to a phenothiazine. However, before switching to another drug, it should be determined whether the lack of therapeutic response is due to failure of the parent to administer the drug or failure of the patient to ingest the medication.

A patient refractory to a phenothiazine or responding to small doses with excessive sedation, should be given a trial of *thiothixene*, *haloperidol*, or lastly *molindone*, in that order.

The use of drugs in the treatment of psychotic children and adolescents has been reviewed by Campbell (1973, 1975) and Werry (1972).

In *chronic brain syndromes*, with or without mental retardation, a trial of drug treatment is indicated when symptoms such as distractibility, impulsivity, hyperactivity, aggressiveness, or explosiveness are present. If diphenhydramine fails, a neuroleptic can be prescribed.

The same drugs can be administered to children with *mental retardation* (biological and intermediate group) and associated psychosis, or with symptoms such as hyperactivity, aggressiveness, self-mutilation, or explosiveness. Drug treatment of the mentally retarded has been reviewed by Lipman (1970), Freeman (1966, 1970), and Sprague and Werry (1971). It has been pointed out that unfortunately neuroleptics are often used as chemical straightjackets in this population (Lipman, 1970).

Minimal brain dysfunction (*MBD*) is a diagnostic category where the efficacy and superiority of stimulants over placebo has been demonstrated in well designed and controlled studies. Stimulants should be tried first: dextroamphetamine or methylphenidate, and if these fail, magnesium pemoline. In the opinion of these authors, a neuroleptic is indicated only if a stimulant does not produce improvement (Werry, Weiss, Douglas, & Martin, 1966; Werry & Aman, 1975). Although imipramine was administered successfully to hyperactive children in controlled studies (Rapoport, Quinn, Bradbard, Riddle, & Brooks, 1974; Waizer, Hoffman, Polizos, & Engelhardt, 1974; Winsberg, Bialer, & Kupietz, 1972), its use remains investigational in this diagnostic category.

It must be remembered that there are many causes of hyperactivity in children and stimulants are useful in only some of them (Fish, 1971). MBD is only one of the conditions which may be associated with hyperactivity. In addition, only about two-thirds of the hyperactive children with MBD respond to drug treatment. Psychotic patients usually show worsening of disorganization and of other preexisting symptoms on stimulants (Campbell, Fish, David, Shapiro, Collins & Koh, 1972; Campbell et al., 1976; Fish, 1971).

Gilles de La Tourette's syndrome (Maladie des Tics) has been treated effectively with haloperidol, according to reports in the literature (Bruun, Shapiro, Shapiro & Sweet, Wayne & Solomon, 1976; Challas & Brauer, 1963; Chapel, Brown, & Jenkins, 1964; Lucas, 1967; Shapiro, Shapiro, & Wayne, 1973). Bruun and associates (1975) treated 34 patients below the age of 18 with this drug. However, there is only one well controlled study, involving four patients, 12 to 14 years of age, showing that haloperidol is statistically significantly superior to both diazepam and placebo in reducing tics (Connell, Corbett, Horne & Mathews, 1967).

Controlled studies are available indicating the superiority of imipramine over placebo in the treatment of *enuresis* (Poussaint & Ditman, 1965), but other studies report no such positive findings (Abrams, 1963). Enuresis, very much like hyperactivity, is a nonspecific symptom found in a variety of disorders; it occurs in children who were never properly trained or, more frequently, as a result of regression due to a conflict. The underlying problems should be explored and dealt with, or if this is not feasible, conditioning techniques may be tried; they produce longer lasting effects than drugs (McConaghy, 1969). Cure rate is high with sympathetic handling alone (Dische, 1971), or even spontaneously (Forsythe & Redmond, 1974). We do not recommend drug treatment for enuresis, particularly for children under six years of age. The use of drugs in mentally retarded enuretics has been thoroughly reviewed by Sprague and Werry (1971).

At the present time there is no specific drug or class of drugs available for any of the behavioral disorders of childhood and adolescence. In addition, classification and diagnosis in child psychiatry has remained an unresolved problem. The same underlying pathology may be manifested in different symptoms at different ages, while a variety of causes may result in the same behaviors, particularly in young children, because of relative lack of differentiation of functions. The same symptom may be considered mild in a four-year-old, whereas in an adolescent it can be one of the first manifestations of schizophrenia (e.g., school phobia).

Drugs should not be used in mild disorders where environmental factors are prominent, if not causative, except when the purpose of drug administration is to break a vicious cycle. Delinquency or reactive aggressiveness will not be altered by a biological treatment. Eisenberg (1964, 1968) has emphasized that giving drug treatment to a child whose symptoms stem from correctable social, familial, biological, or intrapersonal distrubances, without making an attempt to change the factors causing the symptoms, is poor medicine.

Drugs are most effective in reducing certain target symptoms (Freyhan, 1959) or altering target functions of behavior (Irwin, 1968, 1974). For instance, neuroleptics are most effective in diminishing psychomotor excitement. Irwin (1974) pointed out that this is a direct drug effect on a target function of behavior and is usually predictable; the indirect drug effect develops slowly, usually as a result of the modified interaction of the individual with his environment. He suggested that the only enduring effects of drug therapy on behavior are due to the concurrent environmental, psychosocial treatments. Thus, the hyperactive psychotic child with short attention span, when calmed down by a drug, may be able to focus his attention on a task and thus acquire some reading and writing skills. The agitated, assaultive, or self-mutilating patient, when these symptoms are eliminated or reduced with an effective psychoactive agent, may develop more adaptive social interactions which in turn will improve learning.

Drugs themselves do not create learning or intelligence, nor do they necessarily alter parental attitude, but they can make the child more amenable to environmental treatments or manipulations. It is important to institute drug treatment in the early stages of illness rather than after other, frequently inappropriate therapies have failed. In our clinical experience, the patient seems to respond more to drug therapy in the early stages of illness, though this was not systematically investigated.

Clearly, in the formative years of the individual, drugs alone never suffice. The choice of other treatments (remedial education, individual psychotherapy, group therapy, parental counseling), as well as hospitalization, will depend on contributing factors, associated handicaps of the individual patient, and the family. Many patients, even after the cessation of symptoms such as hyperkinesis, agitation, hallucinations—and no longer in need of drug therapy—will require continuation of other treatment(s) and follow-up.

DRUG ADMINISTRATION

It must always be remembered that drug therapy in children and adolescents should be only a part of the total treatment plan for a particular youngster. Drugs are used to decrease certain symptoms in order to promote maturation and to make the young patient more amenable to other forms of therapy. Consequently, any drug or other modality which interferes with these processes should be discontinued.

A careful inquiry into drug allergy or sensitivity, as well as a comprehensive history of prior drug intake (type of drug, dosage, duration, and date of last drug administration) must be obtained. This is of utmost importance, particularly in emergency situations, since drugs interact and potentiation may take place. Therefore, in an emergency, chloral hydrate or paraldehyde (oral or intramuscular) should be used rather than a neuroleptic.

Role of Parents

Since most, if not all, psychoactive drugs are potentially harmful if not properly used, it is essential to have the drug given by a reliable and cooperative parent. If that is not the case, neuroleptics or other potentially harmful drugs should not be prescribed on an out-patient basis. Accidental overdosage in young children and impulsive suicidal gestures in adolescents with medically prescribed drugs are frequent occurrences. As in general pediatrics, when a medication is prescribed, the physician must be sure that the drug will be given in the prescribed manner. The parent must be advised as to what are the expected therapeutic effects, possible untoward effects, and the limitations of drug treatment. It is equally important for the parents, as well as the child's teacher, to be accurate and reliable observers and to report any changes in the child's adjustment. Whenever possible, the child should also be informed, to the degree he is capable of understanding, as to why he is taking the medication and what he can expect to experience both in therapeutic responses and possible side effects.

The availability of the treating physician, even by phone, may prevent serious complications as well as unnecessary anxieties.

Method of Dose Regulation

Because of the great individual differences that are found among some children, it is recommended that a drug be initially prescribed in low and perhaps often therapeutically ineffective dosages. The dose is then increased in a step-wise and regular progression until either the therapeutic result is achieved or untoward effects are reported or observed; only then is the optimal dose determined. Psychomotor stimulants can be increased two to three times a week, a tricyclic antidepressant or neuroleptic once a week. It is a common clinical error not to explore the full dose range of a particular drug before it is considered to be ineffective for the individual patient. Similarly, it is not good practice to maintain a patient on a too high dosage, which may produce negative effects. It is not uncommon to observe worsening of preexisting symptoms on excess drugs. This must be differentiated from the lack of response to an ineffective low dosage. Referral to the most recent PDR (Physicians' Desk Reference) is recommended.

Polypharmacy

It has not been demonstrated that the use of a combination of psychoactive drugs in children is useful. In fact, polypharmacy is poor medicine since it can confound the therapeutic as well as the untoward effects. Routine administration of antiparkinsonian agents is not recommended; there is evidence that they decrease the plasma levels and the efficacy of neuroleptics and that they may worsen the preexisting psychosis (for review, Ayd, 1975). For the treatment of acute dystonic reactions, administration of 25 to 50 mg of diphenhydramine intramuscularly or orally is effective.

Duration of Drug Treatment

The length of drug treatment is dependent upon several factors and the following should be used as guidelines. Obviously, a child who is experiencing a good clinical response to a drug should be maintained on that drug for a time, but no longer than necessary. In mild cases, where the drug was prescribed to break a pathological cycle, the drug may be stopped when the cycle is broken. In acute psychotic episodes, one month of drug therapy may be sufficient. With chronic symptomatology, three to four months of drug therapy should be maintained before the drug is discontinued to see whether the child has acquired positive or more adaptive behavior which he can retain without the need for continued medication. If the symptoms recur, drug therapy should be reinstituted.

Short drug-free periods or "drug holidays" are recommended over weekends or during school vacations. It is believed that such intermittent discontinuation of drug maintenance will reduce both the risks and incidence of adverse reactions. Clinical experience has shown that drug-induced adaptive behaviors and developmental gains can be retained in many youngsters even after drug withdrawal.

Neuroleptics should be discontinued during acute febrile or childhood illnesses. Medication can be reinstituted in gradual increments after the patient's full recovery.

Failure of drug response can be due to various factors: underdosage, overdosage, noncompliance, manner of drug absorption and metabolism, genetic determinants, and polypharmacy. Of course, there are individuals whose symptoms or illness are refractory to drug treatment.

Psychological dependence and addiction to any of the usually prescribed psychoactive agents does not appear to be a problem in the prepubertal child (Freedman, 1971).

CLASSIFICATION OF DRUGS[2]

PSYCHOMOTOR STIMULANTS

Since Bradley's report in 1937 on the effects of benzedrine in children with a variety of behavioral disorders, the superiority of stimulants over placebo in the treatment of hyperactive MBD children has been documented. The results are based on many well controlled studies, in clinically homogeneous populations, and using sophisticated methodology and statistical analysis.

Symptoms such as disruptive behavior, restlessness, hyperactivity, inattentiveness, and short attention span show marked reduction on stimulant drugs (Conners et al., 1967) in about two-thirds of patients. The results in responders are dramatic. In addition to behavioral improvements, data indicate that psychomotor stimulants improve attention span and performance (Cohen, Douglas, & Morgenstern, 1971; Conners et al., 1967; Conners, 1971a, b; 1972b; Sprague & Sleator, 1973), although correlation between change in behavior and psychometric tests was not always found (Gittelman-Klein & Klein, 1975).

There are indications, however, that the stimulants are therapeutic and equally effective in some non-hyperactive, overcontrolled children (Eisenberg & Conners, 1971; Fish, 1971).

[2]Refer to Table 2-1

The precise mode of action of the stimulants is not known, although there are several interesting theories. Gittelman-Klein and Klein (1973b) suggest that stimulants enhance attentional processes which then enable the child to focus on a task. Secondary to improved attention, the child's behavior is more controlled and he is less hyperactive. Whereas Wender (1975) suggests that one of two major abnormalities of the MBD child is an apparent hyperarousal, accompanied by hyperactivity, inability to concentrate and to focus attention, Satterfield and co-workers (1974) found physiological evidence of low CNS arousal levels in responders to treatment with stimulants. Others have not found that hyperactive children with soft neurological signs and abnormal EEG are necessarily good responders to stimulants (Werry & Sprague, 1974).

The two most commonly used drugs are *dextroamphetamine* and *methylphenidate*. As a starting dose for dextroamphetamine, 2.5 mg b.i.d. is recommended, given at breakfast and at noon; the dose can be rapidly increased. Maximum dosages of 40 to 80 mg per day have been reported. However, 10 to 25 mg per day seems to be the average dose, with good clinical results and yielding fewer side effects than higher doses.

Methylphenidate administration can be started with 5 mg b.i.d.; dosage as high as 80 to 120 mg per day has been reported. Sprague and Sleator (1975) have emphasized that daily dosage should be determined in the standardized form of milligrams per kilogram of body weight, and that side effects are dose related. Sprague and Werry (1973) demonstrated that 0.3 mg/kg of methylphenidate was as effective as higher doses but side effects increased with dosage, including weight loss and worsening of behavior.

Magnesium pemoline has been shown to be promising in the treatment of hyperactive children (Page, Bernstein, Janicki & Michelli, 1974; Dykman, McGrew, & Ackerman, 1974). Its advantage seems to be that it can be given in a single morning dose.

Caffeine too has been explored in hyperkinetic children; controlled studies did not show significant differences between placebo and drug (Conners, 1975; Garfinkel, Webster, & Sloman, 1975).

Table 2-1 CLASSIFICATION OF PSYCHOTROPIC DRUGS AND DOSAGE

	Generic Name	Trade Name	Range in mg/day[1]	Number of Divided Doses
		I. PSYCHOMOTOR STIMULANTS		
	Amphetamine	Benzedrine		
	Dextroamphetamine	Dexedrine[2]	10–25	1–2
	Methylphenidate	Ritalin[3]	30–60 (0.3 mg/kg)	1–2
	Magnesium pemoline	Cylert	25–125 (1.9–2.7 mg/kg)	1
		II. ANTIDEPRESSANTS[4]		
		A. Tricyclics		
	Imipramine	Tofranil, Presamine, SK-Pramine, Imavate	6–225[5] (1–5 mg/kg)	2–3
	Amitriptyline	Elavil	10–75	1–3
	Nortriptyline	Aventyl	10–75	1–3
		B. Monoamine Oxidase (MAO) Inhibitors		
	Phenelzine	Nardil		
	Nialamide	Niamid		
	Tranylcypramine	Parnate		
		III. NEUROLEPTICS (ANTIPSYCHOTICS, MAJOR TRANQUILIZERS)		
		A. Representative Phenothiazines		
a. Aliphatics	Chlorpromazine	Thorazine, Chlor-PZ	10 to 200 (oral) i.m. max 40 (up to 5 years of age), max 75 (5 to 12 years of age)	2–4
	Triflupromazine	Vesprin	1 to 150	2–4
b. Piperidines	Thioridazine	Mellaril	10–200	2–4
c. Piperazines	Fluphenazine	Permitil	0.25–16	1–2
	Trifluoperazine[3]	Stelazine	1–20	1–2
		B. Thioxanthenes		
	Thiothixene[6]	Navane	1–40	1–2
	Chlorprothixene[3]	Taractan	10–200	1–2
		C. Butyrophenones		
	Trifluperidol[7]			
	Haloperidol[6]	Haldol	0.5–16	1–2
		D. Dihydroindolones		
	Molindone[6]	Moban	1–200	1–3

[1]Dosage for children under 12 years of age. Dosage for adolescents comparable to adult dosage. See current PDR for available dosage forms.

[2]Not recommended for patients under 3 years of age.

[3]Not recommended for patients under 6 years of age.

[4]Except for the use of imipramine for enuresis in patients over 6 years of age, tricyclics are not recommended for patients under 12. MAO inhibitors should not be given to children.

[5]Recommended dosage for enuresis: 25–50 mg 1 hour before bedtime for patients 6–12 years of age; 75 mg for patients over 12.

[6]Not recommended for patients under 12 years of age.

[7]Withdrawn from investigational use in U.S.A.

The most frequent *side effects* of stimulants are loss of appetite and weight, and insomnia. Headaches, abdominal pain, irritability, tearfulness, aggressiveness were also noted. Increase of blood pressure and pulse rate has been reported (for review, see Aman & Werry, 1975). Hallucinations were described in both dextroamphetamine (Ney 1967; Winsberg, Bialer, Kupietz, & Tobias, 1972) and methylphenidate (Lucas & Weiss, 1971). Gilles de la Tourette's syndrome developed after eight weeks of administration of 20 mg per day of methylphenidate in a 9-year-old child (Golden, 1974). Though long-term administration of stimulants was said to affect growth adversely (Safer, Allen, & Barr, 1972; Safer & Allen, 1975), this has not been confirmed by an anterospective one-year follow-up; body weight and height of children who were receiving methylphenidate did not differ from controls (McNutt, Ballard, Boileau, Sprague, & von Neumann, 1975). Another one-year follow-up of children treated with the same drug showed a significant decrease in growth rate for weight but not for height (Quinn & Rapoport, 1975).

For review on the use of stimulants, a chapter by Eisenberg and Conners (1971) and books by Conners (1974) and Gittelman-Klein (1975) are suggested.

ANTIDEPRESSANTS

Imipramine, a potent tricyclic antidepressant, has been used since the fifties: studies in adults showed that depressed patients with psychomotor retardation respond better to this drug than those who are agitated.

Tricyclic antidepressants and MAO (Monoamine Oxidase) inhibitors were administered to children, as noted earlier, with a variety of disorders. However, their use, with the exception of imipramine in enuretic children over 6 years of age, remains investigational. MAO inhibitors are not recommended for children or adolescents.

In studies of imipramine in enuretics, usually a low (25–50 mg) single h.s. dose is used and therefore side effects are minimal or absent.

The most common *side effects* with imipramine are anorexia, drowsiness, insomnia, dry mouth, constipation, and irritability. Increase in blood pressure and pulse changes (Greenberg & Yellin, 1975), weight loss (Rapoport, Quinn, Bradbard, Riddle, & Brooks, 1974), orthostatic hypotension (Gittelman-Klein & Klein, 1971), and electrocardiographic abnormalities (Winsberg, Goldstein, Yepes, & Perel, 1975) were reported in children. It remains unresolved whether imipramine has epileptogenic effects (for review see Petti & Campbell, 1975). The pharmacokinetics of imipramine may be different in children than in adults (Winsberg, Perel, Hurwic, & Klutch, 1974) and therefore high single h.s. dose is not recommended.

According to new FDA guidelines, investigational protocols will be approved only if the daily doses do not exceed approximately 2.2 mg per lb. body weight (Hayes, Logan Panitch, & Barker, 1975).

For review of the side effects of antidepressants in children, see Saraf, Klein, Gittelman-Klein, and Groff (1974), and DiMascio, Soltys, and Shader (1970).

NEUROLEPTICS

The advent of neuroleptics (antipsychotics or major tranquilizers) has dramatically changed the practice of psychiatry in adult patients. The impact of these drugs has not been as great in the youngest age groups, and their role has not been clearly established in child psychiatry. Perhaps this is partly due to the fact that the purpose of treatment in children and adolescents is not only to decrease symptoms but, in addition, to enhance development.

For adolescents and children who show the clinical picture of acute schizophrenia, the purpose of treatment is to restore normal functioning. The goal for the preschoolage psychotic child is not only correction of deviant behavior, but also promotion of the delayed or retarded development. Emerging or nonexistent functions, such as speech and adaptive skills, have to be created. Whereas in adults and adolescents with acute schizophrenia, diminution in reactivity via neuroleptics is a desirable effect, the same is considered an untoward effect in the young child who is apathetic, anergic, and lacking motor initiative.

Fish (1970) found that the prepubertal psychotic child is comparable to the chronic schizophrenic adult in terms of response to drugs: he is sedated by small doses of the sedative type of neuroleptics, and the more stimulating agents evoke a more therapeutic response. It is conceivable that the excessive sedation of the child at very low doses of chlorpromazine may be a result of the degree of cerebral dysfunction, as noted above.

There is some, though inconclusive, evidence that the sedative type of neuroleptics, such as chlorpromazine and thioridazine lower functioning and therefore interfere with learning and performance in psychotic and retarded children and in children of normal intelligence (Fish, 1960; Freeman, 1966; McAndrew, Case, & Treffert, 1972; Werry, Weiss, Douglas, & Martin, 1966).

These findings led Fish to a series of clinical trials of psychoactive agents with stimulating properties (trifluperidol, thiothixene, molindone, and T_3), found to be safe and effective in the adult counterpart of psychotic children. On the other hand, a small portion of very young and low IQ children responded positively to drugs which cause worsening of psychosis in adult schizophrenics (such as imipramine, lithium, and L-dopa). (For review, see Campbell, 1973, 1975; Campbell et al., 1976).

With the neuroleptics, therapeutic effects most frequently noted are reduction of excitement, hyperactivity, hallucinations, insomnia, and stereotyped behavior. Drugs with greater potency (requiring small doses) are least sedative and have less tendency to lower the seizure threshold; but they also tend to increase the incidence and severity of extrapyramidal symptoms, particularly akathisia and acute dystonic reactions.

The specific antischizophrenic action of neuroleptics is said to be based on their dopamine-blocking activity (Snyder, 1976).

There are five classes of neuroleptic drugs: the phenothiazines, thioxanthenes, butyrophenones, dihydroindolones, and dibenzoxazepines.

The *phenothiazines* are divided into three subclasses: aliphatic, piperidine, and the piperazine derivatives. The aliphatic group (chlorpromazine, triflupromazine) produce sedative-hypnotic effects. This may be desirable in an older child or an adolescent with acute psychosis and associated symptoms of agitation and anxiety. In the young apathetic and hypoactive child, where psychosis is often associated with retarded functioning, a more stimulating piperazine derivative, such as trifluoperazine or fluphenazine, is recommended. Thioridazine is the representative of the piperidine subclass. It has a low incidence of extrapyramidal and autonomic side effects, and seems to be well tolerated by patients with preexisting seizure disorders.

Chlorpromazine or thioridazine can be given orally in 2 to 4 divided doses, from 10 to 200 mg per day in children under twelve years of age. Doses in adolescents are comparable to adult doses.

Fluphenazine and trifluoperazine (FDA approval for patients over six years of age only) can be given in doses of 0.25 mg to 16 mg up to 20 mg daily, in one to two doses.

Of the *thioxanthenes*, chlorprothixene (FDA approval for patients over six years of age only) can be given in a single or divided dose from 10 to 200 mg daily. Thiothixene (FDA approval for patients over 12 years of age only) is given in 1 to 2 doses a day, from 1 to 40 mg daily. This class of drugs is less likely to produce hematopoetic and hepatic damage and photosensitivity reactions than the phenothiazines. Thiothixene has stimulating properties and a wide therapeutic margin.

The *butyrophenones* decrease agitation without the hypnotic effect of aliphatic phenothiazines. However, the incidence of extrapyramidal side effects is high.

Haloperidol (FDA approval for patients over twelve years of age only) was found effective in both withdrawn and assaultive or self-multilating patients by Engelhardt, Faretra, and others. It can be given in a single dose or in divided doses, from 0.5 to 16 mg daily.

Data indicate that molindone (FDA approval for children over 12 years only), a *dihydoroindlone*, is a neuroleptic with some characteristics of antidepressants: it has activating, stimulating properties, like the piperazine phenothiazines. In our study of preschool children (Campbell et al., 1971), optimal doses were 1 to 2.5 mg per day; extrapyramidal side effects were seen at levels of 1.5 to 7.5 times the optimal dose. Loxapine succinate, a tricyclic *dibenzoxazepine* derivative, a new antipsychotic agent (FDA approval only for patients over 16 years of age), was administered to adolescents 13 to 18 years of age, with a diagnosis of schizophrenia, acute, or chronic with acute exacerbation (Pool, Bloom, Mielke, Roniger, and Gallant, 1976). In this double-blind study, the 75 subjects were randomly assigned to loxapine (average daily dose 87.5 mg), haloperidol (average daily dose 9.8 mg) or placebo; both drugs were significantly superior to placebo in reducing psychotic symptoms, as shown on Brief Psychiatric Rating Scale, but the differences between the two drugs did not appear to be significant.

Of the *untoward effects*, particularly in children, the first to be seen frequently are the behavioral. Some of the undesired effects (sleepiness or hypoactivity) are exaggerated forms of desired effects. Overdosage may result in worsening of preexisting symptoms (hyperactivity, irritability), and must be differentiated from too low a dose.

The *immediate untoward effects of neuroleptics*, in addition to behavioral toxicity (alteration of psychomotor and perceptual-cognitive functions and emotional states—for review, see DiMascio, 1970; DiMascio & Shader, 1970; DiMascio, Shader, & Giller, 1970), are hepatic damage, agranulocytosis, extrapyramidal effects, cutaneous and ocular disorders.

The most serious side effects are allergic (idiosyncratic): icterus occurs usually in the early weeks of treatment, and agranulocytosis in the first two months. The latter is unrelated to dosage; temperature elevation, sore throat, and enlarged lymph nodes are the first clinical signs. Both icterus and agranulocytosis rarely occur when children are under careful clinical and laboratory monitoring.[3]

The extrapyramidal symptoms (EPS) consist of Parkinson-like symptoms (tremor, cogwheel phenomenon, excessive salivation) and dyskinetic symptoms (abnormal movements of face, neck, tongue, jaw, torticollis, oculogyric crisis, opisthotonus, difficulty in speech, and swallowing). Reduction of dosage is recommended; administration of antiparkinsonian agents (benztropine mesylate) is rarely required. Diphenhydramine (25 to 50 mg) orally or intramuscularly relieves the acute dystonic reaction.

Convulsive seizures are reported with neuroleptics; chlorpromazine increased the incidence of seizures in patients with a history of convulsive disorders (Tarjan, Lowery, & Wright, 1957).

Skin and ocular reactions are rare in children. (For review of side effects, see DiMascio, Soltys, & Shader, 1970; Shader & DiMascio, 1970).

Information concerning *long-term untoward effects* is limited. Since psychoactive agents affect the neurotransmitters which control the secretion of hypothalamic neurohormones, caution should be exercised in their administration to prepubertal children and adolescents. They may influence growth, central nervous, endocrine, and reproductive systems. Chlorpromazine decreases growth hormone secretion in adults (Sherman, Kim, Benjamin, & Kolodny, 1971); there are no reports on children. Menstrual irregularities, amenorrhea, galactorrhea, aspermia, and particularly marked weight gain, have been noted. Prolonged administration of neuroleptics may adversely affect IQ (McAndrew, Case, & Treffert, 1972).

Reports are available concerning a neurologic syndrome in children resembling tardive dyskinesia in adults (Schiele, Gallant, Simpson, Gardner, & Cole, 1973). McAndrew et al. (1972) found that of 125 hospitalized patients, age 8 to 15 years, ten developed involuntary movements of the upper extremities with akathisia after the abrupt withdrawal of phenothiazines, and six of these ten patients showed facial tics. These neurological effects were first observed 3 to 10 days after drug withdrawal and ceased within 3 to 6 months. Comparison of these ten patients with those who remained asymptomatic showed that the median duration of drug intake was 32 months in the symptomatic group, versus 4 months in the asymptomatic group. The daily termination dose was 400 mg of chlorpromazine equivalents, in accor-

[3]Pretreatment alkaline phosphatase, serum glutamic-pyruvic transaminase (SGPT), serum glutamic-oxaloacetic transaminase (SGOT), complete blood count (CBC), and urinalysis are recommended. These tests are to be repeated weekly during the first two months of treatment, once a month until the sixth month, and thereafter when indicated.

dance with the standard dose conversion table (Hollister, 1970), in the symptomatic and only 99 mg in the asymptomatic group. The median gram intake was 403 in the first and 8.7 grams in the latter group.

Polizos, Engelhardt, Hoffman, and Waizer (1973) found that 14 out of 34 out-patient childhood schizophrenics showed similar symptoms (involuntary movements, primarily in the extremities, trunk, and head, associated with ataxia) after withdrawal of neuroleptics. Both abrupt total withdrawal and gradual, graded withdrawal with weekly reduction of dose by 25% gave the same results. The relationship of this apparently reversible syndrome to persistent, tardive dyskinesia in adults has not been determined (Engelhardt, 1974).

Miscellaneous

Diphenhydramine was used by Fish (1960); Korein, Fish, Shapiro, Gerner & Levidow (1971) in divided doses ranging from 3 to 26 mg per kg daily (200–800 mg/d) in prepubertal children.

Triiodothyronine (T_3) has been tested by Sherwin et al. (1958) and Campbell et al. (1972, 1973) in a small number of preschoolage autistic children. In these studies, T_3 had both stimulating and antipsychotic effects and was viewed as an agent that is potentially effective in the treatment of this patient population. Further investigations in a homogeneous group of patients under more controlled conditions are required.

Data of Gram and Rafaelsen (1972) and Campbell et al. (1972) indicate that *lithium* administration may be effective in decreasing hyperactivity, aggressiveness, and stereotypies in some retarded autistic schizophrenic children. There is some evidence that lithium has a specific antiaggressive effect when aggressiveness is associated with explosiveness and excitability (Dostal, 1972). The efficacy of lithium should be further explored. It may prove of value in certain behavioral profiles of treatment-resistant severe disturbances.

Both acute and maintenance clinical trials were carried out in psychotic children with the *hallucinogens* d-lysergic acid diethylamide (LSD-25) and a methylated derivative of LSD, L-methyl-D-lysergic acid butanolamide bimaleate (for review, see Fish et al., 1969; Campbell, 1973). The results are inconclusive. In some patients these drugs led to improvement in behavior with a decrease in withdrawal. In other children, stimulation resulted in an increase in anxiety and disorganization.

Barbiturates and *diphenylhydantoin* should be used only as antiepileptics; they are ineffective or may cause a worsening of disorganization.

The value of *anxiolytics* has not been critically assessed in children, although in daily practice they are frequently prescribed.

Chlordiazepoxide may worsen the preexisting psychosis or even create a florid psychosis in patients with borderline schizophrenic features (Campbell and Fish, in preparation); it is not therapeutic and may even be contraindicated in certain diagnostic categories or profiles.

Data of DiMascio, Shader, and Harmatz (1969) from studies with adult patients and normal controls suggest that chlordiazepoxide and some other anti-anxiety agents should not be given to individuals with poor impulse control or aggressiveness.

Hoffer's (1970) findings on the superiority of niacinamide and ascorbic acid over placebo in some schizophrenic children were not confirmed in a double-blind study by Greenbaum (1970). Even Rimland (1973), an advocate of *megavitamin* treatment, considers his results merely encouraging.

An American Psychiatric Association task force concluded that megavitamin therapy was of no value in the treatment of adult schizophrenia (Lipton et al., 1973).

REFERENCES

Abrams, A. L. Imipramine in enuresis. *American Journal of Psychiatry*, 1963, *120*, 177–178.

Aman, M. G., and Werry, J. S. Methylphenidate in children: Effects upon cardiorespiratory function on exertion. In Conners, C. K. (Ed.), *Clinical use of stimulant drugs in children.* Amsterdam; Excerpta Medica, 1975, 119–131.

ANNELL, A. L. The prognosis of psychotic syndromes in children. A follow-up study of 115 cases. *Acta Psychiatrica Scandinavica*, 1963, *39*, 235.

ANTHONY, E. J. Psychoneurotic disorders. In A. M. Freedman and A. G. Kaplan (Eds.), *Comprehensive textbook of psychiatry*. Baltimore: Williams & Wilkins Co., 1967.

AYD, F. J. Treatment resistant patients: A moral, legal and therapeutic challenge. In F. J. Ayd (Ed.), *Rational psychopharmacotherapy and the right to treatment*. Baltimore: Ayd Medical Communications Ltd., 1975.

BENDER, L., and FARETRA, G. The relationship between childhood schizophrenia and adult schizophrenia. In A. R. Kaplan (Ed.), *Genetic factors in "schizophrenia."* Springfield, Ill.: Charles C Thomas Publisher, 1972.

BRADFORD HILL, A. *Principles of medical statistics*. New York: Oxford University Press, 1971.

BRADLEY, C. The behavior of children receiving benzedrine. *American Journal of Psychiatry*, 1937, *34*(5), 577.

BRAMBILLA, F., GUERRINI, A., RIGGI, F., and RICCIARDI, F. Psychoendocrine investigation in schizophrenia. *Diseases of the Nervous System*, 1974, *35*, 362–367.

BRAMBILLA, F., and PENATI, G. Hormones and behavior in schizophrenia. In D. H. Ford (Ed.), *Influence of hormones on the nervous system*. Basel: Karger, 1971.

BRUUN, R., SHAPIRO, A., SHAPIRO, E., SWEET, R., WAYNE, H., and SOLOMON, G. E. *A follow-up of 78 patients with Gilles de la Tourette's Syndrome*, American Journal of Psychiatry, 1976, *33*(8), 944.

CAMPBELL, M. Biological interventions in psychoses of childhood. *Journal of Autism and Childhood Schizophrenia*, 1973, *3*, 347–373.

CAMPBELL, M. Pharmacotherapy in early infantile autism. *Biological Psychiatry*, 1975, *10*(4), 399.

CAMPBELL, M., FISH, B., DAVID, R., SHAPIRO, T., COLLINS, P., & KOH, C. Response to triiodothyronine and dextroamphetamine: A study of preschool schizophrenic children. *Journal of Autism and Childhood Schizophrenia*, 1972, *2*(4), 343.

CAMPBELL, M., FISH, B., DAVID, R., SHAPIRO, T., COLLINS, P., & KOH, C. Liothyronine treatment in psychotic and non-psychotic children under 6 years. *Archives of General Psychiatry*, 1973, *29*(5), 602.

CAMPBELL, M., FISH, B., KOREIN, J., SHAPIRO, T., COLLINS, P., & KOH, C. Lithium-chlorpromazine: A controlled crossover study in hyperactive severely disturbed young children. *Journal of Autism and Childhood Schizophrenia*, 1972, *2*(3), 234.

CAMPBELL, M., FISH, B., SHAPIRO, T., & FLOYD, A., JR. Study of molindone in disturbed preschool children. *Current Therapeutic Research*, 1971, *13*(1), 28.

CAMPBELL, M., SMALL, A. M., COLLINS, P. J., FRIEDMAN, E., DAVID, R., & GENIESER, N. Levodopa and levoamphetamine: A crossover study in schizophrenic children. *Current Therapeutic Research*, 1976, *19*(1), 70.

CHALLAS, G., and BRAUER, W. Tourette's disease: Relief of symptoms with R1625. *American Journal of Psychiatry*, 1963, *120*(3), 283.

CHAPEL, J. L., BROWN, N., and JENKINS, R. L. Tourette's disease: Symptomatic relief with haloperidol. *American Journal of Psychiatry*, 1964, *121*(6), 608.

CHRISTENSEN, D. E. *Combined effects of methylphenidate (Ritalin) and a classroom behavior modification program in reducing the hyperkinetic behaviors of institutionalized mental retardates*. Thesis submitted for the degree of Doctor of Philosophy in Psychology, University of Illinois at Urbana-Champaign, 1973.

CHRISTENSEN, D. E., and SPRAGUE, R. L. Reduction of hyperactive behavior by conditioning procedures alone and combined with methylphenidate (Ritalin). *Behavior Research and Therapy*, 1973, *11*(3), 331.

COHEN, N. J., DOUGLAS, V. I., and MORGENSTERN, C. The effect of methylphenidate on attentive behavior and autonomic activity in hyperactive children. *Psychopharmacologia*, 1971, *22*(3), 282.

CONNELL, P. H., CORBETT, J. A., HORNE, D. J., and MATHEWS, A. M. Drug treatment of adolescent tiquers. A double-blind trial of diazepam and haloperidol. *British Journal of Psychiatry*, 1967, *113*(497), 375.

CONNERS, C. K. Symptom patterns in hyperkinetic, neurotic, and normal children. *Child Developement*, 1970, *41*(3), 667.

CONNERS, C. K. The effect of stimulant drugs on human figure drawings in children with minimal brain dysfunction. *Psychopharmacologia*, 1971, *19*(4), 329. (a)

CONNERS, C. K. Recent drug studies with hyperkinetic children. *Journal of Learning Disabilities*, 1971, *4*(9), 476. (b)

CONNERS, C. K. Pharmacotherapy of psychopathology in children. In H. C. Quay and J. S. Werry (Eds.), *Psychopathological disorders of childhood*. New York: John Wiley, 1972. (a)

CONNERS, C. K. II. Psychological effects of stimulant drugs in children with minimal brain dysfunction. *Pediatrics*, 1972, *49*(5), 702. (b)

CONNERS, C. K. Deanol and behavior disorders in children: A critical review of the literature and recommended future studies for determining efficacy. *Psychopharmacology Bulletin*, Special Issue, "Pharmacotherapy of Children," 1973.

CONNERS, C. K. (Ed.) *Clinical use of stimulant drugs in children*. Amsterdam: Excerpta Medica, 1974.

CONNERS, C. K. A placebo-crossover study of caffeine treatment of hyperkinetic children. In R. Gittelman-Klein (Guest Ed.), Recent advances in child psychopharmacology, *International Journal of Mental Health*, 1975, *4*(1–2), 132.

CONNERS, C. K., EISENBERG, L., and BARCAI, A. Effect of dextraomphetamine on children. *Archives of General Psychiatry*, 1967, *17*(4), 478.

CYTRYN, L., GILBERT, A., and EISENBERG, L. The effectiveness of tranquilizing drugs plus supportive psychotherapy in treating behavior disorders in children: A double-blind study of eighty outpatients. *American Journal of Orthopsychiatry*, 1960, *30*, 113–129.

CYTRYN, L., and MCKNEW, D. J. Proposed classification of childhood depressions. *American Journal of Psychiatry*, 1974, *129*, 149–155.

DIMASCIO, A., and SHADER, R. I. Behavioral toxicity. Pt. I: Definition and Pt. II: Psychomotor functions. In R. I. Shader and A. DiMascio (Eds.), *Psychotropic drug side effects*. Baltimore: Williams & Wilkins, 1970.

DIMASCIO, A., SHADER, R. I., and GILLER, D. R. Behavioral toxicity. Pt. III: Perceptual-cognitive functions and Pt. IV: Emotional (mood) states. In R. I. Shader and A. DiMascio (Eds.), *Psychotropic drug side effects*. Baltimore: Williams & Wilkins, 1970.

DIMASCIO, A., SHADER, R. I., and HARMATZ, J. Psychotropic drugs and induced hostility. *Psychosomatics*, 1969, *10*(1), 46.

DIMASCIO, A., SOLTYS, J. J., and SHADER, R. I. Psychotropic drug side effects in children. In R. I. Shader and A. DiMascio (Eds.), *Psychotropic drug side effects*, Baltimore: Williams & Wilkins, 1970.

DISCHE, S. Management of enuresis. *British Medical Journal*, 1971, *2*(5), 33.

DOSTAL, T. Antiaggressive effect of lithium salts in mentally retarded adolescents. In A. L. Annell (Ed.), *Depressive states in childhood and adolescence*, Stockholm: Almquist & Wiksell, 1972.

DYKMAN, R. A., MCGREW, J., and ACKERMAN, P. T. A double-blind clinical study of pemoline in MBD children: Comments on the psychological test results. In C. K. Conners (Ed.), *Clinical use of stimulant drugs in children*. Amsterdam: Excerpta Medica, 1974.

EISENBERG, L. The autistic child in adolescence.

American Journal of Psychiatry, 1956, *112*(8), 607.

EISENBERG, L. Role of drugs in treating disturbed children. *Children*, 1964, *2*(5), 167.

EISENBERG, L. Psychopharmacology in childhood: A critique. In E. Miller (Ed.), *Foundations in child psychiatry*, Oxford: Pergamon Press, 1968.

EISENBERG, L., and CONNERS, C. K. Psychopharmacology in childhood. In N. B. Talbot, J. Kagan, and L. Eisenberg (Eds.), *Behavioral science in pediatric medicine*. Philadelphia: W. B. Saunders Co., 1971.

EISENBERG, L., GILBERT, A., CYTRYN, L., and MOLLING, P. A. The effectivenss of psychotherapy alone and in conjunction with perphenazine or placebo in the treatment of neurotic and hyperkinetic children. *American Journal of Psychiatry*, 1961, *117*(12), 1088.

ENGELHARDT, D. M. *CNS consequences of psychotropic drug withdrawal in autistic children: A follow-up report*. Paper presented at the Annual ECDEU Meeting, Key Biscayne, Florida, May 23–25, 1974.

FISH, B. Drug therapy in child psychiatry: Pharmacological aspects. *Comprehensive Psychiatry*, 1960, *1*(4), 212.

FISH, B. Methodology in child psychopharmacology. In D. H. Efron, J. O. Cole, J. Levine, and J. R. Wittenborn (Eds.), *Psychopharmacology, review of progress, 1956–1967* (U.S. Public Health Service Publication No. 1836). Washington, D.C.: U.S. Government Printing Office, 1968, 989.

FISH, B. Psychopharmacologic response of chronic schizophrenic adults as predictors of responses in young schizophrenic children. *Psychopharmacology Bulletin*, 1970, *6*(4), 12.

FISH, B. The "one child, one drug" myth of stimulants in hyperkinesis, importance of diagnostic categories in evaluating treatment. *Archives of General Psychiatry*, 1971, *25*(3), 193.

FISH, B., CAMPBELL, M., SHAPIRO, T., & FLOYD, A., JR. Schizophrenic children treated with methysergide (Sansert). *Diseases of the Nervous System*, 1969, *30*(8), 534.

FISH, B., SHAPIRO, T., and CAMPBELL, M. Long-term prognosis and the response of schizophrenic children to drug therapy: A controlled study, *American Journal of Psychiatry*, 1966, *123*(1), 32.

FISH, B., SHAPIRO, T., HALPERN, F., and WILE, R. The prediction of schizophrenia in infancy. Pt. II: A ten-year follow-up of predictions made at one month of age. In P. Hoch and J. Zubin (Eds.), *Psychopathology of schizophrenia*. New York: Grune and Stratton, 1966.

FORSYTHE, W. I., and REDMOND, A. Enuresis and spontaneous cure rate. *Archives of Diseases in Childhood*, 1974, *49*(4), 259.

FREEDMAN, D. X. Report of the Conference on the use of stimulant drugs in the treatment of behaviorally disturbed young school children. Washington, D.C.: Office of Child Development and the Office of the Assistant Secretary for Health and Scientific Affairs, U.S. Department of Health, Education, and Welfare, 1971.

FREEMAN, R. D. Drug effects on learning in children. A selective review of the past thirty years. *Journal of Special Education*, 1966, *1*(1), 17.

FREEMAN, R. D. Psychopharmacology and the retarded child. In F. Menolascino (Ed.), *Psychiatric approaches to mental retardation*. New York: Basic Books, 1970.

FREYHAN, F. A. Clinical and investigative aspects. In N. S. Kline (Ed.), *Psychopharmacology Frontiers*. Boston: Little, Brown & Co., 1959.

FROMMER, E. A. Depressive illness in childhood. In A. Coppen and A. Walk (Eds.), *Recent development in affective disorders, a symposium* (Special Publications, No. 2). *British Journal of Psychiatry*, 1968, 117.

FROMMER, E. A. Indications for antidepressant treatment with special reference to depressed preschool children. In A. L. Annell (Ed.),

Depressive states in childhood and adolescence, Stockholm: Almquist & Wiksell, 1972.

Garfinkel, B. D., Webster, C. D., and Sloman, L. Methylphenidate and caffeine in the treatment of children with minimal brain dysfunction. *American Journal of Psychiatry*, 1975, *132*(7), 723.

Gittelman-Klein, R. *Methylphenidate, behavior therapy and their combination in the treatment of hyperkinesis*. Paper presented at the 14th Annual Meeting of the American College of Neuropsychopharmacology, San Juan, Puerto Rico, December 16–19, 1975. (a)

Gittelman-Klein, R. (Guest Ed.) Recent advances in child psychopharmacology. In *International Journal of Mental Health*, *4*(1–2). White Plains: International Arts and Sciences Press, 1975. (b)

Gittelman-Klein, R., and Klein, D. F. Controlled imipramine treatment of school phobia. *Archives of General Psychiatry*, 1971, *25*(3), 204.

Gittelman-Klein, R., and Klein, D. F. School phobia: Diagnostic considerations in the light of imipramine effects. *Journal of Nervous and Mental Disease*, 1973, *156*, 199. (a)

Gittelman-Klein, R. and Klein, D. F. *The relationship between behavioral and psychological changes in hyperkinetic children*. Paper presented at the 12th Annual Meeting of the American College of Neuropsychopharmacology, Palm Springs, California, 1973. (b)

Gittelman-Klein, R., and Klein, D. F. Are behavioral and psychometric changes related in methylphenidate-treated, hyperactive children? In R. Gittelman-Klein (Ed.) 1975, *International Journal of Mental Health*, *4*, 182–198.

Golden, G. S. Case report—Gilles de la Tourette's syndrome following methylphenidate administration. *Developmental medicine and child neurology*, 1974, *16*(1), 76.

Goldfarb, W. *Childhood schizophrenia*. Cambridge, Mass.: Harvard University Press, 1961.

Goldfarb, W. *Growth and change of schizophrenic children: A longitudinal study*. New York: John Wiley, Halsted Press Book, 1974.

Gram, L. F., and Rafaelsen, O. J. Lithium treatment of psychotic children. In A. L. Annell (Ed.), *Depressive states in childhood and adolescence*, Stockholm: Almquist & Wiksell, 1972.

Greenbaum, G. H. An evaluation of niacinamide in the treatment of childhood schizophrenia. *American Journal of Psychiatry*, 1970, *127*(1), 129.

Greenberg, L. M., and Yellin, A. M. Blood pressure and pulse changes in hyperactive children treated with imipramine and methylphenidate. *American Journal of Psychiatry*, 1975, *132*, 1325–1326.

Group for the Advancement of Psychiatry (GAP). Pharmacotherapy and psychotherapy: Paradoxes, problems and progress (Report No. 93). Vol. IX, New York, 1975.

Hayes, T. A., Logan Panitch, M., and Barker, E. Imipramine dosage in children: A comment on "Imipramine and electrocardiographic abnormalities in hyperactive children." *American Journal of Psychiatry*, 1975, *132*(5), 546.

Hoffer, A. Childhood schizophrenia: A case treated with nicotinic acid and nicotinamide. *Schizophrenia*, 1970, *2*, 43.

Hollister, L. E. Choice of antipsychotic drugs. *American Journal of Psychiatry*, 1970, *127*, 186–190.

Irwin, S. A rational framework for the development, evaluation, and use of psychoactive drugs. *American Journal of Psychiatry*, Suppl., 1968, *124*(8), 1.

Irwin, S. The uses and relative hazard potential of psychoactive drugs. *Bulletin of the Menninger Clinic*, 1974, *38*(1), 14.

Klein, D. F. Importance of psychiatric diagnosis in prediction of clinical drug effects. *Archives of General Psychiatry*, 1967, *16*, 118–126.

Klein, D. F. Psychiatric diagnosis and a typology of clinical drug effects. *Psychopharmacologia*, 1968, *13*, 359–386.

Klein, D. F., and Davis, J. M. *Diagnosis and*

drug treatment of psychiatric disorders. Baltimore: Williams & Wilkins, 1969.

KOLVIN, I. Psychoses in childhood—a comparative study. In M. Rutter (Ed.), *Infantile autism: Concepts, characteristics, and treatment*. Edinburgh: Churchill Livingstone, 1971.

KOREIN, J., CAMPBELL, M., and SMALL, A. M. EEG findings in young schizophrenic children: A study of levodopa and levoamphetamine. Manuscript submitted for publication, 1976.

KOREIN, J., FISH, B., SHAPIRO, T., GERNER, E. W., & LEVIDOW, L. EEG and behavioral effects on drug therapy in children. Chlorpromazine and Diphenhydramine. *Archives of General Psychiatry*, 1971, *24*(6), 552.

LIPMAN, R. S. *Methodology of drug studies in children*. Paper presented at the American Orthopsychiatric Meeting, Chicago, Illinois, 1968.

LIPMAN, R. S. The use of psychopharmacological agents in residential facilities for the retarded. In F. Menolascino (Ed.), *Psychiatric Approaches to Mental Retardation*. New York: Basic Books, 1970.

LIPTON, M. A., BAN, T. A., KANE, F. J., LEVINE, J., MOSHER, L. R., & WITTENBORN, R. *Megavitamin and orthomolecular therapy in psychiatry*. Washinton, D.C.: American Psychiatric Association, 1973.

LUCAS, A. R. Gilles de la Tourette's disease in children: Treatment with haloperidol. *American Journal of Psychiatry*, 1967, *124*(2), 243.

LUCAS, A. R., LOCKETT, H. J., and GRIMM, F. Amitriptyline in childhood depressions. *Diseases of the Nervous System*, 1965, *26*(2), 105.

LUCAS, A. R., and WEISS, M. Methylphenidate hallucinosis. *Journal of the American Medical Association*, 1971, *217*(8), 1079.

MCANDREW, J. B., CASE, Q., and TREFFERT, D. Effects of prolonged phenothiazine intake on psychotic and other hospitalized children. *Journal of Austism and Childhood Schizophrenia*, 1972, *2*(1), 75.

MCCONAGHY, N. A controlled trial of imipramine, amphetamine, pad-and-bell conditioning and random awakening in the treatment of nocturnal enuresis. *Medical Journal of Australia*, 1969, *2*(5), 237.

MCNUTT, B., BALLARD, J. E., BOILEAU, R., SPRAGUE, R., and NEUMANN, A. von. *The effects of long term stimulant medication on growth and body composition of hyperactive children*. Paper delivered at the Annual Meeting of ECDEU, NIMH, Key Biscayne, Florida, 1975.

NEY, P. G. Psychosis in a child, associated with amphetamine administration. *Canadian Medical Association Journal*, 1967, *97*, 1026.

PAGE, J. G., BERNSTEIN, J. E., JANICKI, R. S., and MICHELLI, F. A. A multi-clinic trial of pemoline in childhood hyperkinesis. In C. K. Conners (Ed.), *Clinical use of stimulant drugs in children*. Amsterdam: Excerpta Medica, 1974.

PETTI, T. A., and CAMPBELL, M. Imipramine and seizures. *American Journal of Psychiatry*, 1975, *132*(5), 538.

PICHEL, J. I. A long-term follow-up study of sixty adolescent psychiatric outpatients. In S. Chess and A. Thomas (Eds.), *Annual progress in child psychiatry and child development*, 1975, New York: Brunner/Mazel, 1976.

POLIZOS, P., ENGELHARDT, D. M., HOFFMAN, S. P., and WAIZER, J. Neurological consequences of psychotropic drug withdrawal in schizophrenic children. *Journal of Autism and Childhood Schizophrenia*, 1973, *3*(3), 247.

POOL, D., BLOOM, W., MIELKE, D. H., RONIGER, J. J., and GALLANT, D. M. A controlled evaluation of loxitane in seventy-five adolescent schizophrenic patients. *Current Therapeutic Research*, 1976, *19*, 99–104.

POUSSAINT, A. F., and DITMAN, K. S. A controlled study of imipramine (Tofranil) in the treatment of childhood enuresis. *Journal of Pediatrics*, 1965, *67*(2), 283.

Psychopharmacology Bulletin (Special Issue), *Pharmacotherapy of Children*, Spring 1973.

QUINN, P. O., and RAPOPORT, J. L. One year follow-up of hyperactive boys treated with imipramine or methylphenidate. *American Journal of Psychiatry*, 1975, *132*(3), 241.

Quitkin, F., Rifkin, A., and Klein, D. Neurologic soft signs in schizophrenia and character disorders. *Archives of General Psychiatry*, 1976, *35*(7), 845.

Rapoport, J. L., Quinn, P. O., Bradbard, G., Riddle, D., and Brooks, E. Imipramine and methylphenidate treatments of hyperactive boys. *Archives of General Psychiatry*, 1974, *30*(6), 789.

Rimland, B. High dosage levels of certain vitamins in the treatment of children with severe mental disorders. In D. Hawkins and L. Pauling (Eds.), *Orthomolecular Psychiatry*. San Francisco: W. H. Freeman and Company, 1973.

Robins, L. N. *Deviant children grown up*. Baltimore: Williams & Wilkins, 1966.

Robins, L. N. Follow-up studies investigating childhood disorders. In E. H. Hare and J. K. Wing (Eds.), *Psychiatric Epidemiology*. London: Oxford University Press, 1970.

Rutter, M. Autistic children: Infancy to adulthood. *Seminars in psychiatry*, 1970, *2*(4), 435.

Rutter, M., and Lockyer, L. A five to fifteen year follow-up study of infantile psychosis. I. Description of sample. *British Journal of Psychiatry*, 1967, *113*, 1169–1182.

Safer, D. J. and Allen, R. P. Side effects from long-term use of stimulants in children. In R. Gittelman-Klein (Ed.), Recent advances in child psychopharmacology. In *International Journal of Mental Health*, 1975, *4*, 105–118.

Safer, D., Allen, R. P., and Barr, E. Depression of growth in hyperactive children on stimulant drugs. *New England Journal of Medicine*, 1972, *287*(5), 217.

Saraf, K. R., Klein, D. F., Gittelman-Klein, R., and Groff, S. Imipramine side effects in children. *Psychopharmacologia*, 1974, *37*(3), 265.

Satterfield, J. H., Cantwell, D. P., Lesser, L. I., et al. Physiological studies of the hyperkinetic child, I. *American Journal of Psychiatry*, 1972, *128*(11), 1418.

Satterfield, J. H., Cantwell, D. P., and Satterfield, E. T. Pathophysiology of the hyperactive child syndrome. *Archives of General Psychiatry*, 1974, *31*(6), 830.

Schiele, B. C., Gallant, D., Simpson, G., Gardner, E. A., and Cole, J. O. Tardive dyskinesia. *American Journal of Orthopsychiatry*, 1973, *43*(4), 506; 688.

Shader, R. I., and DiMascio, A. (Eds.). *Psychotropic drug side effects*, Baltimore: Williams & Wilkins, 1970.

Shapiro, A. K., Shapiro, E., and Wayne, H. Treatment of Tourette's syndrome. *Archives of General Psychiatry*, 1973, *28*(1), 92.

Sherman, L., Kim, S., Benjamin, F., & Kolodny, H. D. Effect of chlorpromazine on serum growth-hormone in man. *New England Journal of Medicine*, 1971, *284*(1), 72.

Sherwin, A. C., Flach, F. F., and Stokes, P. E. Treatment of psychoses in early childhood with triiodothyronine. *American Journal of Psychiatry*, 1958, *115*(2), 166.

Snyder, S. H. The dopamine hypothesis of schizophrenia: Focus on the dopamine receptor. *American Journal of Psychiatry*, 1976, *133*, 197–202.

Sprague, R. L., and Sleator, E. K. Effects of psychopharmacologic agents on learning disorders. *Pediatric Clinics of North America*, 1973, *20*(3), 719.

Sprague, R. L., and Sleator, E. K. What is the proper dose of stimulant drugs in children? In R. Gittelman-Klein (Guest Ed.), Recent Advances in Child Psychopharmacology. In *International Journal of Mental Health*, 1975, *4*(1–2), 75.

Sprague, R. L., and Werry, J. S. Methodology of psychopharmacological studies with the retarded. In N. R. Ellis (Ed.), *International review of research in mental retardation*, New York: Academic Press, 1971.

Sprague, R. L., and Werry, J. S. Pediatric psychopharmacology. *Psychopharmacology Bul-*

letin (Special Issue), 1973, Pharmacotherapy of children.

STACK, J. J. Chemotherapy in Childhood Depression. In *Depressive states in childhood and adolescence*, Stockholm: Almquist & Wiksell, 1972.

TARJAN, C., LOWERY, V. E., and WRIGHT, S. W., Use of chlorpromazine in two hundred seventy-eight mentally deficient patients. *American Medical Association Journal of Diseases of Children*, 1957, *94*(6), 294.

WAIZER, J., HOFFMAN, S. P., POLIZOS, P., and ENGELHARDT, D. M. Outpatient treatment of hyperactive school children with imipramine. *American Journal of Psychiatry*, 1974, *131*(5), 587.

WEINBERG, W. A., RUTMAN, J., SULLIVAN, L., PENICK, E. C., and DIETZ, S. G. Depression in children referred to an educational diagnostic center: Diagnosis and treatment—Preliminary Report. *Journal of Pediatrics*, 1973, *83*(6), 1065.

WEISS, G. The natural history of hyperactivity in childhood and treatment with stimulant medication at different ages: A summary of research findings. *International Journal of Mental Health*, Spring-Summer 1975, *4*, (1–2), Recent Advances in Child Psychopharmacology, Guest Editor, R. Gittelman-Klein, 213.

WENDER, P. H. Speculations concerning a possible biochemical basis of minimal brain dysfunction. In R. Gittelman-Klein (Guest Ed.), Recent Advances in Child Psychopharmacology. In *International Journal of Mental Health*, 1975, *4*, 11–28.

WERRY, J. S. Childhood psychosis. In H. C. Quay and J. S. Werry (Eds.) *Psychopathological Disorders of Childhood*. New York: John Wiley, 1972.

WERRY, J. S., and AMAN, M. G. Methylphenidate and haloperidol in children, effects on attention, memory and activity. *Archives of General Psychiatry*, 1975, *32*(6), 790.

WERRY, J. S., and SPRAGUE, R. L. Methylphenidate in children—effect of dosage. *Australian and New Zealand Journal of Psychiatry*, 1974, *8*, 9–19.

WERRY, J. S., WEISS, G., DOUGLAS, V., and MARTIN, J. Studies on the hyperactive child, III. The effect of chlorpromazine upon behavior and learning ability. *Journal of the American Academy of Child Psychiatry*, 1966, *5*(2), 292.

WINSBERG, B. G., BIALER, I., KUPIETZ, S., and TOBIAS, J. Effects of imipramine and dextroamphetamine on behavior of neuropsychiatrically impaired children. *American Journal of Psychiatry*, 1972, *128*(11), 1425.

WINSBERG, B. G., GOLDSTEIN, S., YEPES, L. E., et. al. Imipramine and electrocardiographic abnormalities in hyperactive children. *American Journal of Psychiatry*, 1975, *132*(5), 542.

WINSBERG, B. G., PEREL, J. M., HURWIC, J., et al. Imipramine protein binding and pharmacokinetics in children. In I. S. Forrest, C. J. Carr, and E. Usdin (Eds.), *The phenothiazines and structurally related drugs*, New York: Raven Press, 1974.

WORLD HEALTH ORGANIZATION. Scientific group on psychopharmacology: Research in psychopharmacology (WHO Tech. Rep., Series, No. 371.) Geneva: World Health Organization, 1967.

3

BEHAVIOR THERAPY

Anthony M. Graziano

This chapter presents an overview of behavior therapy, and as such is not intended to be a detailed examination of research or clinical cases. Rather we will briefly sketch the development of behavior therapy, its current status within the mental health field, its principal forms, and the major issues that concern their use. Although we limit our task to an overview, the field is complex enough so that any brief discussion remains, in effect, merely an "opening statement."

The terms *behavior modification* and *behavior therapy* are often used interchangeably but should be differentiated. Behavior modification is the more inclusive term, referring to a large area of research and application involving the systematic, empirical study of behavior, its development, maintenance, and change. Focusing on observed data, behavior modifiers use scientific methods, largely patterned after laboratory experimentation, to discover, test, and predict empirically derived relationships among variables. An important feature of behavior modification is the commitment to test continuously its own assumptions and effectiveness through the application of systematic methods that are specified, publicly accessible and, therefore, replicable. Claims made by its adherents can thus be publicly reexamined by others.

Some of the most important assumptions made by behavior modifiers are that (1) human behavior is complex and multiply determined; (2) the immediate stimulation (both discriminative and reinforcing) of the external environment is among the most critical of those multiple determinants; (3) behavior is thus largely a function of its consequences; (4) systematic manipulation of those immediate stimulus conditions will result in predictable behavioral changes; and (5) the most desirable form of behavior modification is self-control, i.e., when the systematic manipulations of the environment are planned and carried out by the person whose behavior is to be modified.

This broad category, behavior modification, includes several subsets, which share the assumptions noted above but focus on different problems, subjects, or settings. Thus a set of behavioral approaches to academic tasks has been termed "programmed instruction," while "behavior therapy" is the application of behavior modification to clinical problems. The subsets are defined not by differences in basic concepts but by the different problem behaviors on which they focus and the specifics of applied strategies appropriate for those problems.

Behavior therapy, then, as the clinical subset of the larger category, behavior modification, assumes that a person's psychological problems are largely determined by current environmental factors; that the most effective intervention for many clinical problems is the careful, systematic manipulation of specified environmental variables; that such manipulation will result in predictable improvement, and that self-control is the general goal of behavior therapy.

HISTORY

However new behavior modification and its subsets might appear, they are descendants of much earlier experimental work, for example, the animal psychology of Thorndike, Hunter, Hamilton, Yerkes, and Small; the Russian objective psychologists Sechenov, Behkterev, and Pavlov (Boring, 1950); and Watson's strongly stated behaviorism. Applied subsets of behavior modification emerged in the 1920s as both behavior therapy in clinical practice and as automated teaching and "behavior modification" in education. Early behavior therapy included work by Haberman (1917), Watson and Raynor (1920), Jones (1924), Jacobson (1929), Kantorovich (1929), Holmes (1936), Weber (1936), and Mowrer (1938), much of it focusing on children's fears, conditioning treatment for enuresis, and relaxation training for adults.

The first usage of the term *behavior modification* as an applied area may have been in J. Stanley Gray's 1932 article entitled "A biological view of behavior modification." Writing to educators, Gray urged them, in good Watsonian tradition, to give up their subjectivism and instead focus on children's behavior, determining for each pupil *what* behavior is to be modified and then, with careful attention to details, controlling all relevant learning variables in that environment. Gray maintained that any child's failure to learn is a failure of the educator to teach—i.e., not effectively manipulating those relevant variables.

Another early form of behavior modification in education was the development of automated teaching machines by Sidney L. Pressey from about 1919 through 1932. Pressey maintained that the development of his teaching machines could lead to an advanced "technology of education." However, few others had Pressey's foresight; thus despite the now obvious promise of his early teaching machines and the continued interest of a few researchers, his development was largely ignored. In 1932 Pressey "regretfully" abandoned his project, still hoping that others would eventually recognize its potential.

The important point here is that by the 1920s two applied subsets of behavior modification had already emerged from its laboratory and animal psychology background: (1) behavior therapy, i.e., behavior modification applied to clinical problems; and (2) programmed instruction, consisting of Pressey's teaching machines and Gray's "behavior modification" in schools. Neither development, however, had significant impact on applied psychology at that time. Behavior therapy was thoroughly overshadowed by Freud's revival and popularization of the "Romantic Psychiatry" of nearly a century earlier; the educational technology foreseen by Pressey was largely inappropriate, particularly in the depression years (Graziano, 1975).

For approximately the next thirty years psychiatry, using mainly psychodynamic and organic models, was the major profession that struggled with the problems of treating mental patients. Applied behavior modification virtually disappeared, but in academia experimental psychologists continued their laboratory study of behavior. Psychologists amassed behavioral data, developed learning concepts and even elaborate and perhaps premature theories of learning processes, and they trained several generations of graduate students. By the late 1950s academic psychologists had educated a large number of professionals, probably a more knowledgeable and sophisticated group than any other professionals in the scientific study of human behavior—but not necessarily sophisticated in the practical application of behavioral science to the solution of common clinical problems.

It was not until the late 1950s and early 1960s

that behavior modification in applied forms would reemerge and begin its still continuing exploration toward an effective technology of human behavioral change in education and mental health. This reemergence occurred as increasing numbers of psychologists entered mental health settings, largely because of the manpower needs of World War II. Among those clinicians were many behaviorally oriented psychologists who introduced a behavioral dimension into the clinical field. By the late 1950s behavioral concepts as well as treatment roles for psychologists were becoming fairly common in the field, although not without frequent, serious conflicts, particularly between psychologists and psychiatrists. The psychological learning views were gradually influential both because of the experimental basis of the learning concepts and a simultaneous weakening of various psychodynamic models. Behavioral explanations, particularly those based on the respondent and instrumental models of Pavlov and Hull were seriously proposed, not only as adjuncts to psychodynamic conceptions (e.g., Dollard & Miller, 1950) but also as clearly alternative models (e.g., Eysenck, 1959; Wolpe, 1958). A number of psychologists who were identified as research workers "... turned their attention to clinical populations and problems so that the distinction between experimentalist and clinician became blurred" (Ullman & Krasner, 1965, p. 58). Quite clearly, behaviorally oriented psychologists were entering the mental health "mainstream" as increasingly active and influential professionals. By 1960 the conceptual "mix" of the mental health field was quite different than it had been just a few years earlier, and the old psychodynamic certainties were no longer secure.

Add to this the "rediscovery" and refinement of Pressey's teaching machines by Skinner (1954) and the remarkable, crisis-toned public demands in the late 1950s for massive "crash programs" to improve our educational system so as to surpass the Russians—and behavior modification, in the form of programmed instruction, was rapidly ushered into schools. This served as an important precedent for the slightly later surge of behavior therapy. With these developments influencing both education and mental health, behavior modification applied to the solution of human problems grew rapidly. It developed its own literature and professional training programs and became a highly visible—and intrusive—part of the mental health field.

CURRENT STATUS

Since its reemergence in the late 1950s and early 1960s behavior therapy has grown rapidly, proceeding through several stages. First, the work of the early sixties largely involved the demonstration of behavior change—i.e., that clinically important behaviors of adults and children can be systematically modified and that the changes are associated with a variety of behavioral treatment "packages." Many early treatment packages were devised and applied to increasing numbers and varieties of clients and subjects—systematic desensitization, implosive therapy, aversive therapy, extinction procedures, parent training, programmed psychotherapy, behavioral counseling, and so on. Generally the majority of those early studies had so many methodological weaknesses that it was virtually impossible to identify the specific variables that were responsible for the measured changes. More importantly, although behavior changes were demonstrated, many critical characteristics of those changes were not evaluated. For example, accepting the notion that demonstrated changes did occur, it must still be asked if those measures of change were valid and reliable; if the changes were successfully generalized from the treatment situation to the natural environment; whether the changes, as generalized, were permanent or at least long lasting and, perhaps most importantly, whether the observed changes were *psychologically* significant, statistical significance notwithstanding.

These earlier studies raised many questions and left many unanswered. Through the 1960s their significance lay not in their research methodology, precise validation, or attempts to answer all questions, but in their repeated and varied demonstrations that systematic behavior change does occur.

Those early demonstrations of successful behavior change were too often uncritically overinterpreted by enthusiastic adherents. They overvalued the significance of the observed changes and prematurely attributed them to particular aspects of their total treatment packages, despite the fact that their research generally lacked sufficient controls to isolate the effective variables. As a result the claims and suggestions of effectiveness of particular procedures were overblown and became easy targets for appropriate criticism. Unfortunately the criticisms, while very well taken, obscured the most significant aspect of that early clinical research, i.e., that systematic behavior change was being repeatedly demonstrated, across a wide variety of problems and clients.

As research continued many other early weaknesses were highlighted and attempts made to correct them. One of the major problems that became apparent in the late 'sixties was that although behavioral change had been amply demonstrated there was little evidence that the changes were permanent or satisfactorily long lasting. Researchers seldom tracked the behavior changes over time. In fact it became clear that all too often when the treatment conditions were withdrawn the original maladaptive behavior was quickly reinstated. Gradually it was realized that behavior change was only part of the therapeutic process, that maintenance systems must be designed into behavior therapy. At the present time the technology of maintaining new, adaptive behavior does not seem to be as well developed as that of behavior change, and a good deal of continued work is needed.

By about 1970 it had been demonstrated that clinically problematic behavior can be systematically changed—although the precise variables responsible for the change were not isolated—and that behavior maintenance systems must be designed as carefully as behavior change systems. Early maintenance systems consisted essentially of continued application of therapeutic contingencies by persons other than the therapist, particularly in work with children. For example, in the late 'sixties and early 'seventies parents were trained to continue the therapists' contingency management of children in the home, and teachers to maintain these methods in the classroom. However, concern was expressed over teaching parents, teachers, and others sophisticated control over children, pointing out that the goals of such control were not necessarily in the child's best interest. Further, adult clients would find it difficult or impossible to accept control imposed by persons other than the therapist. Essentially those maintenance systems would involve a transfer of control from the therapist to other persons in the client's natural environment—and such extended control would create its own problems. Why not, then, teach clients to be in charge of their own behavioral change and maintenance programs? Teaching self-control—to recognize and effectively manipulate the variables controlling one's own behavior—was not a new idea, but for the first time was being considered by many therapists and researchers as a potentially valuable treatment paradigm. By the mid-seventies self-control had become a major and growing area of investigation by behavior modifiers.

In the past two years or so, there has been a marked heightening of the old ethical issues, all grouped around the basic question, What are the conditions under which the various behavior modification subsets can be operative without severe conflict with other value systems in our society? The ethical issues are far from new, but they have acquired new urgency as behavior technology has developed to more sophisticated levels.

Currently behavior modification in general and behavior therapy in particular have high professional and public visibility. The number of articles and books that have appeared surpassed in 1972 the number of publications in psychoanalysis (Hoon & Lindsley, 1974). Benassi and Lanson (1972) reported a striking growth in the number of college courses in behavior modification and Yen (1971) noted that 84% of psychology doctoral programs offered at least one course in behavior modification. Between 1963 and 1970 four new professional journals appeared—*Behaviour Research and Therapy*, *Journal of Applied Behavior Analysis*, *Behavior Therapy*, and *Behavior Therapy and Experimental Psychiatry*. By such measures behavior therapy is our most rapidly growing area of therapy research and writing.

Training of new professionals in behavior

therapy has increased but is still largely concentrated within the discipline of psychology, while psychiatric training settings have largely ignored behavior therapy (Brady, 1972). A recent American Psychiatric Association task force (Birk, et al., 1973) has recommended that behavior therapy be made part of psychiatric training. However, even if medical schools and residency programs were immediately to initiate behavioral training, the influence of their graduates in the applied clinical field would not be apparent for a number of years. It appears that for some time to come psychology will remain the most active, contributing discipline in behavior modification.

It is clear that behavior modification concepts are having considerable influence on the more academic areas of research and publication, where psychologists are particularly active. But its influence in applied clinical practice is still not known. Although at least one national survey has been attempted (Pailler & Graziano, 1972), sufficient information on the use of behavior therapy in clinical settings is not yet available.

Behavior modification has unfortunately also been the recipient of some rather negative comments. Public officials—Spiro Agnew, the former Vice-President in the corrupt Nixon Administration, was one of the first—have flayed "behaviorism"; journalists of such stature as the *New York Times*' Tom Wicker have condemned it, and Jessica Mitford, an able and influential writer, has added her popular book *Kind and Usual Punishment* (1973) to the public criticisms. Legal actions (Martin, 1974) have even been initiated and, clearly, behavior modification is perceived neither lightly nor as a matter limited to private therapist-client interactions. Congressional investigations such as the one conducted by Senator Sam Ervin's committee and special presidential review panels are clear indications that fears of the possible abusive power of behavior modification have gone far beyond writers' criticisms and have reached the level of both congressional and executive federal concern.

Public investigations, debate, and challenges will undoubtedly continue for many years.

Behavior modification is generally perceived by laymen and professionals as a new and perhaps even "revolutionary" development that is categorically "different" from other, "traditional" therapies. However new and revolutionary it may appear, (1) behavior modification has a history of more than fifty years, emerging from fairly well-defined academic areas, and (2) behavior therapy, by virtue of its inclusion in the contemporary mental health mainstream, necessarily shares the same "helping" goals, humanitarian and ethical concerns, and practical limitations imposed by the realities of delivery systems. Since behavior therapy is now an active and interactive dimension within this common professional ground, it can no longer rightly be considered "categorically" different or separate from other therapy models. Viewed in this manner behavior therapy is not only a subset of behavior modification but also a contemporary variation in the common enterprise of psychological "helping."

In summary, behavior therapy, a clinical subset of behavior modification, has a history reaching back into the 1920s, but its most vigorous development began in the 'sixties. It is now a highly visible part of the mental health mainstream, sharing common goals and many problems with all other variations of psychological helping, but making different assumptions about the nature of psychological disturbances and the most effective intervention strategies. Behavior therapy's current status is that of a highly active and still growing area whose major strength is its continuing commitment to critical evaluation of its own assumptions and effectiveness.

MAJOR FORMS OF BEHAVIOR THERAPY

Behavior therapy has been applied to adults and children across virtually all psychological problem areas. Ideally, however active the behavior therapist may be, client participation will be high, with the client's development of self-control skills remaining a major goal. Hopefully the behavior therapist and the client will develop an explicit "contract," sometimes written, that specifies goals, methods of change, maintenance, and monitoring, i.e., a statement of each party's expected commitment to the therapy process.

Some form of baseline behavior evaluation is carried out in all behavior therapy in order to identify (1) the target behavior that is to be modified, (2) the controlling stimuli surrounding those responses, and (3) the specific stimuli that will be best manipulated in order to bring about the planned behavior changes.

Behavior therapy is a constellation of paradigms and clinical procedures rather than a single model, and its diversity of forms can be organized in many ways. A useful organization has been provided in Rimm and Masters' (1974) textbook, and will serve as the basis for the following material.

SYSTEMATIC DESENSITIZATION

Developed by Wolpe (1958, 1974), this form of behavior therapy is used primarily with adults and rarely with children, for anxiety-mediated or generally "neurotic" problems. It is one of the best known and widely applied behavioral approaches.

In Wolpe's view neurotic problems develop through classical conditioning, in which powerful anxiety responses come to be elicited by common stimuli. The conditioned anxiety is a physiological response, a burst of activity of the sympathetic nervous system. When it is of high magnitude or prolonged, the anxiety can seriously inhibit productive alternative behavior and severely impair the person's functioning. Thus the central task in treating problems of a "neurotic" nature is to break those classically conditioned bonds between the conditioned stimuli and the anxiety responses. Systematic desensitization is the therapeutic technique that Wolpe has proposed to bring about that deconditioning.

According to Wolpe, systematic desensitization operates on the principle of reciprocal inhibition, which assumes that incompatible responses tend to inhibit or weaken each other. It follows, then, that when a person emits two nearly simultaneous, incompatible responses of unequal strength, the stronger will tend to inhibit the weaker, and under carefully controlled conditions those inhibiting effects can be maximized and used therapeutically. As the inhibiting response, systematic desensitization employs deep muscle relaxation, a response mediated by the parasympathetic nervous system. The client is trained in deep muscle relaxation and, when sufficiently skilled, is presented with a sequence of imaginal, anxiety-eliciting stimuli, arranged in the order of least to most anxiety producing. At each step in the hierarchy the relaxation response is presumably always maximal, while the anxiety response begins at a minimal level, only gradually increasing in strength. Thus, at each step, the more powerful relaxation response will presumably inhibit anxiety and gradually break the conditioned bonds. At the completion of the desensitization sequence, little or no anxiety should be elicited by even the most powerful stimulus on the hierarchy. Systematic desensitization constitutes a gradual exposure to anxiety-producing stimuli, paired at each step with anxiety-inhibiting, maximum relaxation responses, and resulting in the dissolution of the classically conditioned bonds.

Systematic desensitization is applied to anxiety-mediated problems, typically in a one-to-one therapy setting, and employing imaginal anxiety stimuli. Variations of this basic application include in vivo, group, and automated desensitization procedures. In vivo desensitization has the client using relaxation skills to proceed along a planned hierarchy not in imagination, but in real-life settings. As in the imaginal procedures, gradual exposure in planned sequences, with maximal relaxation at each step, is emphasized. It is generally agreed that in vivo desensitization should be attempted only after the client has had initial success in the imaginal procedure.

Both group and automated desensitization have obvious implications for greater efficiency in a limited-resource field and have been successfully tested across a number of phobic problems. The success of automated desensitization also provides some additional validation for the power of desensitization techniques, since automated presentations largely control for therapist factors.

Wolpe's work has had a powerful systematic and heuristic impact. The research literature indicates that systematic desensitization is effective with a wide variety of adult, anxiety-mediated problems, and generally requires relatively few (16 to 23) treatment sessions (Paul, 1969). While systematic desensitization is clearly an effective and useful clinical technique, it is a complex treatment package where the specific variables that account most for the improvements have not yet been isolated. Research activity in this area proceeds at a fast pace, aimed both at additional validation of the total treatment package and isolating the effective variables within the package. There is every reason to expect continued research to yield even more effective and efficient systematic desensitization procedures.

Some researchers have applied relaxation training, alone or in conjunction with systematic desensitization, to a number of children's problems. For example, Graziano and Kean (1968) reported an early use of relaxation training to reduce "high excitement" responses of severely psychotic children. Alexander, Miklich, and Hershkoff (1972) successfully employed relaxation training to reduce asthmatic responding in children.

Assertive Training

Many clients have serious difficulty asserting themselves, even mildly, in social situations. Their inability may be the result of strong anxiety that inhibits assertive behavior, for example, the person too fearful to express emotion or to refuse unreasonable demands made by others, particularly authority figures. Non-assertion may also be caused by lack of social skill, which results in social failures and consequent anxiety. In either case non-assertive behavior, whether anxiety-mediated or caused by social skill deficits, might be modified by some form of assertive training.

Consistent with overall behavioral approaches, assertive training includes (1) a specification of the conditions under which problematic non-assertive behavior occurs and (2) systematic training to teach specified, alternative behavior, in this instance, assertive behavior. The training might proceed from relatively unstructured discussions of how to deal generally with problem situations, through behavior rehearsal, a role-playing technique much like Kelley's fixed-role therapy. In behavior rehearsal the client practices assertive statements and affective expressions that are appropriate in specific situations, while the behavior therapist assumes appropriate roles. Following such behavior rehearsal, the client might begin applying the newly learned assertive statements and affect in real-life situations. This might be arranged in hierarchical form, proceeding from relatively simple real-life situations that elicit minimum anxiety, through more highly charged settings. As in systematic desensitization, lower levels of mastery are required before proceeding to more demanding situations.

Success in assertive training has been attributed to reciprocal inhibition, a respondent model in which assertive behavior is assumed to be incompatible with an inhibiting of anxiety; to social reinforcement, an operant model in which skill training leads to progressively greater social success, which is presumably of high reinforcement value; and to the combined effects of both. There is growing evidence for effectiveness of assertive training techniques. Generally there is less systematization in clinical approaches and fewer basic data on the effective variables for assertive training than is the case for systematic desensitization. At any rate, assertive training is another very useful clinical tool through which certain problems can be approached, and which does result in reduced anxiety and greater social skill.

Even more than systematic desensitization, assertive training has been used primarily with adult clients. Its appropriateness with shy, unassertive children and adolescents seems obvious, but there has been little work in this area. Such lack of application to children, despite the apparent appropriateness, might reflect a generalized, strong negative value that adults place on children's assertive behavior.

Operant Methods

Behavior therapy approaches that involve operant methods constitute a vast and varied field of techniques applied to virtually all behavior problems. These methods essentially involve the application of operant paradigms in which behavior is understood to be controlled by specifiable antecedent and consequent stimulus events. It has been amply demonstrated that behavior is modifiable through the systematic manipulation of either or both sets of controlling stimuli.

Consistent with general behavior therapy approaches, the therapist specifies the target behavior to be modified and identifies the controlling stimuli. The latter include both discriminative stimuli, which precede and "set the occasion for" behavior, and the reinforcing or punishing stimuli which follow and strengthen or weaken the behavior. The therapist then initiates one or more operant procedures that provide for weakening specified maladaptive behavior and/or strengthening of adaptive behavior, through the systematic manipulation of discriminative and reinforcing stimuli.

The term *contingency management* refers to only part of a total behavior therapy program, the manipulation of *consequent* stimuli, the rewards and punishments that follow or are contingent upon the response. Although contingency management often appears to be the major focus of operant therapy approaches, it is also crucial to control the other end of the paradigm, the antecedent or discriminative stimuli. The planning of an operant treatment program requires knowledge of both discriminative and reinforcing functions and, at least at this point, is still best done by therapists with knowledge of operant theory. Once the program has been planned, contingency management can be carried out in a relatively straightforward manner by closely supervised teachers, ward personnel and, increasingly, parents of child clients. Contingency management can appear deceptively straightforward, and often casual observers and critics mistake some simple contingency management procedure for total behavior therapy programming. This lack of understanding might be one factor in the often heard criticism that behavior therapy is "simplistic."

The details of operant programming are complex, involving the simultaneous integration of many important dimensions, and programs vary greatly from one case to another. In general outline, however, operant programming (1) specifies target behavior and its controlling antecedents and consequents; (2) identifies specific, effective reinforcing stimuli; (3) arranges for systematic manipulation of discriminative stimuli and for systematic contingency management; (4) monitors the program's effects; (5) arranges for the generalization and maintenance of behavioral gains outside the treatment setting; (6) aims throughout therapy for the overall development of client self-control or self-management.

Operant methods have been applied to adults, adolescents, and children in individual and group therapy; in institutional groups such as schoolrooms, hospital wards, and prisons; and in residential settings. They have been applied to virtually all behavior problems; to weaken and remove maladaptive behavior, to strengthen already existing adaptive behavior, and to generate and strengthen new adaptive behavior. Programs have ranged from simple, unidimensional efforts such as reducing a child's severe bedtime crying by withholding parents' attention, to complex operant programming involving entire wards or families. In the latter programs, entire social systems are involved and many complex, interacting factors are simultaneously included.

Overall, operant strategies of behavior change are aimed at the reduction of maladaptive surplus behavior (response decrement) and the development of adaptive behavior (response acquisition and facilitation). Generalization and maintenance of behavior gains entail an extension of those basic strategies. Some of the major operant methods to reduce maladaptive behavior include *extinction* (e.g., withholding social reinforcement for throwing a tantrum); *punishment* (e.g., contingent electric shock to reduce self-injurious behavior); *response-cost*, a contingent punishment procedure (e.g., clients in a weight-reduction program pay a fine each week they post no weight reduction); *response-countingent withdrawal of reinforcement*, (e.g., "time out"); *overcorrection*, (e.g., contingent mouthwashing and teeth brushing following an undesirable oral act such as a child's chewing inedible or dangerous substances); *negative practice* (e.g., standing in front of a mirror and going through prolonged practice of a tic; a fire-setting child being made to complete many trials of lighting innumerable matches in quick succession until satiated).

Methods to increase adaptive responding entail variations in stimulus control and in positive and negative reinforcement. The therapist can manipulate stimulus control to increase the probability that the desired response will occur through *instructions* to the client that might be relatively informal or might be formalized to the degree of a written contract; specific *cueing* of a response will increase its probability; *modeling* the behavior to be imitated is often used; developing social "rules" such as those in token economies and, generally, *modifying the physical environment* so as to maximize the occurrence of certain classes of responses (e.g., reducing distracting auditory and visual stimulation to increase attention to reading tasks in brain-injured children).

Positive reinforcement is seen in many variations of *shaping* procedures, such as in training attentive behavior in retarded children and adults; in *token economies*, applied individually or in whole social groups such as hospital wards; and in *self-reinforcement* where clients reward themselves, contingent upon their own desirable behavior.

Negative reinforcement is strengthening a response through the withdrawal of aversive stimulation contingent on a desirable response. Although common in everyday life (e.g., a child ceases his noxious whining when his mother finally gives in to his demands, thus reinforcing his mother's "giving-in" behavior), negative reinforcement is difficult to manipulate therapeutically and is not a common procedure. One example is from our own work with non-responsive autistic children (Graziano, 1974); to generate responses to the staff we maintained a "barrage" of social stimulation at the child, ceasing only when the child emitted a vocal sound. Another example is provided by Blake (1965) whose aversion treatment of alcoholics included the termination of an electric shock each time the client spit out a mouthful of liquor. Negative reinforcement in an aversion therapy method is difficult to use except under extremely well-controlled conditions and is not a common behavior therapy procedure.

Behavior therapy based on operant paradigms cannot be considered a single approach or model of therapy, but is instead a varied set of strategies. In the final analysis, no evaluation can be made of the effectiveness of "operant therapy." Each operant strategy, as applied to specified classes of problem behaviors, must be evaluated separately.

Modeling Procedures

Modeling procedures in behavior therapy are relatively new, very promising and not yet as widely used as systematic desensitization or the array of operant procedures. Although largely operant in concept, employing social cueing and reinforcement, modeling provides a combination of operant and respondent concepts and employs methods ranging from shaping through systematic desensitization.

The essential paradigm in modeling is the presentation to a client of one or more persons behaving in some specified, desired manner (e.g., speaking out in a group, approaching some irrationally feared animal), followed by the client's reinforced imitation of the modeled behavior. The basic paradigm is then modeling–imitation–reinforcement.

Modeling techniques have been studied as methods to bring about the acquisition of new behavior (e.g., teaching speech to autistic children); to facilitate existing but weak behavior (e.g., increasing the social responsiveness of shy children); to reduce anxiety and to disinhibit behavior that had been inhibited by anxiety (e.g., approach or assertive behavior in a feared situation). Modeling appears particularly well suited for work with children, and much of the literature reflects this.

Modeling can be adapted for many procedures to meet the particular problems of given clients. The models displaying the target behavior might be actually present (live modeling) or on film or videotape (symbolic modeling). Modeling can be carried out for individuals or for groups of clients, can be presented in one session or in a graduated sequence over several sessions, depicting increasingly difficult behavior. Clients may observe and later practice imitation or they can be progressively involved, as in participant modeling. In some fear treatment, for example, contact desensitization can involve a graduated sequence of guided, participant modeling with progressively decreasing body contact with the therapist (e.g., holding therapist's hand).

Modeling involves maximum cueing for the client in a complex paradigm—i.e., attention is paid not only to modeling overt acts but also to illustrating the cues that surround the target behavior. Further, the behavior modeled is not necessarily a unidimensional social or verbal response, but appropriate *affective* behavior is also illustrated. Finally, both imitation by the client and reinforcement is planned into the treatment sequence.

The reinforcement in modeling approaches, particularly those approaches aimed at the acquisition or facilitation of behavior, can be arranged along operant lines, i.e., contingent on the client's imitation of the modeled behavior. For example, in teaching verbal behavior to autistic children, the child is presented a food reward immediately upon each successful imitation of some vocalization modeled by the therapist.

In graduated contact desensitization, modeling procedures are organized in a manner similar to in vivo systematic desensitization. For a child afraid of animals, the therapist might first model appropriate fearless behavior (approaching and petting a dog) as the child observes. Then holding the child's hand or with an arm around a shoulder, the therapist accompanies the child as they approach the animal, maintaining physical contact and soothing the child as they proceed. They stop at any point the child indicates his discomfort is growing too high, in order to calm down and renew their progress. In graduated steps the child moves closer to the animal, touches and pets it, still in body contact with the therapist, and gradually progresses to fearless interaction with the dog without body contact with the therapist.

While a great deal of research has been carried out on the reduction of adults' fears, Graziano (1975) points out that very little has been done with reducing children's fears. Some modeling approaches appear well suited for children's fear reduction, for example, live modeling (Bandura, Grusec, & Menlove, 1967) and symbolic modeling (Bandura & Menlove, 1968). In a review Rachman (1972) predicted that modeling procedures will become increasingly important in children's fear reduction.

AVERSION THERAPY

Aversion therapy entails a variety of techniques predominantly used to treat adult behavior disorders that are highly self-reinforcing (e.g., sexual deviations, alcoholism) and severe behavior that has resisted all other treatment efforts, such as cases of severely self-mutilative psychotic children. Overall, aversion therapy aims at the direct reduction of resistant maladaptive responses and is used when response decrement is the major goal.

Aversion therapy paradigms involve the manipulation of aversive events, in close association with the emitted target behavior and the antecedent cues that occasion or elicit the target behavior. The particular emphasis on and timing of these three events (cue, target behavior, aversive stimulus) may vary depending on the particular goals at that point in therapy; i.e., the aversive event can be presented simultaneously with or immediately following the target behavior, or paired with any antecedent controlling stimuli or with a response anywhere in the chain leading to the target behavior. Further variations are possible in the nature of the aversive stimulus, which can range widely in intensity and duration and can consist of the presentation of a variety of unpleasant stimuli (e.g., electric shock, loud shouting, a slap on the thigh, unpleasant tasting material).

1. Contingent aversive stimulation is the most commonly used strategy in aversive therapy—and it is also, a notably common child-rearing strategy in our soceity (e.g., spanking). It entails the application of an aversive event during or immediately following an undesirable behavior. Response suppression is typically rapid under these conditions but it is extremely important to also strengthen a desirable alternative response.

2. Covert sensitization is a relatively recent technique (Cautela, 1966) and involves *imaginal* pairing of the target behavior with imagined aversive consequences. Typically the therapist attempts to develop imagined aversive events that are truly horrendous for the client. Covert sensitization has been used to treat

a variety of problems including alcoholism, obesity, sexual problems, sadistic fantasies, gasoline sniffing, delinquent behavior, self-destructive behavior, and smoking.

Overall, the research literature reflects reasonably good success with adults in the treatment of sexual disorders and alcoholism, and in reducing self-injurious behavior of psychotic children. As Rachman and Teasdale (1969) conclude, desensitization is preferred over aversion for reducing or eliminating surplus behavior but, where the disorder is not anxiety-mediated, aversion may be necessary.

There are many problems, ethical and physical, in applying aversive techniques. The use of drugs must be clearly medically supervised and sometimes requires hospitalization in order to provide safeguards against negative side effects. Obviously a client's informed consent is particularly important in aversion therapy. Where such consent is problematic, as with child clients, aversive techniques beyond such forms as mild contingent punishment (e.g., verbal punishment) must be considered only in rare and extreme situations where all else has failed. An example is use of contingent electric shock to eliminate severe self-abusive behavior of a child.

Extinction Procedures

Extinction refers to the gradual weakening of a response through its nonreinforced repetition. The operant strategy of withholding reinforcement upon occurrence of an undesired response, e.g., ignoring a child's temper tantrums that had been maintained by social reinforcement, is an example of an extinction procedure. An array of other tactics, operantly and respondently based, such as negative practice and satiation procedures, are not properly extinction processes, but are also used to weaken and eliminate undesirable behaviors. The methods in this group and their theoretical rationales vary but, because their shared goal is one of response decrement, they are generally grouped as behavior "extinction" procedures.

Aversive therapy also includes a heavy, but not exclusive emphasis on response decrement, because of the nature of the major reinforcing stimuli used, however, they were discussed separately.

1. The systematic withholding of contingent reinforcement for undesired behavior is clearly an extinction procedure, one that is frequently used with children. In practice operant extinction is best combined with the systematic reinforcement of desirable alternative behavior, and the extinction procedure actually becomes one of systematic, differential reinforcement.

Problems treated successfully with operant extinction procedures include children's whining and crying, temper tantrums and disruptive behavior in school; excessive scratching, somatic complaints, and psychotic verbalizations in adults.

Although withholding positive reinforcement has aversive properties, it is generally "benign" in nature, but there are cautions for its use. Extinction procedures require many unreinforced repetitions of the target behavior and often also result in a "frustration effect," an immediate upsurge of the target behavior. Thus for certain classes of problems, such as a child's self-injurious behavior, extinction procedures are clearly not appropriate. Although extinction in such instances might eventually prove effective, a child could, during prolonged extinction trials and because of the frustration effect, self-inflict severe physical trauma. Also, in many group settings it is extremely difficult for a teacher or therapist to control and contingently withhold reinforcement. Social reinforcement in particular can be provided by persons other than the teacher or therapist. Other children, for example, can easily undermine an extinction procedure by continuing to pay attention to the class disruptor while the teacher tries to ignore him. A procedure to reduce the effects of such peer reinforcement is "Time-Out," i.e., temporarily and contingently removing the child from the reinforcing setting. Finally, as noted above, it is important to include a response facilitation dimension to any operant extinction strategy, i.e., to add a systematic differential reinforcement of some desirable alternative behavior.

2. Graduated extinction is an approach aimed at the elimination of avoidance and fearful behaviors. Essentially, the child is moved along a graduated hierarchy, usually real rather than imagined, from weak to strong fear-evoking stimuli, and is not allowed

to engage in his characteristic avoidance behavior. In some ways similar to systematic desensitization, it differs in that there is no competing response, such as relaxation, paired with the anxiety-inducing cues. Rather the anxiety reduction presumably occurs from non-reinforcement rather than reciprocal inhibition.

Graduated extinction has been reported in the treatment of fear of going out-of-doors, of public speaking, and of small animals. It is a promising approach, but there has not been a great deal of research or clinical use of the technique.

3. Imaginal, covert variables are employed in a variety of extinction procedures, including covert extinction, flooding and response prevention, and implosive therapy. In covert extinction the clients imagine that they have emitted the target behavior, but the usual reinforcing stimuli do not occur. An adolescent stutterer, for example, is instructed vividly to imagine a scene in which he stutters, but no one becomes upset, laughs, or otherwise reacts negatively. The imagined scenes are repeated, often presented in massed practice, and can also be progressive, along a hierarchy.

4. Flooding and response prevention involve exposing an individual to maximum fear-inducing simuli, while preventing the occurrence of avoidance responses. Flooding has not been widely used in a clinical setting, but animal studies have shown it to be a potentially useful technique that must be considered still tentative and experimental. It is not an appropriate technique for children or adolescents.

5. Implosive therapy is essentially a flooding procedure applied within a psychoanalytic framework. It involves the presentation of highly fear-provoking, imaginal scenes rather than real objects or events, their content determined by the therapist employing psychoanalytic interpretations. In practice they are truly "horrific" scenes, presented in highly dramatic fashion, all designed to invoke maximum anxiety responses by the client.

The research evidence for implosive therapy is at best very mixed and weak (Morganstern, 1973) and the technique is of doubtful effectiveness.

Implosive therapy is inappropriate for children. As we have noted elsewhere (Graziano, 1975) implosive techniques with children or adolescents have been reported in at least three cases. However, "There are obvious ethical and humanitarian issues involved in deliberately, maximally and repeatedly frightening children, whatever the therapeutic goals may be. After all, the child-client is not allowed the option of walking out of a session or of summarily disengaging the therapist, options that are routinely available to adults. . . . Further . . . there is little or no convincing evidence of the effectiveness of implosive therapy. We submit, then, that there are good reasons for *not* using implosive techniques with children, and we strongly urge that their use be discontinued" (Graziano, 1975, pp. 286–287).

It seems clear that behavioral treatments of first choice for anxiety-mediated problems are best developed around systematic desensitization models. Graduated extinction procedures appear to have clinical value but need much more clinical research. Flooding appears promising but must be considered to be experimental, used with caution and then more for research rather than clinical goals. Implosive therapy does not appear useful and, given the available alternatives, is not recommended.

COGNITIVE BEHAVIOR THERAPY

The major emphasis in behavior therapy is on the objective manipulation of overt behavior and its controlling external stimuli. However, internal stimuli including cognitive and emotional variables, are also manipulated in behavior therapy. In systematic desensitization the client attends to such internal stimuli as anxiety and muscle relaxation; imaginal scenes are manipulated as variables in many procedures; and appropriate affective responding is part of many modeling and assertive training sequences. Cognitions constitute a large class of internal responses and controlling stimuli, and this class has been emphasized in virtually all therapy, including some behavior therapy. In a variety of *cognitive behavior therapy approaches*, cognitive variables are included, while the overall behavioral emphasis on overt behavior, structured interviews, present functioning rather than past experiences, and the systematic manipulation and monitoring of stimulus-response relationships, is maintained.

Cognitive behavior therapy approaches assume that disordered thinking is an important variable in a chain of events leading to disordered behavior, that systematic, rational examination and manipulation of the client's thinking patterns can result in goal-directed change in the client's functioning.

The most extensive and continuing work in this area has been that of Albert Ellis (e.g., 1962) in developing *Rational Emotive Therapy.* Ellis and the client systematically examine the rationality and functional power of the client's thinking in terms of "self statements" that are stimulated or controlled by specific events in the client's life and lead to disruptive emotionality (as opposed to appropriate affect) and to maladaptive behavior, which in turn further reinforces the entire maladaptive chain. The therapist attempts to discover and specify each link in the maladaptive chain, that is, precipitating event—disruptive, inappropriate emotions—maladaptive responses. He or she then attempts to examine and alter the irrational or problematic beliefs and thought patterns.

Another cognitive behavior therapy technique is *thought stopping*, in which clients are taught to discontinue and prevent disturbing obsessive thoughts by practicing self commands such as a sharp "Stop!"

Overall, cognitive behavior therapy treatment packages provide convincing validation through case studies and empirical research, and appear to be useful sets of clinical approaches.

Behavioral Self-Control

Although self-control concepts are not new, a technology of behavioral self-control is very recent. Traditionally self-control has been viewed in terms of trait concepts (Thoresen & Mahoney, 1974), as a person's reservoir of inner strength that allows restraint in the face of powerful external forces. Will power is the common term, and people are thought to "have varying amounts of it." There is little functional value in the traditional views, however, since they do not lead to specific procedures to enhance self-control.

The emerging behavioral concepts view self-control as a person's acquired skills in manipulating variables that affect his or her own functioning. Consistent with the basic behavior modification view, it is assumed that human behavior is functionally related to a variety of internal and external stimuli, discriminative, eliciting and reinforcing; that the functional relationships can be discerned and the controlling variables manipulated so as to modify the person's functioning. In essence the behavioral self-control concept asserts that people *can learn to carry out their own functional analyses, to manipulate the controlling variables and thus modify and maintain their own behavior to their own best advantage.*

This is an optimistic concept, for it asserts that people can learn to exercise much greater control over their own lives. Unlike will power concepts the behavioral model views self-control (self-regulation, self-management) as a set of learned skills that can be taught via a specific teaching technology. It also asserts that the effectiveness of both the teaching technology and the self-control skills can be empirically demonstrated.

By and large self-control studies have been carried out with adults. A few quite recent studies have been carried out with children. As we have noted elsewhere, "the development of self-control skills by children has considerable potential importance; the greater the degree to which children can learn to manage their own lives, the more successful they will become in dealing with the variety of unsettling and even destructive controls that beset adults" (Graziano, 1975, p. 531).

The development of some form of self-control has been a general but implicit goal of virtually all therapy models, but, with recent momentum toward development of a behavioral self-control technology, it seems clear that self-control as an explicit goal, bolstered by at least the beginnings of an applied methodology, is currently best developed, and perhaps found only, in behavior therapy.

In addition to its overall and increasingly explicit position as a common behavior therapy goal, self-control technology has been used specifically in behavioral maintenance programs to preserve newly learned adaptive behavior, to treat problems of obesity and smoking, to improve the study behavior of students, to treat homosexuality, test anxiety, social anxiety, and to develop self-control over impulsive behavior in children.

The implications of the development of an effective self-control technology are significant and, as with other behavior modification areas, continued research is necessary if those implications are to become reality.

CRITICAL ISSUES

The present space is too limited to allow more than a brief glimpse at some of the numerous, complex issues concerning the use of behavior therapy. The reader is referred to the more complete recent discussions by London (1972), Mahoney, Kazdin and Lesswing (1974), Graziano (1975), Begelman (1975), and many others.

The strong reemergence of behavior modification stimulated a still growing literature that was critical of the "new" therapies. Among the first discussions were the Rogers-Skinner dialogues (1956), which seemed largely a modern restatement of the philosophical issues raised in the Romantic Protest movement of the late eighteenth and early nineteenth centuries. Ullmann and Krasner (1965) discussed the issues raised by the mid sixties, and Breger and McGaugh (1965) wrote an important critical review that has been followed by many others. As we noted earlier, the critical issues are currently debated not only in professional journals, but also in the courts, and they have provoked federal administrative and legislative action.

Overall the nature of the criticisms has changed as the field has matured (Mahoney et al., 1974), the criticisms and resulting debates, although intended initially to single out behavior therapy, have sharpened issues that apply to the entire psychotherapeutic field (Graziano, 1975); and, in time, behavior therapists and researchers have become their own sharpest critics, thus integrating into the field active and influential self-corrective components.

The major criticisms can be subsumed into two main categories, (1) ethical issues, and (2) conceptual and empirical issues. Another set has not usually been discussed but, because we believe it to be at least as important as the others, we will include (3) political issues.

Ethical Issues

Many important ethical issues are involved in providing therapeutic services, one of the major issues in behavior therapy being that of therapists' control over their clients. Critics have argued that the very concept of "behavioral control" is antithetical to humantiarian goals of "freedom." In the past arguments purporting to dissociate behavior therapy from "humanistic" therapy have been almost ludicrous. For example, "humanistic" psychotherapists supposedly operate in such manner as to "free" their clients and "implicitly guard against control," while behavior therapy "has nothing at its core to prevent practitioners from becoming behavioral controllers" (Portes, 1971, p. 305). We submit that the position of these critics is both misleading and dangerous, because it persists in presenting to the public the idea that such a grossly contradictory situation as a control-free influence system is available in the form of "humanistic" or "traditional" psychotherapy. That position obscures the most important issue: *the clear, honest, recognition that all therapies and mental health systems exert control over their clients!*

The major ethical issue here is not which therapists exert control over their clients but, rather, what are the ethical limits of control over clients that *all* therapists exert? As we have asked elsewhere (Graziano, 1975), "To what degree should a person or professional system influence the lives of people in the name of helping?" This is a general issue, common to all therapies and must be recognized as such. The client is in a vulnerable position and depends for protection on therapy's "moral surround," i.e., on the therapist's integrity, and on legal and ethical constraints on abuse of the power to influence.

Behavior therapy, more than any other system, specifies its controlling operations. In effect it has forced attention back to all other therapy models in which control is implicit and subtle, but no less real. By making the control issue explicit, behavior therapy may have advanced the entire field, not only by sharpening therapists' responsibilities around control issues, but also by providing explicit guides for clients, the mental health consumers, more intelligently to evaluate the services they are receiving.

Conceptual and Empirical Issues

The basic criticism has been that "behaviorism," the theoretical basis of behavior therapy, is "inherently too simplistic" adequately to account for complex human functioning. Its "limited" S-R focus omits the reality of emotional and cognitive factors which, according to other models, account for virtually all significant clinical events. Applied behavior therapy, therefore, *must* suffer major limitations. For example, it can be applied only to discrete problems or, generally, to "simple behavior and noncomplex patients such as children, retardates, psychotic and autistic individuals" (Portes, 1971, p. 304); and it can be used "only analogically" (Breger & McGaugh, 1965), "as if" the therapy methods accurately reflected the theoretical model. Because of their model's conceptual limitations, behavior therapists, according to critics, must implicitly use traditional techniques. For example, Locke (1971) argued that Wolpe's methods "violate" behavioristic tenets by instructing clients to "introspect," to assess "feelings" and "cognitions," in a therapy environment of "reassurance, support and encouragement." According to Locke those mentalistic and emotional sensitivities have no place in behaviorism and, if they do occur, the therapy, by definition, cannot be behavioral.

Critics admit that behavior therapy may be effective, but not for the reasons given by behavior therapists. Rather, they argue, the "action orientation," verbal manipulation, information feedback, and the implicit emotional support that occurs in behavior therapy help to clarify the client's perceptions and self-understanding through cognitive and emotional changes. Those are the events—not conditioning—that supposedly account for whatever success the therapy might have.

It has also been argued that behavior therapy's empirical base is faulty, the evidence having been drawn largely from clinical case descriptions and poorly controlled studies. Where there is evidence for success, it is said to be limited to uncomplicated, discrete problems. However, even the more obvious successes have not been left unqualified, for a common and, surprisingly, still-expressed opinion is that even if behavior change is brought about, if underlying motivation is ignored, then it will be achieved at the cost of symptom substitution.

Our response to those criticisms is not to deny them—indeed, most of them have some validity. Rather, consistent with our response to the ethical issues outlined earlier, we will emphasize that the criticisms reflect common weaknesses that apply to the entire therapy field; that the controversies have considerable potential value in their illumination of major common issues; and, as behavior therapy solves those issues within its own domain, the entire therapeutic endeavor can be enhanced. This may be an extreme position, but it is this writer's view that at least to the "traditional" mental health practitioner, "behavior therapy" has become a metaphor, albeit barely recognized, for all that is wrong with the field; and the implicit challenge seems to say that if behavior therapists cannot solve the problems, then the entire field will remain at its current dubious level of effectiveness.

Our argument, briefly, is as follows: it is a gross disservice to limit the criticisms to behavior therapy, thereby erroneously suggesting that other therapies are free from those failings. For example, behavior therapy has been criticized for the incompleteness of its theoretical base; yet this writer knows of no "complete" or directly applicable theoretical base for any psychological therapy, and to suggest that such completeness exists outside of behavior therapy is a distortion. In truth, any current model of human behavior must be grossly incomplete, providing only symbolized approximations of nature. When applied clinically, all such models can be used only analogically, *as if* they faithfully represented reality; that is, only as guides to assist the clinician to organize observed and inferred events about the client. Any attempts by science to understand the complexities of nature are essentially analogical and limited to incomplete theoretical statements. In this regard the concepts of behavior therapy are no less complete than those of any other current therapy or personality model.

Similarly, the criticisms that behavior therapy is limited to "simple" clinical problems, that it has ignored cognitive and emotional variables, and that it offers limited empirical evidence of success were perhaps valid in the early 1960s but do not apply to modern behavior therapy. Over the past ten years behavior therapy approaches have been applied to an increasing variety of clinical problems that are far more complex than the earlier focus on unidimensional phobias. Behavior therapy now includes socialization and abstraction skills taught to hospitalized psychiatric patients, complex work skills taught to retardates, and the treatment of marital conflicts, depression, a variety of thought disorders and even "existential neuroses" (as reviewed by Mahoney et al., 1974). Clearly, modern behavior therapy cannot be charged with ignoring cognitive variables, since a major trend in the past decade has been the integration of cognitive and behavioral processes, seen most clearly in the emerging self-control technology. Similarly invalid is the criticism that modern research in behavior therapy is limited to single-subject designs or uncontrolled case studies, since the flood of behavioral research in the past ten years has included notable progress toward more sophisticated, better designed studies.

As for the persistent symptom substitution hypothesis, researchers have repeatedly pointed out that this tenacious belief is not based on empirical evidence. Rather, the theoretical statement that symptom substitution must occur under certain common conditions has been considered, apparently, powerful enough to constitute its own evidence. When one searches for support for the hypothesis, very little is found (Meyer & Crisp, 1964; Balson, 1973). If symptom substitution does occur in behavior therapy, it occurs as the exception and not as the general rule. Overall a good deal of evidence indicates that symptom substitution does not occur ordinarily and, to the contrary, that a good deal of generalized improvement can follow behavior therapy.

By and large the major criticisms of behavior therapy over the past ten years have tended toward the general assumption that theoretical limitations, ethical problems, and empirical inadequacy do not apply to "traditional" therapy models. We have argued that such an assumption is wrong and that those criticisms apply to all psychological therapy models. We cannot accept the implicit assumption that because "traditional" therapy models have been used more extensively for a longer time, they must have somehow already solved all of those problems. "The fact is that most of the serious conceptual, ethical, empirical and political problems have not been solved by any therapy model and the solutions are still ahead of us. In this regard behavior therapy, perhaps more than any other model has incorporated empirical means to evaluate its own effectiveness" (Graziano, 1975, pp. 33–34).

POLITICAL ISSUES

It is generally agreed that the current delivery of mental health services is in many ways inadequate to meet the nation's demands. Whatever the theoretical models and applied strategies, a major—and perhaps *the* major—barrier to delivery of effective services and to making a significant contribution to society is the self-serving politics of the mental health profession. Political power distortions of scientific and humanitarian goals have resulted in scarce, expensive, and questionably effective services (summarized in Graziano, 1975).

Behavior modifiers are proposing alternative technologies; but before we become too enthralled with their promise, we must remind ourselves of the deadly political entrapment that is endemic in any complex social area, including mental health service delivery. We must recognize that the social value of behavior therapy will ultimately depend not only on its future technological, empirically validated effectiveness but, to an equally important degree, on *its success in avoiding the political power distortions that have already affected the mental-health field.* Given that reminder, we must ask: Even assuming the overall technical superiority of behavior therapy (an assumption that takes us far from the data), what leads us to believe that our therapy will be any more successful than that of our psychodynamic colleagues in avoiding those political power distortions?

Regardless of how effective the technology might eventually become, it must always be applied in a political context that will determine who is to control the technology. Behavior modifiers are not sufficiently concerned with these issues and are thus ignoring some of the major external factors that will determine the future value of behavior modification.

SUMMARY AND CONCLUSIONS

We have presented an overview of behavior therapy, touching briefly on its development, current status, major forms, and the main critical issues. Behavior therapy is a large, complex, still growing subset of behavior modification. It has a history reaching back into the 1920s, but its most vigorous development has occurred over the past fifteen years. It is now a highly visible part of the mental health mainstream, sharing common goals and many problems with all other variations of psychological "helping," but making different assumptions about the nature of psychological disturbance and the most effective intervention strategies. Behavior therapy offers concepts and strategies that are clear alternatives to psychodynamic therapies, and perhaps its major strength is its continuing commitment to critical evaluation of its own assumptions and effectiveness.

The earlier studies published through the mid-sixties were largely exploratory and suffered from design problems that limited their power as validation for behavior therapy approaches. However, midway through the seventies, we found the research quality had improved and an impressive amount of good research had accumulated. It must be emphasized that behavior therapy is a constellation of paradigms and approaches rather than any single, unified model. Thus one cannot rightly accept or reject behavior therapy in general but must rather consider the research evidence for each of its major forms, and as applied to the various problem categories.

Behavior therapy is subject to all the major ethical, conceptual, empirical, and political problems and constraints that still apply to the entire mental health field. It is our hope that because of their strong research commitment behavior therapists and researchers will be able to solve many of those problems, not only as they apply to behavior therapy but for the entire field.

REFERENCES

Alexander, A. B., Miklich, D. R., and Hershkoff, H. The immediate effects of systematic relaxation training on peak respiratory flow rates in asthmatic children. *Psychosomatic Medicine*, 1972, *34*.

Balson, P. M. Encopresis: A case with symptom substitution. *Behavior Therapy*, 1973, *4*, 134–136.

Bandura, A., Grusec, J. E. and Menlove, F. L. Vicarious extinction of avoidance behavior. *Journal of Personality and Social Psychology*, 1967, *5*, 16–23.

Bandura, A., and Menlove, F. L. Factors determining vicarious extinction of avoidance behavior through symbolic modeling. *Journal of Personality and Social Psychology*, 1968, *8*, 99–108.

Begelman, D. A. Ethical and legal issues of behavior modification. In M. Herren, R. M. Eisler, and P. M. Miller (Eds.), *Progress in behavior modification* (Vol. I). New York: Academic Press, 1975.

Benassi, V., and Lanson, R. A survey of the teaching of behavior modification in colleges and universites. *American Psychologist*, 1972, *27*, 1063–1069.

Birk, L., Stolz, S. B., Brady, J. P., Brady, J. V., Lazarus, A. A., Lynch, J. J., Rosenthal, A. J., Skelton, W. D., Stevens, J. B., and Thomas, E. J. *Behavior therapy in psychiatry.*

Washington, D.C.: American Psychiatric Association, 1973.

BLAKE, B. G. The application of behaviour therapy to the treatment of alcoholism. *Behaviour Research and Therapy*, 1965, *3*, 75–85.

BORING, E. G. *A history of experimental psychology* (2nd ed.). New York: Appleton-Century Crofts, 1950.

BRADY, J. P. Behavior therapy and American psychiatry. *Journal of the National Association of Private Psychiatric Hospitals*, 1972, *4*, 27–34.

BREGER, L., and MCGAUGH, J. Critique and reformulation of "learning theory" approaches to psychotherapy and neurosis. *Psychological Bulletin*, 1965, *63*, 338–358.

CAUTELA, J. R. Treatment of compulsive behavior by covert sensitization. *Psychological Record*, 1966, *16*, 33–41.

DOLLARD, J., and MILLER, N. E. *Personality and psychotherapy*. New York: McGraw-Hill, 1950.

ELLIS, A. *Reason and emotion in psychotherapy*. New York: Lyle Stuart, 1962.

EYSENCK, H. J. Learning theory and behavior therapy. *Journal of Mental Science*, 1959, *105*, 61–75.

GRAY, J. S. A biological view of behavior modification. *Journal of Educational Psychology*, 1932, *23*, 611–620.

GRAZIANO, A. M. *Child without tomorrow*. New York: Pergamon Press, 1974.

GRAZIANO, A. M. (Ed.) *Behavior therapy with children* (Vol. II). Chicago: Aldine Publishing Co., 1975.

GRAZIANO, A. M. and KEAN, J. E. Programmed relaxation and reciprocal inhibition with psychotic children. *Behaviour Research and Therapy*, 1968, *6*, 433–437.

HABERMAN, J. V. Probing the mind, normal and abnormal. First report. Feeling, association and the psychoreflex. *Medical Record*, 1917, *92*, 927–933.

HOLMES, F. B. An experimental investigation of a method of overcoming children's fears. *Child Development*, 1936, *7*, 6–30.

HOON, P. W., and LINDSLEY, O. R. A comparison of behavior and traditional therapy publication activity. *American Psychologist*, 1974, *29*, 694–697.

JACOBSON, E. *Progressive relaxation*. Chicago: University of Chicago Press, 1938.

JONES, M. C. The elimination of children's fears. *Journal of Experimental Psychology*, 1924, *7*, 382–390.

KANTOROVICH, N. An attempt at associative-reflex therapy in alcoholism. *Nov. Refl. Fiziol Nerv. Sist.*, *3*, 436–447. *Psychological Abstracts*, 1929, *4*, 493.

KAZDIN, A. E. Response cost: The removal of conditioned reinforcers for therapeutic change. *Behavior Therapy*, 1972, *3*, 533–546.

LOCKE, E. A. Is behavior therapy behavioristic: An analysis of Wolpe's psychotherapeutic methods. *Psychological Bulletin*, 1971, *76*, 318–327.

LONDON, P. The end of ideology in behavior modification. *American Psychologist*, 1972, *27*, 913–918.

MAHONEY, M. J., KAZDIN, A. E., and LESSWING, N. J. Behavior modification: Delusion or deliverance? In C. M. Franks and G. T. Wilson (Eds.), *Behavior therapy: Theory and practice* (Vol. II). New York: Brunner/Mazel, 1974.

MARTIN, R. *Behavior modification: Human rights and legal responsibilities*. Champaign, Ill.: Research Press, 1974.

MEYER, V., and CRISP, A. H. Aversion therapy in two cases of obesity. *Behaviour Research and Therapy*, 1964, *2*, 143–147.

MITFORD, J. Kind and usual punishment: The prison business. New York: Knopf, 1973.

MORGANSTERN, K. P. Implosive therapy and flooding techniques: A critical review. *Psychological Bulletin*, 1973, *79*, 318–334.

MOWRER, O. H. An apparatus for the study and treatment of enuresis. *American Journal of Psychology*, 1938, *51*, 163–166.

PAILLER, B., and GRAZIANO, A. M. A national

survey of behavior modification in clinical practice. Unpublished paper, State University of New York at Buffalo, 1972.

PAUL, G. L. Outcome of systematic desensitization. II. Controlled investigations of individual treatment, technique variations, and current status. In C. M. Franks (Ed.), *Behavior therapy: Appraisal and status.* New York: McGraw-Hill, 1969.

PORTES, A. On the emergence of behavior therapy in modern society. *Journal of Consulting Psychology*, 1971, *36*, 303–313.

PRESSEY, S. L. A third and fourth contribution toward the coming 'industrial revolution' in education. *School and Society*, 1932, *36*.

RACHMAN, S. Clinical applications of observational learning, imitation and modeling. *Behavior Therapy*, 1972, *3*, 379–397.

RACHMAN, S., and TEASDALE, J. *Aversion therapy and behaviour disorders.* Coral Gables, Florida: University of Miami Press, 1969.

RIMM, D. C., and MASTERS, J. C. *Behavior therapy: techniques and findings.* New York: Academic Press, 1974.

ROGERS, C. R., and SKINNER, B. F. Some issues concerning the control of human behavior: A symposium. *Science*, 1956, *124*, 1057–1066.

SKINNER, B. F. The science of learning and the art of teaching. *Harvard Educational Review*, 1954, *24*, 86–97.

THORESEN, C. E., and MAHONEY, M. J. *Behavioral self control.* New York. Holt, Rinehart & Winston, 1974.

ULLMAN, L., and KRASNER, L. *Case studies in behavior modification.* New York: Holt, Rinehart & Winston, 1965.

WATSON, J. B., and RAYNOR, R. Conditioned emotional reaction. *Journal of Experimental Psychology*, 1920, *3*, 1–14.

WEBER, J. An approach to the problem of fear in children. *Journal of Mental Science*, 1936, *82*, 136–147.

WOLPE, J. Psychotherapy by reciprocal inhibition. Stanford: Stanford University Press, 1958.

WOLPE, J. *The practice of behavior therapy.* Elmsford, N. Y.: Pergamon Press, 1974.

YEN, S. *Survey of courses in behavior modification at higher learning institutions.* Paper presented at the Fifth Annual Meeting of the Association for the Advancement of Behavior Therapy, Washington, D. C., September 1971.

4

PSYCHOANALYTIC TREATMENT

Melvin A. Scharfman

The first attempts to apply psychoanalytic methods to the treatment of an adolescent or a child were made by Freud in two of his early publications. It is of particular interest to note that of the five famous case histories of Freud, one concerns the analysis of an adolescent, a second, the analysis of a child. These cases were, respectively, "Fragment of an Analysis of a Case of Hysteria" published in 1905 and "The Analysis of a Phobia in a Five Year Old Boy" published in 1909. When Freud published these cases it would appear that he had something different in mind than to suggest that psychoanalytic treatment of either adolescents or children should be undertaken. Rather the cases were published as part of Freud's attempt to confirm his basic discoveries, namely those made in the "Interpretation of Dreams" and "Three Essays on Infantile Sexuality," with regard to their application to understanding neurosis. He was interested in studying the nature of human psychic development and these cases afforded him the opportunity to show the application of his understanding to the phenomena that they presented. They served to confirm for him that the roots of adult neurotic disturbances lay in persistences of infantile sexuality in the psychic life of the individual.

The theoretical background was that of Freud's earliest ideas, including the transformation of blocked libido into anxiety. They were written before he formulated the dual instinct theory, which gave weight to aggressive drives, and before he formulated the structural theory, which brought the understanding of ego and superego functioning into the treatment situation as well. From the point of view of method of treatment, these cases are primarily of historical interest and lack practical application to current treatment methods. The technique of direct treatment of children and adolescents had not yet evolved.

These papers did provide the stimulus for a group of analysts to undertake the psychoanalytic treatment of children years later. Most prominent among those who were involved in the early attempts were Anna Freud and Melanie Klein. Both were gifted, perceptive, and intuitive but each approached the question of psychoanalytic treatment of children from her own unique points of view, which eventually resulted in significant differences in theoretical formulations as well as in clinical techniques. While some of Mrs. Klein's formulations have been integrated into psychoanalytic formulations currently held by the mainstream of British child analysts, Miss Freud's formulations have been the major influence on the development of child analysis in this country. This paper will draw most heavily upon her formulations and those of the several generations of child analysts who have attempted to elaborate and contribute to the further development of her ideas.

GENERAL PRINCIPLES IN THE ANALYSIS OF CHILDREN AND ADOLESCENTS

There have been many discussions about the similarities and differences between the analysis of children and adolescents as compared to that of adults, and sometimes the question has even been raised whether child analysis should be considered psychoanalysis at all. It seems useful therefore to consider what are the common bases that constitute designation of a given procedure as psychoanalytic as well as to indicate those areas in which the developmental needs of children and adolescents may lead to differences in the techniques and conceptualizations of psychoanalytic treatment.

1. The basic factor in the designation of a procedure as psychoanalysis is the creation of the psychoanalytic situation and the assumption of a psychoanalytic stance throughout the course of treatment. The maintenance of the psychoanalytic stance involves certain basic assumptions. The analyst sets as few limitations as possible on the direction of treatment but rather follows the free expression of the patient's thoughts and actions as they appear, paying attention to those derivatives of each of the psychic structures as they present in their interaction.

2. The basic technique utilized is that of interpretation. Appropriate attention is given to dealing with defenses as they impede the flow of material and to the manifestations of transference as they appear in the course of treatment.

3. The analyst restricts the use of educative measures or attempts to change the child's environment as much as possible, intervening only where it appears necessary in order to maintain the continuity of the psychoanalytic procedure.

4. The goal of treatment is to allow individuals to fulfill their development as completely as they can by helping to make conscious those unconscious elements which appear to impede the ability to function effectively.

5. The person of the analyst is offered as an object so that the patient can interact and experience any thoughts and feelings past, present, and future such as may present. The analyst does not limit these varying perceptions of him by the patient but does continuously analyse them.

The general goal is to allow for intrapsychic structural changes to occur rather than to limit the treatment to the removal of a symptom, an emotional abreaction, or a change brought about by suggestion.

So long as these conditions are met, the situation that ensues is a psychoanalytic one and it is suitable for conducting a psychoanalysis. They can be met in the treatment of selected children or adolescents. There are, however, many significant areas in which specific aspects of technique are influenced by those differences between the developmental level of the child or adolescent as compared to that of an adult.

DIFFERENCES BETWEEN CHILD AND ADULT ANALYSIS

Free Association

The essential difference between child and adult analysis lies in the child's inability to free associate. What is assumed to take the place of free association is the encouragement in the analytic setting for the child to play. Children's fantasies are certainly expressed in play, often in a manner such that some of the wishes, fears, and fantasies appear easy to understand. This is particularly so with younger children, yet it is misleading. It is the analyst who associates to the play, not the child, and as such the conviction of interpretation arising out of a patient's own associations is lacking. There is, of course, verbal communication of varying types that does take place. Most children, depending upon their age, communicate both by means of play as well as by the verbal recounting of daydreams and dreams, but they are not able to really free associate to these. However, even with children who develop trust in the analyst and attempt to communicate all their thoughts, there are limitations imposed by their developmental level. The extent to which regression to primary process thinking is a threat to the maintenance of secondary process functioning is very much greater in children. They are, to varying degrees, unable to suspend their need to maintain secondary process thinking.

Given this limitation on free association, the analyst can be tempted to engage in more direct symbolic interpretation of the child's play, dreams, or daydreams, as for example, Kleinian analysts tend to do. It must be kept in mind, however, that this bypasses the individual meaning of what is presented and is essentially something which can become parallel to "wild analyses" in adults, namely interpretation of the unconscious based only on the manifest content of the communications. Such a technique bypasses appropriate attention to the ego's defenses and focuses more exclusively on the drives. It also tends to omit appropriate attention to the realities of the child's life situation.

There is still another area in which children's inability to free associate affects technique of treatment. Adults are told that they are free to express whatever they are thinking and feeling and, at least with patients suitable for psychoanalysis, such expressions are largely limited to verbalizations. While the child may be invited to bring up any of his thoughts or feelings, it is a fact that these thoughts and feelings are most likely to be expressed in motor activity to some degree rather than being limited to verbalization. As such, this motor activity may at times have to be restricted where it either endangers the safety of the child or the person or possessions of the analyst. This is particularly likely since motor activity in children seems to be more closely tied to the expression of aggression rather than to libidinal wishes. What children tend to act out in the psychoanalytic situation therefore tends more toward the aggressive aspects of their wishes. To the extent that such behavioral acting out does not lend itself to being interpreted, or when interpretation of it is not accepted by the child, it is not beneficial to analysis but rather represents a cathartic discharge. Such a discharge may, of course, lead to symptomatic relief but does not relate to the achievement of structural change. These difficulties, that is, the child's inability to free associate and the reliance on action rather than verbalization, mean that the analyst may have to restrict certain aspects of expression particularly with young children. The problem of the lack of free association is not easily solved.

We will indicate later how material obtained from the parents is used to supplement those elements of day-to-day reality which the child is not likely to express. While this is somewhat akin to trying to obtain the day's residue for the material emerging in the analysis, it is, of course, not coming from the children themselves and is therefore not as reliable a guide to the meaning of the particular play or dream. The child analyst is, to this degree, handicapped in attempting to ascertain the complexities of the child's inner life. The reliance upon play, combined as the child gets older with reports of daily activities, dreams, and fantasies, never quite approaches providing an equivalent range of material to that available to the adult analyst. An additional technical problem is in the interpretation of such play activities. The child analyst must be aware that in interpreting the meaning of a particular kind of play he can create a situation in which the child inhibits or ceases playing as such, something which would not be developmentally appropriate. We will say more later about what kind of interpretations are made of the child's playing out in the analytic situation.

THE THERAPEUTIC ALLIANCE

The possibility of developing a stable therapeutic and working alliance in child analysis is much less likely than in adult analysis. This is not to say that there are not periods during the analysis in which such an alliance between analyst and child exists, for if there were not very little analysis would get done. It is, however, a much less stable relationship than exists in treating an adult. This occurs for a variety of reasons.

1. At the beginning of treatment the child is frequently not motivated to the same extent that the

adult is. The child is most often brought for treatment by the parents or because of a recommendation from a school, rather than because he or she is suffering from a personally distressing symptomatology. There is certainly considerable contact with the parents in the early part of the treatment and sometimes throughout the analysis. This contact brings into the treatment situation those figures who are of central importance in the child's life. The relationship with the analyst is affected by the presence of the parents and the child may feel torn at times between the relationship with the analyst and that with the parents.

2. Children's sense of time is different, particularly their view of the future. They are less able to anticipate what benefits the treatment might bring to them and feel more burdened by the extent to which the treatment intrudes into their day-to-day life.

3. The child tends to see problems as caused by the external world, whether by parents, school, friends, etc. Children are more likely to seek to change the external environment rather than to look inside themselves and understand their reactions to that environment. They can become intensely disappointed and frequently angry when the analyst expresses an unwillingness to interfere in changing the external environment in one way or another.

4. From childhood through adolescence there are varying degrees of psychic disequilibrium during which the ego feels in danger of being overwhelmed by the drives or is under the threat of the superego or the environment. The ego is often so engaged in defending against these potential threats that it is unable to participate in a sustained way in the therapeutic alliance. At such times the analysis is viewed as potentially putting the child's ego into even greater danger from those forces.

5. That capacity which in adults we call "the splitting of the ego," namely, the experience in which the ego is alternatively able to experience certain aspects in the treatment situation and then shift to being the observer of those experiences, is very difficult for children, often impossible. The self-observing function of the ego does not really appear much before late latency and it is, therefore, much more difficult for the child to join the analyst in understanding the nature and meaning of their interaction.

6. There are periods during which there is a specific turning away from the past. This is particularly true at the end of the oedipal phase and during adolescence. At such times there is a need to defend against certain intense affective experiences with the parents during treatment. The attachment to the analyst during those phases may lead to the experiencing of such feelings toward the parents now directed at the analyst. The youngster may have great difficulty in dealing with a pull toward those earlier feelings which are now viewed as completely unacceptable and threatening. This leads us to a consideration of the nature of transference reactions as they appear in children and adolescents.

Transference

The nature of transference reactions in child analysis has long been of interest to child analysts and has been the subject of many papers and panel discussions. The fact that some analysts would view the development of the transference neurosis and its subsequent analysis as the cornerstone of any analytic procedure has contributed to the preoccupation with this subject. In her earlier writings Anna Freud felt that children developed "transference reactions" but did not develop a transference neurosis. In 1965 she modified this position and wrote, "I am still unconvinced that what is called transference neurosis with children equals the adult variety in every respect." There certainly is no question that children show the tendency to develop transferences to the analyst and these essentially repeat in the psychoanalytic situation the earlier relationships with their parental objects. Whether or not some children develop a transference neurosis seems to depend upon the definition of transference neurosis. If transference neurosis is seen as involving the repetition of specific neurotic conflicts of earlier periods in the psychoanalytic situation with the analyst as their central focus, there have been reports of its appearance in the analysis of children and adolescents. A number of factors make it more difficult to see the development and elaboration of transference, or of a transference neurosis, in child or adolescent analysis. Anna Freud's observations about the limitations of free association in children and her observations about the connection between motor discharge and aggressive drives in the psychoanalytic setting suggest that it would be more difficult to trace the development of libidinal transference components than aggressive ones. Some of the evidence of the transference would also be hidden because of the lack of free association. It is additionally difficult because the analyst appears in multiple other representations more regularly during the course of child or adolescent analysis than he might in an adult analysis. In particular, the analyst is more frequently experienced as a new object in the course of child analysis than with adults. This is in part because the tendency toward repetition present throughout development is paralleled by a hunger for new experience and new objects.

Anna Freud suggested that the analyst is used for repetition insofar as the child's neurosis or other disturbance enters into the treatment situation, and as a new object insofar as ths child's healthy personality presents itself. It is clear that at certain points the analyst is used as a new object and sometimes as the primary object in conjunction with the evolution of a new developmental phase. In certain youngsters oedipal wishes may first appear as centered around the person of the analyst where this level has not been achieved in relationship to the parents. Such an occurrence would be more likely to take place when a parent is absent during the development of that phase. In such cases, as new levels of fantasies and wishes appear they therefore tend to focus on the person of the analyst. This phenomenon appears frequent in other child analyses and not only where the parent is absent or otherwise unavailable during a given phase. The vicissitudes of the relationship between the analyst as a tranference object and the analyst as a new object should be considered in relationship to the specific developmental phases, but both do appear to a varying extent throughout the course of childhood and adolescent analyses. This tends to cloud the appearance and definition of transference as such. In addition, particularly with younger children, there may be displacements from the present relationship with the parent into the psychoanalytic situation with the analyst as their object. Characteristic behavioral patterns and character traits also may appear in the analysis with the analyst as their focus but these are not specific transference reactions. Any analysis involves to varying degrees these multiple representations of the analyst. What is more specific for child or adolescent analysis is that the balance shifts in such a way that *the predominance of transference reactions as the core of the experience with the analyst is less clear.* Reactions to the analyst as a new object or an object of displacement of current feelings about the parents are more prominent. The fact that the parent plays the overwhelmingly important role in the child's life means that there will be ongoing involvements with his original objects throughout the analysis intermingled with the various levels of experience with the analyst.

Having indicated these general considerations about the nature of child analysis and some of the similarities and differences with respect to adult analysis, we will now consider how analysis has developed in relationship to specific developmental phases. The most central idea of recent years may be the awareness of development as an ongoing process.

It has become clear that this is the proper background against which the nature of child or adolescent analysis must be considered. Analysis must be conducted in a different manner and sometimes with different aims, depending upon the developmental stage reached by the person undergoing analysis. To apply the model of adult analysis or to define analysis solely in terms of that which takes place within a more mature psychic organization is not appropriate. Indications for psychoanalytic treatment, the technique of the treatment, and the aim of the treatment all need to be considered in their relationship to the phase of development. It is obvious then that someone undertaking the analysis of children or of adolescents needs to be thoroughly familiar with the developmental processes at each phase. This is essential not only in terms of determining what would constitute the limitations for therapeutic intervention during a given phase, but also in recognizing the range and extent of fluctuations during a given phase. This awareness affects the analyst's view of the flow of the analytic process and also helps in the determination of what constitutes the indications for termination of an analytic procedure. Therefore, any prospective analyst of children or adolescents needs as wide as possible a range of experiences with children at different developmental stages and in different settings as well as a solid conceptual understanding of the developmental process. There are also certain emotional requirements for those who undertake the analytic treatment of children and adolescents (Feigelson, 1974). This is a complicated subject worthy of much discussion, but it will not be possible to do so in this presentation.

The psychoanalytic treatment of a prelatency child, a latency child, or an adolescent differ from one another as much as they differ from treatment of an adult. We will consider analysis during each of those periods separately. It must be borne in mind that great variations also exist within these larger groupings of developmental phases and that these differences also affect the application of psychoanalysis as a treatment modality.

ANALYSIS OF THE PRELATENCY CHILD

Indications for Analysis

While psychoanalytic interventions have been described with even younger children, this section will consider essentially children who are in the phallic-oedipal phase of development. From the author's point of view this choice evolves from several factors. Psychoanalysis deals essentially with internalized conflicts. While certain aspects of internalization may not be complete until the passage of the oedipal phase, there are nevertheless some indications of internalized conflict in children during that phase. Internalized conflicts result in neurotic symptom formation in children during this phase. These internalizations may also allow for the observation of beginning characterological patterns in some children. Thus at least some of the subject matter of psychoanalytic treatment is present. Psychoanalysis also deals with the development of transference. This means that the child should have come at least to the point where there is sufficient differentiation of self and object and a stability of object representations if it is to be possible for that object representation to be transferred onto the person of the analyst. These minimal requirements for the application of psychoanalysis should be present by this phase of development. This is in no way meant to detract from those applications of psychoanalytic knowledge to younger children or to children who have not achieved this degree of differentiation. These interventions have often been extremely helpful in allowing children to resume their developmental potential. But it may be that they should be considered modifications of analysis inasmuch as they go beyond even the minimal criteria that have been described for a psychoanalytic procedure.

What then can be said to constitute the indications for analytic treatment in children during this phase? There are many children who develop symptoms during the phallic-oedipal phase. These are most commonly children who develop phobias, but one also encounters a variety of conversion symptoms, psychosomatic problems, sleep disturbances, and the beginning of obsessive compulsive symptoms. Such symptoms are often expressions of the vicissitudes of inevitable developmental conflicts and may or may not represent an infantile neurosis. A truly neurotic disturbance which gives indications of impeding the developmental process constitutes the ideal indication for psychoanalytic treatment. The assessment of whether or not one is really dealing with an established neurosis is central. More transitory symptom formations are almost ubiquitous in children and do not necessarily represent an indication for any kind of treatment. Such an assessment means that there should be careful consideration of the various aspects of the child's development along the lines described by Anna Freud in her book *Normality and Pathology in Childhood.*

Essentially a childhood neurosis may be described as having occurred where there is indication of a permanently established regression in the drives to an earlier fixation point without any major regression in ego or superego development. This regression constitutes the determining aspect of the diagnosis of a neurosis or of a characterological modification in the developing child. In practice children showing such development may or may not be brought for treatment. It was indicated earlier that children themselves do not often initiate the treatment because they do not suffer to the same extent as adults. While this is true, there are, of course, some children who do suffer from the existence of their neurotic symptoms and communicate this in such a way that a request for treatment is then initiated by the parents. More often treatment is initiated when the parents feel that their own lives are seriously infringed upon by the child's neurosis or where the neurotic symptomatology creates difficulties in the child's ability to function at the level of other children his age, for example, a phobic child who is unable to remain in a nursery school or kindergarten. The intensity and duration of the child's symptoms and some interference with given areas of ego functioning are common factors in determining whether or not a child may be brought for treatment. These factors also play a part in assessing the indications for analysis and affect the parents' willingness to accept the recommendation for psychoanalysis. Let me give just a brief example.

Nancy was a little over five years of age and had been attending kindergarten at the time she was brought for treatment by her parents. They related that she was increasingly fearful of going to school and often missed almost half of the sessions there. In addition, she was very frightened if her parents went out at night although she was left with a competent adult. She demanded to know exactly where they were going, when they would come back, and often would not let them leave. She would cry and have a tantrum at the time of their departure. They felt that their own freedom was seriously infringed upon. This situation combined with the school difficulty led to their deciding to seek help. Actually, Nancy had shown signs of a neurosis for about a year. It first manifested itself when she developed a reaction of fear upon seeing a friend's parent in a wheelchair while she was visiting their home. She become frightened about any subsequent visits to that friend's home. She then developed reactions of fear whenever she saw anyone injured. Soon she reacted even if she saw someone wearing a bandaid. She would become panicky and on several occasions had had such reactions when out with her parents at a restaurant or visiting friends. She also had not infrequent nightmares. These were handled by the parents either by agreeing that one of them would sleep with her or by allowing her to sleep on their bed. Nancy's fear of school had actually begun when her teacher came to school with her arm in a sling. Gradually this intensified to the point that she would feel panic about the thought of going to school. Her initial phobia had not protected her against the development of anxiety. Instead the phobia had extended and other symptoms had developed. The symptoms became more intense and eventually some of her functioning was interfered with significantly. At the time she was brought to see me it was clear that she had a truly established neurosis and that psychoanalysis was indicated. The parents were also ready by that time to accept such a recommendation.

Any evaluation of the indications for psychoanalysis must consider the nature of the child's parents and their willingness to support the treatment. The analyst needs to feel reasonably sure that he will have the cooperation of the parents. This involves not only the fact that it is an infringement upon the family and their freedom to have to bring the child to treatment so frequently and that a considerable financial burden will be imposed, but also that the parents are willing to accept change in their child. This change may go beyond those symptoms which distress the parents and one needs to assess whether or not they may be able to establish a different level of relationship with the child. Most parents are threatened by the fact that their child develops symptoms severe enough to warrant such treatment. Parental guilt may be a factor in accepting a recommendation for treatment, but if this is reacted to by the therapist either overtly or covertly in such a way as to indicate that they should indeed feel guilty, it will not sustain the treatment for very long. One of the important indications of whether to attempt to analyze a child during this phase includes an assessment of the parents. The analyst must feel that he can develop a working relationship with the parents.

TECHNIQUE OF TREATMENT

In the analysis of children the goal is to remove those obstacles that appear to be impeding development, as well as to facilitate the child's development of his progressive potentials. Those essential aspects of the interpretation of resistances and transference and the widening of consciousness by interpretation of unconscious aspects of drive derivatives, ego, and superego—with the hope for greater dominance of the ego—are much the same as they would be in any analysis. Some of the differences were alluded to earlier and will be mentioned here only from the point of view of how they affect the analysis. The prelatency child is less likely to be suffering from their symptoms although some children do indeed suffer. Even with young children who acknowledge distress and who wish help, there will be difficulty in forming the working therapeutic alliance. Children this age are not able to function as observers of their own reactions, and they are therefore not easily able to join the analyst in looking at their reactions. The initial phase of treating a child of this age involves the development of a mutual trusting relationship. The child has to learn what the analysis is all about—that is, that he is going to join with the analyst in trying to understand why he is having difficulties. This is not easily accomplished because prelatency children tend to externalize and see their problems as caused by the people and things around them. They have difficulty in recognizing that some of their problems are created within themselves rather than just by the external world. The basic tools available to the analyst are patience, a willingness to listen, and the capacity to understand. The analyst reacts differently than other adults with whom the child has had contact. Most other adults tell the child what to do or how and when to do it, things the analyst for the most part avoids. The analyst is more willing to let the child choose his own direction. The child is supplied with a setting in which he or she can express thoughts and feelings in a variety of ways. In working with these children the analyst makes available a variety of different play materials and allows the child to choose from them. These materials are quite deliberately kept simple and do not include highly structured or formal games. Rather they include crayons, pencils, paper, paint, family dolls or puppets, some doll furniture, dishes, etc. Their function is to allow the child to express fantasies as well as aspects of day-to-day experiences in dramatic play with these items.

It is not unusual for children to communicate some aspects of their struggles in what seems a transparent manner. The analyst, however, usually chooses not to interpret the unconscious drive derivative reflected in the play. Berta Bornstein (1949) pointed out in a very lucid manner some of the reasons for this approach. She suggested that forcing the ego rapidly to confront unconscious impulses would result in a quick suppression of the phobic symptoms or in an intensification of the phobia with the analyst himself becoming the phobic object. She went further and pointed out that if one refrained from any interpretation, the child would continue to play out the derivatives of his conflict. This would result in a cathartic discharge and the diminishing of the symptoms but would leave the conflict between ego and id untouched. Such an approach is what happens in some of what is called play therapy. Bornstein also pointed to the limitations of reassurance, pointing out that this would also lead to an avoidance of analyzing the conflict. Finally, she pointed out that the therapist could take the part of the superego and assist in the control of certain drives but that this would essentially bypass the child's own ego development. All of these approaches might lead to a rapid diminution in the child's symptomatology. In order to attempt to initiate a process that would lead to an ego change, however, she suggested that early interventions with the child, be directed to pointing out defenses against affects. Helping to make an unconscious affect conscious facilitates the unravelling of genetic and dynamic elements. This remains one of the best avenues to establish emotional rapport with the child and to facilitate the analytic process. This process is related to what Anna Freud terms an important part of the analysis of prelatency children, namely, verbalization and clarification. Helping the child to put into words what he or she is feeling and experiencing facilitates the ego's functioning. It helps the child verbally to identify in a more specific way what he experiences as danger, thereby lessening the anxiety he feels. Such interventions help the child by facilitating secondary process thinking and thus place the analyst in the position of being an ally to an ego which is temporarily having difficulty in dealing with conflicts.

As analysis proceeds the analyst interprets the many different facets of the material presented. The nature of dangerous situations is clarified and interpreted, and the variety of unconscious drive derivatives are made conscious, in alternation with interpretation of defenses. Traumatic experiences as well as other aspects of the earlier interactions with parents may appear in their relationship to the analyst. These aspects are made conscious, facilitating the process whereby the ego can attempt to master them in a different way.

Let us return to the case of Nancy whose presenting difficulties have been described. For a brief illustration: Nancy readily indicated as the analysis began that she was frightened and worried and that she wanted help. In the first few months she also made it clear that the help which she really wanted was in convincing her parents not to go out and leave her alone. She also thought the analyst should get permission for her not to go to school when she felt upset. Her anger toward her mother became obvious in her play with puppets but was not immediately pointed out. The other thing at which she played quite frequently was to create a situation in which she would be very upset when seeing someone who was injured. What could first be pointed out to her was how sad she must feel. She worried about bad things happening to other people and then felt all alone. In the months that followed we were able to elucidate many of the reasons for her worrying about people getting hurt. As part of her oedipal phase experience she was caught up with fantasies of what her parents did when they were alone. The usual childhood confusions between sexuality and aggression were intensified by the fact that she frequently heard her parents arguing in their bedroom. She thought that someone would get hurt, usually her mother. This led to exploring some of her concerns and ideas about sex and childbirth. She worried about another baby being born. Nancy had one sibling, a younger brother age three. He emerged as the object of a mixture of envy and resentment. She hated all boys and would like to kill them. At the same time one of the reasons she was reluctant to go to school was that she said boys were going to make fun of her or beat her up when she got on the school bus.

We were able to clarify the nature of her projection of her own aggressive wishes onto the boys and she began to deal with her own wish to be a boy. Her parents must have liked boys better and been dissatisfied with her or they would not have wanted to have her brother. She herself had feelings of being damaged as a girl and this was one aspect of her horror in looking at anyone who had any kind of injury. She not only felt defective in her female genitals but felt further damaged in that she didn't have breasts. Besides, she couldn't have a baby. It became clear that she also felt unable to win her father's love and affection. She began to play out some of this in the analytic situation, becoming very coquettish and seductive. She expressed all kinds of curiosity about the analyst and looked for indications of her desirability. After a while she became more able to seek her father's attention directly. This brought about a renewed period of dealing with her anger toward her mother. Her mother didn't like her, her mother only liked boys. Eventually she got around to elaborations of the circumstances of her brother's birth and we were able to understand some things of which she had not previously been conscious. In her play and through some of her verbalized fantasies she recreated her visit to the hospital at the time of her brother's birth. When she played out a woman being brought out of the hospital in a wheelchair, I suggested that her mother had been brought out of the hospital in a wheelchair when they came to take her home. She corrected me to say, "No, it wasn't Mommy in a wheelchair. There was another man with bandages all over him. He was in a wheelchair."

We were now able to clarify her anger toward her mother for having left her to go to the hospital and her resentment of her brother. She had missed her mother while she was away but was also angry with her. Seeing the man in bandages and a wheelchair reminded her of her bad feelings toward her mother and her worry that something might happen to her mother. Bandages and wheelchairs now represented her fear of her death wishes and her fear of then being left without a mother. Her oedipal phase development when it occurred had revived these earlier fears of anger toward her mother and her concerns about her mother's death. All of this had been represented in her initial phobic reaction to seeing someone who was injured and in a wheelchair. The phobia also expressed her fear of her aggressive wishes toward her brother and her feelings that she herself was damaged. The formation of the neurosis had essentially led to a regression away from the oedipal level with a return to preoedipal fears and behaviors. The analysis allowed the undoing of this regression and the resumption of a more phase appropriate developmental process. When progressive development seemed to have been securely resumed, the analysis was terminated.

Obviously such a brief outline does not do justice to what takes place in the course of an analysis. It is presented merely to illustrate a few of the points which have been discussed. There are many much more detailed accounts of the analysis of a child available in the literature. These provide the opportunity to study more in depth the nature of the analytic process, the range of different kinds of materials presented by the child, and the type of interventions made by the analyst.

Termination

In general terms there is very little difference in the criteria for the termination of the analysis of a prelatency child than there would be for that of an older child or an adult. One looks for the resolution of those conflicts that have led to the formation of a neurosis and thereby interfered with the progressive developmental movement. Once the phase specific developmental functioning seems securely established, the analysis would be terminated. A more common problem centers around the parents' view of the analysis, particularly if the analyst has not spent appropriate time in educating the parents. They may withdraw the child from the analysis when they see the abatement of some symptoms and a general improvement in functioning. The analyst recognizes that, in spite of these occurrences, certain central conflicts may remain active and that the analysis could continue with further benefit to the child, but the parents may not accept this. Other parents may wish to interrupt the treatment when the child has changed sufficiently to satisfy them. They may be reluctant to accept any further change in the child, particularly when the child is involved in some neurotic gratification of their own needs. Here again, much depends upon the nature of the parental interaction with the analyst. In certain situations it may be possible for the parents to recognize their own need for treatment and to accept such a recommendation. This possibility often depends upon the reality aspects of the family constellation.

As indicated earlier, analysis may represent considerable strain upon the parents in terms of finances as well as of time. It is sometimes appropriate that the child's treatment be interrupted at a less than optimal point in order for the family to lend financial support to another family member in need of treatment. In such a situation the treatment may be interrupted with the idea of there being occasional subsequent visits to see how the child is progressing. It must be borne in mind that no child analysis is ever "completed." The child will for many years be subject to all of the vicissitudes of development. He or she will also be living within the family context and be subject to all the limitations that the nature of the family structure may impose. The child analyst has often to be satisfied that he has done whatever is possible and hope for the best. Of course, the need for analysis may arise at some point later in life, but this does not mean that the analysis has been a failure nor does it indicate success. One would need to know what the development of such a person would have been like without the analytic intervention. It is obviously very difficult even to make such judgments, let alone to collect more securely based data such as would answer the question more convincingly. We can be satisfied if, at the end of the analysis, there are indications that the child seems to be functioning at a better level than he or she had at the beginning of treatment and does so for a reasonable length of time. In recent years there have been a number of papers reporting cases of persons seen in child analysis who were subsequently seen either for further treatment or as part of a planned follow-up. Hopefully, as such data accumulates, we will have a clearer picture of the benefits and limitations of these procedures.

THE LATENCY CHILD

INDICATIONS FOR PSYCHOANALYSIS

Child analysis has been most widely applied to the treatment of children during the latency period. It would be more correct to say that it has involved children whose chronological age suggests that they should be in the latency period, although many of those youngsters who are treated psychoanalytically have failed to establish a real latency. The indications for undertaking psychoanalytic treatment of a child have been most clearly spelled out by Anna Freud in her book *The Psychoanalytic Treatment of Children* and amplified in her later book *Normality and Pathology in Childhood.* Other analysts see a somewhat wider range of disturbances as indications for psychoanalytic treatment but most will agree that she has characterized those children who are the best candidates for psychoanalytic intervention. In other children psychoanalysis has been recommended based on the feeling that it is the best one has to offer at this time although the analyst may be less than optimistic about the outcome. As with younger children, the clearest indication for psychoanalysis is where there is a well-established neurosis which has resulted in libidinal regression and interfered with the forward developmental progress of the child. With the libidinal regression there is a loss of those qualities and achievements which depend upon the level of libidinal development. For example, the child who has regressed to an oral level will "act like a baby" and will present as impatient, demanding, and insatiable. The assessment of whether or not there has been a significant libidinal regression is not easy, but it assumes greater importance than the isolated existence of symptoms. Transient libidinal regressions may occur in a variety of different circumstances. Even what appear to be fairly serious neurotic symptoms may disappear if the libidinal development resumes its own movement. Where there are indications that the regression to a preoedipal level has become fixed and rigid, it is not likely that the neurotic symptomatology will disappear without treatment.

Another area to assess is the extent to which ego development has been hampered by the operation of neurotic symptomatology. A careful assessment of the various ego functions will indicate whether there has been significant infringement on their operation because of the attempts to deal with neurotic conflicts. While all children utilize a variety of mechanisms of defense in dealing with the inevitable developmental conflicts, the excessive operation of particular mechanisms can lead to difficulties in related ego functions. A child with a hysterical neurosis and its concomitant utilization of repression may present with an impairment of the ego function of memory so that such a child has difficulty in learning and studying in school. This is, of course, assuming that other causes for such difficulty have been ruled out. The phobic child who initially avoids a specific situation of danger may develop an inhibition of activity and motility in many areas, seeing an ever widening variety of situations as dangerous. Such children may present as unable to participate in games or sports, having restricted the ego's control of motility. The excessive use of reaction formation and isolation may lead the obsessional child to present as overly polite and compliant with even the ordinary expressions of discharge of aggression unavailable to the ego. They present themselves as emotionally constricted and overly intellectual. The use of denial and fantasy may be so prominent that the ego's reality testing appears impaired in certain areas. Other children's functions may be excessively sexualized or aggressifized to the extent that the ego's control of motor activity is severely impaired. Any of the types of impairment of ego functioning mentioned, along with a wide variety of other such impairments, constitute indications for analytic intervention.

Children, of course, present other problems considered as indications for psychoanalytic treatment. The child who consistently expresses conscious wishes to be of the opposite sex is one such example. Sexual perversions are another indication, although such children are in reality not often seen by the analyst. But rather than describing further those children for whom psychoanalytic treatment is indicated, it may be more pertinent to consider the types of children actually brought to the child analyst.

Many of those children for whom psychoanalytic treatment might be indicated never even see someone for consulatation because of the parental attitude. Parents may be frightened of the prospects of treatment or reluctant to indicate that their child needs help because it signifies to them their own failure as a parent. Many parents go to great lengths to attempt to conceal their child's difficulties. For example, a child's neurotic conflicts may result in difficulties in going to sleep. Some parents will then go through months or years of allowing the child to sleep with the light on or encourage the child to read or watch television before going to sleep. They may allow the child to stay up inappropriately late or to sleep in their room. It is very difficult for most parents to acknowledge that their child is having emotional problems because they automatically assume that it represents failure on their part. The group of children who are actually seen by a child analyst are often the children of persons associated with the psychological field or the children of parents who have themselves had psychoanalytic treatment. It seems easier for such parents both to recognize the child's difficulties and to seek help. There are, of course, other factors that limit such treatment even with children with whom there are appropriate indications. The financial burden on the family and the infringement of the time commitment were discussed earlier. It is somewhat easier for the late latency child to get to appointments on his own. The geographical availability of a child analyst is, of course, another limiting factor.

The indications listed above are in general quite conservative. The undertaking of psychoanalysis is a major one, and careful consideration should be given before it is recommended. The growth of psychoanalytically derived psychotherapy for children has reached remarkable proportions. While such treatment obviously offers help to many children who would otherwise be unable to obtain it, it sometimes has drawbacks. The kind of developmental difficulties discussed above are unlikely to be significantly modified by a psychotherapeutic procedure. Psychotherapeutic procedures are most successful when they are applied by therapists who go through the same kind of careful assessment of the child and who direct the nature of their intervention appropriately. There are also many children seen in psychotherapy for whom treatment is not necessarily indicated, particularly that group of children who experience relatively transient phase specific symptomatic difficulties. Many such difficulties would disappear spontaneously as the child's development proceeded. Much work remains to be done in clarifying the optimum kind of intervention in the wide variety of childhood disturbances.

Technical Aspects

Much of what has been said in that part of the paper dealing with the general principles of child analysis and the differences between child and adult analysis is pertinent here. So is a good part of the discussion of the prelatency child, although there are clearly differences. The latency age child is much less likely to engage in destructive or aggressive play activities, and there is, of course, an increased capacity for verbalization, although particularly in earlier latency, play continues as a prominent aspect of communication with the analyst. Not only is there a change in the degree of verbalization—but the latency age child shows an increasing preponderance of secondary process thinking. Because of the more extensive repertoire of defenses, wish fulfillment is less likely to be directly expressed either verbally or in play without at least some elaboration. When the latency child plays out or talks about a fantasy, he or she is clearly aware of it as separate from reality most of the time. These changes in the latency child are indications that the ego has achieved a greater degree of control over the drives.

In addition, to the extent that oedipal conflicts have been at least partially resolved, there will be some degree of consolidation of the superego. As a consequence of this there are more likely to be clearly internalized intrapsychic conflicts, particularly in the latter part of latency. The development of the superego also means that the latency child is more likely to experience guilt. In some children this provides a greater degree of motivation at least to begin the analysis. There are other children in whom unconscious guilt is so strong that it inhibits their beginning treatment since the persistence of their symptoms satisfies their need to be punished. Such children are in need of analytic treatment and can benefit from it, but the initial phases may be more difficult. While the latency child is certainly still in a state of psychic fluidity, with progressive development alternating with more regressive aspects of their functioning, there has been some degree of consolidation and more specific characterological formations have occurred. Certain typical characterological traits may be quite evident.

All of these developments suggest that the analysis of the latency child should offer somewhat fewer difficulties than that of the younger child. One would expect that the latency child, given the greater capacity to verbalize and to communicate with logical goal-directed thoughts, would be more clearly able to describe some of his conflicts. This would be true except for other aspects of this developmental phase. The repression of recent oedipal conflict carries with it the repression of much of the earlier years. The latency child diverts much energy to defensive struggles against these conflicts when they threaten to emerge into consciousness. Not only is there anxiety connected with an emerging awareness of unacceptable impulses but there is also fear of losing the hard-won dominance of secondary process thinking. It seems that the latency child will not as directly, even if symbolically, communicate the nature of his conflict in play or by verbalization. The need to maintain a defensive position leads many latency children to talk only about the most mundane matters, sometimes for long periods of time. This is particularly true in the early phases of treatment but reappears throughout the course of an analysis. The dominance of ego and superego functioning provides the analyst with the opportunity to observe and understand the operations of these organizations in great detail. With most latency age children, the analyst is somewhat freer to direct the major portion of his attention to such observations and to choose carefully timed appropriate interventions. There is much less need to be a participant in or observer of play, although there are frequently situations where this remains an important aspect of treatment. The latency child is also more likely spontaneously to report dreams. The analyst's ability to work with these is hampered, however, by the difficulties in obtaining free association. Nevertheless, many latency age children do learn to associate to dreams to some degree. The analyst's capacity to understand the child's communications both in play and verbally becomes greater as he knows more about the child's life patterns and family structure, significant earlier events in the child's life, etc.

With most latency age children, information is supplemented by regular contact with one or both of the parents. The role of such contact with the parents is in part to ensure their continuing support of the treatment, but the focus of the contact is to obtain from the parents those events which may be significant in the day-to-day life of the child. There may also be certain educational aspects in the communication with the parents, particularly in helping them to understand the vicissitudes of the child's behavior in the course of the analysis. They must be educated to the fact that symptom removal does not constitute an indication to terminate the treatment nor does a temporary exacerbation of symptoms mean that the treatment is not proceeding satisfactorily. With some parents it is necessary to deal with their fear of the child's attachment to the analyst as that develops. They may feel threatened and jealous of this attachment. They need to be reassured that the analysis will not take their child away from them, or turn their child against them. Many parents may have such concerns. This is particularly marked in situations where the parents may be divorced or estranged from each other. Each parent may fear that the analysis will turn the child toward the other parent. Situations where there has been divorce in the family have become increasingly frequent in recent years.

Parents may have many other concerns about their contact with the analyst. Some are reluctant to broach the subject of their own personal lives or their reactions to the child or other family members. At the other end of the spectrum are those who seek to turn the contact with the analyst into a treatment situation for themselves. For the most part, child analysts attempt to avoid such a situation. If it becomes clear that the parents wish and need treatment themselves, the analyst will usually refer them for treatment to someone else while continuing to see them for the purpose of obtaining information about the child. There have been situations in which an analyst has simultaneously treated both the child and a parent, sometimes for quite specific reasons, but this is not the usual situation. The parents may also be initially quite concerned about the information they communicate to the analyst and may be fearful of what the analyst will tell the child. Usually, as the situation of working cooperation develops with the parents, they are able to accept the fact that the analyst must be free to use such information at his own discretion and that he would only do so where he deemed it appropriate and necessary. The analyst does not accept the parent's stipulation, "Please don't tell this to my child." The parent is instead informed that the analyst must feel free to communicate whatever in his judgment is necessary. On the other hand, the parent must be educated to accept the fact that the analyst may not communicate the content of the child's revelations to him during the course of the analysis.

Many child analyses encounter difficulty because of problems arising in the contact with parents. For this reason, we repeat that an essential aspect of the determination to undertake analysis includes the assessment of both child and parents. Where the decision has been well taken, the contact with the parents contributes significantly to the analyst's ability to understand the child. The analyst is frequently able to gauge the extent of the working relationship with the parents by the fact that they bring in information that correlates well with what the child is communicating in the analysis. Such information allows for greater specificity of intervention by the analyst, helping to elucidate and clarify the impact of present-day reality on the underlying conflicts.

One of the central technical problems facing the child analyst is when and how to utilize certain information which may be obtained through contact with the parents. Sometimes such information is of events that could be assumed to be of central importance in, or even traumatic to, the child's development. This includes reports about the death of close family members, episodes of severe illness of the child or his parents, hospitalization of a family member, etc. The analyst may form hypotheses about the role of such events but must be aware that it is not easy to know what the child's perception of and reaction to such events have been. Such material is only of use in the course of an analysis when the child himself approaches the subject. Immature or artificial introductions of information obtained from parental contact usually lead to sterile intellectualizations or incorrect reconstructions. As in all psychoanalysis it is the patients themselves who lead the analyst to understand the significant experiences in their lives. The child's mental functioning is just as subject to psychic determinism as the adult's. This means that with patience and understanding the meaning of the child's conflicts will be elucidated and the unconscious determinants understood. What replaces the adult patient's motivation to find relief from inner suffering is the child's intense urge to complete development.

Some general remarks were made earlier about the role of transference in child analysis. A complete discussion of the subject is not possible here. Suffice to say that latency children certainly do show transference reactions and some develop what for most child analysts would be viewed as a transference neurosis. While it is more difficult to delineate the transference and separate it out from other aspects of the interaction with the analyst, e.g., as a new object or as an object of displacement for present feelings about the parents, it is possible to do so. The analysis of transference reactions is an integral part of any child analysis. For more detailed discussions of the role of transference and transference neurosis the reader is referred to the reports of three panel discussions on child analysis held by the American Psychoanalytic Association (Herley, 1961; Abbate, 1964; Van Dam, 1966), and to a group of papers on

"Special Problems of Transference and Transference Neurosis" (Kanzer, 1971). Most child analysts agree that the extent to which the transference develops and is subject to interpretation is a reflection of the maintenance of the psychoanalytic stance by the analyst. The interpretations of defenses, as always, occurs before the interpretation of contents. Transference resistances are quite common in child analysis. Many children require some education about the transference manifestations they may develop, just as they may need some education about the unconscious before they can respond to any content interpretation appropriately.

There are a host of other technical problems in the analysis of a latency child which it is not possible to discuss here. Discussions of such matters may be found in *Handbook of Child Psychoanalysis* (Wolman, 1972; Pearson, 1968) and *The Child Analyst at Work* (Geleerd, 1967).

Termination

Much of what was mentioned in the discussion of termination with prelatency children holds true for latency children as well. Basically the criteria for termination include the following: (1) resolution of neurotic symptoms; (2) the forward progression of ego and libido to age appropriate behavior and relationships; (3) the undoing of libidinal and ego fixations and repressions; and (4) stability in the child-parent interaction.

The question of whether a child should terminate at the time when he would be entering prepuberty is sometimes a difficult one. In certain cases the treatment may be extended in order to help the child deal with the conflicts of this new developmental phase. However, unless there are specific indications to continue, if it is felt that the analysis has proceeded satisfactorily, it is usually terminated. At the same time the youngster is made aware of the possibilities of returning if specific difficulties should develop either in connection with puberty or during adolescence. Usually in a case with a favorable outcome, such returns will not be necessary. Knowing that they have had understanding and help in dealing with their problems and that such help would be available in the future if needed is in and of itself of considerable support to most children in dealing with conflicts which may emerge later. No amount of analysis will protect the child from all of the possible vicissitudes of later development. The undue prolongation of treatment or an attempt to do so is often a reflection of a countertransference problem in the analyst.

PSYCHOANALYTIC TREATMENT OF ADOLESCENCE

The psychoanalytic treatment of adolescents can be said to date back to Freud's publication of the Dora case as "Fragment of an Analysis of a Case of Hysteria" (1905). Dora was not discussed as an adolescent at that time but has more recently been (Glenn in press). It has only been within the last two decades that there has appeared in the analytic literature a significant number of publications concerning psychoanalytic treatment for adolescents. There are probably several factors for this relatively late application of psychoanalytic treatment to adolescents and indeed there is still a considerable range of difference of opinion about the efficacy of psychoanalytic treatment during this phase. One influential factor was Anna Freud's (1958) description of adolescence as a time of considerable psychic upheaval with attempts to ward off very threatening infantile libidinal and aggressive feelings toward the parents, feelings that were revived and intensified at the onset of adolescence. She described specific defenses against these threatening feelings and several forms of psychopathology seen in adolescence. She was, however, quite cautious about her recommendations for psychoanalytic treatment during this phase. She felt that the need to ward off these infantile object ties would jeopardize the analysis because of their effect on the possibility of developing a workable transference. Some adolescents might identify the analyst even during the assessment as a representative of the parents and develop intense transference resistance, which would make it impossible for them to enter analysis. Others might first experience the threatening affects as attached to the analyst's person during analysis and would have to remove themselves from the analysis as they were attempting to remove themselves from the parental ties.

In spite of these cautions it was clear that our existing knowledge of developmental processes during the adolescent phase had indeed been derived from adolescent analyses. A considerable number of analysts continued to undertake the analytic treatment of adolescents and in so doing contributed significantly to elaborations and modifications of our conceptual framework of the developmental processes and to our knowledge of how technique could usefully apply that knowledge. Among the many who have made significant contributions are Blos, Eissler, Erikson, Fraiberg, Friend, Geleerd, Harley, Josselyn, Kramer, Pearson, Settlage and, of course, Anna Freud herself. The growing knowledge and application of psychoanalytic ego psychology has been of central importance in being able to apply these developments to this age group. It has become increasingly clear that the developmental level of adolescents, just as that of children, requires adaptation in analytic technique. The word adaptation is suggested rather than parameter because what is involved is a modification of technique due to a difference in developmental level of organization rather than to the nature of specific psychopathology. Many of the early cautions were based upon fear of the adolescent's being overwhelmed by his drive impulses, with the assumption that analysis would increase this danger if the defenses against the drives were analyzed (Geleerd, 1957). As a consequence of this concern it was suggested that part of the technique concentrate on increasing the tolerance of the ego. In a sense this represents the partial carry-over of a much earlier view of the psychoanalytic process, one which emphasized the idea of making the drives conscious by overcoming the resistances.

Psychoanalytic ego psychology has made it clear that the analytic position should be a much broader one and that attention should be directed toward the superego and the ego and its multiple functions and not only toward its defenses against drives. Where there may be some impairment of a given ego function, a modification of technique is undertaken. In the analysis of adults the widening range of patients taken into analytic treatment has led to frequent use of such modifications of technique in dealing with specific problems. These modifications of the adult ego are assumed to have been brought about by neurotic defensive impairment. In the analysis of adolescents certain ego functions may be in similar difficulty, but in their case because of the normal developmental process. Here too, there can be modifications of technique which do not compromise the basic needs of the psychoanalytic method. Settlage (Harley, 1974) discussed the need for adaptations in standard analytic technique in order to fulfill the purposes of the analytic method and described a specific technique of defense analysis as applied to an adolescent. What these recent developments all suggest is that psychoanalytic treatment of at least some adolescent disturbances has been undertaken with increasing frequency and with much less concern about negative outcomes. As our knowledge of the psychoanalytic psychology of the adolescent process has increased, our attempts to treat adolescents have become more successful. We certainly hope that further addition to our knowledge and clarifications of technical approaches will continue this trend. Actually it has been only for a relatively few years that organized psychoanalytic training has been provided for the analyst who wishes to undertake the treatment of adolescents. For many years such treatment, particularly of the older adolescent, was undertaken by analysts who had no special knowledge or experience with the adolescent process. Many of these felt that a 17- or 18-year-old could be treated as an adult. Fortunately our knowledge has been enhanced and we now know that such a chronological determinant has no necessary correlation with the end of the adolescent process. Many young persons of college age are still involved with adolescent conflicts and may require an analyst who has had specific training and experience with that process.

The Indications for Adolescent Analysis

In considering the indications for psychoanalytic treatment of adolescents, we are aware of varying recommendations that reflect the approach of different analysts. As indicated above there are some analysts who feel that adolescent patients are not analyzable without recourse to parameters of technique, some of which go well beyond the maintenance of a psychoanalytic stance. Among those who have worked with adolescent patients there are some who suggest that the optimum indications for psychoanalytic treatment are a classical neurosis of the hysterical or obsessional type. Anna Freud (1958) herself went beyond this and suggested that in certain adolescents who manifested a withdrawal of libido to the self, analytic therapy was not only indicated but urgent. Essentially she described a marked narcissistic withdrawal with grandiose ideas and hypochondriacal preoccupations. Some analysts would feel that the group of patients whom she described represent a very high-risk population in whom analysis may be undertaken out of desperation but with whom the outcome would be indeed guarded. She also saw indications for analysis in what she described as the "ascetic" adolescent but, in general, felt that the indications for analytic treatment were limited.

Pearson (1968) attempted to discuss indications in terms of specific subphases of adolescence. The one group for whom psychoanalysis was indicated regardless of the stage of adolescent development was that which presented with anxiety hysteria, conversion hysteria, or an obsessional neurosis. He felt that the same criteria which constituted indications for analysis during latency were applicable during prepuberty, namely, those who show a regression in the libidinal level, show inhibitions of ego functions or ego constrictions, perverse symptoms, or express wishes to be of the opposite sex. In discussing the indications for analysis during the pubertal period, he discusses one group which shows impulsive behavior and another which shows ego constriction. Within the group showing impulsive behavior it is suggested that those patients in whom the behavior shows as a defense against depression and those in whom it is a reflection of specific neurotic conflicts constitute those youngsters for whom analysis is indicated. With regard to the ego constriction, it is frequently manifested by learning difficulties in school, by social withdrawal, or by lack of interests. He recommends psychoanalytic treatment, or at least evaluation for analysis, in all these situations.

Friend (Wolman, 1972) was quite cautious about the indications for analysis during early adolescence. He suggested that only with those children who had started analysis during late latency can the analysis continue through puberty and into early or middle adolescence. He felt that analysis was much more feasible with the older adolescent and discussed some of the requirements for analyzability. Among these he particularly considered the capacity to verbalize, meaning the capacity to express relationships and the meaning of the self and the object world to another human being, and to delay discharge. Another indication is the capacity for the cathexis of a given interest or activity, whether that be a hobby, an involvement in sports, participation in some social activity, or reading. Whatever the nature of this activity it should lead to enjoyment and satisfaction. He felt that such activity was an index of object cathexis with sufficient investment such that it suggested a capacity for synthesis and communicated the possibility of the sublimation potential. Further, he considered the ability to acknowledge fantasy formation, daydreams, and dreams minimal requirements for analysis. He suggested careful assessment of these functions: (1) the capacity for object constancy; (2) the capacity to tolerate anxiety without disorganization; (3) intellectual capacity for language and problem solving; (4) the capacity for self-observation; (5) some indications of progression along the lines of genital primacy. Where these criteria are met, he recommends essentially a period of trial analysis.

Harley (1974) presents a group of papers which apply analytic treatment to a very broad spectrum of pathological formations in adolescence. There are cases described which certainly show indications of rather marked disturbances in ego functioning or other structural impairment. At least some of the cases presented there go beyond what could be considered adaptations of technique to a developmental phase but represent instead the use of parameters directed against specific aspects of the patient's pathology. Nevertheless, significant analytic work is achieved with positive growth and consolidation in the adolescent.

In summary, one could say that there are reservations among many analysts about beginning analysis during prepuberty or in early adolescence. Where there are indications for treatment during those periods, some modifications in the form of psychoanalytic psychotherapy are generally advisable. In middle and later adolescence there seems to be general agreement that specific neuroses as well as neurotic character formations constitute indications for psychoanalytic treatment which can be undertaken with those adaptations of technique that are appropriate to the developmental phase. Psychoanalytic treatment with more severely disturbed adolescents, those who evidence borderline functioning or may even have had more severe regressive episodes, may be undertaken when it is felt that it offers the best available means or only hope. It is undertaken with a greater number of modifications in technique and with a more guarded prognosis.

Technical Considerations

Some differences in the technique of approaching the adolescent patient are evident from the first contact with the patient. It is quite likely that the period of assessment with an adolescent patient will be somewhat longer than it might be with an adult. In this context the adolescent and the analyst are each assessing the other for the possibility of their working together. The adolescent will be having varying levels of experience, all of which play a part in determining the nature of the psychoanalytic situation that evolves. On the one hand, the analyst may be immediately identified as someone of the parent's generation with whom the adolescent will feel strange and with whom he will expect to find little understanding or common ground. On the other hand, the analyst is also perceived as a new object, and in this context the adolescent looks with great curiosity for clues to indicate the kind of person with whom he is considering becoming involved. The adolescent will be less likely to tolerate any prolonged silence on the part of the analyst and somewhat more interventions must be made. These should not, however, be aimless or merely conversational. Interventions should reflect the attempt to understand, to clear up difficulties in communication, and to facilitate the adolescent's self-observation and self-curiosity. The adolescent will be attempting to see what the analyst might be like as a real person. He will be looking for some indication that the analyst knows something about the world in which the adolescent lives and can understand something of his language and his experiences. The analyst need not respond by attempting to talk the adolescent's language, but some indication that the analyst understands his experience is necessary. The analyst cannot present as being too "uptight" or distant, nor as attempting to get into a close relationship too quickly. Neither approach will be accepted by the adolescent. It is important that the adolescent get some sense of the analyst as a real person. This will be part of what he will draw upon when he later develops transference feelings toward the analyst and has to differentiate them from his conception of the analyst as a real person.

It was indicated earlier that the failure to make this differentiation is one of the frequent causes for disruption of treatment by adolescents. The adolescent who shows some capacity to be curious about himself and who begins to communicate during the assessment will want to know what analysis involves, if that is the procedure recommended. The idea of coming four or five times a week in and of itself creates anxiety in certain adolescents, sometimes conveying the idea that they must be very sick, at other times bringing up fears of dependency, passivity, or submission to authority. Some realistic information about analysis should be communicated and those fears that can be dealt with should be clarified. The more unconscious meanings cannot, of course, be approached at this time. Some adolescents need to move more gradually into analysis and may start out for a brief period of time wanting to come only two or three times a week. There may also be questions about the couch and some initial reluctance toward the use of the couch. In this, as in other areas, the analyst needs to be flexible and allow the adolescent to experiment at given times. Most adolescents eventually use the couch, and it may be an essential part of establishing a full psychoanalytic relationship that they prove able to do so. They may also, however, have times, particularly early in the analysis, when they choose to sit up. At other times they may lie down but turn around much more often than an adult would. The couch represents a regressive threat for the adolescent on many different levels, and its sustained use will only be possible when a more solid therapeutic alliance evolves with less fear of regressive transferences.

Another practical aspect of the analysis that occurs early in the relationship is the role of the parents in the assessment of the adolescent; also what, if any, role they will have in terms of contact with the analyst during the analysis. Some analysts, viewing the central wish of the adolescent as separation from the parents, are concerned about their being viewed as on the side of the parents. They therefore avoid all contact with the parents or limit that contact to a brief meeting with the parents, usually with the adolescent present. It sometimes occurs that the potential adolescent client comes from a family situation where there is familiarity with analysis as a procedure, or sometimes even knowledge of the specific analyst. In such situations the parents may themselves not initiate any contact with the analyst. Rather, the adolescent may call for and make an appointment on his own. Even in such circumstances it is probably advisable that the analyst see the parents and that the parents have a chance to meet the analyst. Such contact with the parents of the adolescent should occur in the presence of the adolescent. Adolescent patients themselves must determine what information they wish to communicate to the parent about their difficulties. The analyst will have to discuss his reasons for recommending psychoanalysis at a level that the parents can comprehend. Usually such matters as the time of appointment can be arranged directly with the adolescent, but the discussion of fees obviously requires the presence of the parents. Friend (Wolman, 1972) feels that such meetings with both the parents and the adolescent may occur not only during the assessment stage but even at later points in the analysis when there are specific indications for such a meeting. One example would be a meeting to discuss the choice of a college or whether college or continuing the analysis would take precedence. After such matters have been explored with the adolescent patient, it may be necessary for the analyst to reinforce the adolescent's decision in a discussion with the parents. An indirect benefit of such meetings is that they may also serve to help the adolescent in differentiating the style and manner of the analyst from that of his or her parents.

When there are felt to be specific technical reasons why there should not be contact with the parents after an initial meeting, this should be communicated and clarified by meeting with them. Some education of the parents not only helps to secure their support of the treatment, but may alleviate some of their distress. They may not only be feeling guilt, but are also being faced with a situation in which they may feel excluded without understanding the reasons. Such an exclusion may lead them to feel that the analyst is blaming them unless it is clarified.

Turning to toe actual technique of the analysis, the central focus is on the systematic analysis of defenses as they occur in the context of the phase specific development. Settlage (Harley, 1974) discussed the concept and technique of defense analysis as applied to adolescents. He stressed the following points:

1. The recognition that the position of the ego and its need for defenses should be respected. As the analysis proceeds and there are gains through insight and mastery over warded off material by means of defense analysis, the ego is strengthened. The strengthening of the ego is particularly important in that adolescent whose ego is greatly threatened by the intensified emergence of instinctual forces.

2. The analysis of the defense and what it defends against are to be undertaken simultaneously. No defense is analyzed without some consideration of its role in the overall balance of intrapsychic forces. At times specific defenses may be avoided because the impulse-defense configuration suggests that this might be temporarily wise. The ultimate goal is to make clear that something is being warded off, how this is being done, what it is that it is warded off, and why. Observations of verbal and nonverbal behavior lead to the inference of defenses and the reasons for the defense. In the usual situation determinants of the patient's current behavior in the analytic situation

precedes that of transference interpretation and genetic interpretation.

3. Attention is focused first on the most superficial layers of defense with the assumption that the ego will have greater tolerance for the exposure of warded off content at this level than at deeper and more highly defended levels. Interpretation proceeds from the surface. In actual practice there can be a movement back and forth from somewhat more superficial to deeper levels rather than a strictly mechanical hierarchical approach.

4. Analysis of defenses neither removes entirely nor destroys the defenses. The patient is not forced to yield defenses. Rather there is a modification and an increased appropriateness of defenses.

Much of what has been discussed above as the technique of defense analysis in the adolescent does not differ essentially from that which is utilized in the analysis of the adult. The adaptation to the adolescent lies in the choice of which defense to approach and what level of interpretation to assign at a specific point. The greater the degree of familiarity the analyst has with the range of adolescent processes, the more appropriate the choice of such interventions will be. One area in which one can clearly see an adaptation to adolescent processes is in the manner of the technical approach to the transference. The author, in a previous publication (Kanzer, 1971), reviewed the literature on the development of transference and transference neurosis in adolescents and added some reflections on its technical application. He pointed out that the clinical transference picture can very often be obscured by the fact that the phase specific libidinal push and the defensive attempts to deal with it involve the analyst in additional roles. The analyst may not only be a transference object or object of displacement but may also be a new object. Adolescence is characterized as a period in which there is a search for new objects or new levels of relationships as a developmental goal. This search manifests itself in the analytic situation and affects the extent to which transference develops in its purest form, i.e., as a repetition of the earlier relationships. The intensity and depth of the transference phenomena in adolescent analysis show great variation. Appropriately timed interpretations aid the ego in synthesis and foster the therapeutic alliance. The extent to which a patient may develop a full transference experience, i.e., transference neurosis, depends largely upon the choices made by the analyst in interpreting the transference representations. There is an adaptive aspect in that the patient uses the analyst as a new object and that a new level of relationship may be established which draws upon the libidinal ties of the regressive aspects of the transference but also adds to them. Sensitively handled, the interpretation of transference furthers some developments of this phase, facilitating differentiation and synthesis. Adolescent analysts may have to be content with the fact that certain aspects of the transference will not be completely analyzed in adolescence.

It is virtually impossible in an article such as this to discuss the technique of adolescent analysis in appropriate detail. There is, of course, no substitute for a carefully reported actual treatment. Fortunately, more and more such reports are beginning to appear in the literature. It is reasonable to expect that there will be refinements of assessment, indications for analysis and technique, as adolescent analysis is more widely applied now that the earlier cautions against it as a hazardous undertaking have been successfully challenged.

Termination

The termination of a good many adolescent analyses differs significantly from that in adults. Some develop a transference neurosis, and its resolution is the indication to terminate, as it would be in an adult analysis. It may be more appropriate to describe many other adolescent analyses as interrupted rather than terminated, the phenomenon that led Friend (Wolman, 1972) to describe the process as "a piece of psychoanalysis." Such interruptions often occur when the adolescent reaches the point where there is a need for functioning apart from family and analyst. Considering that many adolescents who enter analysis do so in the middle or later phases of adolescence, it may be that the analytic work can only be carried on for two or three years, sometimes even less. A high proportion of those adolescents whom the analyst sees are then faced with college and the often accompanying change of geographical location. It sometimes happens that a joint decision is made to continue the analysis and that the choice of where to go to college becomes secondary. Such young people will attend a college within a reasonable distance from the analyst and their home, if that is feasible. Even with such adolescents, there may come a time when, with further progress of the analysis and with better integration, the wish to function independently away from the family and the analyst appears. This may be a phase appropriate development, and it is not possible to generalize that all adolescents who have such an interrupted analytic experience will need subsequent analysis. Many may make sufficient progress so that the normal developmental process continues once it has been initiated. Other adolescents may return for occasional contacts with the analyst. Still others may resume analysis at a later point in their life, either with the same analyst or with a different one.

As was indicated during our discussion of transference, the analyst has to accept the fact that certain aspects of the transference may not be resolved as ideally as one would wish. In spite of this a sufficient amount of success should be attainable in this area with most adolescents. It sometimes occurs that only during the termination phase can certain of the transference reactions, which were too intense and too frightening to be dealt with earlier in the analysis, be approached by the adolescent. The degree of ego and superego consolidation allows some adolescents to look back at affective experiences which might have been unapproachable six months or a year or two earlier. As the analyst is more consistently experienced as a differentiated object, the transference distortions can be put into perspective. What would not have been possible earlier, due to the phase specific intensity of the drives and the transient ego regressions, can now be analyzed.

Friend (Wolman, 1972) discussed the aims of psychoanalysis of adolescents as more limited than those of adult work, yet comprising effective analytic effort. Included among these are the following: genetic aspects of the individual's development are clarified with the revival of visual and affective memories; the ego ideal and conscience are expanded; ego problems in the areas of learning, memory, sexual inadequacy, or other inhibitions in function can be resolved; the nature of anxiety and the responses to it are better understood; and, finally, the ability to maintain a close, understanding and trusting relationship with another person reaches a level beyond a simple identification. There should be an increased sense of oneself as an individual and a better capacity for self-awareness and expression with improvement in the intrapsychic relationships as well as in social functioning. Certainly, if the analysis brings about a reasonable number of these changes, it constitutes a worthwhile therapeutic endeavor.

In attempting to provide the reader with an overview of current psychoanalytic treatment of children and adolescents, we have tried to show how the different developmental phases affect such considerations as the assessment of the child, indications for psychoanalytic treatment, technical management, and indications for termination. The developmental point of view should also be applied to the field of child and adolescent analysis, which is itself involved in a progressively unfolding developmental process. While there has been considerable growth and consolidation, the prospect of maturity is still a long way in the future. For those who work in this field, however, the process of development itself seems an exciting and stimulating challenge.

REFERENCES

ABBATE, G. Panel report: Child analysis at different developmental stages. *Journal of the American Psychoanalytic Association*, 1964, *12*, 135–150.

BERNSTEIN, I. The importance of characteristics of the parents in deciding on child analysis. *Journal of the American Psychoanalytic Association*, 1958, *6*, 71–78.

Blos, P. *On adolescence: A psychoanalytic interpretation.* New York: Free Press, 1962.

Blos, P. The concept of acting out in relation to the adolescent process. *Journal of the American Academy of Child Psychiatry*, 1963, *2*, 118–136.

Blos, P. The second individuation process of adolescence. *The Psychoanalytic Study of the Child*, 1967, *22*, 162–186.

Bornstein, Berta. The analysis of a phobic child. Some problems of theory and technique in child analysis. *The Psychoanalytic Study of the Child*, 1949, *3–4*, 181–226.

Burlingham, D., Golberger, A., and Lussier, A. Simultaneous analysis of mother and child. *The Psychoanalytic Study of the Child*, 1955, *10*, 165–186.

Buxbaum, E. Technique of child therapy. *The Psychoanalytic Study of the Child*, 1954, *9*, 297–333.

Eissler, K. R. The effect of the structure of the ego on psychoanalytic differences. *Journal of the American Psychoanalytic Association*, 1954, *2*, 711–797.

Eissler, K. R. Notes on problems of technique in the psychoanalytic treatment of adolescents: With some remarks on perversions. *The Psychoanalytic Study of the Child*, 1958, *13*, 223–254.

Feigelson, C. Panel report: A comparison between adult and child analysis. *Journal of the American Psychoanalytic Association*, 1974, *22*, 603–612.

Fraiberg, S. A comparison of the analytic method in two stages of a child analysis. *Journal of the American Academy of Child Psychiatry*, 1965, *4*, 387–400.

Fraiberg, S. Transference in latency. *The Psychoanalytic Study of the Child*, 1966, *21*, 213–237.

Frankl, L. A specific problem in adolescent boys; difficulties in loosening the infantile tie to the mother. *Bulletin of the Philadelphia Association for Psychoanalysis*, 1963, *13*, 120–129.

Frankl, L., and Hellman, I. The ego's participation in the therapeutic alliance. *International Journal of Psycho-Analysis*, 1962, *43*, 333–337.

Freud, A. Adolescence. *The Psychoanalytic Study of the Child*, 1958, *13*, 255–278.

Freud, A. *The psychoanalytical treatment of children: Lectures and essays.* New York: Schocken Books, 1964 (Originally published, 1946).

Freud, A. *Normality and pathology in childhood.* New York: International Universities Press, 1965.

Freud, A. Indications and contraindications for child analysis. *The Psychoanalytic Study of the Child*, 1968, *23*, 37–46.

Geleerd, E. Some aspects of psychoanalytic technique in adolescence. *The Psychoanalytic Study of the Child*, 1957, *12*, 263–283.

Geleerd. E. *The child analyst at work.* New York: International Universities Press, 1967.

Glenn, J. Freud's adolescent patients: Dora, Katarina, and "the homosexual woman." In M. Kanzer and J. Glenn (Eds.), *Freud and his patients* (tentative title). New York: Jason Aronson, in press.

Harley M. Panel report: Resistance in child analysis. *Journal of the American Psychoanalytic Association*, 1961, *9*, 548–562. (a)

Harley M. Some observations on the relationship between genitality and structural development in adolescence. *Journal of the American Psychoanalytic Association*, 1961, *9*, 434–460. (b)

Harley, M. The role of the dream in the analysis of a latency child. *Journal of the American Psychoanalytic Association*, 1962, *10*, 271–288.

Harley, M. *The analyst and the adolescent at work.* New York: Quadrangle (The New York Times Book Co.), 1974.

Kanzer, M. *The unconscious today.* New York: International Universities Press, 1971.

Katan, A. Some thoughts about the role of verbalization in early childhood. *The Psychoanalytic Study of the Child*, 1961, *16*, 184–188.

KESTENBERG, J. Problems of technique of child analysis in relation to the various developmental stages: Pre-latency. *The Psychoanalytic Study of the Child*, 1969, *24*, 358–383.

KRAMER, S., and SETTLAGE, C. P. On the concepts and technique of child analysis. *Journal of the American Academy of Child Psychiatry*, 1962, *1*, 509–535.

KRIS, E. Notes on the development and on some current problems of psychoanalytic child psychology. *The Psychoanalytic Study of the Child*, 1950, *5*, 24–46.

LOEWENSTEIN, R. M. Some remarks on defenses, autonomous ego, and psycho-analytic technique. *International Journal of Psycho-Analysis*, 1954, *23*, 194–198.

MAENCHEN, A. On the technique of child analysis in relation to stages of development. *The Psychoanalytic Study of the Child*, 1970, *25*, 175–208.

NEUBAUER, P. B. The one-parent child and his oedipal development. *The Psychoanalytic Study of the Child*, 1960, *15*, 286–309.

PEARSON, G. *A Handbook of Child Psychoanalysis*. New York: Basic Books, 1968.

REXFORD, E. Child psychiatry and child analysis in the United States today. *Journal of the American Academy of Child Psychiatry*, 1962, *1*, 365–384.

SILBER, E. The analyst's participation in the treatment of an adolescent. *Psychiatry*, 1962, *25*, 160–169.

SKLANSKY, M. A. Panel report: Indications and contraindications for the psychoanalysis of the adolescent. *Journal of the American Psychoanalytic Association*, 1972, *20*, 134–144.

SOLNIT, A. Ego vicissitudes of adolescence. *Journal of the American Psychoanalytic Association*, 1959, *7*, 523–535.

VAN AMERONGEN, S. The psychoanalysis of a young adolescent girl. *Journal of Orthopsychiatry*, 1962, *32*, 160–169.

VAN DAM, H. Panel report: Problems of transference in child analysis. *Journal of the American Psychoanalytic Association*, 1966, *14*, 528–537.

WOLMAN, B. *Handbook of child psychoanalysis*. New York: Van Nostrand-Reinhold, 1972.

5

THERAPEUTIC NURSERIES[1]

Eugene Mahon & Delia Battin

The treatment of children in therapeutic nurseries has been possible in the twentieth century because educators and psychiatrists have discovered that preschool children with emotional handicaps have complicated needs that neither group can meet alone. For instance, the 3-year-old schizophrenic child is unmanageable in a regular nursery. In traditional psychotherapies, in clinics and private offices, his educational needs cannot be met appropriately. In hospital treatment, the bond between child and family is often disrupted for long periods of time. The concept of a therapeutic nursery offers a sensible alternative: a preschooler with emotional problems can go to school where he and his family can get help from a team of educators and psychiatrists. After school, he can go home to his family and not be subjected to the trauma of long hospitalization away from his home.

This marriage between psychiatry and education was unknown in previous centuries. Indeed, the whole concept of nursery education is relatively modern, beginning in 19th-century Europe and not really gaining widespread popularity until the 20th century. In 17th- and 18th-century France, as described by Aries (1962) in *Centuries of Childhood* there was a law forbidding children under seven to go to school. As far as therapeutic nurseries are concerned, the historical impetus for their development seems to have been the First World War, which displaced many children from their homes. Siegfried Bernfeld (Ekstein & Motto, 1969) devised a plan for working with these war orphans who were depressed, narcissistic, and deprived. He treated them in "Baumgartens," using educational and psychoanalytic techniques with good results. The Second World War created a similar problem for displaced children which Anna Freud and Dorothy Burlingham have described in their *Infants Without Families*. After the Second World War the psychiatric literature began to reflect the importance of therapeutic nursery education. Since Sante de Sanctis in 1906 described dementia praecoxissima, psychosis in children began to be recognized. Since then, Howard Potter, Lauretta Bender, Leo Kanner, Margaret Mahler, William Goldfarb, Michael Rutter, and others have defined and redefined the

[1]The authors wish to thank the other members of the therapeutic nursery staff who helped shape the ideas expressed in this chapter: Amy Belkin, Josephine Bliss, Amy Bloom, Pierre Boenig, Nancy Cowall, Joe Franzen, Teresa Gardian, Shoshana Mafdali-Goldman, Clarice Kestenbaum, Liz McHugh, Ruth Mollod, Lilo Plaschkes, Cal Sumner, Jerry Wiener, Libby Wolf.

nature of infantile autism and childhood schizophrenia, two of the major emotional disorders in preschoolers. In 1954 Alpert described therapeutic educational techniques she employed at the nursery of the council of the Child Development Center. She introduced the concept of guided regression in a corrective object relationship therapy for severely deprived children. Mahler (1968) described a tripartite design of therapy for autistic symbiotic children, and Pfeiffer (1959) described a modified nursery school in a hospital, for children disturbed enough to be in a hospital, who need diagnostic evaluation and short-term treatment. Margaret Lovatt (1962) described the introduction and treatment of an autistic child, one child at a time, in a day nursery for normal children. Robert Furman and Anny Katan (1969) described the therapeutic nursery school in Cleveland (Hanna Perkins School) where child psychoanalysis and treatment via the mother are offered to a preschool population with emotional disturbances.

THERAPEUTIC NURSERY EDUCATION IN PRACTICE

This brief historical note will serve to introduce the concept of therapeutic nursery education. Now let us try to define the treatment of children in therapeutic nurseries. Obviously the treatment will depend on the need of the individual child and his family, the severity of the diagnosis, and the availability of professionals to meet the needs. The therapeutic nursery brings together a team of experts from varied disciplines who work together from year to year and can become a sophisticated therapeutic instrument to meet the needs of even the most severely damaged youngster. Therapeutic nurseries across this country have opened their doors to children with emotional disturbances as varied as childhood schizophrenia, infantile autism, brain damage with language disorders and perceptual impairments, hyperkinetic children, and children with developmental deviations and character disorders.

For instance, Frank, a 4-year-old boy with symbiotic psychosis and sensory and expressive language disorder, posed a complicated problem for his team of therapists. In addition to the child's severe psychopathology, the family was disturbed also. Frank had replaced his father in the mother's bed, an arrangement that allowed his parents, who were borderline personalities with paranoid features, to avoid each other in bed as well as in every other aspect of their mysterious marriage. The father worked nights, the mother days. The father brought the child to school. The mother was almost impossible to involve in psychotherapy of any duration. However, despite the severe pathology in the child and his parents, a substantial therapeutic regimen was possible. The father brought the child to school every day. The mother made occasional visits. The child was involved in classroom therapy every day, individual psychotherapy twice weekly, and language therapy once weekly. He began his nursery education with no differentiated sense of self or objects, with no communicative language and with perceptual defects involving many aspects of cognition and memory. The perceptual and the emotional defects went hand in hand. He had no sense of parents or teachers or friends as reliable, constant objects—they were out of sight, out of mind. He would have inconsolable tantrums if the teacher left the room. By the same token he could not remember the piece of a puzzle that was missing. He could not get the meaning of peek-a-boo or hide-and-seek games. Language therapy, perceptual training in the classroom, individual psychotherapy, and family therapy all contributed to the establishment of a differentiated sense of self, the internalization of a communicative sense of language, the acquisition of a more reliable memory, and a sense of object constancy. The parents were able to allow him to have his own bed when they began to understand that it was their own separation anxiety they were protecting and not the child's by keeping him in the parental bedroom. We will return to this child and his family in the clinical discussions to follow. At this time we are trying to establish the point that severely damaged children with emotional and perceptual and familial pathology often need comprehensive, sophisticated multiple therapy involving a variety of disciplines. In a therapeutic nursery where family therapist, individual therapist, language therapist, and special educational teacher meet together regularly to discuss the interdigitation of their various approaches, the child can receive the quality and quantity of therapeutic interventions that are necessary.

Let us describe a therapeutic nursery so that the reader can become familiar with the concept. There are many therapeutic nurseries across the country, each one perhaps with a different philosophy and perhaps even different diagnostic criteria for the admission of children. But let us describe an actual therapeutic nursery, how it began, the kind of children who are treated in this nursery, with the full realization that the model about to be described may not represent precisely what other therapeutic nurseries are offering.

The St. Luke's Hospital–Riverside Church Therapeutic Nursery

The Riverside Church weekday school in New York City has been serving the needs of local children since the 1930s when it was built. The school had approximately 200 children between the ages of 2½ and 6. The director, Josephine Bliss, took great pride in her achievements with handicapped children as well as with the 200 other normal children. Since the 1950s she had enrolled handicapped children in the school: for example, a number of children with Down's Syndrome, osteogenesis imperfecta, blindness, and hydrocephalus were integrated into the regular classrooms with great success. Wheelchairs, crutches, and physical deformities became a part of the school atmosphere. The children and the staff overcame their fears and their prejudices together, and the school was the better for it. Handicaps are a part of life, society shouldn't ostracize, these were the attitudes that permeated the classrooms and corridors and the playgrounds of the school.

A few hundred yards from Riverside Church stood St. Luke's Hospital. In 1965 Jerry Wiener, chief of Child and Adolescent Psychiatry at the hospital, devised a plan together with Josephine Bliss. They would set aside two classrooms for autistic and schizophrenic children. The church would provide the classrooms free of charge. The hospital would provide the personnel. Since then these therapeutic nursery classrooms serving the needs of emotionally disturbed children have operated side by side with regular classrooms. At times children from the therapeutic classes "graduated" and were able to make a transition into the regular classrooms. At times, children in the regular classes were discovered to be emotionally ill and could be transferred without any difficulty to the therapeutic classes. Children from the regular classes with emotional conflicts not severe enough to be in the therapeutic classrooms were treated by the therapeutic nursery staff in group therapy twice weekly after school. This particular project (Plaschkes, 1975) was very successful and was an indicator of how well the two staffs, that is, the regular and the therapeutic classroom staffs, could work together.

But it is the work of the two therapeutic classrooms, the therapeutic nursery proper, that this chapter will describe. The staff of the therapeutic nursery is a team that tries to meet every emotional need of the child and the family. A child psychiatrist, a child fellow, a psychiatric social worker, a psychologist, two language specialists, an art therapist, three special education teachers, and a special education intern comprise the staff. All are employed part-time—except the teachers, who are full-time. Children are diagnosed at the Child Psychiatry Clinic of the hospital and referred to the therapeutic nursery for treatment. At this time it is explained to the family that the child and the family will be treated concomitantly in the therapeutic nursery school.

The classrooms open their doors at 9:30 a.m. and end at 12 noon. However, the children may also be seen for individual attention from any member of the staff before or after class. The individual attention could be perceptual training, language stimulation, art therapy, play therapy, psychotherapy, psychological testing, etc. The parents are seen in individual and group therapy by the psychiatric social worker. Group therapy for the parents is once weekly for two hours. Individual therapy for the parents is once, twice, or even three times a week for 45-minute sessions of psychoanalytically oriented psychotherapy.

Let us try to describe the classroom. Let us begin at the door, perhaps the most important area in a therapeutic nursery school. The mother brings her child here every day and the child is expected to leave her and go into the classroom. Let us compare the regular classrooms and the therapeutic classrooms in this regard. Every September at the beginning of the school year, mothers wait in the corridors of the regular classrooms for their 3-year-olds to feel comfortable enough to let them go home. After a few days or maybe weeks, the 3-year-old feels comfortable enough and mother can drop him off and leave promptly. Anna Freud sees this ability of normal children to separate from their mothers and participate in nursery school education as a developmental milestone that can be expected around 3 years of age. This milestone is made possible by the intrapsychic work that the child has been doing on the subphases of separation-individuation during the first three years of his life. Having passed through phases of symbiosis, differentiation, and rapproachement, he has gone on to form a cohesive sense of self and a sense of object constancy. The mental representation of a mother whom he loves and misses and whose absence he can tolerate because he knows she will return, gives him a sense of confidence about himself that allows him to play with his peers and learn.

Let us return to the door of the therapeutic classrooms. The mother arrives here with her handicapped child. The child has schizophrenia or brain damage or aphasia: the child has a poor grasp of who he is or who his mother is; he has no language, no reliable set of inner symbols that he can call on to communicate his needs. When he wants something he may kick or scream; when he walks into the classroom he does not carry with him an inner sense of self or the constancy of self and of objects. When he becomes frustrated, angry, or fearful, he may have to return to the door, the place he last saw his mother. If she is there he can refuel and, having pulled himself together, can return to the classroom. The point we are stressing here is that the mother may have to wait at the door of the classroom for a long time until her handicapped child feels comfortable letting her go. It would be an error to consider the child's travels to the door to find his mother a disruption of classroom cohesion or peripheral in any way to the educational goals of the classroom. In fact the opposite is true: the mother at the door and the child's struggle to leave and to feel comfortable without her because he has a sense of her within him—this is the behavioral axis upon which meaningful education can be built. The mother, the first educator of the child, and the therapeutic nursery teacher cooperate at this early point in the management of the child to create a curriculum of trust and patience so that the child can learn his first lesson: a door doesn't shut you off from your mother, it opens up possibilities of individuation and learning and pleasure.

Once inside the classroom, the child's anxieties will prevent any meaningful psychoeducational work from being done unless the teacher is resourceful and intuitive and unless the curriculum can be geared at any moment to the needs of the child. Any rigid curriculum would make no sense at all. How can you teach an obsessional child to enjoy making a mess; how can you teach an impulsive, messy child to enjoy order and cleanliness; how do you teach an angry child who bites you or bites himself to put his feelings into words; or an aphasic, angry child, to express his feelings in symbolic play or other nonverbal communication? How do you teach a child to make eye contact with you? The teacher is confronted with these difficult tasks—to be the auxiliary ego at all times to children whose egos are immature and fragile. Finding the proper approach to fit the needs of each individual child is a matter of skill, intuition, patience, and perseverance. The teacher is better able to approach this formidable educational challenge when she is armed with all the information about the child that can be made available to her by the rest of the therapeutic nursery team. Teachers, language specialists, social workers, art therapists, psychologist, child psychiatrists, all meet regularly (3 times a week or more) to share their knowledge. The social worker describes her work with the parents, her individual and group therapy. The other specialists describe their work. The teachers describe the classroom progress. In this way the staff shares all of its knowledge; the teacher is aware of the psychodynamics of the parents, the progress of language therapy and other individual therapies. This helps the teacher to understand behavior that might otherwise be baffling.

Typical Experiences of a Child in a Therapeutic Nursery

Let us try to describe a typical child and how the therapeutic nursery classroom must appear to him. If he can tolerate the separation from mother, he will enter a world of other children who seem as perplexed as he is, and adults who seem to want to help. Let us try to imagine the scene from inside the child's head. The teacher is singing a song about the names of all the children and the day of the week it is. The child is sitting on a rug with the others trying to feel comfortable. The song is reminding him where he is, who he is. He is beginning to feel safe. He looks at himself in the mirror. The teacher is in the mirror too, naming the parts of his body for him, helping him to get a sense of himself. Suddenly he becomes sad seeing himself in the mirror without his mother. The sadness quickly turns to anger. He tries to punch the teacher. She says no. But he cannot stop. Now he is running around trying to punch everybody and the children are punching back. The adults are separating child from child trying to restore order. The child climbs up on the shelf and jumps. He repeats this. The teacher encourages him. He enjoys this new game with the teacher. The anger has been rechanneled and forgotten for a while. But now the sadness returns; he is missing mother again. He takes the towel and covers his head with it. The teacher removes it and says peek-a-boo; he laughs—he covers his head again; he enjoys this game too. It is as if he can make the teacher go away and come back again. This makes him feel less helpless. He throws a ball under the table, he retrieves it. He opens and closes the door of the dollhouse. He can make things go away and come back. He can open doors and close them again. Now the teacher wants him to paint. He cannot grasp the brush well with his immature neuromuscular reflexes. He tries to make a circle but the paint splashes all over—he is about to have a tantrum when the teacher begins to admire the splashes. He splashes some more, the teacher applauds. Now he lies down on the brown paper, that the teacher has spread under him. The teacher makes a line of paint all around his body; he stands up. He can see the shape of himself outlined on the paper. The teacher hangs it up on the wall and puts his name under it. He never realized his body could create such an outline. He stands amazed looking at it with his own name written under it. Now the teacher is singing another song, about going home soon and not returning until tomorrow. He hates the transition and change, the separation from the teacher and the children. He is upset by any change, expecting danger not safety. But the teacher is preparing him for it, reminding him that mother will be along soon and that school will reconvene the next day. From this impressionistic vignette, one can hopefully get a sense of a classroom buzzing with activity: children communicating their feelings on a variety of developmental levels with the damaged ego equipment at their disposal; teachers struggling to make sense out of these often perplexing miscommunications. As Eugene O'Neill put it in *All God's Chillun Got Wings*, "Man is born broken, he lives by mending, the grace of God is glue." In a sense the therapeutic nursery teacher searches for a glue to heal the fractured communications of these perplexing children. She will use anything she can find to reach these children. The games, the songs, the paint in the impressionistic vignette just described were used to try to help the children struggle with some of their very painful feelings. These children have a poor sense of body image, a poor sense of identity, a poor sense of their ability to communicate, via any channel, with other human beings. The teacher is therefore forever using paint, water, the mirror, music, or any material she can think of to become a vehicle of communication through which these children can be reached. As mentioned earlier, the teacher is part of a team. She will be discussing her own approaches with the psychiatric social worker, the language specialist, the music and art therapists; the information available to her from the social worker about the parents will help her understand the child better. Similarly the information available to her from all other disciplines (language and art therapy, behavior therapy, and pharmacotherapy) will help her to formulate and modify her own psychoeducational approaches. We cannot do justice to all of these therapies in this chapter; language therapy, behavior therapy, art therapy, and music therapy would require individual explication. Let us focus instead on how these therapies influence the teacher in the classroom.

BEHAVIOR THERAPY IN THE NURSERY

Let us begin with behavior therapy. Since Watson and Rayner (1920) demonstrated the ease with which a fear reaction could be conditioned in a child, behavior modification has been of interest to educators. Mary Cover Jones (1924) described the two most effective methods for eliminating fears in children: (1) direct conditioning; that is, eliciting a pleasant response in the presence of the feared object, and (2) social imitation; that is, placing the child with peers who are not afraid of the fear stimulus. In 1959 Premack articulated a principle which greatly influenced behavioral engineering. Premack's principle suggested an endless range of potential reinforcers (a reinforcer is a stimulus which alters the future probability of the occurrence of the behavior which immediately precedes it; reinforcers can be positive or negative). Premack's principle suggested that given two responses, *a* and *b*, if *b* occurred with a greater frequency than *a*, it could be used as a reinforcer for *a*. By counting behaviors in a classroom, one can become aware of the contingencies and plan behavioral approaches for individual children in the classroom. For instance, Harris, Wolf, and Baer (1967) demonstrated the potency of attention as a reinforcer. They tried to reverse the normal inclinations of teachers to attend to deviant or undesirable behavior, thereby reinforcing it. One child in a laboratory preschool spent 80% of the time crawling on the floor; another child cried or whined 8 times per morning. The modification program ignored problem behavior and gave immediate attention to more appropriate behavior (children on their feet, verbalizing their needs rather than whining). Within 10 days substantial results were evident. A more controversial behavior therapy in the treatment of children is aversive therapy. A few case histories described by Bucher and Lovaas (1968) demonstrate the use of aversive stimulation. John, a 7-year-old boy with an IQ of 25 and psychotic behavior, had been self-destructive since age 2. Without restraints he would hit his head against the crib and strike his head with his fists. Scar tissue covered his head; his ears were swollen and bleeding. Thirty-eight sessions of behavior modification were instituted, the first 15 sessions serving as a baseline. Self-destructive behavior continued at a high level during this period. Twelve one-second electric shocks, contingent upon self-destructive responses were administered over sessions 16, 19, 24, and 30. Self-destructive behavior dropped immediately and was maintained at essentially zero from the 16th to the 38th and final session. The child was able to be released from restraints and join in a normal ward routine.

This brief description of behavioral techniques with children does suggest what an effective instrument it can be in sensitive hands. In a therapeutic nursery one is intuitively manipulating the contingencies of reinforcement as one plans strategies of psychotherapy for each individual child. Teaching an autistic child to make eye contact may require endless patience, resourcefulness, and a repertoire of reinforcers. The child may like being tickled or being sung to: one can make these contingent upon eye contact with the therapist. Primary reinforcers like food may be necessary. Language stimulation may have to rely on a similar contingency of positive reinforcement. It is our experience and conviction that positive reinforcement is a crucial part of any effective therapy in the nursery. It is our equal conviction that negative reinforcement and aversive therapies can modify behavior, but that the negative effects on the object relationship with the teacher are so damaging that the victory over psychopathology is pyrrhic.

LANGUAGE THERAPY AND OTHER TREATMENT MODALITIES

Now let us focus on the language therapist's individual work with schizophrenic children. Again, since we cannot possibly do justice to the scope of this work here, let us focus instead on how the teacher can cooperate with the language therapist in the classroom. Frank, the child whom we mentioned earlier, presented with symbiotic psychosis and a severe language disorder. The teacher and language therapist met together to discuss their work with this child. The teacher found Frank to be clinging, whining, provocative, and intrusive. He could not let her out of his sight without having a tantrum. The language therapist described how Frank's memory was poor. He had trouble remembering the sequence of perceived objects. It was as if he could not hold onto the language symbols. The memory and the words would not stay in place, so to speak. Suddenly the teacher and the language therapist realized they were up against similar problems. The child had no sense of the constancy of mental representations of people in his mind nor did he have a sense of the constancy of the mental representations of words in his mind. Together they could devise mutually reinforcing therapeutic games: peek-a-boo with words as well as peek-a-boo with people. For instance, where is the missing word? Which word is missing from this puzzle? What comes after this word, before that word? Do you remember? Those games with words helped reinforce all the other therapeutic games the teacher provided for the child to help him with perceptual and libidinal object constancy (peek-a-boo; hide-and-seek; you-can-be-angry-with-me-and-I-won't-stop-loving-you games; you-can-be-needy-and-cuddly-and-no-harm-or-humiliation-will-come-to-you games). We can see how the development of reliable internal mental representations in one sphere will assist the development of reliable mental representations in the other. Basic trust in language will foster the growth and development of basic trust in people.

We also cannot convey any idea of the meaningful and exciting work being done in the fields of music therapy or art therapy in this brief chapter. We refer the reader to the many applications of these modalities in treatment as outlined by Podowsky (1954), Heimlich (1965), and Kramer (1971). However, let us make one general statement. Since in therapeutic nursery work we are often dealing with atypical children with damage to their perceptual and integrative ego equipment, who cannot communicate or be communicated with via verbalization or play techniques, *extraordinary approaches become crucial.* The child may be reachable only through (a) tactile sensations (tickling, finger painting, etc.), (b) kinesthetic sensation (dance therapy, etc.), or (c) special sensory modalities, such as music. (One child in our nursery could play songs on the piano and allow human contact to be built up around this one splinter skill, while all other perceptual cognitive avenues seemed to be closed.) It is as if all doors of perception are closed except one or two. It is on this door that the music therapist, art therapist, play therapist, dance therapist, etc. must knock, hoping to be allowed to enter so that with patience, the keys to other doors may be found and more and more of the child's ego can be reclaimed.

PSYCHOTHERAPEUTIC INTERVENTION WITH THE CHILDREN AND THEIR FAMILIES

Having discussed classroom therapeutic interventions with the children, let us now turn to the other psychotherapeutic modalities with the children and their families. As a general rule, all parents receive group therapy and individual therapy. When needed, couple and family therapy can be offered.

We have found it imperative to work as much with the parents as with the children. Emotional disturbance in children takes a toll on all members of the family. The child struggles to communicate. The family struggles to understand. The result, through nobody's fault, is often miscommunication, misunderstanding, grief, and confusion. We disagree with Bettelheim who would solve this dilemma by removing the parents from the scene and treating the child alone. The opposite is our therapeutic stance: everybody needs as much help as possible to understand the child's communications and to avoid miscommunication and perpetuation of pathology.

Outside the classroom, the children may be involved in either individual, concomitant, or tripartite treatment (terms to be explained momentarily) or treatment via the mother. Let us begin to describe these various modalities in the following order: treatment of a child via the mother, tripartite, concomitant treatment of mother and child, group therapy of parents, and management of siblings.

TREATMENT OF AUTISTIC TWINS VIA THE MOTHER

The treatment of the child via the parent owes its origin to Sigmund Freud who treated little Hans via his father. Anny Katan, influenced by Freud, began to treat children via the parents, at first in Europe and later in Cleveland, in the therapeutic nursery school (Furman & Katan, 1969). Katan stresses that the treatment is most useful for children with mild developmental deviations and reactive disorders. However, in our experience, treatment via the mother is a useful auxiliary modality for severely disturbed children in a therapeutic nursery. Let us describe such a case.

Mrs. S., a very concerned mother of autistic twins, talked about treatment of her children with her therapist. Let us listen to her own recollections of the treatment:

> As you recall, when we first came to the nursery, both Sam and John were "out of it." They were 3 years old. They could walk like any other 3-year-old, but they were like young babies: still on the bottle, not toilet trained, no intelligible sounds came out of them, except for screeches. They were not minding people. John could not stay in your arms. Sam could, but it was like he did not feel it.
>
> When you told me that you and I together were going to help my kids, I thought that it was crazy.
>
> I was no expert. You were supposed to be the expert. You explained that I was the one who observed them from day one, and had learned ways of giving them food, dressing them, making attempts at toilet training them, etc.; all this was true. . . . But I felt better when you said that together we would be looking at what I saw, trying to figure out where the kids were at, and with the help of the teacher's observations, we would figure out ways to help the kids to grow.
>
> You got excited when I told you certain things about them: when Sam, who was forever running away from us, seemed to stay around when his father pretended to box with him or tickled him. When you explained that this could be a way for me to enter into Sam's world I thought it was crazy. After we talked about how self-conscious I felt doing these things, and how scared I was of hurting them with the pretend boxing, I could finally do it. Only one year later, I was able to talk about my wishing at times that Sam and John would not "be," and understood then my fear of hurting them. [Here we see Mrs. S. struggling with her hostile impulses towards the children.] And I could also spend time trying to gently direct John's and Sam's head with my hands so they would look at me when I tried to talk to them. That was hard. Sam would screech and run away. John would also try to get away. But we made it! Now they can look at me when I talk.

If there were no problem of space, we could allow Mrs. S. to describe the whole treatment in her way. She worked very hard indeed with her children. Following the therapist's instructions, fully understanding the reasons for doing what she did, she worked at home on making eye contact and affective contact in any way she could, by way of tickling, holding, listing body parts while bathing the children, and in front of the mirror, gently but firmly training them to stay in their room at night, teaching them to touch to say hello rather than to hit or scratch or bite. While the teachers followed a similar approach in the classroom, Mrs. S., as patiently and consistently as possible, would firmly stop Sam and John from biting themselves, trying to use words to describe what they might be experiencing at those times.

In her weekly sessions, while she discussed her understanding of both her observations and her coping tactics, she also spoke about her feelings about having children like Sam and John, the impact this had on her marriage and on her 8-year-old daughter.

After 2 years of work, Mrs. S. had the satisfaction of hearing Sam speak in sentences with expressions of some affect. She could indeed get excited when Sam began having nightmares and called her to his bed, rather than running to her bed in obvious panic, unable to say anything. And again she could report with delight how John would test if he could come out of his room by throwing his shoes from his room into the corridor; if there were no reaction from his mother, he would come out.

At this time Sam and John are toilet trained and eat solid foods on their own. They seem aware of their own bodies, of each other, and of other people. Sam's language is coming along; John can as yet say only single words. John can be very affectionate with his mother, though. This developed particularly after his mother understood that he had reached the stage when he wanted to be involved in almost everything she did; for example, if she wanted to change a T.V. channel, she got John by the hand and guided his hand to change the channel—if she did not do this, he would scream inconsolably. In addition, John has begun to be aware of what is acceptable or unacceptable: if he does something wrong, like having an "accident" in his pants, he goes to his mother asking to have his hand stroked.

Sam began to show signs of superego development also, as we see from the following episode. One night he wet his bed. He called his mother saying, "Bed is cold." Mrs. S. understood that he had wet his bed. He insisted on changing himself without help. That morning again he would not allow his mother to hug him or help him dress as usual. Moreover, when his father greeted him, Sam said, "No good morning." And Mrs. S. was able to say, "We know you do not want to pee in bed. I think you were unhappy last night when I gave special time to John. Maybe you peed because you were angry with me. You can say 'Mummy, I am angry. Read to me' (Sam enjoys books; he has started to read and write and frequently asks his parents and teachers to spell words for him)."

The above material illustrates how a sensitive, concerned mother, open to insight into her own feelings and those of her progeny, can provide treatment for her children in the home beyond the nursery situation.

Treatment via the mother was useful because (1) it helped Mrs. S. to decode the puzzling, chaotic behavior of her autistic twins; and (2) it introduced her to new ways of reaching them (e.g., sparring with them, fostering eye contact, etc.). This treatment modality became a powerful reinforcer of the classroom therapy. The mother is the first educator of the child; treatment via the mother does not ignore the important psychoeducational role that a parent can play in the therapeutic nursery education of the handicapped child.

Treatment of a Schizophrenic Child Via the Mother with the Help of Classroom Observation

Mother and therapist meet weekly in the observation booth, looking into the therapeutic classroom through a one-way mirror. They observe, trying to understand what the child is experiencing, why he reacts the way he does, and why the teachers handle him the way they do.

Mrs. I. was the mother of a schizophrenic child with a major language disorder, isolated, showing no affect. It was decided that Mrs. I. needed this approach because of her initial despair and excessive anxiety when discussing child handling.

A flood of questions opened as Mrs. I. entered the observation booth, not just about the child, but also about the other five children in the classroom. Why was Louis trying to flush toilets all the time (the bathroom is visible from the booth)? Why was Howard obsessed with twirling things as if they all were fans? Why was Derek so involved in dressing up with grown-up clothes? Why was Arie curled up at the window? Why was her son placing his hands on his ears each time someone approached him, or else standing or sitting in one place, apathetic, sucking his sleeve?

Mrs. I. had trouble expressing her feelings. She was obviously tense: she held onto herself with her arms, talking with clenched teeth.

The therapist at first merely focused on Mrs. I.'s observations. Putting together what she had been hearing in the mothers' group therapy sessions and what she was observing, Mrs. I. was able to begin to understand what the children expressed or were unable to express.

Watching the teacher's attempts to penetrate her son's world by way of gentle talk and water play (Bill seemed to watch running faucets with fascination), Mrs. I. began talking about her own attempts at imitating the teachers at home. Soon afterwards, four months into the therapy, Mrs. I. began to use her observations in more creative fashion. She would ask questions about the possibility of using different handling than the teachers used. This received much support from the therapist. Mrs. I. began expressing appropriate praise and criticism of the teachers' actions. If experts like the teachers could make mistakes, maybe she could be more confident about trying out things without feeling helpless, immobilized, about the possibility of making an error.

As she watched Bill getting involved with water play, being helped later to introduce dolls in the water play, and later still to bring these dolls into the dollhouse and begin symbolic play, Mrs. I. became justifiably excited about what this progression meant. Her child was growing; he still had no expressive language, but he was giving evidence of internal language.

The flatness of Bill's affect still bothered Mrs. I. She began to discuss and then initiated games that involved drawing faces, making them happy, sad, angry, and labeling the affects. She showed those same feelings by making faces herself and then by constantly labeling his and her feelings throughout the interactions she had with Bill. For example, if he got hurt, she would say "Ouch! that hurts! Bill is in pain!" and mimic the appropriate facial expressions; or when Bill would eat the only food he liked, she would remark, "It is so good! Bill is happy to eat candy," again with the appropriate facial expressions.

Bill began to smile. His play with dolls became more focused, he selected a mommy, a daddy, a baby boy, and a girl to play with, disposing them in the various rooms of the dollhouse, making them interact with gestures only. Mrs. I. and the therapist continued to try to understand what Bill was expressing and then Mrs. I. would use her understanding at home as well.

Mrs. I.'s self-esteem was obviously growing as a result of her ability to use her work during the weekly observation sessions and the group and individual sessions.

Four years later, Billy is talking, is still in individual and language therapy, and is attending a regular school.

Mrs. I. is continuing individual psychotherapy and is still talking about the help she felt she received through what she calls "observation sessions."

We can see that this modality served an important adjunctive role, side by side with other therapeutic interventions. In particular, it helped the mother to gain some confidence, to be less perplexed. Her observations of the classroom helped her to see that the teachers were not infallible—her child could perplex and baffle the experts. This realization was reparative of her damaged self-esteem. She began to really observe her child and was able to initiate his affective responses: her laughter triggered his. She taught him how to imitate affect. Later, as language developed, she taught him how to express it.

TRIPARTITE TREATMENT OF AN AUTISTIC CHILD

This treatment for psychotic children involves a therapy with a tripartite design to include mother, child, and therapist, as described by Margaret Mahler (1952). We will first describe the clinical material and later discuss the philosophy of treatment.

Presenting Symptoms and Diagnosis. Louis entered the nursery at age 3; a handsome looking boy with enormous black eyes, he seemed removed from the affective world of relationships. When one tried to approach him, he would move away or remain stiff and unresponsive, unable to make eye contact. He had no language; he would only screech, sometimes without apparent reason, at other times when one interfered with his wish to sit at the window or to eat inedible materials. He walked on tiptoes or jumped up and down.

He mouthed and often swallowed anything within his reach, favoring frankfurters and newspaper. Eating paper kept him under constant medical surveillance for lead poisoning.

He always held in his hand a parking lot ticket with numbers; he had been given these tickets when his father had a car; and later, whenever he went near the parking lot next to his house, he screeched until he got one of those tickets.

He was still on a bottle and was not completely toilet trained.

The salient points in his life history were the following: prenatal history included Mrs. M.'s constant kidney trouble; his birth was uneventful;

at one week Louis developed diarrhea, which necessitated his remaining in the hospital for three weeks. Once at home he was brutalized by his father at night. Mr. M., a Vietnam veteran, returned from the war severely traumatized from multiple wounds and from watching his friends die; he woke up nights to attack his wife and son, believing that they were enemies who were trying to kill him. This continued well into Louis' second year of life. Moreover, Mr. M. became violent whenever he drank to excess. Mrs. M., the epitome of passivity, was unable to protect herself or her son. In her own childhood, she had developed this passive style watching her own father brutalize her mother when he was under the effect of alcohol.

Mrs. M. recalled that Louis had always been a very quiet baby, unresponsive to people, except for smiling occasionally at his mother and crying when his father woke him up to play with or to brutalize him. Louis had been able to sit at 4 months, to crawl soon after, and to walk at 11 months. He had rejected pacifiers as substitutes for eating inedible materials and had developed food fads (frankfurters and spaghetti). He had never uttered sounds except for shrill crying and screeching. He had had ear surgery for otitis 3 months before entering the nursery and had remained in the hospital for one night without his mother.

Two months before admission into the nursery, a new baby boy, Tony, was born to the M. family.

The initial diagnosis of Louis' condition was autism, secondary to a symbiotic-type psychosis. It is probable that genetic predisposition existed and the insult was reinforced by the family pathology. It was postulated, therefore, that since Louis' defective ego was not protected against Mr. M.'s assaults by Mrs. M, the symbiotic object, Louis had to withdraw into an autistic shell. In Mahler's terms, he had lost the symbiotic object "which amounts, at the symbiotic stage, to a loss of an integral part of the ego itself, and thus constitutes a threat of self annihilation" (1968, p. 220).

Treatment Plan. In view of the above, treatment for Louis was planned as follows: weekly tripartite sessions with the mother, child, and therapist; classroom therapy to involve close work between child, teacher, and therapist; weekly group and couple sessions for Mr. and Mrs. M.

The plan was effected except for Mr. M.'s peripheral participation (he came to the couple and group sessions only occasionally, and to the tripartite sessions three times during the third year of treatment, once alone with his son).

We will now focus on the tripartite treatment. For our purposes, tripartite treatment is a type of therapy designed for autistic children who have withdrawn from symbiosis. In order to involve the mother in the treatment and to reestablish the symbiotic bond between mother and child, the therapist, mother, and child meet together. Margaret Mahler describes it as a "corrective symbiotic experience" (1968, p. 167). She has outlined the treatment goals as follows: "(1) restoration or establishment of greater body image integrity, which should convey a better sense of entity and identity; (2) simultaneous development of object relationships; and (3) restoration of missing or distorted maturational and developmental ego functions" (1968, p. 170).

Mahler singles out two treatment phases. During the first phase, the therapist focuses on providing for both mother and child a "mothering principle" by creating a soothing, unthreatening atmosphere as protection against the environment, as well as against inner discomfort and distress (Winnicott's "holding environment").

During the second phase, that of treatment proper, "the therapist both leads the child and follows his development from the mother of part-object relationship to an investment of the more differentiated whole human object" (Mahler, 1968, pp. 203–4).

Since the psychotic child in flight from symbiosis deanimates the world (e.g., by attaching to a psychotic fetish) and his psychic efforts are geared to maintain sameness (Kanner, 1943), the therapist's task is to reanimate the child's world so that he can attach to his mother and continue thereafter hopefully along the multiple paths of emotional development.

Let us look at what happened with Louis, at how his deanimated world became reanimated.

Initial Steps in the Treatment Process. After the total treatment plan was discussed with both Mr. and Mrs. M., Mrs. M. and the therapist (the psychiatric social worker) met alone four times to discuss how they would both be working as a team, to try to help Louis out of his shell. Mrs. M.'s knowledge of Louis' reactions, of his history, of his daily life were given a great deal of importance as tools to enter into Louis' world.

In view of Mrs. M.'s expressions of inadequacy and her fears of being "active" during the sessions, she was encouraged initially to imitate the therapist and then, as she gained more confidence, to take initiative whenever she would feel comfortable doing so. The importance of reinforcing at home whatever Mrs. M. and the therapist would be able to accomplish with Louis was also emphasized. It was also explained that the work would be carried on similarly in the therapeutic class. In other words, this was to be a treatment model, which was to operate in three tripartite situations: mother, child, therapist; mother, child, father; child, therapist, teacher.

The tripartite sessions began at the window where Louis spent the initial sessions in a static position, seemingly looking out, fetish in hand. Mother and therapist stood by the window, next to Louis. Initially mother and therapist expressed the awareness that Louis seemed to feel good, ticket with numbers in hand: "Louis feels good holding onto this ticket with numbers." In a calm, soothing tone of voice, the therapist would start and Mrs. M. would follow, mentioning anything one could see from that window that had numbers (e.g., I can see 247 on that door, 2 and 5 on that car, 120 on that street sign).

After six sessions, Louis' eyes seemed to begin following what his mother and the therapist were observing. "Good Louis! You can see 247 on that door, too,!", the therapist would exclaim and Mrs. M. would echo.

Four months later, Louis allowed his mother and the therapist to enter further and enrich his world. He left the window, began sitting at a table looking at a book that had numbers, objects, and people. He began saying numbers in a very shrill voice, with what seemed like anxious excitement. Both mother and therapist began saying, "Louis is number one! Mommy loves Louis!" Mrs. M. mentioned at this point that Mr. M. had started to say at home, "Louis is my number one gorilla."

We can see how during the first four months of treatment we had taken the numbers that the child had used defensively to maintain his deanimated, autistic world and reanimated them. The numbers had taken on a more personal meaning; Louis had become the number one child of his mother and the number one "gorilla" of his father (his father always referred to Louis as "his gorilla").

Discovery of Body Parts. Mrs. M. was encouraged to say all that she liked about Louis. Since he was a handsome boy, his physical attributes were easily picked up by his mother. The therapist encouraged doing this in front of a mirror, as a way of helping Louis to discover his body. "This is Louis' nose. Louis has a nice nose. Mummy loves Louis' nose." Louis began doing the gestures back to his mother and therapist, later using simple words such as "nose" and "eyes". Mrs. M. was encouraged to accompany the game with a song to help Louis get to know his body better. While bathing Louis she would sing, "This is the way we wash Louis' hands, lips, chest, etc."

It was after much playing of this game that Louis at the end of the first year of treatment discovered his penis: he was 4. Mrs. M.'s feelings of discomfort at her son's open handling of his penis and at his wish to go around without pants had to be dealt with in individual, group, and tripartite sessions. She finally came to terms with the notion that Louis' belated penis discovery, an 8-month milestone in normal development (Kleeman, 1965), was all right. The classroom teachers as well had to warmly accept this behavior.

Just as we were able to use the numbers in the early part of treatment to build bridges between child, mother, and therapist, during the second phase of treatment the child's discovery (or rediscovery?) of his own body could be used as an effective bond of symbiotic closeness between child and therapist and child and his mother.

When, during the course of treatment, the autistic child discovers his body parts, including the penis, it is crucial that this behavior be seen as a sign of developmental progression and not as excessive masturbatory play that should be discouraged. To discourage this play at such a crucial moment would discourage the child from his new-found psychic achievements and return him again to the autistic shell.

It is important to point out that while we were reanimating his world, giving more personal meaning to the numbers, helping the child to discover body parts, Louis' capacity for eye contact became established. As he would play out these "symbiotic games" with therapist and mother involving numbers and the parts of his body, he would look at his mother's eyes, at his therapist's eyes, for longer and longer time periods.

Mrs. M. was also encouraged to review during the sessions what Louis' life was like outside the nursery. Mrs. M. would describe the bathing sessions, Louis' special liking for frankfurters and spaghetti. She would also talk about the frequent visits to the doctor involving needles when the lead level in the blood went too high. Mrs. M. was asked to express all the affect she could muster, mainly pleasure, fear, pain so that her child might learn from her. Gradually Louis began to allow his mother to hug him.

Progress in Communication. By the third month into the second year of treatment, Louis began to leave his psychotic fetish in the therapist's handbag. When the therapist would show that it was there at the next session, Louis would take it and put it back in the handbag. "Louis feels good leaving the paper with numbers in Delia's bag and finding it when we meet again," both mother and therapist would say. One month later Louis seemed no longer interested in the fetish.

By the time Louis began dropping the fetish in the therapist's bag, wooden people and dolls and doll furniture had been introduced in his sessions. Louis favored the wooden people. The therapist encouraged the mother to play with the wooden mommy, daddy, and two little boys. Louis began to handle this family too, giving evidence of the beginning of symbolic play. As Mrs. M. reported that Louis and his brother had begun fighting at home, Louis would shriek "Tony," his brother's name. The therapist would say, "Louis at times does not like Tony. Louis wants to be number one all the time, to have Mummy all for himself," and Louis seemed to listen very intently. And then she would add, while handling the wooden dolls, "This boy also wants his Mommy all to himself and wants to push his brother away from his Mommy like this." Louis caught on. He would drop the brother doll on the floor, throw it across the room, and so on.

At this time Mrs. M. reported that Louis began watching Sesame Street with real interest. Within a few weeks, he was saying Susan, Bert, Big Bird, and so on. He brought into the session the wooden Sesame Street figures his mother had bought him. Mrs. M. received a great deal of support for her initiative. She was also encouraged to supply dialogue to the characters Louis would mention by name. Louis seemed to enjoy this a great deal: he would smile.

Since Louis now became interested in letters as well as numbers, having been inspired by Sesame Street, and his mother had mentioned Louis' fascination with books, the therapist introduced papers and pens, announcing that Mommy, Louis, and the therapist would write a book on Louis, for Louis, with Louis. Lo and behold, soon after this was initiated, Louis took one of the Sesame Street characters, Susan, put her on paper, and traced a drawing which he then finished by locating eyes, nose, mouth and hair! The therapist's excitement was transmitted to the mother and both women gave great praise to the new Michelangelo. This may seem grandiose, but if one considers the child's presenting symptoms not quite two years prior to this time, this was indeed a giant step. Then he could not communicate at all, would not talk, draw or write, could not even maintain eye contact with another person.

Louis' language and ability to communicate through drawing and writing were both growing. He became interested in learning about dates in the month and days in the week. He also gave up the bottle.

From drawing and centering communications around Sesame Street characters, on which Mrs.

M. elaborated, 4 months into the third year of treatment, Louis drew his Mommy, writing the word Mommy underneath. About 3 weeks later Louis could tell a story. He came into the session and rushed to the paper and pen, saying "needle." He drew his concept of a needle (it looked pretty thick!), said and wrote "hospital," said "go hospital," drew a bus stop on a street with a 5th Avenue sign, drew another sign, which his mother identified as Mt. Sinai Hospital. Then he drew rectangles with something in it—which his mother identified as the examination room and the lab with the doctor and nurse (Louis always saw the same doctor and nurse). When the therapist and mother responded to Louis' mentioning "needle" by saying, "Yes, it hurt, ouch!" he wrote down "ouchie." And when the therapist said how brave Louis was and wrote down "Louis is brave and good," Louis added to this sentence the words "times" and "Mommy," followed by the therapist's name. The therapist interpreted this to mean that Louis felt good when Mommy and the therapist understood him and that these were good times. His face glowing at this statement, Louis responded with much affection to his mother's hug.

Management of Aggression and Separation Anxiety. Not everything went so smoothly during the course of treatment. Louis would get involved in provocative behavior, like trying to throw objects around, trying to eat paper, switching lights on and off. The same was going on at home. Mrs. M. was crawling the walls because the other boy was apparently going through a similar phase. In front of Louis, the therapist explained to Mrs. M. that to get involved in power struggles would not be productive, so long as he did not hurt himself or others. He had been "thrown around" by his father; perhaps he was trying out being active and aggressive. He was discovering newly acquired "powers" testing out "no's." After a number of sessions Louis came to the table and wrote down "no" first and then when the therapist said, "Yes, Mommy and I understand," he wrote down "yes."

There came a time when this began to take on a different connotation. Four months into the third year of treatment, right after Christmas recess, it became increasingly difficult for Louis to leave the session: he would start flying around the room, throwing down chairs and screaming "no time to go." The therapist interpreted Louis' anger and disappointment at not being with both his mother and the therapist for two weeks, his fears of losing good times; time he felt as especially long in spite of the calendar he had made showing when the next meeting would be. Louis began to take something along from the session, e.g., a crayon. This was allowed after the interpretation was made that he wanted to take some object along that would remind him of the special time with Mommy and the therapist. Louis began saying and writing down 2 or 3 times during each session "time to go" and when told no, he would write "no" in front of "time to go." At the end of the session, he would still experience trouble leaving, but less than before. Finally, about 3 weeks later and after much interpreting of how important it was to be with Mommy and therapist, Louis began writing at the end of the session "the end" and was able to leave with less difficulty.

Louis showed some separation anxiety at the classroom door around the same time. He was allowed to work it through not just during the tripartite sessions but also by keeping Mrs. M. at the classroom door until Louis was ready again to let his Mommy go, about 5 weeks after the Christmas recess. The week before Louis let his Mommy go from the classroom, Mrs. M. had been encouraged to get for Louis the soft Sesame Street dolls. This had been a great success. Bert became Louis' great companion also at nighttime, marking the step of attachment to a transitional object. From a psychotic fetish to a transitional object!

Let us try to define what we mean by relinquishing a fetish and using a transitional object. This phase of the treatment was characterized by Louis' increasing attachment to the therapist and to his mother; he was no longer content to rely on numbers and body games. He had learned to make eye contact. He had learned how to talk to his mother and the therapist even if only in two- or three-word sentences; he had learned to communicate through play, first with wooden people, then through drawing and writing and then combining this with play with soft people. He was finally enjoying being with his mother and the therapist in the symbiotic environment they had created for him. Consequently, separation became a problem for him. Earlier in the treatment his autism had protected him from any sense of attachment to or separation from any object other than his beloved tickets with numbers (fetishes), which he could control at all times anyway. But then he became attached to people, not numbers. So when people would leave him, he would be overwhelmed by anxiety. However, he struggled with his newly acquired human dilemmas by carrying a crayon or some other transitional object. His newly acquired ego functions (e.g., growing sense of time, more reliable memory, language) would allow him to maintain contact with the mental representation of the objects he was separated from.

Louis' treatment is still continuing and we hope to be able to make a later report on his additional steps toward higher levels of development.

We would like to stress at this point how Mrs. M. has "grown" alongside her son; although still a passive type, through identification with the therapist she has become a more "related" human being, able to take pleasure in her son's "attachments." This has freed her so that now she can give attention to herself. She has begun a diet and is taking steps eventually to go back to school to study nursing.

Mr. M. pari passu has been able to take pleasure in his son's growing "attachment" to him. During the tripartite session to which he came alone with his son, Mr. M. spoke about the pleasure he has in taking Louis to the park and to the store where he works, and about the special fun they have when they carry on their habitual contest involving who can say first the numbers on car license plates.

Concomitant Treatment of a Borderline Child and His Mother

Concomitant treatment means the simultaneous treatment of mother and child by different therapists. It is especially useful in a therapeutic nursery setting which allows such simultaneous treatment to occur. Simultaneous treatment allows the child and the mother to work through pathological attitudes and symptoms that are perpetuating mutual problems. For instance, in the case we are about to describe a hidden separation anxiety in the borderline mother was perpetuating separation individuation difficulties in her child. The influence of the mother's pathology on the child could best be understood and corrected in concomitant therapy. The clinical description to follow also outlines the use of family therapy as the initial treatment plan. Family therapy made it possible for the mother to recover her position in the family; only at that point could individual treatment be considered.

Clinical Material. Mrs. E. was the mother of a 3-year-old boy admitted to the nursery because of language and behavior immaturity (he was still on the bottle), excessive temper tantrums, and a pseudo-affective quality to his facial expressions, combined with an undifferentiated seeking out of people, typical of the deprived child. According to GAP nomenclature, he was diagnosed as developmental deviation with a severe language and behavior disorder and borderline features.

Both parents seemed concerned, bright individuals who had raised two daughters, ages 15 and 17, who took what seemed to be excessive responsibility in the care of their little brother. The initial treatment plan included family therapy and therapeutic classroom for Ali.

The family sessions were conducted only during the first 3 months as the need arose; they were geared to discovering family interaction and feelings among the family members, to reconstructing a more accurate history of Ali's three years of life, and to helping Mrs. E. reassume the mother-role she had given up when Ali was 18 months old. At that time Mrs. E. had experienced a "breakdown." Ali had been placed in a nursery where he lived for two weeks without any contact with family members in spite of his continuous desperate, inconsolable crying. Upon Ali's return home, Mr. E. and his daughters became the main caretakers for an Ali who had become at once clinging and aimlessly explosive; this change became in turn a source of anger and guilt for the rest of the family. Mrs. E. saw no choice but to keep away from her son, maintaining her stance of sickness, experiencing, however, tremendous guilt feelings. Another reason for Mrs. E.'s attitude was her hope that her marriage, for years in danger of dissolution because of the unrealistic expectations of both partners, would survive so long as Mr. E. had to take such an active role in the care of Ali. Ali's sisters felt "trapped" as well; the oldest, about to leave the family to go to college, experienced anger at her mother for being "sick" and a mixture of guilt and relief about leaving the situation; the younger one felt depressed because of her inability to express her fury at her mother "dumping on her," at her sister for leaving, her brother for existing, and her father for allowing all this to happen. As all of the above came to surface, changes began to take place; with everyone's support, Mrs. E. expressed and acted on her wish to reestablish herself as a mother.

The treatment plan changed; Mrs. E. was offered individual and group therapy and so was Mr. E.; Mr. and Mrs. E. were to receive couple therapy as the need arose in order to discuss marital discord; the younger daughter was also referred for individual and group treatment at the Child Psychiatry Clinic, and individual sessions were begun with Ali; the oldest daughter decided not to enter individual treatment in view of the proximity of her departure. It had become clear that both Mr. and Mrs. E. had problems related to the parenting each one of them had experienced and these could be better treated in individual sessions. This seemed true as well for the daughters.

Mrs. E. also responded favorably to the notion that it was necessary for her to remain in the classroom with Ali to reestablish the affective bond between her and her son so that he could separate on his own terms. The importance of the door and the need to allow handicapped children to separate on their own terms at their own pace has been alluded to earlier. There is no better way for a child to develop basic trust in his mother and in the school all at once.

The Concomitant Individual Treatment Procedures. We will now focus on the concomitant individual treatment of mother and child. During the first few months, in weekly sessions with Mrs. E., the following unfolded: Mrs. E. was born in the West Indies; her family was poor. She had one older brother and one older sister, and several older half-brothers from her father's former marriage. When she was 2, her mother died of trichinosis at 33 years of age. Between 2 and 5, Mrs. E. remained in the West Indies. Mrs. E. remembered nothing of these years—she had been told about these times but she still experienced the story as belonging to someone else. At five, Mrs. E. was taken to New York to live with one of the older half-brothers and his wife. They had no children. In her mind they have been her parents. When she was 11, her stepfather died. This was a terrible blow. Her relationship to her stepmother became problematic; Mrs. E. felt abandoned when her stepmother went to work or socialized with men. That was the time when Mrs. E. met her present husband; she found solace in his teenage "caring," and decided to go and live with him against her stepmother's wish at age 17. Mr. and Mrs. E. decided to marry one year later. They both finished high school. Mrs. E. had been interested in music, and singing in particular, but she went to work to supplement her husband's income and prepare for having a family. Her daughters were born. She described her involvement with their development as very pleasurable; they were affectionate, bright, and became good students who loved music as well. Mr. E. continued on a successful path despite his lack of a college degree; he became the head of a rehabilitation program. Difficulties in the marital relationship existed through the years in varying degrees (e.g., 8 years ago Mrs. E. slammed the door on Mr. E.'s finger on purpose during a fight). They became intensified when Mr. E. lost his mother. It was then that Mr. and Mrs. E. decided to have another child to "patch up" their union. Ali was born. Both parents were very proud of having produced a boy. They gave him a special name, symbolic of their expectations that he be a "savior" and would grow up "perfect" to satisfy the pride of his parents. Mrs. E. was 33 years old.

During the 18 months following Ali's birth, Mrs. E. became increasingly depressed. Ali was difficult in that he cried a great deal, particularly at night time. Mr. E. became more and more involved with his work. Mrs. E. developed vaginitis; the gynecologist supposedly suggested that sexual intercourse be interrupted. Mrs. E. withdrew to her bedroom, and Ali was sent for a while to the sleep-away nursery.

As Mrs. E. went into the second month of individual treatment, she began to be late for her appointments, which was interpreted as a fear of attachment in the light of her past disappointments whenever she became attached: her natural mother and later her brother-father had died. Mrs. E. responded to these interpretations by being on time again for her appointments and by slowly recalling memories from the first five years of her life.

Mrs. E. missed her first appointment after the therapist returned from her summer vacation. She was able to tell her therapist during later sessions how she had felt abandoned, deserted, and furious. She thought her rage would destroy the therapist so that the therapist would never be back. As Mrs. E.'s feelings surfaced, her memories were surfacing as well. She could at last begin to remember her mother, the aunt who had taken care of her after her mother's death against her husband's wishes and hers, her father, the house where she used to live, details of various painful events of those years.

Ali's treatment proceeded along similar lines. Six months of extreme passivity were followed by peek-a-boo games with the therapist, which then evolved into repetitive hide-and-seek play. These were interpreted along the lines of practicing feelings associated with people going away and coming back. The therapist also related these feelings to Ali's missing his mommy when he was away from home without her. Still unable to use language and play with dolls, Ali began to become more "assertive," to the point where he kicked his therapist's shins when he experienced "missing" feelings. Also at home Ali was showing his newly acquired "assertive" ways: one day, when his mother had failed to respond to his demands that she stay in his room, Ali did not get into a tantrum but took a knife and waved it in front of Mrs. E. in a threatening way.

By the end of the first year of treatment, Ali had been able to let his mommy go away from the classroom (this took about 5 months), had begun to use one-, then two-word sentences which were not echolalic, and seemed to have relinquished his pseudo-affective ways of expressing his feelings; even though his expression of feeling was quite primitive (e.g., kicking his therapist's shins in anger when interpretations of "missing" feelings were offered), it showed Ali's growing confidence that his expression of anger would not destroy the people he was attached to and it allowed him to start trusting again.

Mrs. E. also began to understand how her fears of dying, as her mother had at 33, had contributed to her depression (a depression that made her son experience the abandonment of his mother just as she herself had experienced it). She was identifying with her son in an effort to master her experience by way of repetition compulsion. Then too, she began to analyze how she had ways of pushing people away (e.g., her husband), again in an attempt to use active ways to master her continuous fears of being abandoned, rejected (e.g., she would push her husband away so as to prevent feeling the helplessness of being abandoned that she had experienced when her mother had died). Tremendous guilt feelings toward Ali were expressed, while vague guilt feelings toward her dead mother surfaced.

After 15 months of treatment, the attachment between mother and son seemed solid enough to allow for occasional weekend separations (Mrs. E. went, for example, to visit her elder daughter in college). Ali could also give up his bottle spontaneously and began asserting himself with words and refraining from aggressive behavior to some degree. Also the marital relationship between Mr. and Mrs. E. seemed freer from conflict than ever before.

This case illustrates how a variety of treatments helped this family. The family and couple therapy helped to marshall the family's resources so that later concomitant treatments were possible. The concomitant treatment was especially useful because it allowed the full dissection of the separation problem of the child and the perpetuating borderline symptomatology in the mother. When the mother realized her massive identification with her son whom she had abandoned at 18 months in the same manner as she had been abandoned 34 years earlier, the predestination of a repetition compulsion rooted in the past could finally be undone.

GROUP THERAPY FOR PARENTS OF EMOTIONALLY DISTURBED CHILDREN

Group therapy for the parents of children in a therapeutic nursery is perhaps one of the single most valuable therapeutic modalities we can offer these families. Each parent of a handicapped child enters the group with a similar set of worries. Each one feels low self-esteem for having given birth to a defective child. Each one feels guilty for the unconscious murderous feelings he experiences toward his offspring. Each one feels perplexed and inadequate as he struggles to relate to his bewildering child. Each one feels that he must repress these unspeakable affects. In a group these issues can be dealt with openly and honestly: each parent slowly begins to realize that his plight is shared by others, that his feelings are not unique. As the processes of group identification and group cohesiveness develop, the parents, mostly mothers, grow "together"; they become tolerant of their own guilt and rage and the ubiquitous depression begins to lift, leaving the parent free to manage his child more appropriately and to pursue neglected interests beyond the child (spouse, career, social activities, etc.).

"I never would want my child to die. How can you say that you wish your child did not exist?" Mrs. B. said with horror in response to Mrs. S.'s open expression of anger at the fates for having a "damaged" child who should have never been born that way. Mrs. J., who had already been in the program for three years, explained to Mrs. B. that she had also been frightened at first by the thought that one could wish for her own damaged child not to exist and it had taken some time for her to understand how "natural" a feeling it was. Mrs. D. chimed in, "Yes, it took me some time too to be O.K. with feelings like this. I used to even think that I was so powerful as to make things happen just by wishing: like I thought I had something to do with my mother dying when I was nine, because I wished her dead when she punished me for something." "That's right," said Mrs. E. "I almost felt like a murderer when I found out that my dreaming about my child being dead was really that I wanted him that way." "Remember," added Mrs. M., "how upset you also were when we said how you were damn angry at your son for being born. You did not buy it that a mother could hate and be angry at an innocent baby." "I remember . . . I also felt so badly . . . like I was punished for the bad things I had done." "I think that sometimes," said Mrs. B. "Honey, what went on in your belly had nothing to do with your sins," Mrs. R. joined in, as usual injecting some humor into the session. "You can say that. But you can't stop her feeling like that. Let her talk," said Mrs. M.

It is clear that this is a group of mothers discussing their feelings about having given birth to and having to raise emotionally handicapped children.

From this tiny sample one can appreciate some of the issues this group of mothers is struggling with. Anger toward their child and feelings of guilt are openly discussed by the "seasoned" group members, while those same feelings are still a source of conflict for the relatively "new" mother. At the same time, one can see how the "new" mother is introduced to the notion that her superego is too harsh, and is at the same time encouraged to express whatever is on her mind.

All of these mothers used to be like the "new" one in this vignette. During the time they were part of the program, they learned to trust their therapist and each other. They shared their depression, their feelings of inadequacy, helplessness, when confronted with the day-to-day difficulties of raising their children (e.g., one child hit people indiscriminately, provoking the rage of strangers; another evoked strangers' comments by his bizarre mannerisms; another would smear feces on the parental bed, etc.). Material from individual sessions was also brought up by the mothers during the group time and vice versa.

Discussion of the feelings mentioned above is but one aspect of the mourning process these mothers experience in treatment. As Solnit (Solnit & Stark, 1961) pointed out, parents of damaged children have to mourn the normal child they would have wanted instead of the "damaged" one.

By withdrawing the libido invested in the psychic representation of the "normal" child they would have wished for, these mothers can then proceed to reinvest that libido in the relationship to the damaged child. This is particularly crucial, since most of these children have problems that involve the mother-child bond.

Group therapy seems to facilitate this mourning process. Superego resistances to the emergence of murderous feelings toward the handicapped child are more easily dealt with in a group for the following reasons: (1) delegation of superego power to the group leader (Freud, 1921) lessens the superego resistances; (2) mutual ego support of each group member for the other helps (each member can so easily identify with the dilemma of the other).

As the group works through their grief, self-esteem grows. Discussions around child handling become more effective. As they struggle to accept their feelings about the children's handicaps, they develop an understanding of their own childhood and its effect on their present feelings.

For example, when Louis discovered his penis, as mentioned in the tripartite treatment section, the mothers discussed the meaning of this discovery, its management, sexuality in children, and at the same time associated to feelings around sexuality relating them to their own childhood experiences and fantasies.

As Mrs. R. said, "The group is like a good family; we kvetch (this is a black woman who has learned Jewish terminology from the Jewish mother in the group), we cry for us and our children; we try to understand our insides together; we get excited when we find out things about our insides, when we see we are feeling good and our kids are growing even tiny bits; and we like each other and don't stop even when we get mad."

Siblings

One has an important therapeutic responsibility to the siblings of the handicapped child. The siblings in the family are often neglected, while the "sick" child soaks up all the attention. Preventive interventions by the nursery staff are necessary to protect the siblings from neglect and depression which may manifest itself in a variety of pathological ways. One sibling's reaction was aggressive power struggles with the mother and academic failure in school; she was evaluated by the nursery staff and referred for her own individual psychotherapy. Another 10-year-old sibling, the older sister of autistic twins, was being neglected by the parents who had the awesome responsibility of managing two autistic children 24 hours a day. This sibling was evaluated; no overt psychopathology was discovered. However, she was assigned to a Big Sister, and an important relationship developed between the two, which made up for some of the unavoidable neglect. These are just two examples to illustrate the vulnerability of siblings and the important preventive role that an alert therapeutic nursery staff can play.

SUMMARY AND CONCLUSION

Therapeutic nursery education is designed to meet the emotional and educational needs of disturbed preschoolers. Children with a wide variety of psychiatric disturbances can be managed in therapeutic nursery settings (childhood schizophrenia, infantile autism, brain damage, language disorder, hyperkinetic syndromes, developmental deviations, etc.). A nursery school placement has the advantage of allowing the child to be exposed to a team of experts without breaking up family cohesion. In fact, the child and his family can be treated together. The child returns to his home every day, avoiding the complications of prolonged institutionalization. A variety of treatment approaches have been developed in the past 30 years by pioneers such as Goldfarb, Bender, Alpert, Mahler, Furman and Katan. Clinical examples of these psychotherapeutic approaches with children and their parents were described. Psychoeducational approaches in the classroom were outlined. The role of the special education teacher was described. The contributions of language therapy, music and art therapy, and behavior therapy were noted. Other approaches involving the parents were cited. Treatment via the mother (Furman & Katan, 1969) and the tripartite therapeutic design of Margaret Mahler were both presented, using clinical material from the treatment of autistic children. Group therapy of the parents, concomitant treatment of a borderline child and his mother, and the management of siblings were offered for further thought. In broad terms, the treatment of the child is an attempt to unravel the tangled threads of development so that understanding and communication can replace hatred and confusion in the parent-child relationship. In broad terms, the treatment of the parents is an attempt to help them to mourn the normal child that nature did not grant them (Solnit & Stark, 1961) and to learn to accept the "changeling" and the complicated feelings of hatred and guilt and hope and love they experience toward these emotionally handicapped children. An advantage of therapeutic nursery education is that emotionally disturbed preschoolers can be diagnosed and treated as early as possible, when preventive and therapeutic opportunity is greatest. Whenever possible the child is mainstreamed back into the regular educational channels. The location of the therapeutic classrooms in a regular school setting keeps the doors of communication open between regular education and special education and discourages the ostracism of handicapped children that our institutions sometimes covertly perpetuate.

REFERENCES

ALPERT, A. Observations on the treatment of an emotionally disturbed child in a therapeutic center. *The Psychoanalytic Study of the Child*, 1954, *9*, 334–343.

ALPERT, A., and KROWN, S. Treatment of a child with severe ego restriction in a therapeutic nursery. *The Psychoanalytic Study of the Child*, 1953, *8*, 333–354.

ARIES, P. *Centuries of childhood.* New York: Knopf, 1962.

BENDER, L. Childhood schizophrenia. *Nervous Child*, 1942, *1*, 138–140.

BENDER, L. Childhood schizophrenia. *American Journal of Orthopsychiatry*, 1947, *17*, 40–56.

BUCHER, B., and LOVAAS, O. I. *Use of Aversive Stimulation in Behavior Modification.* In M. R. Jones (Ed.), *Miami Symposium on the Prediction of Behavior, 1964.* Coral Gables, Fla.: University of Miami Press, 1968.

EKSTEIN, R., and MOTTO, R. *From learning for love to love of learning.* New York: Brunner/Mazel, 1969.

FREUD, ANNA. "Infants without families." *The Writings of Anna Freud, Vol III, 1939–1945.* Written in collaboration with Dorothy Burlingham. New York: International University Press, 1973.

FREUD, S. Analysis of a phobia in a five-year-old boy. In *Standard Edition* (Vol. 10). London: Hogarth Press, 1955.

FREUD, S. Group psychology and the analysis of the ego. In *Standard Edition* (Vol. 10). London: Hogarth Press, 1955.

FURMAN, R. A., and KATAN, A. *The therapeutic nursery school.* New York: International Universities Press, 1969.

GOLDFARB, W. *Childhood schizophrenia.* Cambridge, Mass.: Harvard University Press, 1961.

HARRIS, F. R., WOLF., M. M., and BAER, D. M. Effects of adult social reinforcement on child behavior. In S. W. Bijou and D. M. Baer (Eds.), *Child development: Readings in experimental analysis.* New York: Appleton-Century-Crofts, 1967.

HEIMLICH, E. P. The specialized use of music as a mode of communication in the treatment of disturbed children. *Journal of the American Academy of Child Psychiatry*, 1965, *4*, 86–122.

JONES, M. C. A laboratory study of fear: The case of Peter. *Pedagogical Seminary*, 1924, *31*, 308–315. (a)

JONES, M. C. The elimination of children's fears. *Journal of Experimental Psychology*, 1924, *7*, 383–390. (b)

KANNER, L. Autistic disturbances of affective contact. *Nervous Child*, 1943, *2*, 217–350.

KANNER, L., and EISENBERG, L. Notes on the follow-up studies of autistic children. In P. H. Hoch and J. Zubin, *Psychopathology of childhood.* New York: Grune and Stratton, 1955.

KLEEMAN, J. A. A boy discovers his penis. *Psychoanalytic Study of the Child*, 1965, *20*, 239–266.

KRAMER, E. *Art as Therapy.* New York: Schocken Books, 1971.

LOVATT, M. Autistic children in a day nursery. *Children*, 1962, *9*, 103–108.

MAHLER, M. S. On child psychosis and schizophrenia: Autistic and symbiotic infantile psychoses. *The Psychoanalytic Study of the Child*, 1952, *7*, 286–305.

MAHLER, M. S. *On human symbiosis and the vicissitudes of individuation.* New York: International Universities Press, 1968.

PFEIFFER, E. A modified nursery program in a mental hospital. *American Journal of Orthopsychiatry*, 1959, *29*, 780–790.

PLASCHKES, L. *Supportive educational group therapy in a nursery school.* Paper presented at the annual meeting of American Academy of Child Psychiatry, St. Louis, Missouri, 1975.

PODOWSKY, E. *Music therapy.* New York: Philosophical Library, 1954.

POTTER, H. Schizophrenia in Children. *American Journal of Psychiatry*, 1933, *12*, 1253–1269.

PREMACK, D. Toward empirical behavior laws: 1. Positive reinforcement. *Psychological Review*, 1959, *66*(4), 219–233.

RUTTER, M. Concepts of autism: A review of research. *Journal of Child Psychology and Psychiatry*, 1969, *9*, 1–25.

DE SANCTIS, SANTE. "Sopra alcune varieta della demenza precoce" published in *Rivista Sperimentale di Freniatria*, 1906, *32*, 141–165.

SOLNIT J., and STARK, M. Mourning and the birth of a defective child. *Psychoanalytic Study of the Child*, 1961, *16*, 523–537.

WATSON, J. B., and RAYNER, R. Conditioned emotional reactions. *Journal of Experimental Psychology*, 1920, *3*, 1–14.

6

FAMILY THERAPY

Jesse Schomer

SOME HISTORICAL IMPRESSIONS

The modern-day resurgence of family psychiatry, beginning less than 30 years ago on both coasts of the United States through the work of such innovative clinicians and theoreticians as Nathan Ackerman, Theodore Lidz, Don Jackson, Jay Haley, Lyman Wynne, Israel Zwerling, William Goldfarb, and others, continues to generate special interest and concern for child psychiatrists. The interest can be ascribed to a combination of factors: a varying but persistent feeling of dissatisfaction with the efficacy of many of the more established (if no more scientifically based) therapeutic techniques presently available in the field; and the obvious enthusiasm, high promise, and freshness of views observable in practitioners of what has been characterized with mixed feelings as the family therapy movement. The concern seems to be related to fears that perennially beleaguered and grossly insufficient child psychiatry funds and staff would be siphoned off by this new arrival; or worse still, that a hard won, modest, but discernible body of useful knowledge might become less available to children if Procrustean emphases in diagnosis and treatment planning emerged among family therapy enthusiasts.

By the mid-1970s practitioners of child psychiatry in the United States could be arbitrarily grouped in two widely separated camps, with a third (largest) group sharing a good deal of the beliefs but also many of the respective criticisms of the first two about each other. The following description of the two more extreme groupings is to some degree a caricature, unfair to many individual exceptions, but may nevertheless be of overall descriptive value.

"Traditional" child psychiatrists tend to focus diagnostically on the intrapsychic pathology of the child, consider the child as the main, if not the only patient, and view diagnosis of and work with parents and family as adjunctive to their primary child-centered tasks. In a clinic setting, they see themselves as leaders of the tripartite (orthopsychiatric) team classically made up of a psychiatrist, who provides overall direction, diagnoses the child and either treats the child himself or supervises the treatment; a psychiatric social worker, who counsels the parents and does liaison work with schools, residences, camps, and other agencies; and a psychologist, who performs testing. Various counselors, technicians, educational specialists, neurologists, etc. are called in when needed by the team leader. If siblings or parents develop psychiatric symptoms they are more likely to be brought into parallel or sequential rather than conjoint diagnostic and treatment processes. Thus a multiproblem family could and on occasion has ended up with as many therapists as it had individuals with observable problems.

In contrast to the above, child psychiatrists (and other child mental health workers) who most conspicuously identify themselves as family therapists are less likely to have trained and worked (for long) in a traditional child guidance setting organized on orthopsychiatric principles, and have been known to refer to the team as the "holy trinity." They may have moved into family therapy after an earlier period of more child-centered work, but are as likely to have had an early interest, training, and concern with family diagnosis and therapy as it applied to adults and adolescents as well as to children. They are less likely to adhere exclusively or mainly to what they see as a too narrowly conceived medical model of child psychiatric illness. Rather they will feel equally or more at home with other frames of reference to complement or supplement what they view as too strict a reliance on biologic sciences. They may currently work in private practice, in association with a free standing family institute, or if part of a medical school team, with a family-oriented child psychiatry department or one of the fully constituted departments of Family Studies or Family Medicine that have sprung up in some universities and hospitals. Even the more extreme subgroup of family therapists most often do not flatly reject the body of knowledge accumulated by more traditional practitioners. However, in dealing with disturbed families and children, they tend to pay less attention to more subtle manifestations of biologic, neurologic, heredo-constitutional, and psychoanalytic (intrapsychic) frames of reference. Instead they are more comfortable with data derived from the interpersonal, sociologic, behavioristic "outside" observers' stance, seeing the child functioning as a member interacting with others in a structured homeostatic open family system. For example, they would be more likely to view distortions in verbal communications as a cause rather than an effect of schizophrenic pathology in a family. By popularization of concepts implied in such terms as the identified patient, scapegoating, family sculpting, quid pro quo, double binding, parental perplexity, interfamily networks, they have unquestionably extended the intrapsychic and dyadic range of focus of the traditionalists in the field. Members of the more traditional camp might properly add that they have too often lost sight of the special position and therapeutic needs of the individual child in the rush to work within this broader field. (In my own child psychiatry experience, I have made, and I hope have learned, from both types of errors of overemphasis. That is, I have worked on and with disturbed but relatively benign or irrelevant family systems only to see later that a more traditional individual child treatment would have better served a particular child. Conversely, I have wasted unnecessary time and effort with an individual child [play] therapy when more precise diagnosis and earlier therapeutic attention to ongoing family systems that were "feeding the flames" would have made much more clinical sense.)

There is as yet no unified or comprehensive theory of family diagnosis much less of family therapy. This is so despite the impressive and ambitious preliminary efforts of a host of well-known theoreticians and clinicians in the field. Nathan Ackerman came closest. His goal of formulating such a theory and integrating it with what he (controversially) viewed as the enduring and central concepts of psychoanalysis was not attainable in his lifetime. What family therapists have made do with, have been their own best empirical talents in over two decades of trial and error, buttressed and partly integrated with incomplete borrowings from a wide variety of theoreticians in family and allied fields. Most often, these comprised extrapolations and analogies derived from child and adult clinical psychiatry and psychology, psychoanalysis, anthropology, sociology, psychodrama, transactional analysis; systems, field, and communications and game theory, among others.

In this tumultuous and heady atmosphere, there has been in the burgeoning literature of family therapy, no shortage of trees obscuring forests, reductionistic insights heralded as major breakthroughs, wheels ponderously rediscovered, iceberg tips excitedly sighted and promptly named, "as-if" emotions mistaken for genuine, and simplistic or post hoc fallacies promulgated as causal.

In retrospect, it now seems that with regard to any massive effects in secondary and tertiary prevention of mental illness in children, family therapy may have been as naively oversold as were certain aspects of the child guidance movement and of applied psychoanalysis in the 'thirties and 'forties, or community psychiatry mental health concepts in the 'sixties. As with these earlier hopeful experiments, the passage of time and exposure to some harsh realities have been helpful in gaining perspective. We may now be approaching a time for more rigorous selection and refinement of those concepts and therapeutic techniques that have shown some solid promise. In this connection, certain of the family-centered approaches appear to me by the mid-seventies to have earned a worthwhile if more modest and selective place in a comprehensive child psychiatry practice. In the remainder of this chapter, I will attempt to survey these, indicate where I have found them useful in diagnostic or therapeutic work in child psychiatry, and share my experiences as to some contraindications for their use. My first task, however, will be operationally to define what I mean by a "family technique" and further to spell out some of the special and general attributes of this type of work as compared to psychiatric work with individual children.

A WORKING DEFINITION OF FAMILY DIAGNOSIS AND THERAPY

For the purposes of this chapter, I will define family operations in child psychiatry as diagnostic or therapeutic procedures which by design are conducted in the simultaneous presence of at least two members of the child's nuclear or extended biologic family (or its functional replacements). This includes the not uncommon situations where a child is not the only, nor even the most seriously ill member of a treated family, or where the child is seen largely for reasons of primary prevention. I will, however, exclude as beyond the scope of this chapter family therapies where a child is not ill at all and happens to be involved in a family treatment whose main goals are improvements in the family or the mental health of one or both parents. I will also (somewhat more arbitrarily) exclude other common and often valuable treatment modalities which may be designed for, or incidentally achieve, important changes in the child's family, but where the therapeutic work itself is not done *with* the family as defined above. Thus such therapeutic measures as parental counseling, placement of a child in a therapeutic milieu, individual or marital psychotherapies with the child's parents, play therapy using family dolls, or antidepressant pharmacotherapy (or vocational training) for a mother or father will not be covered.

SOME GENERAL CHARACTERISTICS OF FAMILY THERAPIES

Family work can and often does have special and different qualities and impact on the child psychiatrist, the child, and other family members than is the case when the child is seen individually. Perhaps one personal observation may catch some of the flavor of this: I cannot recall a family session where I have noted a nonphysiological attack of (my own) sleepiness. In contrast, this state has afflicted (and I hope informed) me under certain conditions in individual therapies with both adults and children. Family sessions do seem to generate a more vivid, active, charged and exposed atmosphere that, in my experience, has not been conducive to countertransference defenses associated with the therapist's wish to sleep. (I have, however, seen individual family members use sleepiness and falling asleep as a defense and a communication, although not as often as in one-to-one therapies.)

The presence of a whole family, or some of its members, in a room together with the therapist tends to generate an increased emphasis on reality-oriented here and now public interchanges; and there is an associated shift away from observable indicators of more primitive regressive transferences. Even more conspicuous by its absence is the full-blown individual regressive transference neurosis (or psychosis) seen in intensive individual psychotherapies or psychoanalyses. Instead, the simultaneous operation of multiple transferences and countertransferences introduces a much more shifting, complex, voluminous (and at times overwhelming) amount of data for the family therapist to perceive, sort out, understand and, when appropriate, share. Even if specific steps are taken to oppose it, there will be a shift away from nondefensive sharing of deeper fantasies, dreams, and primary process thinking, and this goes along with the change in quality of the transferences. While the child may still be regarded as the (identified) patient, there will usually be a diminution in his (and the family's) perception of him as being singled out, alone, and about to be further exposed, or as the (only) one needing help. Depending on the kind of structure provided by the therapist, it may now be the parents who are more threatened by exposure. But all family members usually will experience an increase in their fear of revelation and potential loss of previously implicit key pleasure and security systems. Even more so than is the case with individual therapies, there may be a prolonged defensive display of noisy symptoms and problems before enough trust is developed to let a therapist in on how and where the family really lives. As one perceptive adolescent ironically put it during a period of relative quiescence marked by silences alternating with parental searching for "topics," "I guess we've run out of nothing to say."

As for the family therapist, the absence of a comprehensive and fairly well laid out body of theoretical knowledge and technique opens up opportunities for experimentation, innovation, and creativity. It also introduces all of the dangers of wild analysis and countertransference behavior, rationalized as being "human," "flexible," "practical," or "active." In my own family work, and in family treatments I've been consulted on (or read about), I've been impressed with the increased hazards of well-known forms of countertransference difficulties: self-aggrandizing exhibitionism (often brought in under the guise of presenting a demonstration model of the therapist's ego functions to not-so-disorganized families), patronizing overcontrol (advice or direction when it's not called for), inappropriate gratification of patient's social, dependency, or parentifying wishes (to adopt the therapist), rationalized as providing a corrective emotional experience. In connection with the last, I have had occasion to look more favorably (and sadly) at the dictum that corrective emotional experiences are most lastingly corrective when they are spontaneous, repetitive, and occurred before age 4. (See the late Augusta Alpert's [1959] work with what she named a corrective object relations therapy for depressed children; good results appeared limited to a critical early intervention period, before entrance into the first grade.)

SOME COMMON INDICATIONS AND CONTRAINDICATIONS

Diagnosis

I routinely schedule an initial home visit followed by an office family session as integral parts of the diagnostic evaluation of children and adolescents unless there is a compelling clinical or logistical reason not to do so. I have found these to be powerful, rapid, and efficient providers of important and occasionally crucial information; and I have a feeling of incompleteness about any diagnostic work-up which has omitted one or both of them. There are surprisingly powerful resistances (by us professionals) to both of these commonsense procedures. This is shown by widespread and persistent tendencies for them to be left out of otherwise comprehensive, painstaking, and time-consuming child psychiatry evaluations. In my experience, this is true today in both clinic and private settings. I consider such omissions somewhat analogous to those of an internist who focuses on the laboratory reports of a cirrhotic liver's histopathology and pathophysiology without supplementing this with relevant information on his patient's other body systems, current and past drinking habits, and life style. My best guess as to some of the irrational resistances to home visiting is that they relate to our own conflicts over intense voyeuristic, erotized, or competitive impulses stirred up by the procedure, in addition to predictable issues such as role diffusion and uneasiness with the new, active, and unknown.

A common sequence that I've found useful in child and adolescent evaluations is to get a brief (5 or 10 minutes) initial history of a presenting situation from the referring source and the parents' first telephone contact, followed by a scheduled home visit of half an hour to an hour. I try to stop in either at the end of the family's dinner (and join them for coffee, dessert and/or a drink, if offered) or an hour before bedtime with younger children; and I arrange this on a day when parents, siblings, boarders, pets, and other important household members will be at home. I view the diagnostic home visit as a semistructured clinical session by a professional participant-observer, charge a regular private (or clinic) fee for it, and encourage myself (or consultees) to summarize the very rich material and include it as part of the written clinical record while it is still fresh in mind. (If I can think of one clinical situation where note taking on the spot would be ruinous, this is it.) When scheduled routinely and early, a home visit is usually very well received by child and family, and I've found can get some otherwise shaky intake procedures off to a good start. If a full study is indicated and feasible, the home visit can be followed by a briefer diagnostic family office session (5 minutes to half an hour) with the symptomatic child patient also seen alone at the end of this appointment. With most adolescents, or any children where distrust, rage, and fear are prominent aspects of the transference, it is often wise to omit or defer an initial history-taking parental session and use the open family sessions as a way to first contact the parents in the child's presence. With very guilty, frightened parents and a reasonably (or unreasonably) compliant child, it is sometimes better to go along with the parents' needs for a prominent identified child patient and see the child alone instead of scheduling a family session too early in a touch-and-go diagnostic alliance. Other parts of the work-up—such as psychological testing, phone consultations with pediatricians, school administrators, and classroom teachers, school or nursery observation visits, neurologic and other medical diagnostic procedures, and additional history taking or individual psychiatric interviews with child or parents—can be fitted in as needed and tolerated.

The diagnostic family interview which is scheduled in the office provides a second opportunity to observe the family in action, this time in a more structured and comfortably familiar setting (for the psychiatrist). This can be reduced if necessary to a 30-second vignette of child and parents as they separate in the waiting room or can be held for the better part of an hour. (Perhaps because of the intensity, richness, and vividness of family work, I've found that I rarely run a diagnostic or therapeutic family session much beyond 45 minutes.) I have been often struck by how much important and reliable information about a family's life style, stable action systems, and interlocking parental characterology can come across in as small a time as the 3 minutes they are seen together before starting an "official" interview with the child. Such waiting room interchanges as eroticized verbal and facial teasing between a 13-year-old girl and her middle-class father as the mother (literally) knits, or a puzzling and depersonalizing maternal instruction to "say hello to the doctor" given to a shy 8-year-old boy with whom I had just exchanged a smile and handshake, are two recent examples of this. More typically a longer family diagnostic interview will yield less compressed but equally valuable information on basic systems of dependency, security, power relationships, techniques of communication, and affectual styles in interpersonal terms of who does what with whom. In addition, because of the simultaneous presence of parents and symptomatic child (also siblings or grandparents, when indicated), history taking from verbal accounts of the current life situation and past events is much less subject to uncorrected distortions by any single family informant. The Rashomon effect, while not eliminated, can thus be gratifyingly reduced. This is particularly valuable in diagnosis with families where more subtle projective, hysteroid, or "as-if" styles of verbal communication exist, in addition to those where grossly misleading, evasive, or delusional material is offered.

Absolute contraindications to a diagnostic home visit or office family session are rare and in my experience limited to extreme schizoid or paranoid pathology, or very special transient disruptive situations in the home. Relative contraindications are less rare, but worth pausing for. I can recall a few such instances where I received clear signals from parents or adolescents that led me to defer planned home visits, or leave them out of the evaluation altogether. On one home visit, I first learned of some less clear but effective signals when I arrived at an apartment to find no one home. The parents had taken everyone out to a Chinese restaurant, having mistakenly expected me the following evening. This mistake was highly overdetermined, but I later had good evidence to associate it at least in part with acute feelings of shame and anticipation of exposure and humiliation from my entrance into their home. On occasions a visit is resisted because of a professed need to "protect" a grandparent or healthy sibling from being involved in (contaminated?) or pained by knowing about severe family troubles. More commonly a threatened family will intuitively unite to keep the diagnostic intruder focused away from the family at home and on the identified child patient in the office. Whether and how long to honor these defenses is a matter of clinical judgment. One useful principle I try to observe is to avoid ultimatums or premature confrontations. Poor timing or lack of tact here can put an end to the consultation and any later chances for learning about and helping a child.

Rapid Triage and Crisis Management

Family techniques can be tailor-made for these, for at least two reasons: the special ability of the diagnostic family interview to gather vast amounts of important here and now information rapidly and accurately; and the high leverage impact of family interviews as a vehicle for transmitting the therapist's influence powerfully, clearly, and rapidly to several family members simultaneously. Thus whenever the clinical situation seems emergent and genuinely cries out for fast evaluation and intervention, family sessions can be a most effective use of precious clinical time. Adolescent psychiatry provides many but by no means all of these crises. Most child psychiatrists working (or consulting) for a busy hospital emergency room, or on weekend or night call for a child psychiatry clinic, quickly learn the diagnostic and therapeutic values of active family interviewing and direction for crisis (or pseudocrisis) situations. Suicide attempts, runaways, acute school reluctance syndromes in pre-adolescence (by adolescence school reluctance is no longer so hopeful a crisis), fulminating psychoses, drug reactions, pregnancies, arson, theft, or other destructive and/or delinquent child and adolescent behaviors can all exert tremendous social and psychiatric pressures for rapid evaluation and decision making, preferably in that order. The knowledge that a trained professional has stepped in and is working with everyone involved in the family can have a powerful stabilizing effect in defusing an otherwise malignant turn of events and buy time for more considered restorative measures to be worked out. Undoubtedly at times this involves a considerable investment of magic belief in the family therapist by child, parents, police, school principals, pediatricians, and hospital administrators. Nevertheless, I have seen timely family work prevent an unnecessary hospitalization, school expulsion, brutal punishment, or distintegration of a fragmenting family enough times for me to accept such faith. It will be followed often enough by a more modest but valued hope about what we can do to ameliorate intrapsychic and interpersonal pathology once the crisis has been successfully survived.

Contraindications here can be fairly clear-cut, i.e., when elements of a crisis situation are already fairly well diagnosed (or become so after one or more initial family interviews) and appear more likely to respond to another treatment modality. A more subtle contraindication exists with certain types of middle-class families who seem to be crisis prone and to persist (but not change) with a course of seemingly interminable family therapy sessions. These require more careful psychiatric diagnosis of the marital relationship and character structure of each parent. Most often if treatable at all they will be best served by an individual psychoanalytically oriented psychotherapy for a parent and a separate treatment, if still indicated, for the child. These families should be carefully delineated from crisis prone multiproblem families suffering from gross or marginal parental incompetence secondary to severe chronic psychopathology. Often these families will have "drifted down" to social classes IV and V and have incurred complex nutritional, neurological, educational, and cultural disadvantages on the way. These compound their children's precarious adjustments. Regular meetings with a family therapist can be the most practical means of providing this type of family with direct guidance, counseling, appropriate role models and, probably more important, a beginning sense of hope and a feeling that someone important cares about them. The family therapist, if a child psychiatrist, can also have (or partly delegate) a key role as ombudsman, social agent, and central coordinator for planning and maintaining continuity among a myriad of adjunctive services needed by these children and their parents.

SYNDROMES WHERE A PARENTAL PRESENCE IS NEEDED FOR TECHNICAL REASONS

Adolescents with Negative Transferences or Reactive Rage. Many of these adolescents are untreatable or barely treatable on a one-to-one basis. They are consciously enraged over perceived parental or societal injustices, and/or they form immediate transference misperceptions of the therapist as an intolerably punitive, dangerous, or seductive parent figure. They defiantly or fearfully protest against scheduled appointments and effectively carry out their needs to avoid therapy by voting with their feet. This kind of stalemate is commonly encountered with a wide range of mild or major delinquency syndromes, neurotic personality disorders, and also (but less often) with the sicker schizoid and schizophrenic illnesses of adolescence. In this connection, when an adolescent is willing to see a therapist, this is more often a sign of either severe integrative pathology or of immaturity, with major fixations at an infantile or at least pre-adolescent level of personality organization. On rarer occasions, I've had the pleasurable surprise of evaluating a much less sick (and much more hopeful) adolescent who did request psychiatric help based on a sense of basic trust, exposure to favorable parental or peer models, and quite possibly a felicitous mix of chromosomes. In any case, if an adolescent, for whatever non-scapegoating reasons, is willing to come to treatment sessions by himself, I consider this a relative contraindication to family therapy. The reasons for this is the greater success that I've had, and believe is possible in general, with use of the individual psychotherapies than with family (or any group therapies) as far as the more ambitious goals of structural characterological change. However, with the larger group of negative transference adolescents, family sessions can be a valued way to get a treatment started. Bringing the parents into the office can both decrease the adolescent's conscious sense of injustice and dilute the frightening or enraging transference due to the shift toward reality that family (and all group) therapies tend to generate. Not that all hostile, cynical or negativistic school underachievers, drug abusers, conduct disorders, shoplifters, or promiscuous angry young men (or women) will come to family sessions; but a gratifyingly larger number can be inducted into treatment involving one or both parents and siblings than would otherwise be reachable by an out-patient psychiatrist. And once regular family sessions are initiated, all kinds of favorable possibilities are then opened up for continuation of the family work, if indicated; or for an even more ambitious shift to individual therapy if the adolescent will tolerate this after several weeks or months of preliminary family work. An additional advantage of a trial of family therapy for these adolescents is that it offers a hopeful, non-coercive alternative to a potentially embittering, always expensive, and possibly regressive forced institutionalization.

Severe Anxiety Reactions. An allied technical indication for family therapy occurs in situations where such relatively overwhelming anxiety exists, or is stirred up by treatment (often in association with immaturity or damaged reality testing), as to preclude establishment of a one-to-one working alliance; and where this anxiety can be specifically diminished by a mother's and/or father's presence. Thus, severe separation anxiety in very young and in emotionally immature older children can be allayed by having the mother sit quietly in the room or be visually present in an adjoining room during an induction period. This is commonly done in play therapy, for example, with a nursery age or latency child. With a terrified schizophrenic child of any age, a smoother induction into therapy can often be arrived at when the child is seen together with both parents than when seen alone, medicated, or hospitalized. Frequently, the child's reaction to the first few office family sessions will indicate whether or not this is going to be the modality of choice. Even when it turns out not to be helping, the trial period will have been brief and inexpensive and will have incurred relatively few risks compared with other alternatives.

Relevant Interlocking Parental Illness (When not Approachable by any More Effective Therapeutic Modality)

By relevant interlocking illness I refer not only to coexistence of child and parental illnesses but also to that aspect of parental illness that has an ongoing etiologic significance in sustaining or exacerbating a child's disturbance. Implicit in this is the concept of critical phases of susceptibility to noxious influences during the child's development, after which little or no further damage (or at least a different kind of damage) will occur, despite continuation of the same parental factor. Thus, ego-syntonic parental pathology that might justify an active family therapy (or other) intervention when seen at the time of a 3-year-old child's developing illness, might safely be left alone once the child's illness and character have more fully crystallized (if first seen) 10 years later. The therapeutic efforts can then best be concentrated on the child's treatment.

Estimating the extent and relevance (or irrelevance) of parental illness is a difficult, time-consuming, but worthwhile task for the child psychiatrist. It involves correlating data best obtained in one or more diagnostic psychiatric interviews with each parent alone with other data from child, family, and marital observations. A decision can then be put together as to what seems the best feasible treatment strategy.

Many parents who bring a child for help will have tightly defended ego-syntonic neurotic or psychotic character illnesses underlying some of their own symptoms. Therefore, it may be advisable to defer or shorten overly threatening individual interviews for one or both parents. In that case I try to arrive at a working diagnosis for each parent based on the wealth of data available about them from the home visit, a marital interview, and other extensive but less threatening clinical contacts with them. While I do not as a rule order psychological testing for a parent, I have found one inexpensive test well worth the 5 minutes or so of their time that it takes to procure. This is a set of figure drawings. These, if selectively and tactfully requested as part of the intake routine, are often well tolerated by parents and can add important data to help with puzzling parental diagnoses.

Diagnosis should include an estimate of the balance of current strengths and weaknesses in important areas of life performance. In my experience, there are two partly overlapping parental impairments, the coexistence of which should lead a child psychiatrist to consider a family therapy. These are:

1. Absence of or severe distortions in the ego capacities necessary for attainment and maintenance of child-rearing competency.
2. Defects in identity sense and in cohesiveness and stability of self-representation.

The first of these two qualifies as relevant interlocking pathology whenever the parental impairment occurs in phase with a complementary need of the child. In general, the younger the children the more dependent they will be on parental functions and the more likely that one or more of these parental deficits will pertain to the current needs of at least one child in the family. However, with less sick parents we are more apt to see relatively pinpointed, partly reactive impairments that can change with life stages in child or parent. For example, a mother may do very well with infants of either sex but have trouble letting a kindergarten daughter separate; or a father can provide much of what his son needs from him during mid-adolescence whereas he interacted in a depressed and competitively destructive manner with the boy during his infancy.

The second type of impairment (in identity and self-representation) can be considered a special case of the first, but I list it separately to emphasize its importance in the choice of family therapy over some other treatment for the parents. The rationale here relates to the clinical need to provide a more realistic exposure to the therapist and to dilute primitive transferences when identity confusion or fragmentation pervades the family. Even when some of these parents can be greatly helped by intensive long-term individual psychotherapies, it is often desirable to conduct a preliminary or parallel course of family therapy. This provides a more rapid impact and greater protection for the children.

With the above two classes of impairment in mind, a number of common syndromes of parents are easily called up. They will be found regularly to provide many of the candidates for family therapy intervention:

1. The schizophrenias, when functioning at an overtly psychotic level, i.e., with major defects in reality testing and/or at a pseudo-defective level (occasionally misdiagnosed as "true" mental deficiency).

2. Borderline personality organizations, with primitive splitting mechanisms toward self and object representations, poor impulse control, or regressive affect regulation in major parental roles.

3. The group of pseudoneurotic schizophrenias. These parents are not overtly psychotic, and often maintain smoothly functioning social, vocational, or parental facades. Included here are the "as-if" personalities so well described by Helene Deutsch over 40 years ago and very commonly seen (if not always diagnosed) today. This group, or a close variety thereof, is also referred to by Winnicott (1960) as the "false-self" personality and by John Frosch (1970) as the psychotic character. All of these parental syndromes can expose children to distorted communications, skewed or conflicting role models, and hollow imitations of genuine feelings.

4. Severe passive-dependent (infantile or "oral") personalities with or without direct addictive complications (alcohol, food, cigarettes, or drugs). These parents sometimes present as "doll-house marriages" with gross overdependency on in-laws and more or less open competition for infantile supplies with their own children. More commonly, and particularly among middle-class parents, these needs will appear in subtler and disguised forms requiring careful individual and family diagnostic approaches for their elucidation.

5. Parental incompetence syndromes secondary to mental deficiency and/or cultural deprivation. These families seldom present without the complex of accumulated difficulties that was discussed in the section on crisis management of multiproblem families. I mention them again here to emphasize how helpable they can be whether or not they are seen in an immediate crisis. Family work with these parents and children should not be limited to helpful educative, directive, and supportive measures. I have recurrently been impressed with my own tendencies to underestimate the value and potential for further growth inherent in some family systems and cultures about which I had much to learn. Furthermore, the tenacious characterological rigidities or severe emotional distortions seen in most parents of the first three categories are much less frequent in these families.

With any of these five parental conditions, family therapy may be the best way to alter (or more likely deflect) or temporarily replace ongoing family systems rapidly enough to meet the growing child's or siblings' needs for effective parenting. Even if, as is common, the family work provides only a partial and transient moratorium, this can be worthwhile in allowing other favorable factors to take effect. One of these is time, with passage by the child out of a critically vulnerable developmental phase; or a simultaneous individual psychotherapy for the child, which can be started under the protective umbrella of a family therapy. I have scheduled family therapy sessions once a week or once every two weeks to help provide a surprisingly effective "holding environment" with chaotic, defective, or malignant home atmospheres that do not appear responsive to amelioration through parental counseling.

CONTRAINDICATIONS

1. Massive but minimally relevant parental pathology. I have been struck by how some children seem to thrive, or at least survive and do well in important life tasks despite what looks like an emotional disaster

area in the home. I can best illustrate this contraindication to family therapy with a clinical vignette:

> Billy, an 8-year-old third grader, and his parents were referred for family therapy by a psychiatrically oriented internist who had treated his mother's migraine headaches and was familiar with her chain smoking, overuse of alcohol, and "somewhat strange" marriage. This was an upper-middle-class family, a late marriage between two moderately sick, talented people who had an only child. Their family life was replete with role reversals, angry tantrums on both parents' parts, long sulking cold wars between them, overt competition, and schizoid retreat on the father's part to his perfectionistically conceived work as senior editor for a publishing house. Billy's mother had achieved much gratification and success as a nonfiction writer and both parents were hurt and worried over Billy's marginal school performance. He was also cited for disruptive outbursts and clowning in class. His history revealed a birth weight of just over 3 pounds with a possible etiology of first trimester maternal smoking. Typical soft neurological signs, behavioral history of the child, and his figure drawings were all highly suggestive of a chronic brain syndrome (MBD). This child did very well on dextroamphetamine medication supplemented by brief counseling for both parents and a monthly relationship visit with me. On 5-year follow-up in mid-adolescence he was an above average student at a rather academically demanding boarding school. He had developed a sense of humor and a sturdy, obsessional character with considerable capacity for pleasure.

2. Divided, separating, or reconciliating marriages. As a rule, family therapy is not, and shouldn't be a substitute for the minimum amount of parental love and dedication that can hold a marriage together. With divorced parents, or those who have taken real steps (in contrast to talk) toward a separation, I prefer to work with the parent who has custody as far as any conjoint sessions; and I specifically try to stay out of any decisions on divorce or reconciliation in line with my conviction that matters as important as romance and psychiatry should be kept as far apart as possible.

3. Dishonest, secretive, or criminal families. Any requirement to conceal major (nonclinical) information from either parent or the children precludes the open communication and trust a family therapy needs to avoid iatrogenic effects. Thus a non-mentionable continuing extramarital liaison, a rigid request never to reveal a child's adopted status or the true nature of a father's livelihood (an inheritance) should raise serious reservations as to a family approach. In addition, parental or adolescent persistence in antisocial activities that are known to the family but grossly out of line with my own values requires their decision to suspend them at least for the duration of treatment, or discontinue the work.

4. Defensive misuses of family therapy. These are not uncommon and usually take the form of eagerness to plunge into a family- and/or child-centered approach in order to deny individual responsibility for a major personality or character illness of one or both parents. In this connection, the early hopes that intensive family therapy might be a definitive treatment for achieving structural characterological change have not been realized. Despite the fascination of, and insights gleaned from the application of general systems theory to clinical psychiatry, in my opinion this difficult task remains still in the province of therapies more closely approximating the one-to-one relationship of the mother-child dyad.

REFERENCES

Ackerman, N. W. *The Psychodynamics of Family Life*. New York: Basic Books, 1958.

Alpert, A. Reversibility of pathological fixations associated with maternal deprivation in infancy. *The Psychological Study of the Child*, 1959, *14*, 169–185.

Bateson, G., and Ruesch, J. *Communication: The social matrix of psychiatry*. New York: Norton, 1951.

Bateson, G., Jackson, D., Haley, J., and Weakland, J. Toward a theory of schizophrenia. *Behavioral Science*, 1956, *1*, 251–264.

Bertalanffy, L. von. *General system theory*. New York: George Braziller, 1968.

Deutsch, H. Some forms of emotional disturbance and their relationship to schizophrenia. *Psychoanalytic Quarterly*, 1942, *11*, 301–321.

Frosch, J. Psychoanalytic considerations of the psychotic character. *Journal of the American Psychoanalytic Association*, 1970, *18*, 24–50.

Goldfarb, W. The mutual impact of mother and child in childhood schizophrenia. *American Journal of Orthopsychiatry*, 1961, *31*, 738–747.

Jackson, D. Family interaction, family homeostasis and some implications for conjoint family psychotherapy. In J. Masserman (Ed.) *Individual and family dynamics*. New York: Grune and Stratton, 1959.

Jackson, D. (Ed.). *The etiology of schizophrenia*. New York: Basic Books, 1960.

Kernberg, O. Borderline personality organization. *Journal of the American Psychoanalytic Association*, 1967, *15*, 641–685.

Lidz, T., Fleck, S., and Cornelison, A. R. *Schizophrenia and the family*. New York: International Universities Press, 1965.

Liebowitz, B., and Black, M. The structure of the Ravich Interpersonal Game/Test. *Family Process*, 1974, *13*, 169–183.

Meyers, D., and Goldfarb, W. Studies of perplexity in mothers of schizophrenic children. *American Journal of Orthopsychiatry*, 1961, *31*, 551–564.

Papp, P., Silverstein, O., and Carter, E. Family sculpting in preventive work with "well families". *Family Process*, 1973, *12*, 197–212.

Weakland, J. H. "The double-bind theory" by self-reflexive hindsight. *Family Process*, 1974, *13*, 269–277.

Winnicott, D. W. Ego distortion in terms of true and false self. In Khan, M. (Ed.), *The Maturational Processes and the Facilitating Environment*. New York: International Universities Press, 1960.

Wynne, L. C., Ryckoff, I. M., Day, J., and Hirsch, S. I. Pseudomutuality in family relationships of schizophrenics. *Psychiatry*, 1958, *21*, 205–220.

7

COMMUNITY APPROACHES TO INTERVENTION[1]

Emory L. Cowen & Ellis L. Gesten

The relative ineffectiveness of past efforts to deal with children's disorders (Levitt, 1971) raises several serious questions: (1) How does a child reach the point of being labeled a "casualty"? (2) When a child's problems crystallize to a certain point, how restricted is even the most effective intervention? (3) What can be done to avert pathological childhood end-states? (4) What does a "community approach" offer in this regard? These questions frame the present chapter.

PROBLEMS IN CHILD MENTAL HEALTH

The Existing System: Brief Overview

Children enter the formal mental health system after significant others (e.g., parents, teachers) perceive a deficit, failure to meet standards, or the inability to cope. It takes time for such impressions to jell to the point of being labeled as "real" problems. Moreover, people use idiosyncratic personal assessment barometers to make these judgments. Problems that are obvious and persistent, that resist first-line ameliorative efforts and radiate to new areas, are more likely to be seen as "for real." When that happens, the child may be brought to an agency or practitioner, with a cry for help.

Next, the child is likely to be evaluated leading to recommendations or an action-plan. The latter might involve suggestions to parents or teachers, changing the child's environment, starting him in treatment, or recommending institutional care. Subsequent developments are monitored, largely at a clinical-intuitive level. If things work out, fine! If not, other forks in the road can be followed or the entire process can be recycled through another agency or practitioner.

Though grossly oversimplified, the above resume nevertheless reveals several mainstays of our past orientation to child pathology and treatment. Although these ways have served some children well, they harbor two major types of problems: (a) mechanical and (b) conceptual. Mechanical problems pertain to a system's vulnerability or breakdown points; conceptual problems implicate

[1]This chapter was done with grant support from the NIMH Experimental and Special Training Branch, MH 11820-06, for which the authors express sincere gratitude.

aspects of the system that would be socially inefficient, even if it were working with 100% effectiveness, mechanically.

Mechanical Limits

Several factors restrict a child's entering the service system. Significant others may not, for many reasons (e.g., naiveté, denial, or the belief that difficulties will go away with time), recognize that he has a psychological problem. Even recognizing such a problem does not guarantee that help will be sought. Some avoid that step because it is stigmatizing or an admission of failure. Others do not make the connection between an evident problem and the mental health system. The net result in each case is much the same, i.e., a child who needs psychological help fails to enter the mental health system. Failing to do so, his problems remain to simmer or spread.

System mechanics falter in other ways. Families lack sufficient means to get help or they face impossible geographic, transportation, or logistic problems. Helping resources even if requested are not always available. Such resources are inequitably distributed in ways that favor the wealthier, more highly educated, more verbal segments of the urban population (Hollingshead & Redlich, 1958; Sanua, 1966; Lorion, 1973). Moreover, traditional "middle-class" ways of delivering mental health services may not match the life styles of some people and may even turn them off (Riessman, Cohen, & Pearl, 1964; Reiff & Riessman, 1965; Cowen, 1967; Cowen, 1973; Zax & Cowen, 1976).

Entering the system doesn't guarantee success in it. There are also post-entry mechanical breakdowns. Children's assessment and diagnostic procedures are far from foolproof. Diagnostic tools are global and imprecise. Skilled clinicians, using the same observations and test data, come up with very different diagnoses (see, for example, Nathan, Andberg, Behan, & Patch, 1969). Even good diagnostic agreement doesn't assure agreement about an optimal treatment strategy. Nor does the latter guarantee a postitive treatment outcome. Reviews of the effectiveness of child psychotherapy (Levitt, 1971) are less than encouraging; indeed the most informed current view of psychotherapy in general (Bergin, 1971; Bergin & Suinn, 1975) is that it is at best a moderately effective approach.

Given these ponderous mechanical problems, it is a tribute to the system that it works at all. But it does! At the same time, it is a socially insufficient system because so many children who need help can't enter it, and many of those who do are not materially helped by its best intentioned, most skillful efforts. In the final analysis, the existing system cannot deliver anywhere near the amount of service needed by the aggregate of children with problems.

Conceptual Limits

Conceptual limits are on a different plane than mechanical ones. By challenging a system's pivotal assumptions they point to entirely new ways of engaging problems. Sarason (1971) uses the term "regularities" to describe a system's defining practices. In principle, regularities are as they are to promote the system's goals (Lorion, Cowen, & Kraus, 1974). But things don't always happen that way. Sarason argues that a system's regularities must continually be reviewed to see how well they are serving its objectives. He says:

> . . . when any programmatic regularity is no longer viewed in terms of (the) universe of alternatives, rational thought and evaluation of intended outcomes are no longer in the picture, overwhelmed as they are by the power of faith, tradition and habit. (1971, p. 71).

Current practices in child mental health can be viewed as a system with its own special regularities: (1) identifying malfunctioning children; (2) assessing their problems; (3) intervening to alleviate their dysfunctions. How essential are these steps? What are the alternatives? The next section lists, and raises questions about, several key assumptions in child mental health.

Several Key Assumptions in Child Mental Health

Children's Psychological Problems are Much Like Their Physical Problems. There are important structural parallels in the methods of child mental health and those of pediatric practice (Cowen, 1973; Zax & Cowen, 1976). For the modal referral, both begin by trying to identify specific causes of a current problem and, on that basis, to intervene remedially. How justified is this? Are there significant differences between modal cases in the two spheres? On the surface, it would seem that psychological problems, compared to most physical problems, have longer standing histories, more complicated networks of interconnections and are more influenced by people and settings. Certainly they are less current and circumscribed than colds, earaches, the chicken pox, or broken bones. Moreover, they are harder to diagnose and interdependencies between diagnosis and treatment are less precise than for physical problems. Paying closer attention to these real differences might help significantly to expand the universe of alternatives for engaging children's psychological problems.

Children's Psychological Health is Best Promoted by Getting Rid of Their Symptoms. Mental health specialists work reactively with children's problems. The problems per se and the grief they cause the child and others are the foci of their interventions. Unfortunately, however, long standing symptoms have adaptive-protective value and hence are hard to give up. Moreover, symptoms often spill over adversely into other areas of a child's functioning. Interventions mounted under such circumstances start with two strikes against them.

Although symptoms are the things that get people uptight and impel them to action, two related assumptions of child clinical practice bear review: (1) that there *is* a reciprocal relation between symptoms and health, and (2) that reducing symptoms builds health. To the extent that these are unfounded, we must raise alternative possibilities about when, where, and how children can best be helped.

Direct, Person-to-Person Interventions Are the Best Way to Deal with Children's Problems. A child's problem comes to the attention of a professional, cast in the role of a knowledgeable expert. His task is to wave the problem away. But because so many problems are already well rooted at referral, the cards are loaded against quick and easy cures. Is the face-to-face rehabilitative mode the only way to help children? Can health better be promoted from a perspective other than that of the knowledgeable expert stamping out illness by sagacious individualized repair?

These conceptual problems are not independent of each other. Their most important common thread is that too much of child mental health's effort has been directed to crystallized dysfunctional "end-states" (Cowen, 1973; Zax & Cowen, 1976)—conditions which, by definition, most resist repair.

To this point, we have avoided defining "community approaches." The concept is delightfully vague and that vagueness has well served our purposes. The word "community" (whether followed by psychiatry, psychology, mental health, or approaches) means different things to different people. These are often defined operationally by whatever the defining person happens to be doing. One reason for reviewing current problems in children's services is to provide a framework that may help to clarify the term *community approaches*.

Mechanical limits of children's services, such as lack of reach, fallible diagnosis, and imperfect treatment, are important to be sure. Solutions for some of those problems may be found in the community, because it harbors richer possibilities than the practitioner's office, clinic, or hospital for reaching more children and providing them with more appropriate, effective services. Activities so generated would, by our definition, be community mental health—i.e., using community settings and resources to do a better job than we now do. The problems addressed by community mental health may be quite similar to those handled by traditional practice, but they can be engaged earlier, and in settings closer to the action. Such work is secondary prevention.

A shift in emphasis from repairing casualties toward building health and competence in all children challenges the system's assumptions and raises serious questions about past givens in practice. It means new ways of doing things, by new cadres of personnel, in new settings, and it calls for different training, skills, and behaviors than those emphasized in current professional training. Such activities are close to a pure concept of primary prevention and can help to define the fields of community psychology and psychiatry. As the terms are used in this chapter community mental health and community psychology (psychiatry) taken together comprise the broader entity "community approaches."

EVOLVING RESOLUTIONS

One reason why child mental health practices have evolved as they have is that there have been few good alternatives. Although some are now starting to surface, few could argue that we have sufficient experience or data bases to justify wholesale reform. More realistic is the view that we need to budget child mental health priorities. Since child mental health resources are finite, doing new things may mean giving up *some* current practices.

A continuing emphasis on young children (Smith & Hobbs, 1966) is certainly warranted. Because of the young child's flexibility, because his problems, however severe, are still less rooted and spread than adults', work with children promises richer payoffs for finite mental health investments. Indeed, the younger the better! The search for more effective diagnostic and remedial approaches cannot be dropped. Children who need help will be around for a long time to come; they cannot simply be repressed. But *some* portion of our effort must go into cutting down the flow of future problems. Practically, then, the task is to assign priorities to a large pool of potential activities (i.e., alternatives) in child mental health.

Emerging strategies and programs considered below under the embracing rubric "community approaches" are diverse. They include examples of both community mental health and community psychology or psychiatry approaches. Target children run the gamut from 100% "end-state" conditions (e.g., childhood schizophrenia) to those who are entirely problem-free. Together, these approaches broaden the options available to child mental health.

RESTORATIVE APPROACHES: COMMUNITY MENTAL HEALTH

Systematic Early Detection. The present child-serving system has been described as "passive-receptive" (Cowen, 1967). Problems are not actively sought out because more than enough find their way into the system spontaneously to exhaust its resources. Because this is so, the problems of many children remain to eat away and to spill over into new areas. These problems are often expressed later as demands on the mental health or related system (i.e., as problems of delinquency, criminal justice, welfare, or addiction). Community approaches can help to change this classic passive-receptive stance toward more active, seeking directions by using community settings and resources to identify children's problems earlier and more systematically. Rather than waiting for rooted troubles to show up, problems can be located before they have crystallized, when less than drastic actions can make a difference.

Family and school are the two systems that most strongly influence young children. That's where the child spends his time. Those are the systems that significantly shape him, his coping styles and adaptive mechanisms; they also furnish his main identification models. Although early identification could, in principle, be done both through families and schools, parsimony favors the latter. Schools are the main setting in Western society that communally affect all children during their formative years (Bardon, 1968). They house many youngsters under a single roof and administrative structure. They are committed to approaches to facilitate children's development, *and* they have become more and more aware of the critical interfaces between educational and psychological growth. A child must acquire certain skills and competencies in school. Failure to do so defines failure in the system. Children who can't "cut it" in school are at a great disadvantage in achieving later life goals. Thus, schools have been loci for important recent developments in active, systematic early detection and remediation of children's adaptive problems.

The St. Louis County Project (Gildea, Glidewell, & Kantor, 1967; Rae-Grant & Stringer, 1969), dating from the late 'forties, was among the earliest of these efforts. Initially, this program used teacher observations and ratings of children's emotional states, as well as sociometric and semiprojective measures, to evaluate school adjustment. Later (Rae-Grant & Stringer, 1969) an objective early detection instrument, the Academic Progress Chart (APC) was developed. This grid depicts a child's academic and psychological development graphically, according to chronological age expectancies. Using the APC retrospectively, they found that 60% of the children eventually referred to school mental health services could have been detected anywhere from 1 to 8 years earlier. The issue raised by this finding is the extent to which unattended children's problems solidify and fan out over the years.

A second influential approach to school screening was carried out by the California State Department of Education in the late 'fifties and early 'sixties (Bower & Lambert, 1961; Bower, 1969). This group developed early detection procedures that have been very useful to later workers and have identified some important correlates of early-detected school dysfunction. Their early detection measures include: the Thinking About Yourself (TAY)—a self-concept measure; the Class Play (CP)—a sociometric measure of peer-perceived adjustment; and the AML—a quick screening device used by teachers. The two main findings of their large-scale study based on 5,500 California school children (Bower, 1969) were that (1) there was marked overlap between children that teachers and clinicians considered to be disturbed, and (2) identified children, compared to nonidentified classmates, had more negative behaviors, poorer self-concepts, and were seen less positively by peers. The PACE ID Center in San Mateo (Brownbridge & Van Vleet, 1969) used Bower's early detection methodology, particularly the AML, to identify a large sample of young maladapting school children, within a larger group of 6,000. On this basis a preventive program was mounted to strengthen their adjustment.

The Rochester Primary Mental Health Project (PMHP) (Cowen, Trost, Lorion, Dorr, Izzo, & Isaacson, 1975) has for many years used systematic early detection procedures; i.e., group intellectual and personality tests, social work interviews with mothers of primary grade children, and several teacher rating-measures of children's school adjustment status (Cowen et al, 1975). PMHP found that about one of three primary grade children had moderate to severe school adjustment problems (Cowen et al., 1975). Consistent with PMHP's growing interest in *positive* mental health, Gesten (1976) recently developed a new screening device that measures children's resources and competencies. PMHP used early detection data both to identify children who need help and to guide specific interventions. The project has developed mathematically based procedures to describe the predominant nature of a child's school adjustment problem (Lorion, Cowen, & Caldwell, 1974). This "pure-types" approach identifies acting out–aggressive behaviors; shyness, timidity and withdrawal; and learning difficulties as the three most common types of school maladaptation.

Systematic early detection procedures have also been used in a ghetto environment (the Woodlawn area in Chicago) with rampant school adjustment problems (Kellam, Branch, Agrawal, & Ensminger, 1975). These detection procedures included: (1) teacher interviews, plus the "Teachers' Observation of Classroom Adjustment" (TOCA) scale—a measure of children's academic and social adaptation; (2) direct classroom observation; (3) a behavior-problem inventory submitted by mothers of first-grade children; and (4) a brief self-report measure called "How I Feel." Even though 80% of Woodlawn's teachers were black and teacher judgments were central to the screening proceudre, 70% of Woodlawn's young school children were judged to have school adjustment problems.

Although the early detection programs thus far cited are all school based, the process is not wedded to the schools per se. The Sumter Child Study Project (Newton & Brown, 1967), set in a geographic area with few mental health services, used a systematic *preschool* check-up with more than 500 children. This two-session check-up included structured observations and testing of the preschool child, plus an interview with the mother in the first session, and a pooling of data and information and formulation of plans in the second. Children judged to be at-risk in screening were later found to have poorer attendance, reading rates, performance and promotion records than those seen as developing satisfactorily. The Sumter program moves systematic detection back earlier in time—a theoretically attractive step, if, as argued, the young child's flexibility and the likelihood that his problems have spread less, improve intervention prognosis.

Early detection approaches have been applied even earlier, with disadvantaged ghetto infants and toddlers, in the first two years of life (Stendler-Lavatelli, 1968; Cowen, 1973; Gottfried, 1973; Jason, 1975). Often, assessment of such youngsters has identified weaknesses in the cognitive and social skills needed for later school adjustment. Hence, in this area too, early detection methods provide a base on which to build constructive intervention.

Systematic early detection offers a bona fide community-based contrast to traditional ways of engaging children's psychological problems. As an active approach, it can identify large numbers of children, from all social strata, before their problems pass a point of no-return. Methods for identifying problems rapidly and accurately have been developed. Early detection findings provide a stark measure of reality that social planners cannot ignore. Illustratively, one task force (Glidewell & Swallow, 1969) of the Joint Commission on the Mental Health of Children, in a comprehensive survey of school maladjustment detection-studies, found that currently 30% of American school children experience moderate to severe school adjustment problems. For roughly 10%, those problems are sufficiently severe to require immediate professional help. The magnitude of that problem dwarfs resources to deal with it, even if we define helping in terms of semi-traditional definitions of child mental health services. This discrepancy dictates that alternative, scope-expanding helping approaches be developed. Community options must be considered for that to happen.

Alternative Delivery Systems. Early detection data raise the question of how transitory or stable children's problems are (Cowen, 1973; Zax & Cowen, 1976); obviously the greater their stability, the greater the need for early remedial follow-through. Although this remains a controversial issue, some findings are well established: (1) serious childhood problems endure (Robins, 1966); (2) aggressive and acting out problems last longer than those of shyness and undersocialization (Clarizio, 1969); and (3) whereas some problems dissipate over time, many persist and fan out.

Critics of early detection procedures (e.g., Caplan, 1964) note, with some justification, that they are limited by our ability to follow up constructively. What, for example, would be the value of lung X-ray procedure that accurately detected prodromal pretuberculous signs if there were no meaningful follow-through? Indeed, without follow-through early detection can do more harm than good. If children at-risk were identified for a third-grade teacher who was then told that helping resources were regrettably not available, she would have good reason to feel frustrated and resentful.

AUGMENTING RESOURCES

Professional manpower shortages have sharply limited constructive follow-through of early screening and detection findings (Albee, 1959; Arnhoff, Rubenstein, & Speisman, 1969). There are far more people—adults *and* children—who need psychological help than can be handled by mental health professionals now or in the foreseeable future. The clarity of this gap prompted the original Joint Commission (1961) to formulate influential proposals to liberalize views of "who may treat whom." Thus necessity, more than philosophical conviction, led to exploring the use of nonprofessional manpower in mental health. Pressures made it essential to reconsider critically, personnel regularities of the delivery system, and to try out new possibilities from the universe of alternatives. Questions that were important in this process included: (1) To what extent do such factors as IQ, advanced degrees, and prior clinical training and experience determine the help that a person in the helping role brings to a distressed "other"? (2) Might personality, life experiences, and stylistic variables be more important factors than credential-related criteria in determining whether interpersonal help-giving behavior is genuinely effective? If nothing else, the Joint Commission legitimized exploration of such questions.

The growth and diversity in the use of nonprofessionals in mental health in the past decade have been enormous (e.g., Arnhoff et al., 1969; Gartner, 1971; Guerney, 1969; Sobey, 1970). Helper groups have included students, housewives, inner-city residents, retired folks, and many others. Parents have been trained to work with their own children, especially using behavior modification approaches (Guerney, 1969). Recruitment and training practices with nonprofessionals have also been diverse, and their helping efforts have spanned a broad range of actions and settings. Children have been important targets for these interventions—inner-city toddlers in infant stimulation programs, children in settlement houses and residential settings, and particularly school children with adjustment and/or learning problems.

One pioneering program (Rioch, 1967) trained housewives to function primarily as therapists in a variety of settings, including schools and clinics. Carefully selected for their helping qualities, these women were found to be very effective clinically. They also equalled or surpassed beginning psychiatrists in their knowledge of content on standard Psychiatric Board Exams. Extensive performance data (from employers, supervisors, and co-workers, plus self-reports) collected three years after their training had ended (Magoon, Golann, & Freeman, 1969) showed that they had done a highly competent job in areas previously seen as exclusive professional turf.

Another case in point is the Rochester school mental health project (PMHP) cited above. Following early identification of school adjustment problems, PMHP uses nonprofessional child-aides as the prime direct help-agents for maladapting children (Cowen et al., 1975). Aides are selected primarily for interpersonal and life experience qualities, rather than for their education or advanced degrees. Both clinical impressions and research data show them to be warm, facilitating people (Sandler, 1972; Cowen, Dorr, & Pokracki, 1972). The initial aide training is focused and time-limited and, although they receive further on-the-job training and supervision, the program is built primarily around what they can offer as people. The child-aide model markedly expands the reach of early helping services (Cowen, Lorion, Kraus, & Dorr, 1974). A single part-time child-aide can see 10 to 12 children at a time. Hence the system brings helping services to about 10 to 15% of primary grade children—a substantial fraction of those known to have school adjustment problems (Glidewell & Swallow, 1969). Moreover, available data—school record measures, teacher ratings, aide judgments, and test measures—indicate that these services are effective (Cowen et al., 1975).

Cost-benefit analysis of PMHP (Dorr, 1972) indicates that an approximate 40% cost increment extends the reach of effective services by more than 1000%. The average cost of an aide contact-session with a child is around $8.00, varying somewhat with the school's pay schedule. Measured against going market rates, the per session cost for a PMHP child is about 20 to 25% of that of private professional services. Effectiveness data for the child-aide program are as strong and systematic as those for professional services. And beyond extending reach, the aide program offers a flexible structural model that can be applied to a wide range of problem areas (e.g., learning disabilities, incipient socioemotional problems, etc.) and to population sectors with the greatest need for help.

Child-serving programs that use nonprofessionals encourage new, appealing, socially utilitarian professional roles (e.g., in recruitment, training, and supervision)—not professional obsolescence (Cowen & Lorion, 1976). These evolving uses point toward a delivery system with geometrically augmented reach, an attractive prospect in the light of current shortages. All communities harbor large, untapped pools of nonprofessional help-agents—paid or volunteer. This is a potentially invaluable, if historically underused, helping resource. Some nonprofessionals, disenfranchised by age, social class, or role-typing, can personally benefit from the chance to engage in ego-enhancing, socially beneficial new careers.

Riessman (1965) calls this the "helper-therapy" principle. Using nonprofessional help-agents does not per se change the assumptions of child mental health services (though one can imagine uses that *would* do so). Rather, it attempts to deal more realistically with a critical breakdown point in the current system; i.e., its limited, biased reach. The roots of the nonprofessional approach lie within the community. Although the development has outpaced its evaluation, early returns, on balance, are favorable. Currently, this low-cost, reality-born development stands as an important step in community mental health toward improved child mental health services.

CONSULTATION

As with the use of nonprofessionals, consultation is justified by several limitations of current child mental health services. In this case, the realities are these: Whether due to failures to interpret children's problems correctly, misgivings about mental health services, poor trust relations, or lack of resources, children's psychological problems find their way into systems other than mental health. Gurin, Veroff, and Feld (1960), for example, report that clergymen and family physicians field many more emotional problems than do mental health professionals. It has been estimated that one-third of all problems brought to pediatricians are psychological rather than physical. Classroom teachers, too, know that many learning problems of children have important psychological roots. Sarason et al. (1966) use the term "professional preciousness" to describe the conviction of many mental health people that they stand alone as society's bulwark against maladaptation. Traffic patterns do not bear out that view.

The truth, like it or not, is that many (most) children's psychological problems go first to social agents who lack mental health training—either people trained in other professions (e.g., medical, legal, and educational) or informal helpers with no professional training at all. This isn't necessarily all bad. Often such contacts benefit from an established prior base of trust that facilitates interpersonal helping. However, the person whose help is sought in a natural context may lack the understandings and skills needed to deal with a problem. This is one entry point for mental health consultation—an approach that joins, rather than fights, reality.

Through consultation (Caplan, 1970; Mannino, MacLennan, & Shore, 1975) mental health professionals try to broaden consultees' understandings of the determinants of psychological problems, and to suggest alternatives for dealing with situations that go beyond their background and training. Consultation thus seeks to strengthen the caregiver's hand and to provide him resources and backstopping that allow him to be more effective with people in distress. Much consultation work has been directed to children, especially through the schools (e.g., Newman, 1967; Beiser, 1972). Many child mental health projects designed to expand the reach of children's services (Cowen et al., 1975; Brownbridge & Van Vleet, 1969) have consultation components.

Mental health consultation programs are not limited to schools. Caplan (1964) correctly notes that pediatricians are important psychological caregivers because of their regular, enduring interactions with children and their families. Both through direct child-contacts and within-family radiating effects, a consultation program with a dozen pediatricians could potentially touch several thousand people. That one-third or more of pediatricians' time is invested in psychological, rather than medical, dialogue underscores the potential value of consultation with them. Knowing norms and base-rate expectancies for cognitive and social development in the first several years of life may be just as important to a pediatrician's effective functioning as knowing when to start a child on Pablum or strained spinach (Murphy & Chandler, 1972).

The effects of consultation are not easy to evaluate. The most accessible criterion—i.e., how much the experience changes consultees' knowledge and attitudes—is not the most important. The key issue is the extent to which the process ultimately facilitates children's behavior and development. Even so, consultation addresses major mechanical flaws in existing delivery systems. It reaches out, rather than waits for crystallized problems to enter a formal system. It provides access to psychological problems sooner. It capitalizes on existing entry points and climates of trust. And group consultation offers an attractive option for expanding the reach of helping services. Certain types of consultation, for example, to social planning bodies or agencies, can help to develop settings and approaches that promote positive mental health in children.

Crisis Intervention

Most interventions with children, we have suggested, do not occur at an ideal time. What *is* a favorable time? Beyond the principle "the sooner (i.e., the younger) the better," Caplan (1964) argues that crisis is an ideal time for parsimonious intervention. He views crises as crucial turning points which, depending on how they are handled, lead either to more effective future coping or greater vulnerability.

A crisis is a relatively brief, transitional period characterized by acute disturbance, discomfort, preoccupation, and emotional upset. In crisis, the person often doesn't know what to do or where to turn for help, vacillates, and is subject to the influence of others. Various investigators (Lindemann, 1944; Cumming & Cumming, 1966) suggest that there is a specific sequence of crisis reactions, including initial turmoil, disruption or immobilization of normal thought and bodily processes, a sense of preoccupation and ill-being, and efforts to mobilize coping resources.

All children experience crises. Some can be anticipated—before surgery, school entry, or the birth of a new sibling; others, for example, the death of a family member or a sudden, severe accident, cannot. Some theories of child development (e.g., Erikson, 1959) consider growth to be characterized by progressions through stages, with each step marked by a predictable series of crises characteristic of that stage. Within such a framework, effective mastery of epigenetic crises is seen as a necessary prerequisite for further healthy growth. Working with children in crisis has appealing features such as the child's susceptibility to inputs during such periods and the disproportionately high impact that successful crisis resolution can have. Hence, relatively small time investments during crisis can benefit both the individual and society. It is a judicious allocation of scarce resources.

Crisis intervention principles can be applied to other than current, florid crises. Several authors have suggested that prior training and rehearsal of children in crisis-coping skills can ease adaptation to anticipatable crises and strengthen the child's repertoire of long-term adaptive skills. Cumming and Cumming (1966) proposed that children be given graded crisis situations to work through under sheltered conditions that help them to learn constructive resolutions and sound coping skills. Caplan (1964) also speaks of training children, before-the-fact, in crisis coping, i.e., "anticipatory guidance" or "emotional inoculation." His approach calls for vivid anticipation of an impending crisis experience and its associated affects. Opportunities to cathart fears and negative feelings are followed by support, guidance, provision of alternatives, and a chance to rehearse behavioral options. Practice under such favorable, sheltered conditions seeks to build immunity against the real McCoy.

There is evidence to suggest that this approach is more than just a theoretical pipe-dream. Melamed and Siegel (1975) report a study in which 60 children about to undergo surgery were shown a film of a child's hospitalization for surgery. The film provided a before-the-fact way of working through the anxiety of surgery. Compared to control presurgical cases who saw a neutral film, the inoculated group had significantly lower preoperative anxiety on behavioral observations, self-report, and palmar sweat measures, as well as less postoperative anxiety. Moreover, parents of the prepared children reported significantly fewer postoperative behavior problems than control parents. Apparently the chance to engage the impending crisis under sheltered conditions and thereby to dissipate anxiety helped children to cope with the real crisis. (Related studies are reviewed in Chapter 17.)

Crisis intervention, to be effective, should be rooted in community settings (such as schools and hospitals) where there is a high probability of encountering crisis in its natural unfolding process. Efforts, so based, can (1) capitalize on ideal timing for intervening, (2) improve the potential pay-off of time-limited interventions, and (3) implant a critical skill in children that gives them a sounder base for meeting later adaptive demands.

END-STATE ALTERNATIVES

This section provides several examples of community approaches targeted to serious, end-state dysfunctions of childhood. Each program addresses an unresolved mechanical failing of the present order. Several, in their use of atraditional settings or personnel, also challenge its assumptions.

Mental Deficiency. Sarason, Zitnay and Grossman (1971) wrote a penetrating essay on community approaches to mental deficiency. As a consultant for a state agency, Sarason encouraged critical reexamination of classic assumptions about the care and treatment of defectives. Often, programs for defectives start with a plan for a new building, as if a building per se could solve all problems. Sarason's group did *not* assume that a new building was necessarily desirable. Indeed, they thought of some powerful arguments against such a structure (1) it would be geographically isolating and separate children from their natural homes; (2) it could well finesse a community's responsibility for, and involvement in, engaging the problems of mental deficiency. As Sarason et al. put it:

> . . . a program that purports to be community-oriented is not consistent with its purposes if it accepts cases in ways which absolve the community of continuing responsibility. (p. 29)

Sarason often asks a hypothetical "what-if" question to get people to reexamine their assumptions (e.g., "What if Congress passed a law tomorrow making the practice of psychotherapy illegal?"). Even though he is not arguing that such things *should* happen, he believes that the question is useful because it forces people to consider how well a program's qualities support its goals. Answering the what-if question helps to identify alternatives that can lead to more productive ways of doing things. Sarason (1972) believes that the chances of developing effective new settings are improved when people identify, and ponder, a universe of alternatives, *before* the fact. A new building for defectives, however elegant, might have sharply restricted the universe of alternatives (particularly community-based ones) for the target group. Settings are thus "created" long before they are built.

In this case, Sarason and co-workers (1971) asked the "what-if" question:

> What if you were given the responsibility to develop residential facilities with the restrictions that they could not be on "institutional land," no one of them could house more than 12 individuals, and no new buildings could be erected? (p. 38)

This question moved people's thinking toward new community-care alternatives. It led to a three-pronged community-based program including (a) a day-care center run by the parents' association, (b) an Independent Living Unit to house retarded youth while they worked in the community, and (c) a Family Involvement Program to accommodate young retardates with difficult family situations, five days a week. Parents in this program agreed beforehand to a time-limited stay for the child, and to spend time in the unit observing the child's behavior and interactions and how they were handled (i.e., largely with behavior modification approaches). Problems that could not be accommodated by these three programs were referred to other agencies and settings. Each of the three programs had deep community roots. Collectively, they offered an alternative community solution to a community problem, based on assumptions and practices that differed substantially from past approaches.

Hard-Core Youth. Goldenberg (1968, 1971) developed a community program for hard-core inner-city youth. He doubted that individual therapy significantly changed such youth. He believed that the problem required settings that were situationally realistic and capable of potentiating positive change. His setting, the Residential Youth Center (RYC), a short-term treatment facility, reflected this view. The RYC challenged several past assumptions: (1) that problems of disadvantaged youth are best solved in locales other than their own; (2) that mental health professionals are best qualified to provide services for the poor; and (3) that a setting for youth should reflect the values and technologies of its professional leaders.

The RYC was set up in the heart of the inner-city. Its staff consisted mostly of young people, born and raised in that area. Staff responsibilities were defined "horizontally." Thus, *all* staff members, not just professionals, had across-the-board responsibility for a certain number of residents. Conversely, all staff people, including professionals, did their share of program-maintenance activities (e.g., cooking). The Center's atmosphere was homelike, with open internal access lines and fluid communication to the surrounding community. The program emphasized educational and vocational training plus personal counseling.

Admission to the RYC was voluntary. Residents were youth between the ages of 16 and 21. The average duration of a stay was 5 months. Residents were active in the Center's operation and governance; all had daily responsibilities to meet. Comprehensive research evaluation, including comparison studies with a nonprogram control group, showed that RYC living led to significantly higher employment rates, better work attendance, more income, and fewer arrests and incarcerations. Attitude and personality measures also favored residents. The average cost of stay, per resident, was about $3000. Contrast that with the estimated cost of $4000 to process a single youth through juvenile court (Duggan, 1965).

Fishman, Denham, Levine, and Shatz (1969) describe another program for hard-core inner-city delinquent youth conducted by the Howard University Institute for Youth Studies (IYS). The IYS program was built around skill training, establishing competencies, and placing trainees productively in jobs. Training included both generic skills (i.e., learning more about oneself, one's community, the world at large; how to observe, record, and use supervision; and knowledge of community services) plus specific job-related learnings. Trainees were prepared for a dozen different jobs including work in day-care, welfare, recreation, geriatrics, and counseling. Training was broad enough to allow trainees to move across areas if specific jobs dried up. The more than 100 program youth included delinquents, dropouts, and the unemployed. Almost all were black inner-city residents, most under 21 years of age. Comprehensive evaluation of the program showed major gains in employment and job stability and reductions in delinquent and criminal behavior.

Programs with documented effectiveness, such as the RYC and IYS, suggest that imaginative community-based solutions that bypass traditional assumptions and settings can be very useful even in situations that some have regarded as unreachable.

Severely Disturbed Children. Hobbs (1966) reports that about 1-$\frac{1}{2}$ million children in this country are so profoundly disturbed that they cannot progress in normal family, school, and community situations. Traditional "treatment" is neither available for these youngsters, nor is it necessarily an approach of choice for them. As a member of the original Joint Commission, Hobbs was influenced strongly by experiences he had in Europe where, under less affluent conditions, appealing alternatives (e.g., the French éducateur) for working with severely disturbed children had developed. The resultant Project Re-Ed (Hobbs, 1966, 1967; Lewis, 1967) is a short-term residential facility for young (ages 6 to 12) seriously disturbed children, based on two assumptions: (1) that round-the-clock education, rather than traditional treatment, is an approach of choice for such youngsters, and (2) that actual behavior, especially adaptation within Re-Ed, is more important than psychodynamics.

Although children live in at Re-Ed five days a week, their home and community contacts are maintained during residency. Precipitous separations are avoided. Re-Ed's philosophy is "to provide an engaging goal-oriented educational climate during the child's working hours" (Lewis, 1967, p. 354). Re-Ed's main help-agent is a new breed of worker, the "teacher-counselor," i.e., former teachers with interest in, and talent for, this exacting work. After receiving didactic and practicum training, they live and work, 24 hours a day, with the children. Re-Ed attempts to establish a climate of trust and understanding, to build children's skills and competencies, and to encourage group esprit and expression of feeling. It also uses limit-setting constructively to help children learn to manage their impulses effectively. Behavior, not dynamics, is paramount.

Re-Ed evaluations (Hobbs, 1966; Weinstein, 1969) cite encouraging findings. The project's success rate with these difficult children was about 80%—a figure that compares favorably to psychotherapy outcome data for children in general (Levitt, 1971). Negative behaviors such as tantrums, bedwetting, and aggressiveness decreased and the children improved in school adjustment, social maturity, and competence. Re-Ed children did significantly better than controls, both in formal test measures and on ratings by parents, teachers, peers, and community agents. One impressive outcome was that *all* Re-Ed alumni were functioning adequately in regular schools at the 18-month follow-up point. Re-Ed costs per child were less than 50% of the costs of state hospital placement, and less than 25% of the cost of private residential treatment.

The Elmont Program (Donahue, 1967; Donahue & Nichtern, 1965) is also designed for profoundly disturbed (e.g., schizophrenic) young children—the "sure" candidates for school exclusion. Although Elmont shares Re-Ed's assumption that education, not treatment, is the natural vehicle for growth in children, it is a day-care, not a residential, program. Elmont well illustrates how a community can broaden intervention options.

Elmont planners accepted responsibility for educating all children but recognized that a small fraction could not profit from regular classroom placement. Facing the usual personnel and budgetary shortages of a school district, they developed an innovative program for profoundly disturbed children. The key help-agents in the new program were "teacher-moms"—warm, empathic, giving women, who donated their time as volunteers. The program's limited professional time was used to train these women and to support their direct help-giving services. Teacher-moms worked intensively in one-to-one interactions with program children based on individualized study plans.

Evaluation of the first 21 children in the Elmont program revealed important signs of intellectual and interpersonal growth. Eleven of the 21, initially destined to deeply troubled lives, returned successfully to their normal classes where they were doing well educationally and personally. Elmont was a very *in*expensive program. Thanks to its community roots and services, its per child cost was only $38 more than the district's standard annual per capita educational cost.

Although, superficially, the foci and problem orientations of the programs reviewed in this section vary, all deal with difficult end-state problems that have not been well handled by past practice. Each starts by reconceptualizing a classic problem and from that base develops an innovative alternative. The documented effectiveness of these "solutions" points to attractive new community options that may help to circumvent several nasty mechanical problems of past child mental health services.

BUILDING-APPROACHES: COMMUNITY PSYCHOLOGY and PSYCHIATRY

This section considers an evolving set of concepts and approaches that differ sharply both from traditional child mental health practice *and* from the community mental health alternatives described above. In fact, conceptually and operationally, the latter two approaches are closer to each other than either is to the so-called *building-approaches*. With a focus on engineering health and competence from the start, building-approaches do not directly engage children's problems. The two main building-approaches considered, social systems analysis and modification, and competence acquisition, are bona fide examples of primary prevention. Although their focus is specific and they avoid nebulous constructs such as "improving the quality of life," they retain prime interest in such dependent variables as adjustment, self-realization, and personal satisfaction—that is, mental health's core goals.

SOCIAL SYSTEMS ANALYSIS AND MODIFICATION

The mental health fields are slowly relinquishing the once dominant view that children's problems are necessarily rooted in their personal psychodynamic histories. Striking associations between poverty and lack of opportunity on the one side and psychological misfortune on the other support the possibility that social system qualities themselves significantly affect a child's psychological adaptation. In the past we have been inclined to overlook system effects. Now, under closer examination, these seem to be anything but neutral in their impact on child development. If psychological strengths are to be built into children from the start, social system effects must be understood and constructively harnessed. This view suggests the need for three major interrelated thrusts.

First, we need frameworks that well *describe* the major impact dimensions of social systems and sensitively reflect differences in individual settings. Although this sounds simple and straightforward, it is a deceptively complex challenge for which we still lack sufficient know-how and tools. Comprehensive, reliable frameworks for describing social systems would permit studying the effects of systems on children exposed to them and identifying those components that encourage and those which impede health. This step is a vital prerequisite to engineering systems that favor positive outcomes (Sarason, 1972). Finally, since systems don't affect all people in the same way, we need also to understand the consequences of specific person-environment combinations (e.g., "ecological-matches"). Examples of these three thrusts are cited in the sections to follow.

Attempts to describe high-impact social systems ranging from communities (Barker & Schoggen, 1973; Price & Blashfield, 1975) to schools and families (Barker & Gump, 1964; Lennard & Bernstein, 1969) have recently been increasing. Moos and his co-workers (Moos, 1973; Moos, 1974; Insel & Moos, 1974; Moos & Insel, 1974; Price & Moos, 1975) have spearheaded this approach. They have developed scales to measure the properties of nine different types of social environments—from mental hospital wards to military, work, and educational settings. Of much interest is their finding that several basic dimensional clusters recur repeatedly in describing what seem, on the surface, to be diverse environments. These clusters include (1) *relational* dimensions reflecting, for example, people's involvement and affiliative patterns; (2) *goal orientation* dimensions such as the environment's competitiveness and task orientation; and (3) *maintenance* dimensions such as the environment's orderliness and rule-clarity (Moos, 1974).

An application of this approach in educational settings can be cited. Moos and Trickett (1974) developed a Class Environment Scale to measure nine separate dimensions of junior high and high-school class environments. They first showed (Trickett & Moos, 1973) that specific class environments varied substantially along these dimensions and, next, that different environments had different consequences (Trickett & Moos, 1974). For example, class environments with good interpersonal relations and clear rules yielded high scores on student measures of satisfaction and positive mood. To the extent that the latter are desirable goals or preconditions for effective learning, this finding suggests that we should try to create class environments with positive interpersonal relations and articulated rule-systems.

Barker and Gump (1964) studied a physical aspect of school environments and its consequences by contrasting how children from large and small (i.e., "overmanned" and "undermanned") schools are seen. Children from small schools compared to those from large schools became involved in more, and more varied, activities, were less sensitive to individual differences, had sharper identities and greater visibility. Other investigators have studied correlates of different educational environments. Illustratively, Minuchin, Biber, Shapiro and Zimiles (1969) and Zimiles (1967) contrasted the effects of "modern" (i.e., emphasizing the development of thought and learning processes) versus "traditional" (i.e., oriented to fact-acquisition) school environments. Modern and traditional were operationally defined in terms of three criteria: (1) how much a school used the surrounding environment as part of the educational experience; (2) how much it focused on current social events and problems; and (3) to what degree it encouraged innovative teaching approaches. Interpersonally, children from modern schools were found to have more differentiated self-images, greater acceptance of negative impulses, stronger investment in their status as children, and more openness about their sex role images. Cognitively, they were more independent, analytic thinkers, who pursued ideas more seriously.

Similarly, Reiss and his co-workers (Reiss & Dyhdalo, 1975; Reiss & Martell, 1974) examined correlates of open-space versus contained educational environments. They found open-space children to have greater oral fluency, to persist longer, and to be more imaginative. But it was not entirely a one-way street. Children entering self-contained classes during the school year found it easier than those coming into open classes to be accepted and to make friends.

Knowing a system's properties and effects are key stepping stones to its constructive modification. Susskind (1969) documents this point. He studied children's curiosity behavior, an end that educators universally value (as an abstraction). Since children's curiosity shows up in the questions they ask in class, Susskind explored question-asking behaviors in third- through sixth-grade social studies classes. He found that an entire class, on the average, asked less than two questions during a 30-minute observation unit. During that same period, teachers averaged 50 questions. These "facts" differed sharply both from teachers' prior estimates of the actual frequency of children's questions and their opinions about what was ideal in this area. Thus, there was a sharp discrepancy between de jure and de facto question-asking practices. A system that highly valued children's curiosity, as an abstraction, failed to produce it. Moreover, content-analysis showed that most teacher questions called for fact and memory rather than reflection and thought.

Pinning down a hidden regularity of the educational system helped Susskind to formulate a program to align behaviors with expressed values. He trained a small group of teachers to modify their question-posing and discussion-leading techniques to encourage children's curiosity. As teachers shifted from fact-oriented to process-centered questions children came to ask more questions. A system flaw had been detected and corrected and, as a result, children's curiosity behavior was freed.

Although the discussion has thus far emphasized school environments, similar thinking can be applied to family environments. Jacob's (1975) review summarizes recent knowledge about interaction patterns in normal and pathological families. Lennard and Bernstein (1969) studied a variety of healthy and pathological family environments and interaction patterns as they relate to children's development. Illustratively, they compared interaction dimensions in families of normal and schizophrenic children. The former, contrasted with the latter, showed (a) greater emphasis on self-initiated, as opposed to responsive, behaviors; (b) socialization, learning, role-expectancy, and behavior standards that were more age-appropriate; (c) better, and more open, lines of communication; (d) more support; and (e) less discord and stress. Lennard and Bernstein's findings suggest that patterns of family interactions have distinct child correlates. Such linkages must be established for planful, informed efforts to promote health-favoring family structures, through education, consultation and other approaches. Understanding family structures and their effects, and how to modify them, offers an intriguing route for promoting well-being and positive adaptation before disaster strikes.

Social environments thus have differentiating properties that affect how children behave and perform in them. But these aren't always simple. A facilitating environment for one child may be chaotic for another. This complication defines the "ecological-match" problem, i.e., the goodness of the child-environment fit. Edney's (1974) review suggests that we know more about such ecological matches in plants and animals than in humans. Even so, several examples of informative applications of the ecological approach to children can be cited. Grimes and Allinsmith (1961) found that compulsive-anxious school children compared to age peers without such qualities, fared better in a highly structured educational environment than in an unstructured one. Reiss and Martell (1974) report a similar finding. Children educated in open-space classes persisted more on difficult tasks than those educated in contained environments; moreover, persistence and academic achievement correlated more closely for them. Yet, *non*persistent (i.e., distractible) children had *higher* educational achievement scores, when educated in self-contained, compared to open classes. Findings such as the latter prompted Reiss and Martell to conclude that multitracked educational options were needed to meet children's diverse needs and styles.

Kelly (1968, 1969) has been an active spokesman for an ecological approach in mental health. He and his colleagues have focused on the types of adaptations generated by stable and fluid school environments (Kelly et al., 1971) defined operationally by annual pupil turnover rates of less than 10% and more than 42%, respectively. They assumed that a given student's characteristics could be adaptive in one environment and maladaptive in another. Differences consistent with an ecological view were found. New students were more readily accepted in the fluid environments where student groups were permeable. Whereas personal development factors were highly valued in the fluid environment, status and achievement were more important in the stable one. Kelly's findings suggest the need for social engineering that maximizes the adaptation of, and benefits to, system members.

The main points established by the work reviewed are that (1) attributes of social systems that affect development can be identified; (2) system qualities seem to be associated with beneficial or detrimental person-outcomes; and (3) the person-system ecological-match is an important determinant of outcomes. Since systems have important effects on people (especially on young children in their formative periods), the more we can develop and use skills to understand them and their consequences, the more likely it is that health-promoting social environments—a key goal of primary prevention—can be created. The proposed pathway illustrates a valid, thus far underutilized, community-anchored alternative to traditional and/or community mental health approaches to children's services, that calls for new skills and training.

Competence and Adjustment

Many eminent military strategists and athletic coaches have argued that, in *their* spheres of operation: "A good offense is the best of all defenses!" Unhappily, that view has not yet made major inroads in child mental health, where past efforts and resources have been invested in trying to comprehend and contain casualty. It is appealing, conceptually, to think that a child who acquires core adaptive skills from the start might thereby also build in the best of all the defenses against problems (Murphy & Chandler, 1972). That position puts a higher priority on educational approaches (e.g., training adaptive skills) than on treating dysfunction; it harbors the intriguing possibility that maladjustment might best be engaged by never engaging it at all. The potential savings in human misery and ineffectiveness, let alone dollars, from this approach more than justifies its consideration. To realize it would go beyond prevention. With truly competent, adapted children, little would remain to be prevented.

Key questions that this view poses include: (1) What "gut" adaptive skills underlie effective adjustment? (2) Are there linkages between specific skill deficiencies and types of maladjustment? (3) Can curriculum be developed in these skill areas and taught effectively to young children? (4) Does skill acquisition improve interpersonal adjustment and/or reduce maladjustment? Positive answers to these questions would richly document the efficacy of primary prevention.

Ojemann's (1961, 1969) program to develop a "causal" teaching approach is an early example of this approach. Causal education, as the name suggests, emphasizes an orientation to causes, understandings, and analytic processes in contrast to a "surface" approach that seeks to impart facts. Ojemann believes that causal teaching helps the child to acquire analytic skills and competencies needed to cope effectively with later adaptive demands. Thus, he perceives linkages between curriculum and skill acquisition on the one side, and adjustment on the other. A variety of "effects" of causal teaching programs have been tracked, by comparing matched groups of children who did and did not participate in them, on many criteria. Children exposed to the approach clearly acquired the causal mode, were better able to generalize knowledge and weigh alternatives, became more sensitive to the factors that underlie behavior, and had lower scores on measures of arbitrary punitiveness and authoritarianism.

Several studies (Bruce, 1958; Muuss, 1960; Griggs & Bonney, 1970) have looked at personal adjustment consequences of causal teaching. Bruce (1958), for example, found that sixth-grade students in a causal teaching program had lower anxiety, and higher security, scores than nonexposed control peers. Similarly, Muuss (1960) found that a "causal" group of fifth- and sixth-graders had healthier adjustment profiles than a matched control group and significantly lower anxiety and insecurity scores. Griggs and Bonney (1970) found that a fourth- and fifth-grade group of pupils in a causal thinking program significantly exceeded controls on sociometric and self-ideal congruence measures and on an overall adjustment index. Thus, data based on an educational (curricular) approach suggest that acquiring analytic, problem-engaging skills establishes a basal competence in the child that can radiate positively to adjustment. However, as Zax and Specter (1974) note, only a minor segment of Ojemann and his followers work includes dependent measures of adjustment.

Spivack and Shure (1974) have taken a further dramatic step in that direction. On the basis of a long line of prior research, their own and others, they argue that children's social problem-solving skills are critical mediators of adjustment. In the past psychologists have been more concerned with *impersonal* problem solving (e.g., how we do puzzles and anagrams, how we reason and form concepts) than social problem solving. Spivack and Shure suggest that the latter skills (e.g., sensitivity to human problems, ability to perceive alternatives, ability to "read" means-end relations and the effects of one's behavior on others) are largely unrelated to impersonal problem solving but are indispensable for effective adaptation.

Hence, they reasoned that if young children could really acquire social problem-solving skills, such knowledge should generalize to other interpersonal situations and improve their overt behavior. The authors developed a two-stage curriculum for teaching social problem-solving skills to young children, based on interesting, enjoyable games and dialogues designed to impart word concepts and cognitive skills. The 46 daily lessons, each requiring 5 to 20 minutes, were taught over a 10- to 12-week period. Early lessons emphasized requisite skills, i.e., listening, attending, and such instrumental concepts as negation, similarity and difference, and amount. Later lessons directly taught prime social problem-solving skills—e.g., alternative, causal, and consequential thinking. Teachers taught the lessons to small ($N = 6$ to 8) mixed-sex groups including both responsive and nonresponsive children. The main study included more than 200, 4-year-old inner-city, Head-Start children from Philadelphia, half experimentals who received the social problem-solving training and half demographically matched nonprogram controls.

Without question, the teaching "took," i.e., at the end of the program the social problem-solving skills of the experimental subjects were significantly superior to those of the controls. They also had fewer superfluous, irrelevant responses or forceful, aggressive problem solutions. These positive program effects were found in children of low-average intelligence as well as the very bright. Follow-up, in kindergarten six months later, showed the gains to be stable (Shure & Spivack, 1975a). A program extension, in which inner-city mothers were trained to teach their own children social problem-solving skills (Shure & Spivack, 1975b), also yielded encouraging preliminary findings.

The first hint at a linkage between social problem solving and adjustment came from behavior ratings submitted by teachers. Based on preprogram ratings, children were classified as adjusted or maladjusted, the latter including inhibited and impulsive subgroups. Maladjusted children, particularly inhibited ones, gained the most in social problem-solving skills. This did not happen with initially maladjusted control children. Equally interesting, program children, compared to controls, showed significant competence gains in several areas not directly related to the program (e.g., concern for others, taking initiative, and autonomous behavior). On those measures, too, initially maladjusted children gained the most. Finally, a significant relation between acquiring social problem-solving skills and improved adjustment was found.

Since Spivack and Shure represented their program to teachers and school administrators as educational, rather than adjustment-related, their findings are even more striking. The competence base established in children by acquiring social problem-solving skills apparently radiated positively to other important life adjustments. Without directly engaging symptoms, they were reduced by training a critical competence. This approach models a brand of primary prevention that merits extensive future investment. Can a competence-building approach loosen the shackles that have fettered the mental health profession to an unyielding reactive stance?

A related conceptual thrust is reflected in a recent, phenotypically distant, but genotypically related, project with the inner-city poor. Rappaport, Davidson, Wilson, and Mitchell (1975) describe the Community Psychology Action Center (CPAC), a setting designed to identify existing competency bases in the community and to strengthen their development. These workers eschew a "blaming-the-victim" view of the poor (Ryan, 1971) and carefully avoid shaping poor people to fit an existing system. Instead, the styles and cultural values of inner-city folk are accepted as they are and an attempt is made to amplify the culture by broadening its competency bases to new areas. Problems, as traditionally defined, are not dealt with. The goal is to foster independence and positive behaviors. Implicit is the view that developing people's strengths is the best way for them to engage problems.

Stamps (1975), in a further experimental application of this view, used self-reinforcement methods to teach 37 inner-city fourth graders realistic goal setting behaviors. Through this training, the children learned to set more accurate goals. One consequence was that their achievement test scores improved significantly. Important gains were also found in behavior and personality. Teachers observed fewer behavior problems in program children after the new skill was acquired. On a locus of control measure, the children took greater responsibility for negative outcomes and they showed growth on test measures of openness, awareness, and self-acceptance. These gains remained after two school years. Rooting a gut competence in disadvantaged children thus contributed to better academic performance and radiated positively to adjustment.

The way we have thus far presented various approaches may unintentionally imply that they are incompatible with each other. That is not so. Community mental health (restorative) and community psychology (building) programs can exist side by side—indeed, they can be mutually supportive and enhancing. This is shown in a recent comprehensive report by Allen, Chinsky, Larcen, Lochman and Selinger (1976), who developed a three-tiered program to address a single elementary school's problems in a realistic way. The program included (1) primary prevention via social problem-solving training, (2) a student-companion project (secondary prevention) for identified, socially isolated, maladapted youngsters, and (3) a consultation program for teachers to improve classroom handling of children with acting out and/or learning problems.

Social problem-solving training for 9- and 10-year-olds covered six main areas, among them generating alternative solutions and considering consequences. Videotape modeling, shaping exercises, follow-up (practice) exercises, and classroom assessment were used as training devices. Children readily acquired these new skills. Several adjustment-related variables were also studied for potential spill-over effects from the problem-solving training. Some changed, others didn't! For example, children who went through problem-solving training, when compared to controls, became more "internally oriented" on a measure of locus of control. In addition, they developed more positive expectancies about future school experiences.

Secondary prevention was approached through a college-student companion program, for children identified by teachers as deficient in social skills. In a marriage of behavioral and community approaches, companions were trained in social reinforcement and modeling techniques. Target behaviors relating specifically to the child's class maladaptation were selected and interventions to improve these behaviors were designed. Program children increased their social interactions in playground recreational situations. Changes on other adjustment measures were not consistent. Student companions who were *not* impartial observers reported significant increases in the children's positive behaviors (e.g., warmth, cooperativeness) and decreases in negative behaviors (e.g., withdrawal, fearfulness) following the program.

The third program component, done in workshop style, was a behaviorally oriented training and consultation program for teachers. Both program and control teachers were asked to identify the six most disruptive and/or study-skill deficient children in their class. Half became target children on whom the intervention focused and the others became in-class controls. Ten 1-½-hour teacher training workshops were held, emphasizing behavior modification and classroom management techniques. The workshops also gave teachers a chance to discuss their program experiences.

Direct classroom observation showed, first, that teacher behaviors changed in anticipated directions (e.g., more verbal reinforcement, less nonverbal attention). Moreover, target children's "on-task" appropriate behaviors increased significantly compared to controls, an improvement that was still evident at follow-up. Target children also decreased in passive "off-task" and aggressive behaviors. Teachers were able to reduce specific negative target behaviors, for example, inappropriate verbalizations and incomplete assignments. An interesting secondary finding was that designated within-class controls *also* improved significantly, compared to nonprogram controls. Although the program was not directed to these youngsters, the teachers' newly acquired behavioral technology and class management skills apparently radiated positively to them. Behavioral measures again showed more improvement than secondary test measures.

Allen and co-workers' (1976) comprehensive program is a fluidly interconnected network, anchored in reality and addressed to real-world problems. Its components, ranging from bona fide primary prevention to helping visibly maladapted children, offer a multi-tiered package that differs qualitatively from other programs in this field. Although their study is not without problems, it models future community approaches and offers a genuine alternative to traditional delivery modes.

Primary prevention and competence training are not new ideas. The difference today is that instead of just talking reverently about them, we have begun to develop the methodologies and research base needed to anchor them more firmly. Consistent with mental health's past inclination to define its mission as combating pathology, Hollister (1967) noted that the English language doesn't even *contain* a concept to describe the antithesis of trauma—that is, a strength-producing experience. He has therefore coined the term *stren*. Finkel (1974) showed that strens could be studied empirically and argued that the concept was important for primary prevention. Beyond further development of the language and concepts of competence, we need supporting methodologies. We are far more skilled at measuring children's problems and maladaptive behaviors than their resources and competencies. A paradigm for the latter is Gesten's (1976) recent development of a five-factor measure of young children's school-related competencies. This measure can be used: (1) to study relations between children's strengths and school performance; (2) as a metric for establishing positive intervention goals; and (3) to evaluate growth following intervention, in other than symptom-reduction terms.

It would be a good thing for mental health if our concepts, language, and programs—some major portion of our total investment—could move toward primary prevention and the establishment of competencies in children. Important modeling steps have been taken in that direction, with gratifying outcomes. This development provides the sharpest contrast yet identified to past-traditional diagnostic-therapeutic approaches in child psychopathology. Its doubtless illusory but nevertheless intriguing ultimate goal is to render the area of child psychopathology obsolescent.

SUMMARY

Community approaches in child mental health do not start in a vacuum. They are part of a groping, evolving effort to deal with the serious problems and insufficiencies of existing child mental health serving systems. The community is not an end. Rather it offers a means to augment the scope and effectiveness of past efforts and to develop and evaluate genuine conceptual alternatives to past approaches.

The term community approaches is too broad to be useful. It has been broken down into two main components—i.e., community mental health (restorative) approaches and community psychology or psychiatry (building) approaches. Community mental health's broadening options include systematic early detection and intervention, widespread use of nonprofessional and atraditional help-agents, changing professional roles, consultation, and crisis intervention. Community psychology approaches are based on different assumptions and methodologies, as, for example, social system analysis and modification and building competencies. Its activities, much closer to primary prevention, differ sharply from what mental health people have been trained to do, and have done, in the past.

Individually or together, these community approaches provide a real alternative to past ways in child mental health. Weaknesses in the existing system, the conceptual appeal of the community approach, and the slow accumulation of effectiveness data for these approaches converge to suggest that children's well-being may better be served in the future by a substantial reallocation of effort, within a resource-limited child mental health portfolio, to these newly evolving alternatives.

REFERENCES

ALBEE, G. W. *Mental health manpower trends.* New York: Basic Books, 1959.

ALLEN, G. J., CHINSKY, J. M., LARCEN, S. W., LOCHMAN, J. E., and SELINGER, H. V. *Community psychology and the schools: A behaviorally oriented multi-level preventive approach.* Hillsdale, N.J.: Lawrence Erlbaum Associates, 1976.

ARNHOFF, F. N., RUBENSTEIN, E. A., and SPEISMAN, J. C. *Manpower for mental health.* Chicago: Aldine Publishing Co., 1969.

BARDON, J. I. School psychology and school psychologists. *American Psychologist*, 1968, *23*, 187–194.

BARKER, R. G., and GUMP, P. *Big school, small school.* Stanford, Cal.: Stanford University Press, 1964.

BARKER, R. G., and SCHOGGEN, P. *Qualities of community life.* San Francisco: Jossey-Bass, 1973.

BEISER, A. R. *Mental health consultation and education.* Palo Alto, Cal.: National Press Books, 1972.

BERGIN, A. E. The evaluation of therapeutic outcomes. In A. E. Bergin and S. L. Garfield (Eds.), *Handbook of psychotherapy and behavior change: An empirical analysis.* New York: John Wiley, 1971.

BERGIN, A. E., and SUINN, R. M. Individual psychotherapy and behavior therapy. In M. R. Rosenzweig and L. C. Porter (Eds.), *Annual Review of Psychology*, 1975, *26*, 509–556.

BOWER, E. M. *Early identification of emotionally handicapped children in school* (2nd ed.). Springfield, Ill.: Charles C. Thomas Publisher, 1969.

BOWER, E. M., and LAMBERT, N. M. *A process for in-school screening of children with emotional handicaps.* Sacramento, Cal.: California State Department of Education, 1961.

BROWNBRIDGE, R., and VAN VLEET, P. (Eds.). *Investments in prevention: The prevention of learning and behavior problems in young children.* San Francisco: Pace ID Center, 1969.

BRUCE, P. Relationship of self-acceptance to other variables with sixth grade children oriented in self-understanding. *Journal of Educational Psychology*, 1958, *49*, 229–238.

CAPLAN, G. *Principles of preventive psychiatry.* New York: Basic Books, 1964.

CAPLAN, G. *Theories of mental health consultation.* New York: Basic Books, 1970.

CLARIZIO, H. F. Stability of deviant behavior through time. In H. F. Clarizio (Ed.), *Mental health and the educative process.* Chicago: Rand McNally, 1969.

COWEN, E. L. Emergent approaches to mental health problems: An overview and directions for future work. In E. L. Cowen, E. A. Gardner, and M. Zax (Eds.), *Emergent approaches to mental health problems.* New York: Appleton-Century-Crofts, 1967.

COWEN, E. L. Social and community interventions. In P. Mussen and M. Rosenzweig (Eds.), *Annual Review of Psychology*, 1973, *24*, 423–472.

COWEN, E. L., DORR, D., and POKRACKI, F. Selection of nonprofessional child-aides for a school mental health project. *Community Mental Health Journal*, 1972, *8*, 220–226.

COWEN, E. L., and LORION, R. P. Changing roles for the school mental health professional. *Journal of School Psychology*, 1976, *14*, 131–137.

COWEN, E. L., LORION, R. P., KRAUS, R. M., and DORR, D. Geometric expansion of helping resources. *Journal of School Psychology*, 1974, *12*, 288–295.

COWEN, E. L., TROST, M. A., LORION, R. P., DORR, D., IZZO, L. D., and ISAACSON, R. V. *New ways in school mental health: Early detection and prevention of school maladaptation.* New York: Human Sciences, Inc., 1975.

CUMMING, J., and CUMMING, E. *Ego and milieu: Theory and practice of environmental therapy.* New York: Atherton, 1966.

DONAHUE, G. T. A school district program for schizophrenic, organic and seriously disturbed children. In E. L. Cowen, E. A. Gardner, and M. Zax (Eds.), *Emergent approaches to mental health problems.* New York: Appleton-Century-Crofts, 1967.

DONAHUE, G. T., and Nichtern, S. *Teaching the troubled child.* New York: Free Press, 1965.

DORR, D. An ounce of prevention. *Mental Hygiene*, 1972, *56*, 25–27.

DUGGAN, J. N. An example of secondary prevention activities in the schools: Talent searching in a culturally deprived population. In N. M. Lambert (Ed.), *The protection and promotion of mental health in schools.* Bethesda, Md.: U. S. Dept. of Health, Education and Welfare, Public Health Service Publication No. 1226, 1965.

EDNEY, J. J. Human territoriality. *Psychological Bulletin*, 1974, *81*, 959–975.

ERIKSON, E. H. *Identity and the life cycle.* New York: International Universities Press, Psychology Issues Monograph No. 1, 1959.

FINKEL, N. J. Strens and traumas: An attempt at categorization. *American Journal of Community Psychology*, 1974, *2*, 265–275.

FISHMAN, J. R., DENHAM, W. H., LEVINE, M., and SHATZ, E. O. *New careers for the disadvantaged in human services: Report of social experiment.* Washington, D.C.: Howard University Institute for Youth Studies, 1969.

GARTNER, A. *Paraprofessionals and their performance.* New York: Praeger, 1971.

GESTEN, E. A health resources inventory: The development of a measure of the personal and social competence of primary grade children. *Journal of Consulting and Clinical Psychology*, 1976, *44*, 775–786.

GILDEA, M. L., GLIDEWELL, J. C., and KANTOR, M. B. The St. Louis school mental health project: History and evaluation. In E. L. Cowen, E. A. Gardner, and M. Zax (Eds.), *Emergent approaches to mental health problems.* New York: Appleton-Century-Crofts, 1967.

GLIDEWELL, J. C., and SWALLOW, C. S. *The prevalence of maladjustment in elementary schools: A report prepared for the Joint Commission on the mental health of children.* Chicago: University of Chicago Press, 1969.

GOLDENBERG, I. I. The Residential Youth Center: The creation of an assumptions-questioning rehabilitative setting. In *Criminal corrections in Connecticut: Perspectives and progress.* West Hartford, Conn.: Connecticut Planning Committee on Criminal Administration, 1968.

GOLDENBERG, I. I. *Build me a mountain: Youth, poverty and the creation of new settings.* Cambridge, Mass.: M.I.T. Press, 1971.

GOTTFRIED, N. W. Effects of early intervention programs. In K. S. Miller and R. M. Dreger (Eds.), *Comparative studies of blacks and whites in the United States: Quantitative studies in social relations.* New York: Seminar Press, 1973.

GRIGGS, J. W., and BONNEY, M. E. Relationship between "causal" orientation and acceptance of others, "self-ideal self" congruency and mental health changes for fourth and fifth grade children. *Journal of Educational Research,* 1970, *63,* 471–477.

GRIMES, J. W., and ALLINSMITH, W. Compulsivity, anxiety, and school achievement. *Merrill-Palmer Quarterly,* 1961, *7,* 247–261.

GUERNEY, B. G. *Psychotherapeutic agents: New roles for non-professionals, parents and teachers.* New York: Holt, Rinehart & Winston, 1969.

GURIN, G., VEROFF, J., and FELD, S. *Americans view their mental health: A nationwide interview survey.* New York: Basic Books, 1960.

HOBBS, N. Helping disturbed children: Psychological and ecological strategies. *American Psychologist,* 1966, *21,* 1105–1115.

HOBBS, N. The reeducation of emotionally disturbed children. In E. M. Bower and W. G. Hollister (Eds.), *Behavior science frontiers in education.* New York: John Wiley, 1967.

HOLLINGSHEAD, A. B., and REDLICH, F. C. *Social class and mental illness: A community study.* New York: John Wiley, 1958.

HOLLISTER, W. G. Concept of strens in education: A challenge to curriculum development. In E. M. Bower and W. G. Hollister (Eds.), *Behavioral science frontiers in education.* New York: John Wiley, 1967.

INSEL, P. M., and MOOS, R. H. Psychosocial environments: Expanding the scope of human ecology. *American Psychologist,* 1974, *29,* 179–188.

JACOB, T. Family interaction in disturbed and normal families. *Psychological Bulletin,* 1975, *82,* 33–65.

JASON, L. Early secondary prevention with disadvantaged preschool children. *American Journal of Community Psychology,* 1975, *3,* 33–46.

Joint Commission on Mental Illness and Health. *Action for mental health.* New York: Basic Books, 1961.

KELLAM, S. G., BRANCH, J. D., AGRAWAL, K. C., and ENSMINGER, M. E. *Mental health and going to school: The Woodlawn program of assessment, early intervention, and evaluation.* Chicago: University of Chicago Press, 1975.

KELLY, J. G. Towards an ecological conception of preventive interventions. In J. W. Carter (Ed.), *Research contributions from psychology to community mental health.* New York: Behavioral Publications, 1968.

KELLY, J. G. Naturalistic observations in contrasting social environments. In E. P. Willems and H. L. RAUSH (Eds.), *Naturalistic viewpoints in psychological research.* New York: Holt, Rinehart & Winston, 1969.

KELLY, J. G., EDWARDS, D. W., FATKE, R., GORDON, T. A., MCGEE, D. P., MCCLINTOCK, S. K., NEWMAN, B. M., RICE, R. R., ROISTACHER, R. C., and TODD, D. M. The coping process in varied high school environments. In M. J. Feldman (Ed.), *Studies in psychotherapy and behavior change, No. 2: Theory and research in community mental health.* Buffalo, N.Y.: State University of New York, 1971.

Lennard, H. L., and Bernstein, A. *Patterns in human interaction.* San Francisco: Jossey-Bass, 1969.

Levitt, E. E. Research on psychotherapy with children. In A. E. Bergin and S. L. Garfield (Eds.), *Handbook of psychotherapy and behavior change: An empirical analysis.* New York: John Wiley, 1971.

Lewis, W. W. Project Re-ED: Educational intervention in discordant child rearing systems. In E. L. Cowen, E. A. Gardner, and M. Zax (Eds.), *Emergent approaches to mental health problems.* New York: Appleton-Century-Crofts, 1967.

Lindemann, E. Symptomatology and management of acute grief. *American Journal of Psychiatry*, 1944, *101*, 141–148.

Lorion, R. P. Socioeconomic status and traditional treatment approaches reconsidered. *Psychological Bulletin*, 1973, *79*, 263–270.

Lorion, R. P., Cowen, E. L., and Caldwell, R. A. Problem types of children referred to a school based mental health program. *Journal of Consulting and Clinical Psychology*, 1974, *42*, 491–496.

Lorion, R. P., Cowen, E. L., and Kraus, R. M. Some hidden regularities in a school based mental health project. *Journal of Consulting and Clinical Psychology*, 1974, *42*, 346–352.

Magoon, T. M., Golann, S. E., and Freeman, R. W. *Mental health counselors at work.* New York: Pergamon, 1969.

Mannino, F. V., MacLennan, B. W., and Shore, M. F. *The practice of mental health consultation.* New York: Gardner Press, 1975.

Melamed, B. G., and Siegel, L. J. Reduction of anxiety in children facing hospitalization and surgery by use of filmed modeling. *Journal of Consulting and Clinical Psychology*, 1975, *43*, 511–521.

Minuchin, P., Biber, B., Shapiro, E., and Zimiles, H. *The psychological impact of school experience.* New York: Basic Books, 1969.

Moos, R. H. Conceptualizations of human environments. *American Psychologist*, 1973, *28*, 652–665.

Moos, R. H. *The social climate scales: An overview.* Palo Alto, Cal.: Consulting Psychologists Press, Inc., 1974.

Moos, R. H., and Insel, P. M. *Issues in social ecology: Human milieus.* Palo Alto, Cal.: National Press Books, 1974.

Moos, R. H., and Trickett, E. J. *Manual for the Class Environment Scale.* Palo Alto, Cal.: Consulting Psychologists Press, Inc., 1974.

Murphy, L. B., and Chandler, C. A. Building foundations for strength in the preschool years: Preventing developmental disturbances. In S. E. Golann and C. Eisdorfer (Eds.) *Handbook of community mental health.* New York: Appleton-Century-Crofts, 1972.

Muuss, R. E. The effects of a one- and two-year causal learning program. *Journal of Personality*, 1960, *28*, 479–491.

Nathan, P. E., Andberg, M. M., Behan, P. O., and Patch, V. D. Thirty-two observers and one patient: A study of diagnostic reliability. *Journal of Clinical Psychology*, 1969, *25*, 9–15.

Newman, R. G. *Psychological consultation in the schools.* New York: Basic Books, 1967.

Newton, M. R., and Brown, R. D. A preventive approach to developmental problems in school children. In E. M. Bower and W. G. Hollister (Eds.), *Behavior science frontiers in education.* New York: John Wiley, 1967.

Ojemann, R. H. Investigations on the effects of teacher understanding and appreciation of behavior dynamics. In G. Caplan (Ed.), *Prevention of mental disorders in children.* New York: Basic Books, 1961.

Ojemann, R. H. Incorporating psychological concepts in the school curriculum. In H. F. Clarizio (Ed.), *Mental health and the educative process.* Chicago: Rand-McNally, 1969.

Price, R. H., and Blashfield, R. K. Explorations in the taxonomy of behavior settings: Analysis of dimensions and classification of settings. *American Journal of Community Psychology*, 1975, *3*, 335–357.

PRICE, R. H., and MOOS, R. H. Toward a taxonomy of inpatient treatment environments. *Journal of Abnormal Psychology*, 1975, *84*, 181–188.

RAE-GRANT, Q., and STRINGER, L. A. Mental health programs in schools. In M. F. Shore and F. V. Mannino (Eds.), *Mental health and the community: Problems, programs and strategies*. New York: Behavioral Publications, 1969.

RAPPAPORT, J., DAVIDSON, W. S., WILSON, M. N., and MITCHELL, A. Alternatives to blaming the victim or the environment: Our places to stand have not moved the earth. *American Psychologist*, 1975, *30*, 525–528.

REIFF, R., and RIESSMAN, F. The indigenous nonprofessional: A strategy of change in community action and community mental health programs. *Community Mental Health Journal*, Monograph No. 1, 1965.

REISS, S., and DYHDALO, N. Persistence, achievement, and open-space environments. *Journal of Educational Psychology*, 1975, *67*, 506–513.

REISS, S., and MARTELL, R. Educational and psychological effects of open space education in Oak Park, Ill.: Final Report to Board of Education, District 97, Oak Park, Illinois, 1974.

RIESSMAN, F. The "helper" therapy principle. *Social Work*, 1965, *10*, 27–32.

RIESSMAN, F., COHEN, J., and PEARL, A. (Eds.). *Mental health of the poor*. New York: Free Press, 1964.

RIOCH, M. J. Pilot projects in training mental health counselors. In E. L. Cowen, E. A. Gardner, and M. Zax (Eds.), *Emergent approaches to mental health problems*. New York: Appleton-Century-Crofts, 1967.

ROBINS, L. N. *Deviant children grown up*. Baltimore: Williams & Wilkins, 1966.

RYAN, W. *Blaming the victim*. New York: Random House, 1971.

SANDLER, I. N. Characteristics of women working as child-aides in a school based preventive mental health program. *Journal of Consulting and Clinical Psychology*, 1972, *36*, 56–61.

SANUA, V. D. Sociocultural aspects of psychotherapy and treatment: A review of the literature. In L. E. Abt and L. Bellak (Eds.), *Progress in clinical psychology* (Vol. VIII). New York: Grune and Stratton, 1966.

SARASON, S. B. *The culture of the school and the problem of change*. Boston: Allyn-Bacon, 1971.

SARASON, S. B. *The creation of settings and the future societies*. San Francisco: Jossey-Bass, 1972.

SARASON, S. B., LEVINE, M., GOLDBERG, I. I., CHERLIN, D. L., and BENNETT, E. M. *Psychology in community settings*. New York: John Wiley, 1966.

SARASON, S. B., ZITNAY, G., and GROSSMAN, F. K. *The creation of a community setting*. Syracuse, N.Y.: Syracuse University Press, 1971.

SHURE, M. B., and SPIVACK, G. *A preventive mental health program for young "inner city" children: The second (kindergarten) year*. Paper presented at the American Psychological Association, Chicago, 1975. (a)

SHURE, M. B., and SPIVACK, G. *Training mothers to help their children solve real-life problems*. Paper presented at the Society for Research in Child Development, Denver, Colo., 1975. (b)

SMITH, M. B., and HOBBS, F. The community and the community mental health center. *American Psychologist*, 1966, *21*, 499–509.

SOBEY, F. *The nonprofessional revolution in mental health*. New York: Columbia University Press, 1970.

SPIVACK, G., and SHURE, M. B. *Social adjustment of young children*. San Francisco: Jossey-Bass, 1974.

STAMPS, L. W. *Enhancing success in school for deprived children by teaching realistic goal setting*. Paper presented at Society for Research in Child Development, Denver, 1975.

STENDLER-LAVATELLI, C. B. Environmental intervention in infancy and early childhood. In M. Deutsch, I. Katz, and A. R. Jensen (Eds.), *Social class, race, and psychological development*. New York: Holt, Rinehart & Winston, 1968.

SUSSKIND, E. C. *Questioning and curiosity in the elementary school classroom.* Unpublished Ph.D. dissertation, Yale University, 1969.

TRICKETT, E. J., and MOOS, R. H. The social environment of junior high and high school classrooms. *Journal of Educational Psychology*, 1973, *65*, 93–102.

TRICKETT, E. J., and MOOS, R. H. Personal correlates of contrasting environments: Student satisfaction in high school classrooms. *American Journal of Community Psychology*, 1974, *2*, 1–12.

WEINSTEIN, L. Project Re-Ed schools for emotionally disturbed children: Effectiveness as viewed by referring agencies, parents and teachers. *Exceptional Children*, 1969, *35*, 703–711.

ZAX, M., and COWEN, E. L. *Abnormal psychology: Changing conceptions* (2nd ed.) New York: Holt, Rinehart & Winston, 1976.

ZAX, M., and SPECTER, G. A. *An introduction to community psychology.* New York: John Wiley, 1974.

ZIMILES, H. Preventive aspects of school experience. In E. L. Cowen, E. A. Gardner, and M. Zax (Eds.), *Emergent approaches to mental health problems.* New York: Appleton-Century-Crofts, 1967.

II

TREATMENT OF SPECIFIC PROBLEMS

8

MINIMAL BRAIN DYSFUNCTION

Gail E. Solomon

Minimal brain dysfunction (MBD) is not a disease but a syndrome with various manifestations including many learning disabilities and behavioral abnormalities, such as hyperactivity, distractibility, and low frustration tolerance. These symptoms are associated with central nervous system signs. The constellation of nervous system signs usually includes poor fine motor coordination, increased adventitious movements, awkward gait, and visual-motor and auditory perceptual difficulties. These children have near average to above average intelligence and are not mentally retarded.

Historically, in the 1920s, after the epidemic of encephalitis lethargica of Von Economo, some children who recovered had a syndrome of hyperactive behavior as well as personality and learning difficulties that were not present before the illness (Leahy & Sands, 1921; Ebaugh, 1923; Bond, 1932). In 1934, Kahn and Cohen described such children as having "organic driveness." Strauss and his colleagues (Strauss & Lehtinen, 1947; Strauss & Kephart, 1955) noted that such children often had visual-motor perceptual problems, hyperactivity, distractibility, impulsiveness, emotional lability but were not mentally retarded. He suggested an educational approach to help these children. In 1962, Paine considered these symptoms as part of the entire spectrum of brain damage. Maximal damage to the motor area results in cerebral palsy, while minimal brain damage presents itself as clumsiness, poor fine motor coordination, and choreoathetoid movements. In 1962, Clements and Peters coined the term "minimal brain dysfunction." In 1966, Pincus and Glaser deemphasized the term "brain damaged" as "merely a label for certain kinds of aberrant behavior." Although still imperfect, brain dysfunction is a better term than brain damage, since there is no known specific pathology correlated with the clinical findings. Clements (1966) defined minimal brain dysfunction as we recognize it today in the monograph of the National Institute of Neurological Disease and Blindness (NINDB). The ten characteristics of minimal brain dysfunction most often cited in order of frequency in the NINDB monograph include:

Ten Characteristics of Minimal Brain Dysfunction

1. Hyperactivity
2. Perceptual motor impairment
3. Emotional lability

4. General coordination deficits
5. Disorders of attention (short attention span, distractibility, perseveration)
6. Impulsivity
7. Disorders of memory and thinking
8. Specific learning disabilities
   (a) Reading
   (b) Arithmetic
   (c) Writing
   (d) Spelling
9. Disorders of speech and hearing
10. Equivocal neurological signs and electroencephalographic irregularities

INCIDENCE

Epidemiological information is meager in regard to MBD. Wender (1971) analyzed studies from Holland (Prechtl & Stemmer, 1962), St. Louis (Stewart et al., 1966), Vermont (Huessy, 1967), Montgomery County, Maryland. The diagnosis was based on minor neurological signs, teachers' reports of over-activity, short attention span, and school questionnaires. Wender found approximately a 5 to 10% incidence of serious symptomatic cases of MBD. Racial, ethnic, and socioeconomic factors were not taken into consideration in these studies. Males were affected more than females with a sex ratio of about 4 to 10 boys to 1 girl using hyperactivity as the criterion. Other studies also show a similar sex differential with between 75 and 80% of cases being males (Paine et al., 1968). This syndrome is more often seen in the first born than those later in the birth order.

DIAGNOSTIC WORK-UP: HISTORY

In the evaluation of such a child, a thorough medical history is perhaps the most important element in establishing the diagnosis and origin of the MBD syndrome. Often there is no known predisposing factor, but from the history, one can surmise a possible cause and also confirm that the symptoms may be on an organic basis rather than an emotional one.

Prenatal history should include genetic factors (Omenn, 1973). In a Swedish study by Hallgren (1950) searching for the presence of dyslexia in relatives of dyslexic children, 94 of 116 probands had one parent who was dyslexic and the other normal. Seven probands had another close relative other than a parent who was dyslexic; 3 probands had 2 dyslexic parents; whereas, 12 probands had no dyslexic relatives. Hallgren suggested an autosomal dominant inheritance pattern with stronger expressivity in males. In patients with dyslexia on a hereditary basis, 30% of the dyslexics and 9% of their siblings without reading problems have behavior problems suggestive of MBD children. Safer's study (Wender, 1973) of fostered-away full siblings and half siblings of children with MBD showed 50% of the fostered-away full siblings had MBD and 15% of half siblings were diagnosed as having MBD. The number of patients is small and the results are preliminary, but are provocative enough to urge the accumulation of more data. The other reports of possible genetic origin of the MBD syndrome are mostly anecdotal, and further epidemiological and genetic studies are necessary to establish if there is a significant genetic factor. Children with hereditary disorders may have learning problems and behavioral deviations as part of the syndrome and a detailed family history is therefore essential.

The birth history might show the infant was small for gestational age, a post-mature baby or a premature baby. Was the pregnancy complicated by drug ingestion, bleeding, toxemia or other maternal complications such as malnutrition, diabetes, or infection? At birth, was there any perinatal anoxia or low Apgar, which is felt to be a contributing factor in some cases? Was there prolonged or prominent jaundice? Was there any neonatal meningitis or hemorrhage or birth trauma?

MBD syndrome has many different causes but it is only by accumulating such data that the relative importance of each can be understood.

In the developmental history, was there a lag in achieving motor milestones? Was the child very active or very quiet, even from birth? Was there a problem in sucking? Although such landmarks as talking and walking may have been met on time, more thorough questions can be contributory: Can the child tie his shoelaces by the age of 6-½? Can he ride a two-wheeler without training wheels by 7-½? Can he perform tandem gait by the age of 7 to 8 without difficulty? Awkwardness, clumsiness, poor ball playing may be clues to some underlying neurological dysfunction early in life. A history of head trauma or meningitis or chronic ear infection should also be sought. A history of febrile seizures may be contributory.

Another essential part of the evaluation is the social history, which focuses on significant family problems, school pressures, or fears which suggest an emotional cause or at least a contributing factor toward worsening the syndrome. School reports from teachers are valuable and allow another source of information; for example, the child is compared to his peers in a situation where stimuli differ from those at home.

The Physical Examination

On the general examination, most of the children with minimal brain dysfunction (MBD) are perfectly normal. One should look very closely, however, for signs or stigmata of a generalized condition which can predispose to MBD. A classic disease which has a higher incidence of MBD is neurofibromatosis. Other neurocutaneous syndromes may also show signs of MBD. Look then for café au lait spots on the examination. Head circumference is important since a head larger by more than 2 standard deviations raises the possibility of arrested or slowly progressive hydrocephalus, which may present with poor coordination and gait disturbance. Macrocephaly or microcephaly can be indicative of organic pathology as can asymmetry of the head. Eyes are examined for pupillary asymmetry, reactions to light, strabismus, nystagmus, visual fields, and acuity. Hearing patterns should be assessed. Although all the classic signs of the neurologic exam are usually normal, "soft" neurological signs may be present. Schain (1972) states that "normative data are lacking for most soft neurological signs." The information that is available shows a wide range of variation. Motivation and experience also affect the performance. When the "soft" neurological signs are present in the child after the age of 8 years, they raise the possibility of cerebral dysfunction but are not themselves diagnostic. The soft signs referred to include awkward gait, clumsiness, increased adventitious choreiform movements of the outstretched hands, associated mirror movements of one extremity when an action is done with the other, minimal reflex asymmetry, difficulty with rapid alternating movements (dysdiadochokinesia), ocular apraxia, finger agnosia, graphesthesia, and extinction of double simultaneous stimulation.

An essential part of the exam is the assessment of the child's mental status including his speech patterns, behavior, and habits. The speech patterns should be assessed as to syntax, enunciation, and appropriate replies. It is helpful to perform screening tests for graphic skills. Problems in visual perception can be seen when a child tries to copy geometric figures. Accepted norms include being able to reproduce a circle and cross by 3 years; a square, by 4 to 5 years; a triangle, by 6 years, and by 7 to 8 years, a diamond. The Bender test for Visual Motor Gestalt, in which the child copies the figures seen on each of the nine cards, often shows a high incidence of perseveration, distortion of spatial arrangements, and rotation as well as the characteristic "dog ears" on the diamond in children who have MBD (Figure 1). The Draw-a-Person test will be helpful in establishing some estimate of intellect and the child's concept of body image with expected scores for each age. Verbal IQ is often better than performance IQ in these children. A general assessment of intellectual ability in the verbal sphere can be obtained by the Peabody Picture Vocabulary test in which the child is asked to recognize a specific picture from the test manual. It is helpful to have grade appropriate reading material available. A child with MBD may read one or two years below grade level. He should be asked to write a few sentences from which the examiner can then see if there are reversals—e.g., *b* for *d* or *p* for *q*. Mirror writing could also be seen at this time. The tendency to omit letters or substitute letters or numbers can also be seen when a child is asked to read or spell out loud as well as write.

With an older child, drawing a clock is helpful

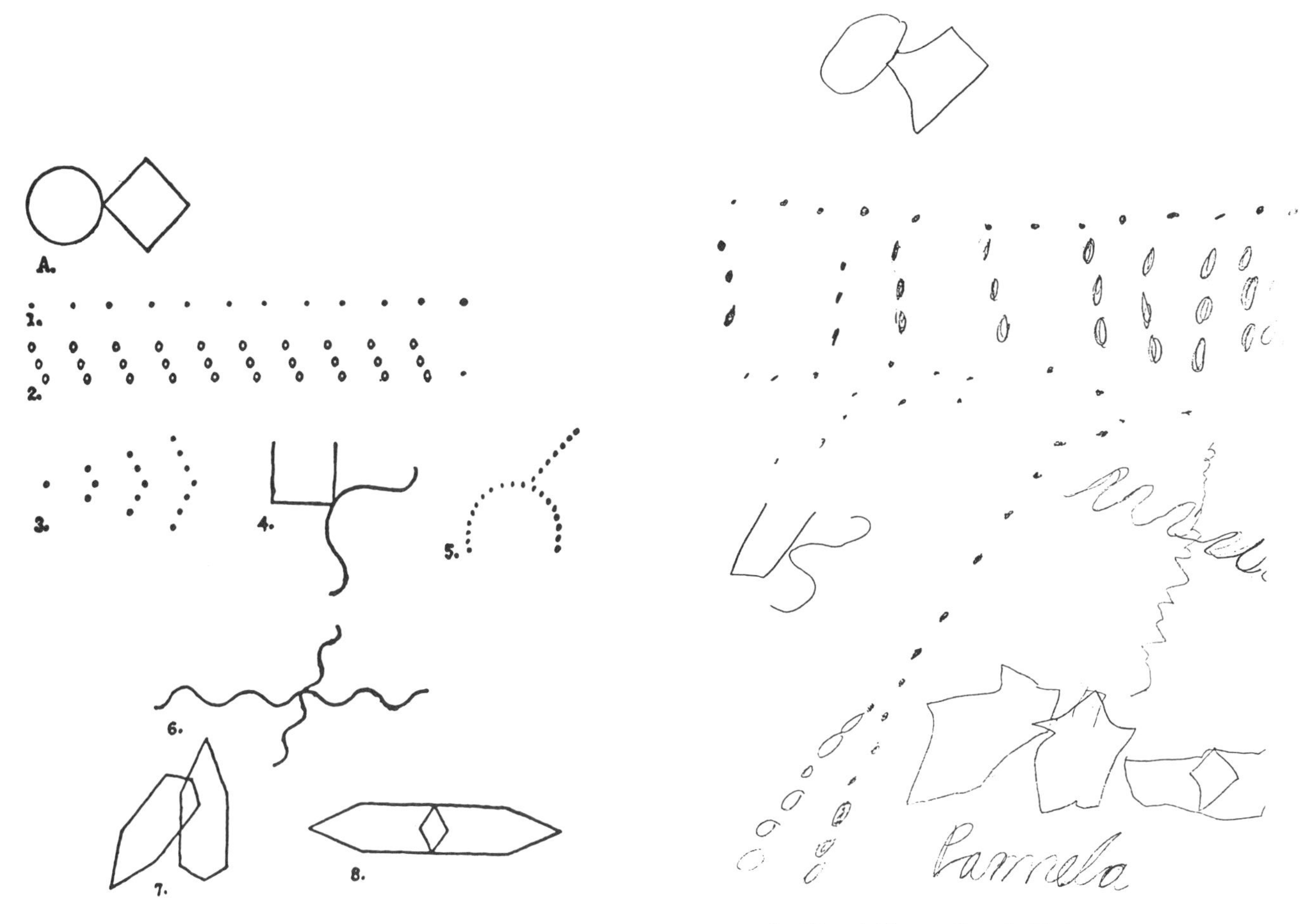

Figure 1 On the left are shown figures from the Bender Visual Motor Gestalt Test. On the right is shown an attempt to copy these figures by a 9-year-old child with MBD. (The Bender figures on the left are reproduced with permission. Bender, L. A. Visual Motor Gestalt test and its Clinical Use: Research Monograph #3, New York. American Orthopsychiatric Association, 1938).

to see if the child puts the numbers in the correct sequence and if the hands are placed appropriately for the time asked. Figure 2 shows a clock drawn by a 7-year-old child with MBD. The numbers are interchanged with letters and are on one side of the clock.

At 7 years, right-left discrimination of the child's own body parts is well established. The appearance of handedness, i.e., the preferential use of one hand is usually seen by age 5; consistent handedness is definitively established by the age of 9 years. Although delay in right-left awareness has been reported in children with reading disorders, a fixed relationship of handedness to reading disabilities has not been firmly established (Belmont & Birch, 1963).

Tests of auditory perception and auditory processing during the office examination might include the Weber and Rinne tests for hearing, and also listening to a watch. Identifying the source and the sound, localizing it, and discriminating between sounds and words is helpful. Reproducing sounds of a melody or combining speech sounds into words and understanding the meaning of different environmental sounds can test central auditory function.

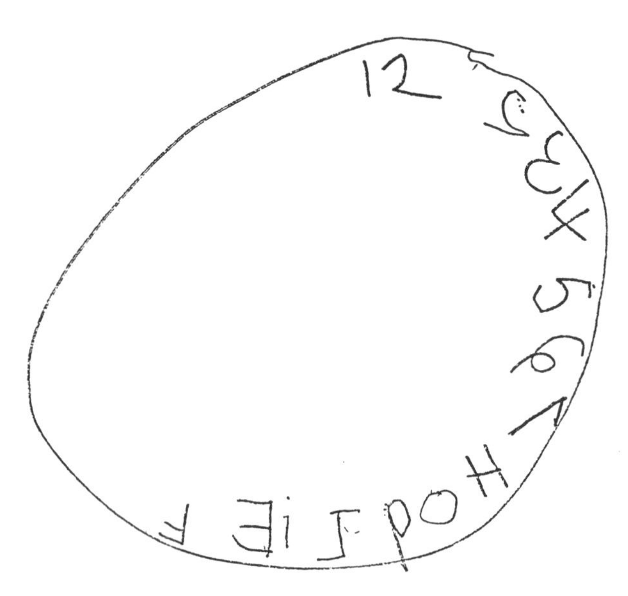

Figure 2 Clock drawn by a 7-year-old child with MBD.

Although a child is hyperkinetic in school, his behavior in the office on a one-to-one basis may be different; therefore, the history is very important. Usually, however, such a child is extremely distracted and hyperactive during the office examination. He may, for example, be putting on the water tap, getting into the instruments and constantly going from one part of the room to another without sticking to a task. Also a low frustration tolerance and a poor self-image may show through when a child is asked to do a task. Sequencing and auditory perceptual factors (remembering and localizing sounds) can be assessed by asking the child to repeat numbers.

The history and physical examination should allow the physician to rule out or consider the possibility that this syndrome might be the first sign of a more significant progressive neurologic illness. For instance, failing school work or abnormal behavior may be the first sign of a degenerative disease in the central nervous system, and in such a case, one would have a history of further neurologic signs. Follow-up visits would certainly show a progressive pattern. There might be a change in the soft signs or reflex asymmetries or changes in the fundi. Furthermore, if school or behavior problems were the first sign of a brain tumor, one might obtain a history of headaches and vomiting and see papilledema or focal neurological signs on physical examination. A child referred because of hyperactivity, inattention, or daydreaming may be having seizures such as petit mal. As part of the physical examination, therefore, the child should be hyperventilated to see if he has any clinical petit mal spells. The electroencephalogram would confirm clinical petit mal by demonstrating 3 cps spike wave discharges. A history of unprovoked stereotyped abnormal behavior with confusion afterwards raises the possibility of temporal lobe seizures and an awake and sleep EEG would be helpful in such children.

The purpose of the neurological exam in the diagnosis of MBD is twofold—to identify a child with organic brain disease who requires further diagnostic evaluation and therapy, and to eliminate the possibility of a slowly progressive organic brain disease needing immediate therapy. These include metabolic problems such as hypoglycemia, hyper- or hypo- thyroidism, chronic lead intoxication (Needleman, 1973), brain tumor, demyelinating disease, or seizure disorder.

A complete psychological evaluation is valuable; this would include intelligence testing (both verbal and nonverbal mental ability scores), academic achievement evaluated from school records, auditory and visual perceptual skills, language skills—both receptive and expressive—and fine motor abilities, as well as social and emotional performance. The basic tests in the psychometric battery usually include the Wechsler Intelligence Scale for Children (WISC). Often MBD children show a spread between their verbal and nonverbal (performance) skills of more than 15 or 20 points. In most MBD children, the verbal will be higher than the performance; however, the pattern may be reversed. To assess perceptual difficulties or "central processing dysfunction," the Bender Visual Performance Gestalt exam as well as the Frostig Developmental Test of Visual Perception and certain parts of the WISC, such as block design, help test visual perception functions and will facilitate identification of children with visual-motor perceptual difficulties. Tests for auditory perceptual problems and language ability include the Wepman test of Auditory Discrimination and subtests of the Illinois Test of Psycholinguistic Abilities (ITPA). When there is a specific learning disability suspected, educators or psychologists with experience in the area of learning disabilities may have to do further testing. In cases where a strong emotional component is suspect, either as a major contributing factor or as a complication secondary to MBD, projective testing for psychiatric illness should also be included in the battery of tests.

An electroencephalogram (EEG) is a helpful diagnostic tool but there is no specific pattern in minimal brain dysfunction. About 35 to 50% of children with MBD have an abnormal EEG compared to at least 15% of the general population (Stevens et al., 1968; Capute, Niedermeyer, & Richardson, 1968). Abnormalities usually noted include mild background disorganization, more slowing than expected for age, and mild paroxysmal features. One of the major reasons for doing an EEG is to rule out the possibility of an underlying seizure diathesis such as petit mal or psychomotor seizures. Over the past year, two children brought to our clinic with a diagnosis of minimal brain dysfunction actually had petit mal epilepsy and one child had psychomotor seizures. The diagnosis of a seizure disorder was confirmed by the EEG after the clinical evaluation. The EEG can suggest a focal structural lesion by a slow-wave focus or raise the possibility of a degenerative disease by severe diffuse slowing. It is paramount that the EEG be critically evaluated. Many normal variants which had previously been termed abnormal, such as occipital slow waves of youth (Aird & Gastaut, 1959) or 14- and 6-per-second positive spikes (Lombroso et al., 1966) have now been shown to occur in normal children.

The role of the EEG, therefore, is mainly to identify focal lesions, and to help diagnose paroxysmal disorders such as petit mal or a localized seizure focus.

THERAPY

Once the diagnostic evaluation has been completed and the findings have been discussed with the parents and with the child (if he is old enough), emphasis on therapy in the home environment, in the social setting, and at school should be discussed. The emphasis of therapy should be on establishing routines. Parents are urged to (1) try to encourage the child, not frustrate him, (2) have a firm consistent approach, (3) reduce outside stimuli which could lead to fatigue and further frustration, (4) play noncompetitive games, (5) establish adequate patterns and specific hours of sleep and meals. Chores should be assigned to give the child a sense of responsibility and to encourage the establishment of self-esteem. The self-image is often very poor in these children.

In school there is a need for special education for a child with significant learning problems. Small classes with teachers trained to handle children with normal intelligence but specific learning problems are essential. Some children are so minimally affected that they can be in a regular class and get special tutoring for certain periods of the day. If the child has particular problems in visual-motor perception, he can obtain more practice in kinesthetic learning by writing in sand, or auditory training by listening to tape recorders to reinforce these learning processes. In special classes or schools, there are generally fewer stimuli, with blank walls and a more consistent approach from trained teachers. Denotative language is used. Specific commands are given since many of the children think mainly in concrete terms; for example, go to the kitchen, open the tap, put water in a glass, and bring it back.

The social worker must work with the family and help alleviate their problems by finding resources, such as camps in the summer and special afternoon programs to work with the child and help him find acceptance in his peer group. The psychologist is needed to perform the necessary tests, evaluation and often counseling.

The psychiatrist is needed for children who have such poor self-images that they develop phobias and other secondary symptoms. Also in some children, counseling by the psychiatrist can help the entire family. Psychotherapy as the sole mode of therapy is not indicated (Wender, 1971). Its main thrust is toward helping identify and assist the child and his family in managing secondary problems.

DRUG THERAPY

THEORIES OF MBD

What about the question of medication? Since the neuropathology of this entity is not really known, there is no specific therapy. We do not have one specific lesion to treat. Bradley (1937, 1950) noted the parodoxical calming effect of the amphetamines on children who had hyperactive behavior. Similarly, it was noted that barbiturates would have a parodoxical effect by making these children even more hyperactive. (Hyperactivity effects from barbiturates and the calming effect from amphetamines, however, does not establish the diagnosis of minimal brain dysfunction.) The therapeutic challenge began with the discovery of a possible agent to help the MBD child and further studies ensued.

The pathophysiology of hyperkinesis is mainly based upon experimental work in animals, in which specific brain lesions are made and their sequelae observed. Bilateral removal of the prefrontal area of the monkey causes a very marked increase in motor activity. Destruction of the subcortical structures such as the corpora striatum also induced hyperactivity (Mettler & Mettler, 1942).

The frontal areas of the brain, the hypothalamus, the reticular activating system, the limbic system, all are implicated in motor activity and behavior.

In studies in monkeys asphyxiated at birth, Sechzer, Faro and Windle (1973) showed an interesting behavior which is similar to that seen in some children with MBD. Developmental studies in infant monkeys asphyxiated for 15 minutes revealed that functioning of adaptive behavior such as visual depth perception, visual placing, and locomotor development which all involve the integration of visual information are significantly delayed. Acquired behavior of memory and learning are severely impaired. Neuropathology of asphyxia in the monkeys showed bilateral symmetrical focal lesions in the thalamus, inferior coliculi, auditory relay nuclei, and vestibular nuclei. The major structural defects were in areas needed to process signals from the environment and associate and integrate information. Although the human brain is less mature at birth than that of the monkey—which may render it more resistant to brain damage—some of the findings in the behaviors of the monkeys simulated some of those seen in children with MBD. The possibility of hypoxia as one of the causative factors is certainly a consideration.

Further investigators have observed certain neuropathology based upon the gestational age at birth. The prematures are particularly susceptible to hypoxia showing periventricular atrophy around the germinal matrix, whereas an anotic full-term baby usually shows cortical damage from hypoxia (Towbin, 1971).

There is a higher incidence of MBD among first-born children and males. Some believe that passage through the birth canal for the first time with a large head can cause damage. It has been postulated that the relatively large head circumference of males compared to females may account for the male preponderance. This explanation seems unlikely since there is such a minimal difference in head circumference (MBD Compendium, 1974). Others feel the syndrome may be on the basis of a neurodevelopmental lag (Kinsbourne, 1973). It may be more apparent in males because they have slower neurologic maturation until adolescence. None of these explanations has been documented.

Wender (1973) posits three possible theories to support a biochemical basis for MBD. The first is the possibility of genetic transmission in certain families (Omenn, 1973), as, for example, previously described in Hallgren's work. The second derives from the historical perspective. Here MBD is seen as the sequela of Von Economo's encephalitis in children, whereas post-encephalitic Parkinsonism is viewed as the sequela in adults. Since this post-encephalitic Parkinson's disease is associated with the destruction of dopaminergic neurons, Wender suggests that perhaps there may be a similar pathology in the MBD child but that it is expressed differently. No corroborative neuropathology is available. The third piece of suggestive evidence is that many of the children with MBD respond well to amphetamines. Responsiveness in some children not only means that the medication calms them, but that they may improve their functioning on psychological testing.

Baldessarini (1972) states that the amphetamines act on catecholamine containing neuron terminals by releasing transmitters and by interfering with the receptor, thus increasing the availability of the transmitter to post-synaptic receptors and enhancing the synaptic transmission along such pathways. Another theory is that children with MBD have decreased dopamine in the caudate nucleus and no neurohumor mediating transmission of nerve impulses in the reticular activating system. Amphetamines then stimulate the release of neurohumor in the caudate, thereby increasing synaptic transmission, thus calming the patient. In normal children, amphetamines usually stimulate the recticular activating system, causing an excitatory reaction (MBD Compendium, 1974).

Some children, after successful treatment with amphetamines, become more sensitive to positive and negative reinforcements. Correlating the anatomic studies with the biochemical data in other experiments, reinforcement behavior had the greatest response with electrode placement in the medial forebrain bundle and certain areas of the hypothalamus and septum (Olds & Milner, 1954; Olds, 1962). Through histofluorescent staining techniques Hillarp et al. (1966) identified ascending monoaminergic neurons whose cell bodies are located in the limbic system and ascend in the medial forebrain bundle to reach the lateral hypothalamus and cortex. This monoaminergic system demonstrated by staining techniques corresponds to Olds' positive reinforcement system (Stein, 1966). The limbic system, diencephalon, and medial forebrain bundle are important in behavior, particularly for appetite, drive, and affect and can also influence learning. Norepinephrine-containing neurons are also involved in the regulation of alertness and consciousness via the ascending reticular activating system.

Although many of the children with MBD appear to be "hyper-aroused" because of their motor activity, the EEG studies by Stevens (1968) show more slowing suggesting hypoarousal. Studies by Satterfield and Dawson (1971) examining the galvanic skin response (GSR) show less of a response, i.e., smaller fluctuations with higher skin resistance, in the children with MBD—again indicating low arousal. Hypoarousal raises the possibility of underactivity of one or more of the monoaminergic pathways such as the ascending reticular activating systems (ARAS). However, hypoarousal cannot be the only explanation because two of Satterfield's and Dawson's 24 children were hyperaroused according to GSR criteria but clinically were suffering from MBD.

The neurophysiological basis for MBD has also been explored by means of electroencephalography and extended by the use of evoked auditory and visual cortical potentials. Satterfield and his colleagues (1973) studied 31 children with MBD as compared with 21 normal controls matched for age and sex. Auditory-evoked cortical potentials in the MBD group had significantly lower amplitudes and longer latencies than those in the control groups. They suggested a theory consistent with delayed maturation of the central nervous system.

SPECIFIC DRUG THERAPY

If after optimal school placement is achieved and the home situation has been modified to help the child gain a better self-image, hyperactivity, distractibility, and low frustration tolerance still persist, then a trial of medication is started. There are no definite criteria to suggest which children will do well. However, in a study of 57 MBD children diagnosed on the basis of the EEG and neurological examination, those MBD children with both an abnormal EEG and an abnormal neurological exam obtained a significantly better response to methylphenidate than did the group with normal EEGs and normal neurological examinations (Satterfield et al., 1973). Of the total 57 MBD children, 70% obtained a good response with methylphenidate and 21% got worse. If one sorts out those with both abnormal EEG and neurological exam, 90% of this group obtained at least 30% or greater improvement. Of those children with both abnormal EEG and normal neurological findings, 60% showed 30% or more improvement. Most of the ratings of the efficacy of medications are those by parents and teachers against checklists. This is very important since this is the way the child performs. Very few studies, however, document objective data revealing change in performance after the medication.

Conners' study (1972) of the psychological effects of stimulant drugs in children with MBD showed improved behavior as judged by clinicians, parents, and teachers plus tests of cognitive, perceptual, and achievement measures. However, he points out that there are very striking inconsistencies. By means of psychological tests and analyses, he was able to divide these MBD-diagnosed children into six groups, using the visual-evoked response as one of the modes of characterizing the children. These groups responded to therapy in different ways. *Group I* is characterized by very poor visual motor coordination and attention. These children showed significant drug effects of amphetamines on the perceptual motor deficit. In electroencephalographic studies, asymmetry in the visual-evoked response was more pronounced with the left side than with the right. In *Group II*, the children were very poor in both perceptual and spatial orientation, but tended to improve with medication, primarily in their attention to tasks and academic ratings. *Group III* was quite poor in spatial orientation but was in fact good in visual motor coordination. Their improvement pattern in the attention sphere was similar to Group II's but they did not show improvement in academic ratings. *Group IV* was low in perceptual integration but quite good in spatial orientation. They showed improvement only in the Bender-Gestalt type tests but not in academic achievement. The EEGs in this group also show marked hemispheric-evoked response asymmetry, with a larger left-than right-sided amplitude. In *Group V*, which included about 20% of the children, patients showed no drug treatment effects whatsoever. Their profile was essentially flat, with some disturbances of conduct in the classroom but no test deficits. *Grup VI* children, whose EEG showed marked hemispheric asymmetry of the evoked response with a very small left-sided amplitude, were very low in achievement and received poor conduct ratings from their teachers. Academic performance, spelling, and arithmetic improved significantly from drug treatment. *Group VII* was low in verbal IQ but very good in parent ratings. Their EEGs showed an extremely asymmetric response with a small left-sided amplitude. On drugs, they improved mainly in their reading tasks.

SPECIFIC THERAPY AND DOSAGE

When the decision is made to begin medication, either with dextroamphetamines (Dexedrine) or with methylphenidate (Ritalin), the usual procedure is to give a divided dose of either drug in the morning and at noon. Methylphenidate is considered the drug of choice (Millichap, 1973) because in some studies there is less anorexia produced than with dextroamphetamine. The dose of methylphenidate is generally two times that of dextroamphetamine. A longer acting dextroamphetamine preparation is available; whereas, methylphenidate has to be administered in two doses. For some children, the morning dose is adequate but others require a third dose. The major contraindication to a dose later than noon is that it may keep the child up at night. A starting dose of either drug is generally 5 mg twice a day. In a young child, or one who attends school on a half day basis, a single dose may be tried first. The dose may be increased by 2.5 to 5 mg to a maximum of 40 mg per day of dextroamphetamine (Dexedrine) or 60 mg per day of methylphenidate (Ritalin). A guide to dosage suggested by Millichap (1973) is to begin with 0.25 mg/kg/day with gradual increase to a maximum of 2 mg/kg/day. Very often an inadequate trial of a low single dose leads to stopping the medication before beneficial effects can be determined.

Each of the two drugs has a short activity period with a rapid onset of effect (1 hour) and a disappearance by 4 to 6 hours. The major undesirable side effects of each include insomnia, anorexia, and gastrointestinal disturbances. Less often with very large doses, idiosyncratic reactions such as psychotic behavior and/or dyskinesias can occur. If one of the medications is ineffective, then the other can be tried. With prolonged use of methylphenidate or dextroamphetamine, the dose may have to be increased.

Safer and Allen (1973) reported significant suppression of height and weight in 49 children taking either dextroamphetamine or methylphenidate with doses above 20 mg a day for more than two years. A follow-up study by Safer, Allen and Barr (1975) revealed that those children whose stimulant medication was stopped at the beginning of the summer subsequently grew in height and weight at a significantly greater rate than those who continued to receive medication during the summer. A dose of 20 mg of Methylphenidate or less per day given throughout the entire year showed no suppressant effects on growth. Serial measurements of height and weight therefore are important to maintain in such patients. The concept of "drug holidays" is an important one, since during long school or summer vacations a period of eliminating the medication may allow rebound growth. If the symptoms of MBD are seen principally at school, some physicians prescribe the medication on school days only. Generally, if hyperkinesis, distractibility, and low frustration tolerance are present in school, there is often a degree of such difficulty at home and it is advisable to take the medication daily and then discontinue it in the summer time. Some children will require medication for their behavior all year, especially if they are in a summer camp with demands similar to those at school. If the medication is discontinued in the summer, the child may be able to start the school year without medication to see if he really needs it in the subsequent year.

Gross (1976) treated 100 children with hyperkinetic syndrome for a minimum of two years, with an average of 5 years, and an average follow-up of 6 years from the onset of treatment. The medications the children received included: 60 with Methylphenidate, 24 with Dextroamphetamine and 16 with either Imipramine or Desipramine. Initially, there was a diminution in expected weight, but not height. Within a few years there was no stunting of growth from long term use of any of the three medications. Contrary to the findings of Safer et al. (1973, 1975) growth took place both in patients still taking medication and those who discontinued therapy.

The average length of treatment is from about 6 months to as long as 3 to 5 years. Few children require medication after 11 to 12 years of age. Hyperkinetic behavior is less prevalent and the neurologic signs become even more subtle after that age (Millichap, 1973). There are some adolescents, however, who do benefit from methylphenidate for MBD.

To date, no long-term deleterious effects have been noted except for the possible growth slowdown in some children, but one should use the medication only if it is absolutely essential. For example, medication is indicated for the MBD child who, despite optimal school environment, home and educational facilities, is still hyperactive, has a short attention span, is distractible, and can't learn or function in the social and family situation. Of those children with soft neurological signs and abnormal EEGs, 66 to 75% who are hyperkinetic show a marked to moderate beneficial effect from methylphenidate (Satterfield et al., 1973) The benefit is often unequivocal.

Once the child has responded dramatically, if a single dose is omitted, he often will return to baseline behavior and the change becomes immediately apparent to teacher and parents (Eisenberg, 1972). To find out if the improvement may be due in part to placebo effect, Conners (1972) compared children on placebo with methylphenidate and magnesium pemoline (Cylert), another medication used for MBD. He found by the end of 4- and 8-week periods of drug treatment that MBD children showed a marked 86% improvement with amphetamines. Those on magnesium pemoline (Cylert) showed a moderately high 77% improvement. There was some improvement in 37% of those on placebo, but the effects were minimal. Although methylphenidate and dextroamphetamine are the chief drugs used, many others have been employed and in certain cases are very beneficial.

Recently, magnesium pemoline (Cylert) has received clinical trial (Page et al., 1974) with some success. Magnesium pemoline is a mild central nervous system (CNS) stimulant, first studied clinically in 1956. It has been used as a psychostimulant and mild antidepressant in other countries. Magnesium pemoline is structurally different from the amphetamines and methylphenidate but has certain similar pharmacological effects without sympathomimetic activity. Page et al. studied 413 children, aged 6 to 12 years, in 21 medical facilities. The study was a double-blind study with magnesium pemoline versus placebo. The medication, which is not a Class II drug, was given on a once a day basis. Generally, the effects were first noted by parents and teachers only after three weeks and by the physician within six weeks, much later than that observed with dextroamphetamines or methylphenidate. Magnesium pemoline studies showed "impressive improvement" in behavior as well as "some improvement" in cognitive and perceptual functions. The minimal side effects included insomnia and anorexia. Dosage recommended is 37.5 mg with increases each week of 18.75 mg with the usual maximum dose of 112.5 mg per day. Clinical trials will be helpful in assessing full potential of this medication. The medication is available in scored tablets of 37.5 mg, 18.75 mg, or 75 mg.

A wide variety of other medications have been investigated to evaluate the effects of abnormal behavior, including major and minor tranquilizers, antidepressants, and anticonvulsants (Millichap, 1973). Diphenhydramine (Benadryl), an antihistamine which has sedative qualities, was one of the first tried. Some success was achieved, but it is not a first choice medication. Hydroxyzine (Atarax, Vistaril) has also been tried and may help to relieve anxiety. Very agitated children or those with emotional problems have been given a benzodiazepine such as chlordiazepoxide (Librium) or diazepam (Valium). These agents mainly calm or tranquilize, but are not specific for the MBD child.

Phenothiazines, mainly chlorpromazine (Thorazine) and thioridazine (Mellaril), have been found to be helpful in certain patients with significant aggressive, hostile, anxious behavior disturbance as part of the MBD syndrome. Phenothiazine is generally given 2 to 4 times a day, starting with 10 mg b.i.d. and increasing the dosage weekly by 10 mg per day until optimal effect or toxicity. Although hyperactivity is diminished, the other behavioral abnormalities such as distractibility and short attention span are not affected. With large doses, learning and performance may in fact be impaired possibly on a sedative basis.

Thioridazine has a somewhat lower incidence of phenothiazine side effects which include skin rash, jaundice and dyskinesia, and in large doses, a lowering of the seizure threshold. Many of the studies of thioridazine and chlorpromazine have been done in children with mental retardation and hyperactivity. Of 308 such patients treated with thioridazine, 57% were benefited and 2% experienced side effects with drowsiness being the most prominent. Millichap (1973) evaluated 15 patients with MBD given thioridazine and found significant improvement in the Jastak reading test and conduct ratings, and ratings of maturity and behavior as well as finger coordination, but found drowsiness a troublesome side effect limiting the use of the drug in a high proportion of patients.

Imipramine (Tofranil) was noted to improve behavior in some children who were given the medication for enuresis. Rapoport (1965) reported improvement in alertness, handwriting, reading, and arithmetic in children with behavior disorders and tantrums. Huessy and Wright (1970) studied the effect of imipramine in 52 children, ages 3 to 14 years, referred for hyperactivity and learning disabilities. Medication is given in one dose, 1 hour after the evening meal. Dosages used were 12.5 mg as a starting dose in those under 5 years and 25 mg in those over 5 years. The optimal dose ranged from 25 to 125 mg with 50 mg on the average. Marked improvement in behavior occurred in 67% of children studied. Rare side effects included mild hypertension, leukopenia in one, irritability, and dry mouth. The tricyclic antidepressants are similar to methylphenidate pharmacologically in that they facilitate synaptic effects of the brain catecholamines as do the amphetamines. The action of the tricyclic compounds is probably similar to the amphetamines and methylphenidate in this condition in that they probably act via the putative neurotransmitters in the brain. More controlled studies, however, are necessary to assess the full value of imipramine in children with MBD.

Anticonvulsants have been used in children with hyperactivity whose behavior and learning problems are complicated by convulsive disorders (Millichap, 1969). When the patient's EEG is mildly paroxysmal and there is no history to suggest a clinical seizure, anticonvulsants generally have no effect and are not recommended (Pasamanick, 1951; Pincus & Glaser, 1966). If a child presents with a great deal of inattention and daydreaming and the EEG shows 3 per second spike and wave pattern, medication for petit mal epilepsy is indicated, and ethosuximide (Zarontin) would be the drug of choice. In certain patients where the EEG is very paroxysmal and the history is suggestive of psychomotor seizures or atypical staring spells, then anticonvulsants should be prescribed. In patients with psychomotor seizures, a trial of diphenylhydantoin would be the drug of choice. If this was ineffective, primidone (Mysoline) could be added or later substituted. Primidone, however, is metabolized in part to phenobarbital and some children do have a hyperkinetic paradoxical behavior effect even with primidone but this is less marked generally than with pehnobarbital. Barbiturates in general are contraindicated since they produce hyperkinesis in these children.

Recently, Schackenberg (1973) has done a limited study on 11 children using caffeine in coffee as a substitute for methylphenidate or dextroamphetamine in hyperkinetic children. He found some improvement in these children, which, in this small group, he claimed was similar to that seen with methylphenidate.

Youngsters treated with stimulant drugs in long-term studies to date have shown no greater tendency to drug addiction than children not so treated (Eisenberg, 1972). Theories to explain these observations include: (1) increase in child's ego strength through the use of the drug, (2) less curiosity about drug experimentation, (3) no feeling of elation from the medication.

Other treatment programs that have been tried include behavior therapy with positive reinforcement for quiet behavior. This has had some success in younger children as part of the general management.

Optometric treatment, based on the theory that deficiencies in various visual functions may be the cause of learning difficulties seen in hyperkinetic children or MBD children, has led to visual-motor training (Getman, 1965). The American Academy of Pediatrics (1972) and other professional academies emphasize that visual training alone is an inadequate approach to the treatment of learning disabilities.

The orthomolecular approach (Cott, 1972), which uses large doses of vitamins (megavitamins), and stresses the importance of low glucose levels and trace minerals in hyperactive children, is unproved.

A diet which omits food additives and salicylates has been proposed for the treatment of hyperactive children by Feingold (1975). In specific patients where there were allergies, the diet may play a role, but there have been no large well controlled studies to suggest that this is an established treatment for MBD. Conners (1976) conducted a double blind crossover trial involving a control diet and a diet eliminating artifical flavors, colors and natural salicylates as recommended by Feingold in 15 hyperkinetic children. Children were rated by parents and teachers. The teachers noted a reduction of symptoms on the diet as compared to control diet but parents did not. As indicated by the author, the study lacked objective measures of change. Guidelines were put forth for controlled studies which are necessary to assess such new therapies.

PROGNOSIS

Although many of these children become better coordinated and are less hyperactive with time, some of the problems do persist. If a child has a very poor self-image and meets with frustration and failure, the psychological impact of this syndrome will take its toll in the growing adolescent and adult. Very few long-term follow-up studies are available specifically focusing on the child with MBD. The few studies that are available in children with learning disabilities and/or hyperkinetic behavioral syndromes suggest a guarded prognosis. Many of the children with dyslexia who receive instruction can eventually read but few ever read at an average or above average level. Certain prognostic factors were cited by Koppitz (1971), who reported that those children with an IQ of 85 or less and auditory and visual perception defects probably would need special education until the age of 21. Poor socioeconomic background correlates with a poorer response.

Most of the follow-up studies are in children who present with hyperkinetic behavior disorder rather than MBD. In a 5-year follow-up study by Weiss et al. (1971), 64 hyperactive boys were followed from age 10 to age 18. During this time span, 46% were distractible, 70% were emotionally immature, 30% lacked ambition or an inability to maintain goals, 30% had no steady friends, and 80% performed poorly academically. Many features of the follow-up were left unsettled and a 10-year reassessment was considered necessary before any final decision about prognosis could be made.

Menkes (1967) studied 12 hyperactive children in a 25-year follow-up. None of these children had received medication for their hyperkinesis. Of the 11 children followed, 36% were psychotic, 18% retarded, and 45% self-supporting. Of the five self-supporting, four had been previously institutionalized.

More optimistic data are derived from Laufer's and McCarthy's follow-up of 60 MBD patients treated with amphetamines (Laufer, 1971; Denhoff, 1973). The average age of onset of treatment was age 8 and the average follow-up was 20 years. Amphetamines had been prescribed in 23% of the cases for 5 years or more. Of the 48 cases for which complete data were available, 76% were receiving or had received higher education, 30% were abnormal in temperament. This study does seem to suggest that the use of medication may improve the ultimate prognosis in children with the MBD syndrome.

Denhoff describes the natural history of children with MBD from compiling many studies. It is important to outline the natural life history so that one can identify these children early and be prepared to help them as soon as possible. In infancy, many of these children are labile in their mother-infant reactions. They are usually very active. In the toddler age, often their exploration activity is exaggerated. In the preschool age, their behavior may be turbulent with frequent temper tantrums and easy frustration and distractibility. Some of these children are not diagnosed until school age, at which time comparison with peers and demands to meet certain standards make hyperkinesis most apparent. If the MBD syndrome is not handled educationally, socially, and in certain cases with medication, the preadolescent becomes further frustrated and gains a poor self-image, which in turn leads to further academic failure. In adolescenec, uneven and unpredicable behavior can ensue. Within the MBD group, Denhoff also noted that the hyperactive children tend to come from lower social classes and have a higher number of visual-perceptual problems and secondary emotional problems. They respond best to psychostimulant medication. In his opinion the hypoactive children had more language-based academic difficulties, were clumsier, and came from the higher social classes. They had, in general, a higher IQ score but a poorer response to medication.

Although more data are necessary, most clinicians will agree that MBD children who receive early appropriate educational help and psychological support, plus medication when indicated, tend to do better and reach adulthood with fewer problems.

REFERENCES

Books

Clements, S. D. *Minimal brain dysfunction. Terminology and identification* (NINDB Monograph No. 3, U.S. Public Health Service

Publication No. 1415). Washington, D. C.: U. S. Government Printing Office, 1966.

FEINGOLD, B. F. *Why your child is hyperactive.* New York: Random House, 1975.

KOPPITZ, E. M. *Children with learning disabilities: A five-year follow-up study.* New York: Grune and Stratton, 1971.

MILLICHAP, J. G. Management of hyperactive behavior in children with epilepsy. In J. G. Millichap (Ed.), *Modern treatment.* New York: Hoeber Medical Division of Harper & Row, 1969.

NEEDLEMAN, H. L. Lead poisoning in children: Neurologic implications of widespread subclinical intoxication. In S. Walzer and P. H. Wolff (Eds.), *Minimal cerebral dysfunction in children.* New York: Grune and Stratton, 1973.

OMENN, G. S. Genetic issues in the syndrome of minimal brain dysfunction. In S. Walzer and P. H. Wolff (Eds.), *Minimal cerebral dysfunction in children.* New York: Grune and Stratton, 1973.

SCHAIN, R. J. *Neurology of childhood learning disorders.* Baltimore: Williams & Wilkins, 1972.

SECHZER, J. A., FARO, M. D., and WINDLE, W. F. Studies of monkeys asphyxiated at birth: Implications for minimal cerebral dysfunction. In S. Walzer and P. H. Wolff (Eds.), *Minimal cerebral dysfunction in children.* New York: Grune and Stratton, 1973.

STEIN, L. Psychopharmacological substrates of mental depression. In S. Garattini and M. N. G. Dukes (Eds.), *Antidepressant drugs* (International Congress Series). Amsterdam: Excerpta Medical Foundation, 1966.

STRAUSS, A. A., and KEPHART, N. C. *Psychopathology and education of the brain-injured child.* Progress in theory and clinic, Vol. II. New York: Grune and Stratton, 1955.

STRAUSS, A. A., and LEHTINEN, L. E. *Psychopathology and education of the brain-injured child.* New York: Grune and Stratton, 1947.

WENDER, P. H. *Minimal brain dysfunction in children.* New York: Wiley-Interscience, 1971.

JOURNALS

AIRD, R. V., and GASTAUT, Y. Occipital and posterior electroencephalographic rhythms. *EEG and Clinical Neurophysiology*, 1959, *11*, 637–656.

American Academy of Pediatrics (joint organizational statement). The eye and learning disabilities. *Pediatrics*, 1972, *49*, 454–455.

BALDESSARINI, R. J. Symposium: Behavior modification by drugs. I. Pharmacology of amphetamines. *Pediatrics*, 1972, *49*, 694–701.

BELMONT, L., and BIRCH, H. G. Lateral dominance and right-left awareness in normal children. *Child Development*, 1963, *34*, 257–270.

BOND, E. Postencephalitic, ordinary and extraordinary children. *Journal of Pediatrics*, 1932, *1*, 310–314.

BRADLEY, C. The behavior of children receiving benzedrine. *American Journal of Psychiatry*, 1937, *94*, 577–585.

BRADLEY, C. Benzedrine and dexedrine in the treatment of children's behavior disorders. *Pediatrics*, 1959, *5*, 24–36.

CAPUTE, A. J., Niedermeyer, E. R. L., and Richardson, F. The electroencephalogram in children with minimal cerebral dysfunction. *Pediatrics*, 1968, *41*, 1104–1114.

CLEMENTS, S. D., and PETERS, J. E. Minimal brain dysfunctions in the school age child. *Archives of General Psychiatry*, 1962, *6*, 185–197.

CONNERS, C. K. Symposium: Behavior modification by drugs. II. Psychological effects in minimal brain dysfunction. *Pediatrics*, 1972, *49*, 702–708.

CONNERS, C. K., GOYETTE, C. H., SOUTHWICK, D. A., LEES, J. M., and ANDRULONIS, P. A. "Food Additives and Hyperkinesis: A controlled double blind experiment," *Pediatrics* 1976, *58*, 154–166.

COTT, A. Megavitamins: The orthomolecular approach to behavioral disorders and learning disabilities. *Academic Therapy*, 1972, *7*, 245.

DENHOFF, E. The natural life history of children

with minimal brain dysfunction. *Annals of the New York Academy of Science*, 1973, *205*, 188–204.

EBAUGH, F. G. Neuropsychiatric sequelae of acute epidemic encephalitis. *American Journal of Diseases of Children*, 1923, *25*, 89–97.

EISENBERG, L. Symposium: Behavior modification by drugs. III. Clinical use in children. *Pediatrics*, 1972, *49*, 708–715.

GETMAN, G. The visuomotor complex in the acquisitions of learning skills. *Learning Disorders*, 1965, *1*, 49.

GROSS, M. D. Growth of Hyperkinetic Children Taking Methylphenidate, Dextroamphetamine or Imipramine, *Pediatrics*, 1976, *58*, 423–431.

HALLGREN, B. Specific dyslexia (congenital word blindness). *Acta Psychiatrica et Neurologica Scandinavica Supplement*, 1950, *65*, 1–287.

HILLARP, N. A., Fuxe, K., and Dahlstrom, A. Demonstration and mapping of central neurons containing dopamine, noradrenaline and 5-hydroxytryptamine and their reactions to psychopharmaca. *Pharmacological Reviews*, 1966, *18*, 727–741.

HUESSY, H. R. Study of the prevalence and therapy of the choreatiform syndrome or hyperkinesis in rural Vermont. *Acta Paedopsychiatrica*, 1967, *34*, 130–135.

HUESSY, H. R., and Wright, A. L. The use of imipramine in children's behavior disorders. *Acta Paedopsychiatrica*, 1970, *37*, 194–199.

KAHN, E., and COHEN, L. H. Organic driveness: A brain stem syndrome and an experience. *New England Journal of Medicine*, 1934, *210*, 748–756.

KINSBOURNE, M. Minimal brain dysfunction as a neurodevelopmental lag. *Annals of the New York Academy of Sciences*, 1973, *205*, 268–273.

LAUFER, M. W. Long term management and some follow-up findings on the use of drugs with minimal cerebral syndrome. *Journal of Learning Disabilities*, 1971, *4*, 55–58.

LEAHY, S. R., and SANDS, I. J. Mental disturbance in children following epidemic encephalitis. *Journal of the American Medical Association*, 1921, *76*, 373–377.

LOMBROSO, C. T., SCHWARTZ, I. H., CLARKE, D. M., and MUENCH, H. Ctenoids in healthy youths. Controlled study of 14- and 6-per-second positive spiking. *Neurology*, 1966, *16*, 1152–1158.

Minimal Brain Dysfunction. Compendium, Vol. 2, No. 15, CIBA-Geigy Pharmaceutical Company, Summit, New Jersey, 1974.

MENKES, M. M., ROWE, J. S., and MENKES, J. H. A twenty-five year follow-up study on the hyperkinetic child with minimal brain dysfunction. *Pediatrics*, 1967, *39*, 393–399.

METTLER, F., and METTLER, C. The effects of striatal injury. *Brain*, 1942, *65*, 242–244.

MILLICHAP, J. G. Drugs in management of minimal brain dysfunction. *Annals of the New York Academy of Sciences*, 1973, *205*, 321–334.

OLDS, J. Hypothalamic substrate of reward. *Physiological Reviews*, 1962, *42*, 554–604.

OLDS, J., and MILNER, P. Positive reinforcement produced by electrical stimulation of septal area and other regions of rat brain. *Journal of Comparative and Physiological Psychology*, 1954, *47*, 419.

PAGE, J. G., JANICKI, R. S., and BERNSTEIN, J. E., et al. Pemoline (Cylert) in the treatment of childhood hyperkinesis. *Journal of Learning Disabilities*, 1974, *7*, 498–503.

PAINE, R. S. Minimal chronic brain syndromes in children. *Developmental Medicine and Child Neurology*, 1962, *4*, 21–27.

PAINE, R. S., WERRY, J. S., and QUAY, H. C. A study of minimal cerebral dysfunction. *Dev. Med. Child. Neurol.*, 1968, *10*, 505–520.

PASAMANICK, B. Anticonvulsant drug therapy of behavior problem children with abnormal electroencephalograms. *Archives of Neurology and Psychiatry*, 1951, *65*, 752–766.

PINCUS, J. H., and GLASER, G. H. The syndrome of "minimal brain damage" in childhood. *New England Journal of Medicine*, 1966, *275*, 27–35.

Prechtl, H. F. R., and Stemmer, C. J. The choreiform syndrome in children. *Dev. Med. Child. Neurol.*, 1962, *4*, 119–127.

Rapoport. J. Childhood behavior and learning problems treated with imipramine. *International Journal of Neuropsychiatry*, 1965, *1*, 635–642.

Safer, D. J., Allen, R. P., and Barr, E. Growth rebound after termination of stimulant drugs, *Pediatrics*, 1975, *86*, 113–116.

Safer, D. J., and Allen, R. P. On two stimulant drugs for the growth of hyperactive children. *Pediatrics*, 1973, *51*, 660–667.

Satterfield, J. H., and Dawson, M. E. Ectodermal correlates of hyperactivity in children. *Psychophysiology*, 1971, *8*, 91.

Satterfield, J. H., Lesser, L. I., Saul, R. E., and Cantwell, D. P. EEG aspects in the diagnosis and treatment of minimal brain dysfunction. *Annals of the New York Academy of Sciences*, 1973, *205*, 274–282.

Schackenberg, R. C. Caffeine as a substitute for schedule II stimulants in hyperkinetic children. *American Journal of Psychiatry*, 1973, *130*, 796–798.

Stevens, J. R., Sachdev, K., and Milstein, V. Behavior disorders of childhood and the electroencephalogram. *Archives of Neurology*, 1968, *18*, 160–177.

Stewart, M., Ferris, A., Pitts, N., Jr., and Craig, A. G. The hyperactive child syndrome. *American Journal of Orthopsychiatry*. 1966, *36*, 861–867.

Towbin, A. Organic causes of minimal brain dysfunction. Perinatal origin of minimal cerebral lesion. *Journal of the American Medical Association*, 1971, *217*, 1207–1214.

Weiss, G., Klaus, M., Werry, J. S., et al. On the hyperactive child: VIII. Five-year follow-up. *Archives of General Psychiatry*, 1971, *24*, 409–414.

Wender, P. H. Speculations on biochemical basis of MBD. *Annals of the New York Academy of Sciences*, 1973, *205*, 18–28.

9

ULCERATIVE COLITIS

Thornton A. Vandersall

Treatment is most effective when it is based upon a clear understanding of the pathogenesis and pathology of a disorder. The lack of agreement regarding the psychopathology of ulcerative colitis could lead to many differing treatment approaches, with differing effects. Accordingly, I will begin with a discussion of the physical pathology and psychopathology associated with ulcerative colitis. Following that I will go into treatment proper. Besides considering the dynamics and usual intervention techniques, I will pay particular attention to the evaluative, early phases of treatment, the problems of evaluating patients in hospitals (where many ulcerative colitis patients are first seen by psychiatrists), the need to collaborate with other physicians caring for the patient, and the role of the psychiatrist when surgery is undertaken.

ETIOLOGIC CONSIDERATIONS

Jackson and Yalom (1966) characterize well the confusion about the psychopathology of ulcerative colitis when, in discussing families of patients with ulcerative colitis, they label as "unlikely" the possibility that ulcerative colitis is "the specific etiologic result of certain family interactional patterns," while they say it is "more likely" that it is "a disorder produced under stress where certain genetic factors already exist." Jackson and Yalom also suggest it is "possible" that the ill child with ulcerative colitis is the "source" of the family stress rather than "one of its products."

In a leading pediatric textbook, Silverberg and Davidson (1972) characterize the etiology of the disease as multidetermined, with family histories suggesting a genetic basis for this disease of the gut. Psychological factors are considered important and changes in emotional states are "often associated" with exacerbations and remissions of the disease. In stating that psychological factors are of importance in the course of the disease, the authors backed away from a position they had taken in an earlier edition of the same text wherein they said there was "no question" that emotional factors influenced the course of the disease. Regarding the role of psychotherapy in the treatment of ulcerative colitis, Silverberg and Davidson plead for an individualized approach. They believe the psychological aspects of the disorder can be well handled in most cases by the pediatrician, with referrals to the mental health specialists reserved for the more difficult problems.

In discussing the psychotherapy of ulcerative colitis, it is essential to distinguish ulcerative colitis from other bowel disorders producing pain and diarrhea. Many patients with pain and diarrhea as presenting symptoms do not have demonstrable organic disease. A large group of such patients are classified as manifesting the Irritable Colon Syndrome. There is a higher degree of correlation between symptoms and life stress in the Irritable Colon Syndrome patient than in the ulcerative colitis patient (Mendeloff, Monk, Siegel, & Lilienfeld, 1970; Chaudhary & Truelove, 1962; Hislop, 1971). The association is so prominent that Almy (1957) has suggested a better term for the Irritable Colon Syndrome would be "adaptive colitis." Once adequate medical work-up has identified the irritable colon patient as free of organic pathology, the patient frequently consults a psychotherapist. The task of treatment of the Irritable Colon Syndrome is simplified by the absence of organic, serious bowel pathology and the clear association of symptoms, in many cases, with life stress. Treatment with these patients should thus proceed along traditional lines with the possible added "advantage" that the therapist has a somatic indicator of emotional stress.

By contrast, the patient with ulcerative colitis has significant bowel pathology. Ulcerative colitis is one of the group of disorders labeled "Inflammatory Bowel Disease." Ulcerative colitis primarily affects the inner lining (mucosa) of the large intestine, and can be distinguished from granulomatous colitis, which affects the entire wall of the large intestine (trans-mural disease) and regional enteritis which is a trans-mural disease of the small intestine primarily. There is similarity and overlap in the pathology and symptoms of these disorders, so that it is often difficult to distinguish medically between them. Furthermore, our experience thus far has not shown any set of distinctive psychological characteristics that could separate one subgroup of inflammatory bowel disease from another. Patients with ulcerative colitis are expected to have more emotional problems related to their physical disorder than are patients with granulomatous disease or regional enteritis, however.

THE PSYCHOLOGIC FACTORS

Our approach to understanding psychosomatic disease has changed over the years, primarily in response to the failure of one theory after another to provide a single, consistent answer to the riddle. This evolution is reviewed in the earlier companion volume of this book (Purcell, Weiss, & Hahn, 1972). While we now have no unified approach to all psychosomatic illness, from each attempt to create a single theory we have gained insights and methods. We thus have the tools to visualize psychosomatic disorders such as ulcerative colitis as a multi-determined process.

Engel (1955) stresses that ulcerative colitis is a disease of the lining surface of the bowel, a surface continuous with the outside of the body, a kind of inner skin and part of the individual's contact with the environment. Engel describes a distinctive mother/child relationship in children with ulcerative colitis that, when disturbed or ruptured, leads to the tissue reaction of the disease. The disturbance in the relationship may be real or fantasied; onset or relapse of the disorder results when the affect associated with the loss of the relationship is one of hopelessness and despair.

Prugh (1951), in an early study to delineate the emotional components of ulcerative colitis in children, found the children to be "passive, rigid, quite dependent on parent figures, particularly the mother, socially inhibited, often narcissistic and emotionally immature." While there was a suggestion of correlation between emotional stress and exacerbations of the disease, it was not possible to establish such relationships in all cases. The parents in the Prugh study were characterized as "rigid, at times overindulgent, and often inconsistent." In play therapy, the children were stereotyped, unimaginative, and reluctant to express any aggression toward adult figures. Play centering around toilet behavior indicated feelings of resentment associated with these functions, but the children continued to manifest a pattern of obediently performing upon parental urging.

Sperling (1946) has described a specific and pathological mother-child relationship beginning very early in life, characterized by great ambivalence and destructive urges. Her articulate and strong views about the psychopathology in ulcerative colitis have influenced the thinking of many therapists and tended to cast all mothers of colitis patients in a bad light. She states that since psychoanalysis is difficult in such cases, "prophylaxis would be the best treatment," starting with the prospective mother.

Finch and Hess (1962) found families with dominating mothers and passive, ineffectual fathers, but could not delineate any patterns with regard to sex, race, religion, number of siblings, ordinal position, or socioeconomic status. Their child patients demonstrated many significant emotional problems including early feeding and toileting difficulties, strong sibling rivalry, and a predominance of obsessive-compulsive, constricted, rigid, and sado-masochistic character traits with a brittle pseudo-maturity as their main adaptive facade. In treatment, these children developed intense dependent relationships that were, however, easily ruptured. They had difficulty dealing with feelings and tended to view things in terms of good and bad polarities.

The literature of childhood ulcerative colitis reveals, amid some dissension and many protestations of ignorance, certain points of agreement. There is often a family history of bowel disease and a strong suggestion that a genetic-constitutional predisposition to bowel disorder is present. The relationship between the child and the mother is often problematic, the father is a nonparticipant, and an unhappy tie is formed. The child remains ambivalently and dependently enmeshed in the family until some disruption of the relationship heralds the onset of ulcerative colitis.

Our own series of cases reveals some measure of congruity with aspects of this formulation but also some glaring incongruities. While we have found many positive family histories for bowel disease in almost all our cases, and strongly support the view that there is a genetic-constitutional predisposition, we have often not been able to find real or fantasied disruption of relationships coinciding with the onset or exacerbations of the disease. Nor have we been able to uniformly indict the families, either as fitting a stereotype or as having a narcissistic investment in producing the pathological tie postulated so often in the literature. We thus are in agreement with Feldman, and co-workers (1967) who found a "normal" distribution of emotional problems in ulcerative colitis patients and who question the characterization of ulcerative colitis as a "classic" psychosomatic disease.

We approach patients and families with the implied assumption, usually openly expressed, that ulcerative colitis is an organic disease of the bowel, with a constitutional basis and a course that is influenced by emotional stress, personality, and the adaptive skills of the patient. The task of treatment is to increase the patient's awareness of his emotions and adaptive style, so that he can more effectively experience emotions and adapt in a more positive manner. If a pathological tie exists between the patient and the mother, or if we suspect it exists, we would not elect initially to focus upon that, preferring first to engage the child and then work with the parents insofar as that appears necessary. While the presence of family pathology might encourage one to search for a qualified family therapist to take on the entire problem at once, in our experience the motivation of these families for psychotherapy is so quixotic as to insure rejection of such proposals. During the course of treatment, however, family sessions are frequently useful, and a family therapy approach may be of value and acceptable to the family after an initial phase of working with the presenting patient and obtaining the family's confidence and cooperation.

Many parents bring their child to treatment with the idea that they have produced the disorder by their interaction with the child. A companion view often held by these parents is that, since this disease is emotional in origin, it can be cured by psychotherapy. Upon making this "discovery," families that would have hesitated even to think about psychotherapy, let alone talk of it, come running to embrace it. Needless to say, such a situation should prompt modesty in the therapist. It is helpful in such cases to point out the basic organic nature of the disorder, while acknowledging the significant role played by emotional factors and offering to help as much as possible in the betterment of that one variable.

CASE EXAMPLE

An 18-year-old girl with recent onset of ulcerative colitis had been hospitalized for over a month to control her symptoms with steroid treatment and supportive measures. That hospitalization was accompanied by a marked depression and very reluctant agreement to see a psychiatrist after discharge. The patient appeared to make her own decisions, her mother being anxious, quiet, and attentive, but almost intimidated by both her daughter's illness and intense personality.

After discharge from the first bout of bleeding, and when she was rehospitalized shortly thereafter for a second exacerbation, the patient "read up" on the disease and found it was caused by faulty emotions. She became most eager to find the emotional causes of her disorder and she, and her family, searched insistently for the most qualified psychiatrist to treat her. When psychotherapy did not produce the desired results, the patient read further to discover that the "only cure for the disease is surgery." The patient then pushed for an early colectomy, which was reasonably indicated. She has done quite well physically and emotionally since that surgery. Her personality, however, still retains its distinctive pre-ulcerative colitis characteristics of intensity, naiveté, impatience, and demandingness.

RELATIONS WITH THE GASTROENTEROLOGIST

The therapist working with ulcerative colitis, or any psychosomatic disorder, must establish a trusting and communicating relationship with the physician primarily responsible for the patient's care. Most ulcerative colitis patients, and their families, are closely tied to the gastroenterologist caring for them. Before the psychotherapist has been called in, the primary physician was the person turned to for both medical and social direction. He has arbitrated many decisions as to what stresses the patient can tolerate in regard to sleeping and eating schedules, school choice, and work load, as well as physical activity, vacations, and so forth. A strong, positive relationship exhibiting many transference qualities often exists between the patient and the gastroenterologist, and usually includes the family. It is essential that the entering psychotherapist become identified with, or allied with, this powerful figure, or the therapist's efforts will be degraded, debunked, and soon discarded. Most gastroenterologists are eager to have a psychotherapist as an ally who can aid them with their most difficult problems. Their main concern about the therapist, in my experience, is that he be realistic and clear in his perception of the patient and the family and free of jargon and preconceived ideas about the psychopathology of this disorder. Gastroenterologists also desire a psychotherapist who is able to plan a treatment program that is acceptable to the family in terms of time and money and who is willing to keep up an ongoing communication with them. This may sound like a big order for a therapist accustomed to working exclusively and confidentially with one patient in the privacy of his own office. While a smaller, selected group of ulcerative colitis patients may eventually be benefited from a traditional treatment setting, the greater majority will require the kind of flexible teamwork suggested above.

EVALUATION PHASE OF TREATMENT

Once the contract with the child and the family has been established, a thorough evaluation must be undertaken. A developmental history obtained from both parents will supply the basic background information and may give insights into the interactions of family members and possible pathological mother-child relationships.

I have not found any unique differences in the developmental history of ulcerative colitis patients from other patients. Toilet training histories vary from a complete lack of information to such blunt facts as "he was toilet trained at 2.8 years." Feeding and weaning histories are not distinctive, except in unusual or rare situations. There are some difficulties discovered at times of separation and new beginnings such as school entry. Again, a larger sampling of ulcerative colitis patients does not reveal a clear pattern of avoidance of such tasks with dependent, angry clinging to mother. In fact, most of our patients have been successful in school and reported entry and progress to new classes uncomplicated. Less than 10% of our cases demonstrate the close, ambivalent, pathological tie with the mother described in the literature. Many demonstrate instead a number of psychological problems developing after the onset of the disease, and often in association with hospitalization and steroid therapy. We choose not to interpret this as a final overt manifestation of pathology, but view it more as a response to the realistic stress of a severe physical illness, or hospitalization, or the personality-altering effects of steroid medications well known for their effects on mood and personality organization.

While some children seen with ulcerative colitis are rigid and prematurely fixed in personality patterns, showing little insight into feelings (as described in the literature), a large percentage of these patients do not fit into that particular personality pattern. Some children in our series were verbal, adaptive, and had healthy responses to their disability. These children generally do not get into psychotherapy. *Thus the child with ulcerative colitis seen by the therapist is not the typical child with ulcerative colitis, but rather the typical child with ulcerative colitis who comes to psychotherapy.* In a large series of children with ulcerative colitis reviewed by Hijmans and Enzer (1962), they found "no consistent pattern of behavior." They called attention to the "secondary maladjustments because of the chronicity of the disease" as one of the indicators for supportive psychotherapy. Their findings on personalities of the children agree with our experience.

The initial evaluation by the therapist usually takes place in a hospital. Privacy is not readily available. The parents may not be available, or may anxiously spend a large amount of time at the child's bedside. The mother may be irritated at the introduction of another specialist who does not come bearing a cure, or too tired and distracted to give any helpful attention to emotional processes being played out along with the physical pain and difficulties of hospitalization. The father is often preoccupied with his work, perhaps working longer hours to pay the extra bills engendered by the hospitalization, and more unavailable than usual for consultation. This is hardly a conducive setting to a careful evaluation, yet one in which the therapist must somehow collect information, appraise the situation, and make a decision about treatment interventions.

The main problem may be a depressed, uncooperative, and whiny patient. In that situation frequent short visits to the bedside, offering a listening ear, perhaps even the use of antidepressant medication, will hold out positive support and hope to the patient while permitting the therapist to evaluate the child's or adolescent's ability to introspect and work toward personality change.

In another situation, the therapist may find it necessary to become involved at once with the mother-child relationship, helping the anxious and hovering mother withdraw enough to allow the staff to work and the patient to breathe. The patient may seem to cooperate but frequently can only undermine the separation process because of his own ambivalent desires for the mother's closeness. Two case examples may illustrate some of the differing approaches necessary.

Case Example

A 10-year-old boy, hospitalized for abdominal pain, was seen at the request of his mother while undergoing diagnostic work-up that later revealed he had ulcerative colitis. The mother believed the child was overly dependent and not working up to his ability in school. She was frankly eager to have him in treatment so that he would be more serene, self-sufficient, and have more friends. The mother had been in intensive psychotherapy for several years and was in the process of separation and divorce from her husband. It was her hope that the therapist could substitute for the lost father and cushion the blow to the child.

The boy himself was verbal and articulate. He used sessions to ventilate his feelings of rejection, loneliness, and inadequacy. He was able to accept, with continuing therapy, the divorce and a move from a suburban home to a city apartment. In this case the child was the only patient proferred or available to the therapist and he was able to work profitably with the therapist.

CASE EXAMPLE

Another 17-year-old adolescent had been in treatment some years previously, but the parents had reportedly "sabotaged" the treatment. They had been excluded from the treatment situation, could not understand what was being done, felt they were being accused of causing the disorder, and, accordingly, withdrew the child.

The patient was a superficially compliant, dependent, and immature boy, with unrealistic expectations about himself. He was the focus of much polarization of feelings and bickering between the two parents. The patient used individual sessions to discuss concrete problems and sought advice that would extricate him from demanding or difficult masks. As it became clear that little could be done with the patient alone, and as the parents asked more questions and indicated a desire to seek some escape from their angry arguments about the boy, the trio was moved toward family therapy (with the patient somewhat opposed) as the most appropriate and helpful treatment modality.

PSYCHODYNAMICS AND TREATMENT

MacKinnon and Michels (1971), discussing the psychiatric interview with the psychosomatic patient and the patient seen in the ward consultation, offer many insightful and instructive comments regarding the psychodynamics of these patients and approaches the therapist can utilize. They note the dependency patterns frequently adopted and the use of regression and denial. The patients focus upon the physical aspects of their disorder and need quiet, minimally confronting, help in finding relationships between their symptoms and their emotional life or in discovering how "talking can help." The idea that they have an "emotional" illness increases their concern and makes them wary of the psychiatrist as one who might find they are "crazy." MacKinnon and Michels approach these patients by asking them about others they have known who might have the disorder, acknowledging their pain and difficulty, inquiring about the reactions of family members to the disease, and being careful not to amateurly attempt to make premature connections between their symptoms and stressful life events. They seem to work with the present behavioral and feeling derivatives of long standing emotional conflicts of the patient which the therapist can understand and use to guide him, but which are not thrown up to the patient in a confronting way during this initial phase.

Finch and Hess (1962) characterize children with ulcerative colitis as dependent and demanding, speaking of feelings only with difficulty, and polarizing and judging each situation in good/bad, guilt/atonement terms. Anger and hostility were rarely expressed. The children had a poor self-image and saw themselves as damaged and degraded. As noted above, this description does fit our experience of some children referred for therapy, but surely not all children with ulcerative colitis. Finch and Hess suggest that in such situations treatment should be based on teamwork with the various specialists involved in the care of the child. Treatment will be long and must involve the families. They believe treatment should be supportive, active, and can rarely follow strict psychoanalytic principles. They suggest that the patient be invited to accept a less dependent role and more openly express his resentment and anger.

I can strongly endorse these principles on the basis of our experience. The therapist must certainly be active, pragmatic, and flexible. A real presence is required to meet the dependent needs of the patient. Many carefully worded, sympathetic, and firm suggestions have to be made to families so that they will permit the independence they ambivalently wish for the child. If the therapist is too confronting or judgmental, the patient or family backs away. The therapist is then caught between a sense of powerlessness and inertia if he does not take an active enough role and the loss of the patient or an opportunity to help if he becomes too active.

Even though we are not able to categorize children with ulcerative colitis under one emotional rubric, we have noted that the children coming into treatment tend to share some mechanisms and ways of adapting. Their dependent needs and demands are usually quite evident and, particularly with exacerbations or hospitalization, they regress and are demanding and withdrawn. They are quiet with little to say, their expressions blank or glum, and they deny or cannot articulate much about the emotions we assume they must be experiencing. Anxieties about loss, helplessness, abandonment, damage, or death are surely not expressed. Instead the child patient seems focused upon pain, the response of those about him to this pain, and methods of release from the pain and incapacity. We are thus forced to deal with the day-to-day operation of the ward or the home and "what they are going to do about" the discomfort of the patient.

Most of the patients we have seen do not complain about the frequent bowel movements or the loss of blood. These seem to be borne quietly, as even the pain is by some patients. They do deal with it by a restriction of social life, immobilizing themselves near a toilet and justifying, often appropriately, their social and emotional position by the severity and nature of their symptoms. Thus a kind of somatization takes place. Their life is controlled by their gut. The gut comes to be viewed almost as another personality, a bad part.

The time with the patient often centers about the day's events with attention to pain and diarrhea. The therapist must show an inquiring and reasonable concern about these most immediate problems of the child. Where demandingness and withdrawal seem to persist to extents beyond that demanded by the symptoms, suggestions about activities and changes can be offered without telling the patient he is behaving immaturely. Many sessions have to be carried by the therapist's energy.

We have not found children who will talk about a sense of being defective, who will openly betray any rage or anger about their plight, or who articulate concern about the loss of a part of themselves as they contemplate surgery. To the extent that these dynamics are present, they seem to be repressed and/or displaced in some way, again onto a concrete concern about the physical processes. The therapist finds himself working from physical reality toward emotional derivatives rather than the other way around. In our opinion, this is the only satisfactory way to approach therapy with these patients.

Transference and countertransference issues have some unique characteristics in these patients. It is rare to sense closeness and intimacy with these patients. They often keep us at arm's length, concerned that we won't believe their pain or will have nothing concrete to offer. At the same time they indirectly seem to ask something of us that they assume we will not or cannot give. This tends to characterize the psychotherapeutic process as a useless charade. Their glorifying comments about the physician as healer are often so excessive as to betray their true evaluation of us as powerless. Through all this many patients continue to avoid any introspective look at themselves or to join us in the venture. The therapist inclines toward communicating to the patient his feelings that the patient is not fulfilling his part of the therapy contract. If this is done prematurely or pejoratively, little benefit will ensue. It may be done indirectly or inadvertently through mannerism and inattention, and this is even more damaging. It is best handled with directness and care at that point in the treatment when the relationship has some history and dependability and the patient has some resilience and objectivity.

CONSIDERATIONS ABOUT SURGERY

A phrase often quoted by those working with ulcerative colitis patients is that "surgery is the only cure." Children whose growth is arrested by severe ulcerative colitis usually show significant growth spurts and maturation when their colons are removed. Furthermore, the threat of malignant change in the gut is diminished and rendered manageable by colectomy. This has led to earlier consideration of surgery. The therapist is often asked to play a role in deciding about surgery by evaluating the emotional consequences of the proposed operation. Some patients seek surgery as a cure, others shun it out of fear of surgery itself or concern about the problems created when the end of the intestinal tract is on the outer wall of the abdomen. While there is some promise that internal pouches may be devised, surgery still has the drawback of being a massive removal of body contents and of creating an unusual and at best unpleasant toileting situation. Prediction is very difficult for the mental health professional, and in such cases where we are asked to consult about surgery, we must confer carefully and at length with the patient, the family, the gastroenterologist, and the surgeon before our tentative impressions can be ventured. Surprisingly enough, it is often the parents who resist the idea of surgery, seeing it as an expensive and massive assault upon the body of their child. The patients are often so concerned with symptom relief and the desire to be free of the debilitating and confining aspects of the disease that they push for surgical intervention. We have not observed any children or adolescents who had unfavorable emotional reactions after surgery, even though most of the patients going to surgery have not given us any verbal assurance that they have a mature emotional understanding of what is going to happen and have worked it through.

While the emotional issues may not be worked through prior to surgery, the patients still experience much preoperative anxiety—centering around pain and the ileostomy rather than loss and change. Talking with a patient who has had a colectomy and now has an ileostomy is often a great aid to children or adolescents prior to surgery. We now arrange such meetings whenever possible.

Since surgery is undertaken only when clearly necessary for the management or survival of the patient, the psychiatrist is usually asked to provide opinions about timing of surgery or to help patients or families work through their feelings or fears about surgery. These tasks are necessary, but not that difficult in view of the positive benefit expected and usually realized from surgery. If the psychiatrist believes colitis to be a disease of the gut, he can counsel positively about surgery. However, if the psychiatrist believes the disorder is predominantly emotional, he can only regard the surgery as an aggressive or masochistic acting out of the patient's deepest emotional pathology and something that should not be countenanced.

SUMMARY

Psychotherapy with the child who has ulcerative colitis should be undertaken with the recognition that the disorder is most likely a multiply determined, genetic-constitutional disease of the bowel with emotional factors playing a significant role in the course of the disorder, perhaps more as effect than cause. Therapists must be prepared to work non-judgmentally with the family as well as with the patient. The evaluation and beginnings of therapy may well take place in the hospital with an ill child and distraught parents. It will be essential to work together with physicians treating the child and to involve the family in the treatment program. The patient will likely be immature, dependent, cautious, and perhaps minimally communicative while at the same time focusing upon physical processes, disbelieving in help, yet expecting magical results. The parents will frequently experience difficulty in allowing the child to individuate, and their relationship with the therapist may range from cooperative to blatantly hostile.

The therapist must be prepared to take an active role around reality issues, stay with the case for a long period of time, and help the child and family work through such real and difficult issues as total surgical removal of the large intestine, while settling for only small gains in insight and personality reorganization. The therapist who views this task as challenging can experience a significant measure of success and satisfaction in the treatment process with these patients.

REFERENCES

ALMY, T. What is the "irritable colon?" *American Journal of Digestive Diseases*, 1957, *2*, 93–97.

CHAUDHARY, N., and TRUELOVE, S. The irritable colon syndrome. *Quarterly Journal of Medicine* (New Series), 1962, *31*, 307–322.

ENGEL, G. Studies of ulcerative colitis, III. The nature of the psychologic processes. *American Journal of Medicine*, 1955, *19*, 231–256.

FELDMAN, F., CANTOR, D., SOLL, S., and BACHRACH, W. Psychiatric study of a consecutive series of 34 patients with ulcerative colitis. *British Medical Journal*, 1967, *3*, 14–17.

FINCH, S., and HESS, J. Ulcerative colitis in children. *American Journal of Psychiatry*, 1962, *118*, 819–826.

HIJMANS, J., and ENZER, N. Ulcerative colitis in childhood, a study of 43 cases. *Pediatrics*, 1962, *29*, 389–403.

HISLOP, I. Psychological significance of the irritable colon syndrome. *Gut*, 1971, *12*, 452–475.

JACKSON, D., and YALOM, I. Family research on the problem of ulcerative colitis. *Archives of General Psychiatry*, 1966, *15*, 410–418.

MACKINNON, R., and MICHELS, R. *The psychiatric interview in clinical practice*. Philadelphia: W. B. Saunders Co., 1971.

MENDELOFF, A., MONK, M., SIEGEL, C., and LILIENFELD, A. Illness experience and life stresses in patients with irritable colon and with ulcerative colitis. *New England Journal of Medicine*, 1970, *282*, 14–17.

PRUGH, D. The influence of emotional factors in the clinical course of ulcerative colitis in children. *Gastroenterology*, 1951, *18*, 339–354.

PURCELL, K., WEISS, J., and HAHN, W. Certain psychosomatic disorders. In B. Wolman (Ed.), *Manual of child psychopathology*. New York: McGraw-Hill, 1972.

SILVERBERG, M., and DAVIDSON, M. Ulcerative colitis. In H. Barnett (Ed.), *Pediatrics* (15th ed). New York: Appleton-Century-Crofts/Merideth Corp, 1972.

SPERLING, M. Psychoanalytic study of ulcerative colitis in children. *Psychoanalytic Quarterly*, 1946, *15*, 302–329.

10

ENURESIS

John A. Sours

"... she used to like to urinate into the cold sea when bathing and so produce a little warm self-created world to enclose her."

Marion Milner, *The Hands of the Living God*

Enuresis continues to be one of the more baffling problems in childhood psychopathology (Freud, 1893, 1905; Gerard, 1936; Hawkins, 1962; Jekel, 1962; Kim, 1959; Lourie, 1959; McLeod, 1959; Silberstein, 1962; Tunioli & De Ritis, 1961). Medical treatment of enuresis, as far back as ancient Egyptian medicine, has been confounded by a plethora of etiological theories, usually biased by the medical *Zeitgeist*. Since the time of Pliny various treatments, ranging from wood lice to swine's urine, were recommended for enuresis, even through the 19th century. And countless causes of enuresis have been postulated, vigorously acclaimed, and then rejected by counterclaims. Collectively, etiological theories of enuresis are too numerous, disjointed, and internally inconsistent for experimental validation. Few have stood the empirical test of time.

Throughout the vast literature of enuresis, epidemiological and clinical facts have often been collected apart from theory; and, conversely, theories have been advanced and multiplied, either without empirical evidence or without regard for known facts. Differences of opinion abound in regard to the definition of enuresis, its critical cutoff age, frequency, sex morbidity risk, and the relative clinical significance of the symptom from preschool to late adolescent years. There is little agreement whether enuresis is a specific clinical entity, a symptom, or a syndrome. Controversies exist over the importance of genetic-constitutional determinants, the role of parental training for bladder control, the interplay of psychosexual, psychosocial and neurophysiological factors, and the association of enuresis with longitudinal development and psychopathology. There are few studies that indicate the natural history of enuresis. Recent research, however, demonstrates that a history of enuresis does not per se predict future neurotic symptomatology, psychotic behavior, or borderline disorganization. Hallgren (1950, 1961) Tapia, Jekel, & Domke (1960), and Bakwin (1961) have even questioned whether enuresis is a sign of an emotional disorder.

Pierce (1967) indicates that 88% of enuretics stop wetting by 4-½ years, 93% by 7-½ years, and the remaining 7% by age 17. Statistics from military psychiatric studies reveal that up to 2% of enlisted men are enuretic and must, like somnambulists (Sours, 1963), be discharged from military duty.

Nocturnal enuresis refers to children who, according to Kanner (1957), continue to wet themselves at night after the age of 3 years or to children who after achieving bladder control by the third year relapse into persistent bedwetting. (Diurnal enuresis, daytime wetting of clothes, is less frequent and more apt to be associated with organicity.) Earlier bladder control, if it is achieved, is actually early "conditioning" by the mother and should not be mistaken for actual acquisition of bladder control. From the statistical-classificatory standpoint enuresis is listed as a habit disturbance under special symptom reactions and considered a transient reaction with the manifestation of the repetitive symptom of wetting.

The incidence of enuresis is higher among boys (2 : 1) (Christoffel, 1944; Sperling, 1965). Despert (1944) attributes the difference in gender and morbidity to the fact that boys have to learn the sitting and standing position for defecation and urination. But also important is the fact that girls submit more easily to toilet training and experience more maternal pressure. The prevalence of enuresis is assumed to be ubiquitous but is impossible to pinpoint because of the indeterminate age at which enuresis becomes pathological (ages 3 to 8 years in the literature) as well as the frequency of wetting. These figures depend on the clinical setting in which children are evaluated. Hospital psychiatric clinics, for example, report the highest rate since enuretics with organic pathology are referred there for evaluation. On the other hand, enuretics seen in the pediatrician's office are less numerous and less severe. But generally enuresis is more prevalent in socioeconomically and culturally disadvantaged people, particularly poor black children who score low on psychometric testing.

Associated with enuresis are other habits and behavioral disturbances, such as stealing, overeating, fire setting, and delinquency (Michaels, 1961) as well as the consequences of regression, particularly of the aggressive drive: nail biting, nose picking, stammering, teeth grinding, withdrawing, thumbsucking, rocking, and genital handling (Michaels, 1961; Murphy, 1971; Vandersall & Weiner, 1970). All these clinical phenomena are related to aggression, impulsivity, and regression. Rarely is enuresis an isolated symptom.

Enuresis is sometimes accompanied by a learning problem, especially when the child is convinced for psychodynamic reasons that his genitals are damaged. Imagined genital damage sometimes manifests itself as "head" damage; i.e., feelings of mental incapacity. Other children may react with denial and activity—believing that they can do anything they set their minds to. These children display the defensive ambition of the enuretic (Katan, 1946).

The purpose of this chapter is to summarize the literature on the causes and effects of nocturnal enuresis, both primary and acquired. A classification of nocturnal enuresis is then suggested, and the various therapeutic approaches to the symptom are examined. Developmental and neurophysiological aspects of enuresis are also reviewed since it is essential that they be kept in mind in the assessment of the enuretic child and in planning for treatment.

Epidemiological and clinical studies strongly suggest that *primary* and persistent enuresis is a symptom with heterogeneous causes, often multidetermined by coexistent psychological and social factors, which later become, in some instances, part of major behavioral disturbances and maladaptive character formation. Primary enuresis is often a symptom which develops within a family—particularly when the family cannot remain objectively detached from the symptom. On the other hand, *acquired* enuresis is usually associated with an environmental, transient factor or a developmental crisis. Less multidetermined, acquired enuresis tends to be short-lived, except for several small groups with internalized conflict, and is relatively amenable to treatment and less likely to be associated with later psychosexual and psychosocial sequelae.

A CLASSIFICATION OF NOCTURNAL ENURESIS

PRIMARY and PERSISTENT ENURESIS: 75 to 80%

Organic:

1. Lesional causes of nocturnal enuresis include genitourinary infections and genitourinary neurologic anomalies. Genitourinary causes of enuresis include

infections, meatal stenosis in boys, vulvitis in girls, trigoneurethritis, and congenital defects of the posterior urethra and urethral valves. Rarely is phimosis involved in enuresis. These make up about 3 to 10% of all cases of enuresis (Sarrouy, 1959; Weber & Genton, 1958; Murphy & Chapman, 1970). Often the pattern of wetting is diurnal. Involuntary passage of urine associated with states of unconsciousness, epilepsy, and drug intoxications also occur (Poussaint & Greenfield, 1966).

The incidence of enuresis in mental retardation is not significantly higher than in the general population; its frequency in this group depends on the attitude of those people who care for the retarded and the adequacy of the environment in which they live (Christoffel, 1944).

2. Genetic-constitutional causes of enuresis relate to neural developmental failure or maturational delay in the substitution of cerebral for hypothalamic-spinal bladder control. Developmental deficiency results in inadequate cortical inhibition of the detrusor leading to lower effective bladder capacity. The terms "irritable bladder" or "detrusor hyperirritability" are ones often used to describe this type of developmental failure or maturational lag. The high morbidity risk among parents and siblings of enuretics (52% according to Kanner, 1957); the high concordance of enuresis in monozygotic twins and enuretic children raised apart from parents in kibbutzim; and the genetic studies of Hallgren (1950, 1961) suggest a genetic group of enuretics whose pattern of genetic transmission is by a dominant gene with polygenic influence, the manifestations of which are affected by exogenic factors (Young, 1963; Bental, 1961). The genetic-constitutional group of enuretics is thought to be the largest organic group and, it is believed, has a high spontaneous remission rate in the second decade.

Heredity may be, for some children, a predisposing factor to nocturnal enuresis, but it also provides the child and parents with a ready-made rationalization for enuresis and absolves the child and family of responsibility. Both parents and the enuretic child are quick to seize upon the fact that other members of the family, both nuclear and extended, have also had enuresis.

However, enuresis is not necessarily an inherited disorder; instead, the tendency to give vent to the pleasure of urinary impulses—an attitude passed down from parent to child, from generation to generation (Johnson, 1953; Nilsson, 1973; Blum, 1970)—may be transmitted through family communication and identifications. A parent who has had enuresis as a child is less effective in helping his enuretic child.

In the last decade it has become more apparent that the neurophysiology of micturition is not clearly understood. Developmental variations in bladder control need further clarification. Muellner (1960) points out that the preschool child learns how to control the voluntary mechanisms of micturition through coordination of the thoracic diaphragmic and abdominal musculature, levator ani, and pubococcygeus. The child learns to push down the vesical neck of the bladder and initiate contraction of the detrusor. By gaining additional voluntary control of the bladder, the child enlarges the capacity of the bladder. Further developmental studies of genitourinary structure and function are needed.

Constitutional factors have been studied from the standpoint of sleep neurophysiology. Electroencephalographic studies suggest a high frequency of dysrhythmic patterns in nocturnal enuretics (Anders & Weinstein, 1972). Sleep studies have shown that enuresis occurs in deep sleep, specifically stage IV, and that enuresis is not a dream equivalent. Deep sleep of the enuretic is related to a physiological dysfunction in the reticular activating system which results in a dissociation of behavior and electroencephalographic sleep, a disorder akin to the electrical abnormalities of somnambulism (Bental, 1961; Boyd, 1960; Broughton, 1968; Hartmann, 1970). The enuretic child is said to sleep deeply,[1] and during enuretic episodes there can be tachycardia, compensatory bradycardia, and tachypnea. Often the enuretic boy has an erection during his night wetting. Dreams during an enuretic night's sleep tend to be aggressive and hostile, although enuretic adults usually dream of passive-dependent situations.

In the management of the young enuretic, specifically the child who appears to have stage IV sleep enuresis with onset early in the evening, guidance and reassurance of the mother may be sufficient. Often this kind of enuresis is monosymptomatic, uncomplicated by neurotic elaboration and family psychopathology. Frequently, stage IV sleep enuresis diminishes and finally ceases when maturational lags in development are no longer present. But in clinical situations where the symptom is persistent and troublesome to the family, Tofranil can be used or an electrical conditioning device can be employed.

Psychogenic:

This type of nocturnal enuresis is traceable primarily to failures in toilet training. Cortical

[1]Not all night wetting, however, occurs during sleep. Often enuretics, particularly deprived and affectively hungry children, wet themselves while fully conscious seeking the pleasure and comfort of a consistent maternal support.

inhibitory control of the bladder has not been established because of failures in training and habit learning. Or the pleasure of wetting during full wakefulness dissuades a child from accepting the responsibility of caring for his bladder function.

1. The lower sociocultural group makes up the majority of enuretics in this group. These enuretics can be viewed as "conditioning" failures. In social classes IV and V multiple deprivations, inconsistent and improper toilet training, and inadequate toilet facilities are often responsible factors. It has been found that institutionalized children, or children who change foster homes frequently, are often enuretic, but the frequency of enuresis depends in large part on the care and attitude of the staff and foster parents. The incidence of enuresis in these circumstances is inversely proportional to the quality of maternal care given these children (Christoffel, 1944). In social classes I and II the causative factors in nocturnal enuresis are permissiveness by the parents rationalized by an intellectualism often hiding maternal detachment and neglect. Bladder control is often ignored until the child enters nursery school at which time control suddenly becomes mandatory, forcing both child and parent into a situation of pressure and frustration.

2. Disturbances in the mother-child relationship account for another variety of psychogenic nocturnal enuresis. In this group the enuresis is related to difficulties in the dissolution of the symbiotic mother-child unit. Such children may wet while fully conscious as a way of entering a pleasurable sea of undifferentiated being. In the symbiotic dyad, tension is acted out by both members and impulse control is not achieved (Pierce et al., 1969). In other disturbances in the mother-child relationship enuretics are apt to be encouraged to play out the role of "Peter Pan" and accept infantilization. Boys may be encouraged to continue their enuresis by a mother who deprecates men and wants her son both ineffectual and rebellious. Such an enuretic boy becomes passive and avoids masculinity in order to please the mother. His father supports the mother-son relationship and thus protects himself from any threat from his son. Although the parents quarrel, this type of male enuretic paints a serene picture of his home and seeks to remain there safe from adult responsibilities. In some instances the disturbance is connected with psychosis or borderline faulty ego structuralization (Blum, 1970).

In another type of enuresis, one sees the symptom occurring as a result of vicarious parental gratification. Often a family history will suggest a traditional attitude toward toilet training; yet it is apparent, on closer scrutiny of the family, that an implicit permissiveness toward bladder dyscontrol is present. Urinary guilt and shame have not been sufficiently communicated to the child; and, in addition, enuresis for some of these children has become erotized (Johnson, 1953).

A variant of this group of enuretics is described by Michaels (1961). He found that persistent enuresis beyond the age of 10 is often associated with a clinical triad consisting of delinquency or sociopathic personality, inability to tolerate anxiety, and the impulsive need for immediate gratification. He related these disturbances to a psychosocial deficiency in learning inhibition and controls.

Treatment of enuresis resulting from various types of failures in toilet training must be decided in terms of etiology. In many instances treatment is aimed at correcting the toilet training attitudes of the parents or the deficiencies of the child's environment. When there is vicarious parental gratification, family therapy is useful; and, for those enuretics with a persistent enuretic symptom associated with sociopathic behavior, individual psychotherapy is necessary. This combined treatment approach may also be necessary for enuretics whose punitive toilet training combined with coercive measures has led to rage and fear during the early stages of the child's superego formation. Here enuresis can serve as an aggressive expression of the child's resentment to his parents (revenge enuresis).

Persistent nocturnal enuresis, sometimes coexisting with diurnal enuresis, may be found with encopresis. Pierce (1967) estimates "that 1 out of every 1,000 enuretics" is encopretic. For these children the prognosis for the enuresis is worse. Encopresis complicates the clinical situation since the deficit in impulse control is much more serious than in enuresis (Shane, 1967).

Acquired, Secondary Transient and Neurotic Enuresis: 20 to 25%

Acquired enuresis is a neurotic reaction to trauma and strain resulting in the child's giving up bladder control and reverting to behavioral immaturity. The symptom, one of low family incidence, may be a reaction to a disappointment in the mother-child relationship after the birth of a sibling. Here the enuretic identifies with his newborn sibling.

Acquired enuresis can in general be divided into two groups:

External Stress: Acquired enuresis can occur without unconscious conflict and be simply a response to the birth of a sibling, physical illness, loss of a parent, or change of nurses. In late adolescence enuresis can occur in going off to college or military service. It is usually transitory and spontaneously remits. If it is persistent, however, the symptom is an indication of an internalized conflict.

Internal Stress: This smaller group in which the symptom results from internal stress can be divided into three subvarieties:

1. The first group consists of children with unresolved Oedipal strivings and conflicts leading to castration anxiety and regression.
2. Children in the second group struggle to cope with a developmental phase. This group is well described by Nagera (1966).
3. Enuresis in the third group is one symptom of a psychosexual crisis following a traumatic sexual experience or erotized stimulation. The traumatic experience can be a primal scene or simply cumulative strain resulting from overstimulation (Berezin, 1954; Ferenczi, 1916). The male enuretic displays ambivalence and confusion over gender identity, fears genital damage, and may harbor wishes to be feminine.

Acquired enuresis may respond to brief goal-defined play therapy permitting the child to reexperience the affect of the trauma and master it. If characterological change has followed the traumatic experience, intensive treatment is required. The therapist should proceed with short-term play therapy for the young child if he believes that the enuresis is the result of a recent trauma and not past traumas that have led to fixations and deviations in psychosexual development and early character formation.

Internal stress acquired enuresis is most common in boys with castration anxiety and fear of genital injury. Enuresis can unconsciously substitute for masturbation with gratification of forbidden wishes and concomitant punishment. For girls, this kind of enuresis is often a part of "tomboyism" with outbursts of temper tantrums and manifestations of repressed aggression (Sperling, 1965; Fraiberg, 1963).

TREATMENT OF ENURESIS

The need for clinical research in the treatment of enuresis is apparent, as are the methodological problems entailed.

A spectrum of drugs has been tried including anticholinergics (belladonna, atropine), antidiuretics, CNS stimulants (amphetamines), hormones (chorionic gonadotropins, methyltestosterone) and psychotropic drugs (chlorpromazine), and imipramine hydrochloride (Tofranil).

An investigative drug-approach to enuresis is suggested by Poussaint and Greenfield's double-blind study of Tofranil (1966), which demonstrates that the drug is clinically and statistically superior to a placebo in the treatment of enuresis. They postulate that Tofranil is effective because its anticholinergic activity relaxes the detrusor and thereby increases bladder capacity; its stimulant action lightens sleep, and its antidepressant action perhaps has an effect on central autonomic mechanisms. It appears that Tofranil-responders are primarily enuretics with genetic-constitutional dysfunction or children who were poorly toilet trained. After gradual withdrawal of Tofranil, a large proportion continue to remain dry at night.

This research raises several questions pertinent to all drug studies: What are the differences between Tofranil-responders and non-responders? How do Tofranil-responders compare with enuretics who become dry after treatment with electrical conditioning devices? How do the two groups of Tofranil-treated enuretics compare in terms of bladder capacity (before and after treatment) and sleep electroencephalograms during treatment? Are there differences in terms of individual and family psychodynamics? Perhaps further drug studies will provide a better delineation of the etiological groups and intergroup responses. What is also needed is a better understanding of the untoward effects of drugs on children during critical phases of growth and development (Parker et al., 1969).

The therapies for enuresis are extremely difficult to assess. Since the very first treatment plan is often successful in 50% of enuretics—merely the physician's interest may suffice for some children—enthusiastic acclaim for one treatment technique is apt to be made. Drug trials are very difficult to evaluate in that therapeutic results do not readily lend themselves to clear-cut interpretation and conclusion. The difficulties in gathering a sample population of enuretics with adequate controls are enormous.

It is also difficult to determine the effect of enuresis itself on character development and adult psychopathology. This is especially true for retrospective studies. Unfortunately, longitudinal studies of enuretic groups are lacking, except for Hallgren's work (1950). Nevertheless, there is clinical evidence that failure of bladder control does damage a child's sense of mastery, impair his self-esteem, and lead to a defective body image, psychosexual dysfunction, and faulty interpersonal relationships (Abraham, 1917; Katan, 1946).

Fluid restriction is not an effective measure in the management of the enuretic child. Neither is awakening the child during the night to have him urinate a useful approach to symptom removal, even for children who wet early in the evening during stage IV sleep. Awakening the child is experienced as both gratification and punishment. Picking the enuretic child up and walking or carrying him to the bathroom is not only ineffective but also fosters the regressive potential and negates his responsibility. Furthermore, the child must be made aware that his wetting is connected with feelings and that wetting involves impulsive gratification.

Behavioral modification techniques (Yates, 1975) are useful for specific types of enuresis, as well as life-endangering anorexia nervosa and monosymptomatic tics. In using an electrical conditioning device, theoretically based on the principles of operant conditioning, the parent rewards the enuretic child when he surrenders his symptoms or, on the other hand, punishes him when the child retains them. A conditioning treatment also mobilizes the parent's activity and approach to the child in such a way that the parents are forced to perform the normal parental role of encouraging age-specific and appropriate behavior and values. Conditioning techniques are effective in certain types of enuresis; it is important to keep in mind, however, that if they are used for the neurotic or psychotic enuretic, or if used by angry, rejecting parents, behavioral modification can provide the child with a very artificial and inhumane environment as well as subject him to a variety of sadomasochistic punishments and gratifications.

In cases where persistent enuresis is related to a disturbance in the mother-child relationship and in cases of acquired and unrelenting enuresis complicated by internalized conflict, psychological treatment of the child is mandatory. Whether the child requires psychotherapy or child analysis is determined by a number of factors, related both to the child and to his family, and takes into consideration the results of the overall assessment of the child (Sours, 1976). Whatever the extent of analytic treatment, therapy for the enuretic child must seek to modify maladaptive defenses, develop structures, strengthen the ego, make "adjustments" in the superego, "tuning" the conscience to instinctual need, and foster neutralization of energy. By introjection of and identification with the therapist the child is able to diminish his sense of emptiness. In both child analysis and therapy, the enuretic child employs the therapist as a real object, learning from him new adaptive styles of behavior and thought. Particularly for those children whose parents have not fostered ego development—or, for that matter, have derailed adequate superego structuralization—the therapist helps the child control impulsivity and adjust his frustration tolerance. In addition, treatment can heighten the child's ability to interact with adults, both in the home and outside the family situation, in a constructive and adaptive way.

REFERENCES

Abraham, K. Ejaculatio praecox. In *Selected papers.* London: Hogarth Press, 1942. (Originally published, 1917.)

Anders, T., and Weinstein, P. Sleep and its

disorders in infants and children: A review. *Pediatrics*, 1972, *50*, 312–324.

BAKWIN, H. Enuresis in children. *Journal of Pediatrics*, 1961, *58*, 806–819.

BEHRLE, F. C., ELKINS, M. T and LAYBOURNE, R. C. Evaluation of a conditioning device in the treatments of nocturnal enuresis. *Pediatrics*, 1956, *17*, 849–856.

BENTAL, E. Dissociation of behavioural and electroencephalographic sleep in two brothers with enuresis nocturna. *Journal of Psychosomatic Research*, 1961, *5*, 116–9.

BEREZIN, M. A. Enuresis and bisexual identification. *Journal of the American Psychoanalytic Association*, 1954, *2*, 509–13.

BLUM, H. P. Maternal psychopathology and nocturnal enuresis. *Psychoanalytic Quarterly*, 1970, *39*(4), 609–619.

BOYD, M. M. The depth of sleep in enuretic school children and in non-enuretic controls. *Journal of Psychosomatic Research*, 1960, *4*, 274–281.

BROUGHTON, R. J. "Sleep disorders," disorders of arousal?, *Science*, 1968, *159*, 1070–1078.

CHRISTOFFEL, H. *Trieb und Kultur*. Basel: Benno Schwabe, 1944.

DANIELS, M. Enuresis, body language and the positive aspects of the enuretic act. *American Journal of Psychotherapy*, 1971, *25*, 564–578.

DESPERT, L. Urinary control and enuresis. *Psychosomatic Medicine*, 1944, *6*, 294–307.

FERENCZI, S. *Contributions to psychoanalysis*. Boston: Badger, 1916.

FISHER, C. BYRNE, J., EDWARDS, A. and KAHN, E. A psychophysiological study of nightmares. *Journal of the American Psychoanalytic Association*, 1970, *18*, 747–783.

FRAIBERG, S. Some characteristics of genital arousal and discharge in latency girls. *Psychoanalytic Study of the Child*, 1963, *27*, 439–475.

FREUD, S. Ueber ein Symptom, das haeufig die Enuresis Nocturna der Kinder begleitet. *Centralblatt*, 1893, *12*, 735–737.

FREUD, S. Three essays on the theory of sexuality. *Complete Works* (*Vol. 7*). London: Hogarth Press, 1953. (Originally published, 1905.)

FREYMAN, R. Follow-up study of enuresis treated with a bell apparatus. *Journal of Child Psychology and Psychiatry*, 1963, *4*, 199–206.

GREARD, M. W. Enuresis: A study of etiology. *American Journal of Orthopsychiatry*, 1936, *9*, 48–58.

HALLGREN, B. Enuresis. *Acta Psychiatrica et Neurologica Scandinavia* (Suppl. 114), 1950, *32*, 1–158.

HALLGREN, B., LARSSON, H. and RUDHE, U. Nocturnal enuresis in twins. II: Urethro-cystographic examinations. *Acta Paediatrica* (Uppsala), 1961, *50*, 117–126.

HARTMANN, E. (Ed.) *Sleep and Dreaming*. Boston: Little, Brown, 1970.

HAWKINS, D. N. Enuresis: a survey. *Medical Journal of Australia*, 1962, *49*, 979–980.

JEKEL, J. F. The natural history of an unnatural phenomenon: Enuresis. A review. *Hartford Hospital Bulletin*, 1962, *17*, 49–63.

JOHNSON, A. Factors in the etiology of fixations and symptom choice. *Psychoanalytic Quarterly*, 1953, *22*, 475–496.

KAFFMAN, M. Toilet-training by multiple caretakers: Enuresis among kibbutz children. *Israel Annals of Psychiatry*, 1972, *10*, 341–365.

KANNER, L. *Child psychiatry* (3rd ed.). Springfield, Ill.: Charles C. Thomas Publisher, 1957.

KATAN, A. Experiences with enuretics. *Psychoanalytic Study of the Child*, 1946, *2*, 510–534.

KIM, H. W. Enuresis: A literature review. *Clinical Proceedings of Children's Hospital* (Washington) 1959, *15*, 153–172.

LOURIE, R. S. Enuresis: a psychiatrist's view. *Clinical Proceedings Children's Hospital* (Washington) 1959, *15*, 175–79.

MCLEOD, J. W. Enuresis: a pediatrician's view. *Clinical Proceedings of Children's Hospital* (Washington) 1959, *15*, 172–75.

MICHAELS, J. J. Enuresis in murderous aggressive children and adolescents. *Archives of Genetic Psychiatry*, 1961, *5*, 490–493.

MILNER, M. *The Hands of the Living God*. New York: International Universities Press, 1969, p. 28.

MUELLNER, S. R. Development of urinary control in children. *Journal of the American Medical Association*, 1960, *120*, 1236–1261.

MURPHY, S., and CHAPMAN, W. Adolescent enuresis: a urologic study. *Pediatrics*, 1970, *45*, 426–431.

MURPHY, S. and CHAPMAN, W. Behavioral characteristics of adolescent enuretics. *Adolescence*, 1971, *6*, 1–18.

NAGERA, H. Early childhood disturbances, the infantile neurosis and the adulthood disturbances. *Psychoanalytic Study of the Child* (*Monograph No. 2.*). New York: International Universities Press, 1966.

NILSSON, A., Enuresis: The importance of maternal attitudes and personality. *Acta Psychiatrica Scandinavia*, 1973, *49*, 114–130.

PARKER, D. C., and TAD, E. Human growth hormone release during sleep: Electroencephalographic correlation. *Journal of Clinical Endocrinology and Metabolism*, 1969, *29*, 1468–1470.

PIERCE, C. M., WHITMAN, R. M., MAAS, J. W., and GAY, M. L. Enuresis and dreaming, experimental studies. *Archives of General Psychiatry*, 1961, *4*, 166–170.

PIERCE, C. M. Enuresis. In A. M. Freedman and H. I. Kaplan (Eds.), *Comprehensive Textbook of Psychiatry*. Baltimore: William & Wilkins, 1967.

PIERCE, M. & Whitman, R. M. Mothers of enuretic boys. *American Journal of Psychotherapy*, 1969, *23*, 283–292.

POUSSAINT, F., and GREENFIELD, R. Epilepsy and enuresis. *American Journal of Psychiatry*, 1966, *122*, 1426–1427.

SARROUY, C., LEGEAIS, G., and SANPEREZ, R. Association of cranial dysostosis, occult spina bifida and enuresis in the same family (French). *Pediatrie*, 1959, *14*, 551–555.

SHANE, M. Encopresis in a latency boy. *Psychoanalytic Study of the Child*, 1967, *22*, 296–314.

SILBERSTEIN, R. M. The problem of enuresis. *Bulletin of the Philadelphia Association for Psychoanalysis*, 1962, *12*, 137–148.

SOURS, J. A. The application of child analytic principles to forms of child psychotherapy. In J. Glenn (Ed.), *Child Analysis: Technique, Theory and Applications*. New York: Jason Aronson, in press.

SOURS, J. A., FRUMKIN, P. and INDERMILL, R. R. Somnambulism: Its clinical significance and dynamic meaning in late adolescence and adulthood. *Archives of General Psychiatry*, 1963, *9*, 400–413.

SPERLING, M. Dynamic considerations and the treatment of enuresis. *Journal of the Academy of Child Psychiatry*, 1965, *4*, 19–31.

TAPIA, F., JEKEL, J. and DOMKE, H. H. Enuresis: An emotional symptom? *Journal of Mental and Nervous Diseases*, 1960, *130*, 61–66.

TUNIOLI, A. M., and DE RITIS, L. Results of a psychosomatic investigation made in a group of enuretic children of school age. *Clinical Pediatrics* (*Bologna*), 1961, *43*, 440–449.

VANDERSALL, T. A., and WEINER, J. M. Children who set fires. *AMA Archives of General Psychiatry*, 1970, *22*(1), 63–72.

WEBER, A., and GENTON, H. Problem of enuresis: Psychopathological and urological examination of a large series of enuretics. (German and French). *Acta Helvetica Paediatrica*, 1958, *13*, 275–291.

YATES, A. J. *Theory and Practice in Behavior Therapy*. New York: John Wiley, 1975.

YOUNG, G. C. The family history of enuresis. *Journal of the Royal Institute of Public Health*, 1963, *26*, 197–201.

II

ENCOPRESIS

Jules R. Bemporad

Perhaps the most pertinent aspect of treatment with encopretic children is that the therapeutic process is frustrating, prolonged, and far from uniformly successful. Almost half a century ago, the pioneer child psychiatrist D. A. Thom wrote of encopretic children: "One can say that these cases call for a careful psychiatric examination by the best qualified person available. And it will often test all his skill and ingenuity to understand the mental processes at work that result in such conduct" (cited in Kanner, 1966). This prophetic statement is still valid today. The reason for the difficulty in treating encopretic children is that fecal soiling is rarely the sole symptom but rather the surface expression of an entrenched personality disorder often complicated by organic problems and reinforced by disturbed family relationships. This situation is particularly true of older children with repeated, frequent soiling. However, as a symptom, encopresis may occur in a variety of children, each requiring different forms of therapeutic intervention. Therefore, before describing the problems involved in the therapy of the "neurotic" encopretic child in whom the symptom has become a form of communication with an environment that is perceived as hostile and ungratifying, a description of the various types of childhood fecal soiling may be warranted as well as a brief discussion of the current theories regarding the developmental aspects of sphincter control.

TYPES OF ENCOPRESIS

Encopresis has been succinctly defined by Kanner (1966) as an act of involuntary defecation which is not directly due to organic disease or deformity. Within the confines of this definition there exists a variety of children who may exhibit fecal soiling for a multiplicity of reasons. While most children are expected to attain fecal continence by age two or three at the latest, in some children training is greatly delayed while in others it is never achieved.

Into this group would fall children with severe intellectual impairment whose soiling is part of an overall retardation of developmental functions. In an early paper on encopresis, Hale Shirley (1938) found that of seventy encopretic children (using 2 years of age as the cut-off limit), 21 had an IQ under 50, and an additional 5 had an IQ between

50 and 70. Ten more had an IQ between 70 and 80. Therefore, over half of Shirley's cases had an IQ under 80. In profoundly retarded children encopresis is simply another manifestation of an overall defect and cannot be truly considered a psychiatric symptom. Furthermore, one suspects that with better facilities for such children and more extensive utilization of behavior modification techniques, soiling would be much less frequent in this group of children than it was 30 years ago.

Another type of impaired child who may present with encopresis is the youngster whose soiling appears secondary to a minimal brain dysfunction (MBD) syndrome. These children are often so distracted and hyperactive that they do not attend to body cues such as the need to defecate. When MBD children are involved in pleasurable activities, they do not want to take the time to stop to go to the toilet and so soil themselves. One such 10-year-old boy who presented with hyperactivity, distractability, and emotional lability occasionally soiled while playing football with his friends where there were no convenient toilet facilities. He was markedly different from the neurotic type of encopretic in that he was cheerful, outgoing, and extremely open and talkative, and his parents appeared unconcerned about his occasional soiling. As with most of these children, his encopresis stopped with amelioration of his primary condition through chemotherapy, parent counseling, and superficial psychotherapy. Medication helped "slow" him down so he could attend to bodily needs and he responded to suggestions that aspects of his behavior (the soiling included) were beneath his more mature capacities. In these children, the soiling does not appear to serve any interpersonal or intrapsychic purpose.

In a study of 76 encopretic children, Anthony (1957) stressed a crucial difference between continuous children, who had never been trained, and discontinuous children, who began soiling after a period of fecal continence. The continuous child is described as "a dirty child coming from a dirty family, burdened with every conceivable sort of social problem." On the other hand, the discontinuous child is a "compulsive child of a compulsive family. He is over controlled and inhibited in his emotional life and scrupulous with regard to his habits." Anthony concludes that the discontinuous child is emotionally disturbed and requires extensive psychotherapy but that the continuous child has not developed the socially expected disgust reactions because of laxity in training and a high familial tolerance for dirtiness. The continuous child simply needs to be retrained to develop a "normal" degree of repugnance to fecal products. This division of encopretic groups has not been overly helpful clinically nor has it been confirmed by other studies. Often it is difficult to distinguish continuous from discontinuous children, since many achieve a marginal form of continence with frequent "accidents" prior to the onset of daily soiling and others alternate between soiling and continence at varying intervals depending on environmental pressures. Anthony also stresses that the continuous child comes from lower socioeconomic families where overwhelming social problems overshadow the relatively minor problem of a child's soiling. Experience with economically deprived families in the New York area has actually yielded the opposite result: that infants from poverty homes are trained early because the mother does not have the time nor luxury for leisurely training, being burdened with other responsibilities. Since Anthony's study was researched in England, there may well be cultural differences, especially if his "continuous" group came from rural areas. Nevertheless, in clinical experience the "continuous" children appear as disturbed as the "discontinuous." Therefore, this distinction does not appear as helpful as a general evaluation of the numerous other factors which could have elicited and maintained the symptom.

Another group of children who exhibit encopresis are those who automatically react to fear or gross stress with evacuation of the bowels. Usually they are quite young (3 to 5 years of age) and their soiling is sporadic and random, except for its association with stress. Sometimes these children also show mild organicity of the MBD variety, although this type of soiling may occur in intact children as was demonstrated by the increase in soiling which occurred in English children removed from their London homes to the countryside during World War II bombardment (Freud & Burlingham, 1943).

One four-year-old boy would soil whenever he was severely scolded by his father. The child was a shy, sensitive boy who truly felt panic when reprimanded. He had signs of neurological immaturity so that it was difficult for him to dampen his emotions and he was easily overwhelmed. His soiling promptly ceased when his father understood his son's overreactions and stopped his scolding as a corrective measure. This boy could not account for his soiling except to concede that it occurred when he was "very scared." Another young child, who had a learning disability and other neurologic problems, began soiling when his divorced father moved away and remarried. At the time, his mother was working and his grandparents, of whom the boy was very fond, had also moved away. Clinging to his mother, the child presented as emotionally immature and generally apprehensive. He could not explain the onset of his soiling but was frightened of never seeing his father again. His soiling stopped when the mother temporarily quit her job and spent more time with him but then recurred 1 month later. It stopped permanently a few weeks later when the grandparents moved back to his home town and were able to offer him sources of security and gratification.

While these children do not require extensive treatment for their soiling, if the source of their fears can be identified and eliminated, therapy should he continued in order to have the parents appreciate the child's apprehensive orientation toward change and to bolster the child's sense of security. Such children may also provide clues for delineating the triggering event in cases of "neurotic" encopresis. Those children who soil more and more frequently until the symptom becomes part of a parent-child power struggle and the soiling itself becomes an expression of a hostile dependent relationship with significant others may first develop encopresis after a traumatic separation or frustration that was never set right. It is this group of children who are so difficult to treat and whose encopresis is a central determinant of their behavior as well as a powerful mode of eliciting responses from others.

In a previous study (Bemporad, Pfeifer, Gibbs, Cortner, & Bloom, 1971) of 17 encopretic children who were randomly selected as they presented for treatment, 14 could be described as "neurotic" in the sense that the soiling was utilized in the service of psychic needs and was stubbornly and irrationally defended despite familial rewards and punishments. These 14 children and their families exhibited a surprising number of common characteristics. In terms of family structure, there was an unusually high rate of divorce (57%). In those cases where the parents had not divorced or where the mother had remarried, it was found that the father was emotionally and physically absent from the home. These men often held two jobs or simply found excuses to absent themselves from family life. Personality assessment of the fathers or father surrogates of encopretic children showed them to be depressed and afraid of social contact.

In sharp contrast to the fathers, the mothers of these children were domineering and intrusive. They showed a peculiar vacillation between infantilizing overprotectiveness and cold, critical rejection toward the children. This inconsistency also was manifested in their ignoring gross deviations in behavior while stubbornly insisting on having a perfect performance in trivial matters. In therapy, they presented the facade of an efficient, unemotional, capable adult; however, in due course, another powerful yet submerged aspect of their personalities surfaced. Beneath their "top sergeant" exterior, they often expressed a romantic yearning of an almost adolescent quality in its idealization and poignancy. It appeared that these individuals were ambivalent in their own personal identities as women as much as in their roles as mothers. They seemed to have given up even on being loved as they desired to be and had resentfully adopted a defensive attitude that such romanticism was trivial and life should be lived with efficient and unfeeling practicality.

In evaluating the histories of the mothers, many disappointments in past relationships were noted. They did not get along with their own mothers but, of greater importance, they had been either rejected or neglected by their fathers who had been distant and had not encouraged their daughters' femininity. While secretly longing for an ideal mate, they had "settled" for unsatisfying husbands whom they could control and who did not challenge their defensive superstructure. Often their disappointment was so great that they became perfectionistic and angry, sensing their everyday responsibilities (children included) as unfair burdens and sources of frustration.

The internal dynamics of these mothers may help to explain a uniform and glaring characteristic: an incredible lack of sensitivity to the feelings and desires of others. The paucity of empathy in otherwise intelligent individuals was at times difficult to believe until the reasons for their self-involvement and their need to block feelings became more understandable. This lack of empathy took the form of openly reporting humiliating things about their children in their presence. They would also disparage their husbands without regard for feelings. One mother began a tirade about her husband and son in a crowded clinic waiting room embarrassing not only her family but the other waiting patients. She loudly made statements such as, "Men have it easy. They just run off and leave the mother stuck with the children." Another expression of this insensitivity is the mothers' shameless intrusion into the private affairs or property of other family members and then the public announcement of secrets that were either discovered or divulged. Quite often these mothers were unable to appreciate the fears of their children and unable to provide the needed sense of security or support. Sometimes, the mothers were so involved with their own dissatisfaction or so depressed that they simply were emotionally unavailable. Other mothers, despite capabilities in other areas, seemed unable to cope with their children's needs.

Despite this lack of attention to the children's emotional needs, all of these mothers reacted strongly to the child's soiling. This was the one activity which prompted them to bribery, punishment, and ultimately an angry sense of defeat. It was not surprising that in 10 of our 14 "neurotic" encopretic children, the soiling occurred only at home and in the mother's presence. It was our impression that if the child felt defeated by his mother's overpowering criticism or impregnable insensitivity, the mother felt equally defeated by her child's embarrassing soiling.

If this description of the encopretic child's mother seems harsh and unfair, it should be tempered by an understanding of her situation. Her husband was either absent or unable to fulfill any emotional demands. The burdens of the household fell almost entirely on her. In addition, the neurotic encopretic child about to be described eventually develops a personality that, quite frankly, is difficult to relate to in a warm manner. He becomes an angry, sullen oppositional child who silently harbors hostile desires or who has aggressive outbursts at the slightest provocation. A vicious cycle seems to be initiated—the soiling enrages the mother, whose subsequent behavior makes the child angry with her, so that he continues to soil, which further enrages the mother and so on. By the time such children are seen for therapy, an almost uniform relationship of hostile dependency exists, one in which the child resists separation from the mother or behaves in an infantile manner while trying to irritate her through soiling or passive-aggressive maneuvers. In return, the mother feels furious and defeated by a child who is a constant source of embarrassment.

The 14 children, all of whom were latency-age males, could be summarized as angry, unhappy, and oppositional. They were noncommunicative and shallow in their relationships. They first denied soiling, then refused to acknowledge any awareness that they soiled, and eventually became sullen and silent if their symptom were discussed. In sessions they appeared bored and were difficult to engage in conversation or in play activities. Sometimes they would complain of having few friends or of how they were mistreated by other children. Most showed poor social judgment and a tendency toward solitary antisocial behavior of an angry, destructive type. Psychological testing revealed a predominance of aggressive fantasies as well as feelings of deprivation and inadequacy. Most expressed a sense of hopelessness over ever being able to communicate with their mothers. Common remarks were "you can't win with her," or "you just have to ignore her." This was part of a pervasive sense of defeatism regarding the assertion of one's will. Most of the boys had an idealized view of their fathers and wanted to spend more time with them, sometimes blaming themselves for the father's lack of attention.

From our clinical experience with these children, we concluded that the soiling was a family problem and represented a distorted, hostile communication toward the mother who allowed no overt form of assertion and was impervious to appropriately expressed needs or feelings. We shifted our therapeutic model to family therapy, insisting on greater participation from the fathers. We were surprised to find that in half of our cases the soiling stopped after the father took a greater role in family life. In one other case, the soiling stopped when the divorced mother remarried and in two additional cases when the father returned to live at home after being on isolated military tours. In these latter cases the soiling stopped without any concurrent movement in treatment and seemed unrelated to what was occurring during the sessions. The importance of an available father figure in the household seemed to have a dramatic effect on the soiling. It could be speculated that the greater participation of the father altered the mother's own feelings of resentment and allowed her to be a more responsive parent. Another possibility is that the father gave the child more emotional support or became his ally in the chronic mother-child power struggle. Whatever the reasons, it became clear that encopresis should be conceptualized as a transactional behavior that involves the entire family unit and seems to respond best to alterations in family equilibrium.

Other studies have subsequently confirmed some of our findings. Hoag and co-workers (1971), in a study of 10 encopretic boys, found the mothers to be compulsive, rigid, and hostile persons who were prone to use intellectualization as a defense and to deny emotions. They also complained of feeling trapped and unfulfilled by their life situations. As for the fathers, "they were all away from home extensively and consistently, i.e., holding two jobs, establishing self-owned businesses, attending many political or scientific meetings, working long distances from home."

The encopretic children were found to feel unloved and unwanted but were unable to express any resentment. They were lonely, depressed, dependent youngsters who longed for acceptance. They were difficult to engage in treatment and resistant to relinquishing their soiling. A successful outcome appeared highly correlated with alterations in familial behavior patterns.

In an article on family relationships and encopresis, Baird (1974) concludes that parent-child interaction is the core problem. Based on her clinical experience with approximately 40 encopretic children, Baird characterizes the families of the patients as demonstrating four major pathological interaction patterns: (1) withholding of information, (2) infantilization of the patient, (3) mishandling of anger through repression and denial, and (4) miscommunication about essential family affairs. It is further significant that Baird cites cases in which the soiling stopped after therapy involving only the parents.

These contributions are relevant in that they shift the emphasis for both a dynamic understanding and a therapeutic approach from the child and his symptom to family transactions. Rather than attempting to interpret and to treat encopresis as symbolic of unconscious fantasies or as a regression to an anal-libidinal organization, the cause, persistence, and cure of encopresis appears more comprehensible as part of a total family situation, with the child's pathology being both a response to and an elicitor of aberrant parental behavior.

Nevertheless, an elaboration of the particular family structure, while pointing the way to treatment, is not very helpful in clarifying the choice of soiling as a symptom. The fact that a child is angry with his mother and that soiling is a powerful way of upsetting her may help explain the persistence of the symptom but not why encopresis was chosen in the first place. Actually, many families seen clinically present with a similar pattern, yet the child does not exhibit soiling. For example, a lonely, angry nine-year-old boy was seen for poor school performance. His father was rarely home and unavailable when in the house. His mother alternated between infantilization and critical rigidity and was lacking in empathy. This little boy would lock himself in the bathroom and threaten to swallow the entire contents of the medicine cabinet as a way of "getting even" with his mother but he did not soil himself. Similarly, we found non-encopretic siblings of soiling children to have varying degrees of pathology also based on feelings of anger and hopelessness. It may be worthwhile, therefore, to consider briefly the problem of symptom choice while remaining aware that any conclusion must remain purely tentative at this time.

Predisposition to Encopresis

The logical choice in the search for a crucial life event that could predispose a child to fecal soiling would be the period of toilet training. In the series of 14 cases mentioned above, we did find evidence of traumatic bowel training in 11 children, training that was initiated in the first year of life and was described as difficult, prolonged, and coercive. Six of the 14 children had never truly achieved continence, continuing to have sporadic "accidents" prior to the onset of frequent, persistent soiling. An additional factor these children commonly shared was some degree of subtle organic defect, particularly in the area of language development. Some children had obvious reading disabilities, others were slow to develop language skills, almost all displayed some degree of incoordination and neurological immaturity—independent of often superior intelligence. It could be hypothesized that the early, rigid toilet training was complicated and made more traumatic by the fact that the child may have been neurologically not yet ready or able to achieve sphincter control. Some of the children were described as bewildered by the initial attempts at toilet training, which were nonetheless continued. The exacting demands of the mother (or in some cases the mother's inability adequately to structure the toilet training procedure) further blocked the usual mastery of the ego over bodily functions.

The normal process of control over wetting and soiling has been carefully documented by Anna Freud (1965) in her theoretical conceptualization of developmental lines. She mentions four stages in this progression: (1) complete freedom to wet and soil; (2) a placing of value on bodily products, which are either surrendered to the mother as a sign of love or expelled from the body as a sign of anger; (3) acceptance of the mother's standards of cleanliness as part of a positive relationship; and (4) autonomous control independent of relationships with others. Freud makes it clear that a secure and continued relationship with the mother is a prerequisite for mastery of this developmental line. She believes that the internalized attitudes toward cleanliness are not stable until latency and that "a child who is severely disappointed in his mother, or separated from her, or suffering from object loss in any form, may not only lose the internalized urge to be clean but also reactivate the aggressive use of elimination."

The children with chronic, neurotic forms of encopresis do not appear to have progressed beyond stage 2 or to have later reverted to it. As a result of the rushed or coercive nature of a too early training, the impeding effect of an organic defect, and the overwhelmingly unempathic attitude of the mother, it appears doubtful that these children were able to internalize or develop autonomous controls over excretory functions but rather regard excretory functions as part of a power struggle which involves their own feelings and the reactions of others. Because of this emotional over-valuation of defecation, there is often a tendency to deny control over evacuation since this would imply conscious responsibility. And to some extent, there may be some truth in the child's denial of responsibility, since it is questionable to what degree the child ever felt mastery over his own body. The whole process of sphincter-control becomes so emotionally laden that it cannot be treated autonomously (stage 4).

Morton Shane (1967) has described his treatment of an encopretic 8-year-old boy utilizing Frend's developmental lines as a theoretical model. As a result of maternal ambivalence and inconsistency, toilet training begun at the age of 8 months was never accomplished. During the course of therapy, the child displayed severe aggressive behavior and motor outburst instead of verbalization of feelings. Beneath the barrage of aggressive activity was a frustrated longing for protection and love from the mother who, because of her own difficulties, had been unable to respond to her son's needs. Shane is able to document how, for 3 years, the boy progressed through Freud's developmental stages as a result of his therapeutic alliance. The gradual control over bodily functions coincided with improvement in other areas, including a better relationship with the mother.

Utilizing Freud's model of developmental lines, we gain the insight that encopretic children have not progressed for several possible reasons. Of greatest importance are the consistent findings that defecation is still closely related to relationships to others and that there has not been an internalization of parental attitudes toward bodily products.

The above discussion of the familial characteristics, interpersonal problems, and intrapsychic distortions of encopretic patients, as well as the emphasis on a close interrelationship between toilet training and mother-child interaction, may serve as a way of placing the aims and problems of therapy in perspective. In the following section, cases of encopretic children and their treatment will be presented as a means of exemplifying this theoretical structure.

APPROACHES TO THERAPY

From the foregoing discussion, it becomes apparent that psychotherapeutic intervention in encopresis should be directed toward altering the interpersonal processes that serve to trigger and maintain soiling. In my own experience, a search for a symbolic meaning underlying the soiling has been uniformly fruitless. Rather, it is better understood as a semi-autonomous act that is elicited by certain environmental frustrations in susceptible children and afterward serves both to arouse reactions in others and to express unacceptable feelings. As will be surmised from the cases to be presented, soiling is often the only act to which the parents respond, despite other, more serious signs of pathology in the child or evidences of chronic unhappiness that go ignored. Therefore, the therapy of the encopretic child usually involves therapy of the entire family.

When the child is brought for therapy, there usually exists a long standing family struggle over the encopresis, in which the child realizes the power of his symptom in upsetting the parents and the parents are furious with the child for refusing to meet their demands for continence. While acutely aware of the soiling, these families are blind to their pathological modes of relating to one another and to the circumstances which elicit and maintain the symptom. It has been my experience that the soiling "mysteriously" disappears with an amelioration of the family atmosphere and interrelationships.

The prime task of the therapist, in my opinion, is to determine what is lacking in the child's everyday life, what is causing him to feel frustrated and angry, what is blocking an appropriate expression of his feelings—in short, the causes of his having to resort to soiling as a method of expression—and then to attempt to rectify these sources of discontent. Obviously, this is not an easy task, since the child often suffers from other emotional defects which make it difficult to engage him adequately in therapy. In addition, the family situation, which is integral with the child's soiling, usually resists change; parents prefer to focus on the encopresis rather than discuss possibilities which might force them to alter their own modes of behavior. As I have described above, the most common feature of the relationships in encopretic families is a lack of empathic understanding. Each parent seems so involved with his or her own disappointments, that there is little or no attempt to appreciate the experiences of the child. The child will interpret this self-involvement and lack of gratification of his needs as parental hostility and eventually will retaliate in the limited ways available. Some children will select acting out or even psychosomatic symptoms. Encopretic children, for some yet unknown predisposing defect, will select soiling and find that it works well to gain attention and punish the depriving parent. Most children, in the course of therapy, will eventually admit that the soiling was utilized to provoke the parent.

The child's unmet needs may not be discovered for some time in therapy or they may become immediately apparent. For example, one nine-year-old boy, who had begun soiling when his parents became involved in arguments over a possible divorce and thus created an unrewarding, hostile home environment, stated during the first session that he did not know why he soiled. Yet when asked to draw some pictures, he spontaneously drew a boy who was angry and frightened because his mother was coming to hit him, and a picture of woman who represented his mother. The woman was smiling because she liked to hit her son because "she hates him" and because "he's bad." When the mother was seen, she presented as resentful that her husband had deserted her and left her in poor financial straits so that she had to work and also to care for the children, who had now become a burden to her. She was depressed regarding her circumstances and her future. This boy interpreted the changes in his household to mean that his mother hated him and enjoyed hitting him, unaware (because of his immature cognitive equipment) that the mother herself was greatly stressed and troubled and unable to respond to his needs as she had previously. It became clear that he was retaliating against her harsh treatment by soiling after verbal protest and other signs of unhappiness were ignored. Once again it appeared to be this lack of responsiveness to the child's needs that finally prompted the soiling as a desperate maneuver.

While most often the parents ignore quite clear and appropriate messages of distress in their children, who then resort to soiling as a powerful mode of communication, it must be admitted that sometimes encopretic children are difficult to understand or empathize with. This is especially true of those children who have marked organic defects, children who are explosive, impulsive, and nonverbal. In these cases the mother is frequently bewildered and intimidated by her child and, while honestly desiring to respond appropriately, is so enmeshed in an everyday struggle with the child's behavior that she cannot see an overall pattern nor her own rejection of this child who has become so troublesome and frightening.

Encopresis Resulting from a Need for Structure and Security

A child who exemplified this latter type of family situation was Michael, a nine-year-old boy who had soiled sporadically since infancy but who had begun to soil daily for the past few months prior to his parents' seeking therapy for him. In addition to his soiling, Michael had problems with hyperactivity, impulsivity, and attention span, as well as extreme emotional lability with frequent angry outburts. He had previously been treated with Ritalin. Michael was described as a very active, friendly infant and toddler but in the past few years had become alternately fearful and inappropriately aggressive. Attempts to toilet train him at age 24 to 34 months were unsuccessful, although gradually he "trained himself" around 4 years of age while continuing to have occasional accidents.

Michael's parents were somewhat elderly, both in age and manner. Both had difficult lives, being uprooted from their country of origin and having to start over in the United States. The mother had had two miscarriages before Michael was born and could not have any more children. The parents presented as well-meaning individuals but there was an air of depression and helplessness about them. The father had suffered from frequent depressive episodes during which he took to his bed and withdrew from involvement with his family. In addition, he was frequently away on business. About the time that Michael began soiling regularly, the parents were considering divorce because of the father's constant depression. While it is doubtful that they truly planned to divorce they threatened each other with separation in front of Michael.

Neither of Michael's parents could assert him or herself with the child. The father had encouraged Michael's aggressive behavior because he wanted Michael to be outgoing rather than shy and withdrawn as he was. However, when Michael became older, the father no longer considered him "cute" and tried unsuccessfully to curb his acting out through moralizing. When the father failed, he would withdraw from the child. At other times, the mother would interfere and accuse him of being too strict. Michael's mother seemed intimidated by her son and could not take a stand against him. She had found it easier to give in to his demands and then withdraw, seemingly willing to pay any price to be left in peace. In taking the history, it seemed as if the parents had unconsciously used Michael to brighten their gloomy existence and unintentionally reinforced his inappropriate behavior. As Michael grew in stature and his pranks became dangerous to himself and others, the parents did not know how to curb his aggression and withdrew from Michael all the more. Both wanted to deny Michael's pathology and had tried to rationalize his angry outbursts whenever he caused trouble in school or with his peers.

In the initial sessions, Michael showed a superficial air of joviality and rambunctious self-confidence, which was the way he usually presented himself to strangers. As therapy progressed, Michael produced material which indicated he was constantly afraid: he reported nightmares, he drew pictures of crashes and accidents, if he made a mistake he would overly reproach himself. He eventually verbalized his numerous fears: that his parents would divorce and abandon him, that his father would die in a plane crash on his numerous business trips, that due to his clumsiness he would hurt himself, or that because of his uncontrollable anger he would hurt someone else and suffer terrible retaliation. Michael saw himself as damaged, he hated himself for not being able to read as well as his peers, he did not understand why other people reprimanded him or avoided him. His anxiety was increased by his parents' inability to set limits for his behavior or to acknowledge that he really had organic difficulties. Rather, they tended to minimize his problems (so that he felt guilty for his performance at school) and to avoid their responsibility for producing structure in his everyday life. Michael was being asked to participate in a parental system of denial of his own difficulties—which were everywhere clearly evident—and to take upon himself responsibility for behavior which he felt he could not control. He seemed angry with his parents for not giving him a sense of security from himself and for not being strong figures. Finally, the prospect of divorce terrified him since it made him feel all the more insecure and vulnerable.

In his own manner, Michael described himself as flying into rages without being able to control himself and then becoming afraid of being punished or of having committed some damaging action. It was in these situations that the soiling occurred. It appeared as though the encopresis was the automatic counterpart of the experience of rage and fear, being compounded by his feeling that he could not turn to his parents for help during these times. He needed someone to reassure him realistically and to control him.

In therapy, the parents as well as Michael were seen regularly. In the sessions with the parents, the mother's fear of Michael and her refusal to set limits were pointed out as well as her need to maintain calm at any price. The father became aware of the effects that his being depressed had on Michael and that he could not relinquish his responsibility as a parent because of his own problems. Michael's difficulties were clearly discussed with his parents as was his need for limits and structure. Gradually, the father began to assert himself more in the sessions and at home, which gave the mother more support in her dealing with Michael.

In Michael's sessions, various themes were discussed. Primarily, Michael's difficulties were realistically assessed and accepted by the therapist and himself without pretense. He was told that he could discuss his fears without embarrassment or shame, and eventually was able to talk about his lack of assuredness and his need to "bluff" by acting like a "big shot." At the same time, he was made aware of the effects of his aggressive behavior on others and how others disliked him for it. The sessions centered on his own attempts to control his behavior as well as his asking his parents for help. Michael would attempt to test the limits of controls by making lists of "bosses," with his father and the therapist at the head of the list, then himself and then his mother. These lists were taken up in a family session in which it was explained that Michael was only nine years old and that he could have the pleasures but also the limitations of childhood, meaning that his mother was the "boss." During this session, Michael protested in clowning manner but appeared reassured that his mother would assume responsibility.

As the parents felt secure to punish Michael and to also spend constructive time with him—not simply gratify him and then leave him—his soiling markedly decreased. On one occasion the father became angry over Michael's destroying property and punished him by "grounding" him and restricting his T.V. viewing time. To the parents' surprise Michael did not complain about the punishment but rather improved his behavior and stopped soiling for a long period of time. These and other incidents were used to convince the parents to supply the structure and reassurance that Michael needed. In time they became more certain of their right to discipline Michael and less reluctant to accept him as a child with moderate but not disabling organic problems. The father's greater involvement seemed pivotal in the therapy, since he gave his wife more security in dealing with Michael and was able to become an idealized model for Michael. Coincident with his greater involvement, the father's depressions disappeared and the marriage improved. At this stage of therapy, the soiling was no longer a problem although it still occurred on rare occasions. From this point therapy took a new direction, centering on Michael's confiding that he was afraid to grow up because he felt he could not compete in an adult world. This basic sense of inferiority which had been present all along had expressed itself in Michael's bravado and aggressiveness; now, however, it was out in the open and could be dealt with directly.

In Michael's case, the encopresis appeared due to his unfulfilled need for structure and security. As the parents became able to recognize and respond to these needs, the soiling essentially ceased. Michael was fortunate in that his parents were eager to help and to become engaged in the therapeutic process, rapidly responding to suggestions and alternative points of view. Both were concerned with Michael's interests, and their own problems did not create excessive therapeutic resistance. They were typical of parents who are bewildered by their child's behavior and react by unconscious denial and withdrawal. Some other parents of encopretic children are neither so well meaning nor so cooperative, making therapy a much more difficult and frustrating process.

Encopresis as Part of an Unresolved Family Pathology

A more usual type of patient was James, a ten-year-old boy who had had infrequent soiling since age four but who in the past year had soiled daily. James presented as a shy, withdrawn child who was small for his age. He had difficulty reading and showed other evidence of neurological immaturity. His mother described him as having no interests, no friends, no ambitions, and no abilities.

He was silent in the initial sessions although he did answer questions tersely. He had to be greatly encouraged to draw pictures or to participate in games. While not directly oppositional, James was difficult to engage in a therapeutic relationship, possibly because he had never really related to others in his life. He showed a pathetic lack of enthusiasm as well as a poverty of inner fantasy life. His main activities seemed to be sorting his collection of random papers and rocks that he had accumulated and playing with his dog. His peers often ridiculed him because of his poor athletic ability, and he had difficulty in school because of his reading disability. There appeared to be nothing positive or gratifying in his life and James seemed to have resigned himself to his fate.

James' mother was a domineering, cold woman, who openly berated her son and her husband in their presence. She was greatly upset by James' soiling and had tried a variety of quasi-punitive measures without success. She additionally blamed James for soiling because she believed this prevented her husband from taking the family on weekend outings. Actually, the father was a shy, seclusive individual, who used his spare time to construct furniture in their basement and probably used James as a convenient excuse to withdraw to his workshop. James' older sister, whose life centered outside the home, was equally content to spend her weekends with her friends. Finally, James disliked these outings, since when the family was together the parents would bicker and his sister would tease him. While it seemed perfectly obvious that the outings were unpleasant events for the family, the mother had no awareness of the feelings of others and insisted that families *should* do things together. The mother went through her day organizing the lives of those around her and would not tolerate any dissension. It appeared that the rest of the family had found it easier to go along with her than openly to oppose her. Actually, she was the driving force of the family and got little support, or even attention, from her spouse. Both parents were afraid of feelings, the mother utilizing a posture of self-righteous intellectualization and the father simply escaping into solitude. Like other families with encopretic children, there was little in the way of socialization with friends or relatives, although the mother did participate in some organizational charity work.

At home the atmosphere was of mutual alienation with almost no interaction between family members. The older daughter spent as little time at home as possible while the father worked in solitary hobbies and the mother "kept busy" in an obsessive manner. Whenever James had tried to approach her she chided him, stating that he was interrupting her and to come back later, except that later he would get the same reaction. Most of the mother's communication with James was critical—in terms of his schoolwork, his laziness, his social ineptness, and later his soiling.

Both the patient and his parents were seen in therapy in an attempt to demonstrate that James' soiling was a result of problems involving the entire family and in the belief that individual therapy could not succeed as long as the home environment remained unchanged. There was great resistance on the part of all family members to experiment with new modes of behavior. During sessions the mother was found to be able to carry out specific suggestions but to miss the point of their purpose in terms of making others feel more worthwhile or less deprived. She continued to be cold and lacking in empathy, although she was able to curb her verbal criticism. The father grudgingly agreed to spend more time with James, although he had difficulty finding things to talk about with his son. Here it must be admitted that James gave back very little in terms of affect or feedback to the overtures of others and seemed indifferent to their attention. However, he did respond favorably to small outings with his father, even simply going to the local drive-in for ice cream. In time they discovered a mutually satisfying activity, going to look at antique cars in a specialty store in a neighboring town. James was encouraged (by the therapist) to make drawings of these cars and later to construct models of them with his father. Later, it was suggested that a schoolmate be asked to accompany James and his father, since James was uncomfortable being with friends, and this proved a fairly safe way to get James to begin socializing.

In the individual sessions, James contributed little at first beyond reporting recent events in a bland manner. Slowly, he began to express anger at his parents, especially toward his mother whom he saw as ungratifying and bossy. He disparaged her manner and complained that he could never get his way at home; however, he was unwilling to make any strong effort on his own behalf. He reported that she randomly threw out his collections of papers and rocks without consulting him and that when he mentioned this to her, she simply said his room needed cleaning. While James came regularly for sessions, he seemed indifferent to therapy and expressed neither pleasure nor annoyance at being in therapy. He seemed passively to "let therapy happen" to him as many other things had occurred without his volition. Attempts to engage him in activities such as board games, darts, or drawings in lieu of talking, which he found difficult, were met with equal indifference. He denied knowing why he soiled or that he had any control over his bowels but acknowledged that his soiling occurred almost exclusively at home near his mother. His self-representation seemed to be one of passive helplessness. For example, when he complained of boredom and it was suggested that he think of some things he might want to do for enjoyment, he replied he could not think of anything he would like. Similarly, he did not know what he wanted to be when he grew up nor could he give an answer to the three wishes question. He would follow through when activities were suggested but with little enthusiasm. He did join the Cub Scouts and appeared to enjoy this activitiy but would never volunteer information about it unless asked.

While James never established a true therapeutic rapport, he was able to utilize therapy as a place where he could verbalize his feelings of failure and frustration as well as his resentment against his mother. The question of more serious pathology often arose, but both testing and continued contact failed to reveal any truly pre-schizophrenic trends beyond a low self-esteem and nongratifying expectations from others. The latter quality changed somewhat as he was able to do more with his father, which became evident when James would discuss the cars he had seen and draw sketches of them in the sessions.

At this point in the therapy, the family relocated because of the father's transfer to another job. While the basic family pathology had not been significantly altered, James' soiling had been greatly reduced because of his closer relationship with his father, and this in turn allowed the mother to be less critical of him. The cycle of soiling causing mother's anger causing child's resentment causing more soiling had been broken. James had begun socializing and seemed to find life somewhat more satisfying. He was now ready to consider going to camp and his schoolwork had improved. Another major future change was the mother's decision to return to work to give her something meaningful to do and to find an acceptable outlet for her considerable clerical abilities. The family was advised to seek further therapy. A few years later I received a request for information from a clinic which stated that James had not resumed therapy and that he had started soiling regularly again.

This case demonstrates the difficulty of altering ingrained familial patterns so often found in families of disturbed children. James presented as a shy, frightened child who was further hampered by reading problems and organic difficulties which prevented him from engaging in sports or other socially acclaimed activities. In reconstructing his history, he appeared to have been cowed by the overwhelming demands of a rigid mother who did not understand his difficulties. She stated that he seemed bewildered by toilet training, but this did not prevent her from continuing the training. Throughout early childhood, James was overwhelmed by his mother, ignored by his father, and teased by an unhappy older sister. His mild verbal complaints went unheard and he eventually seemed to begin soiling more regularly and frequently as a result of his being frightened at school and at home. Once the mother began reacting to his encopresis, he was reluctant to give up such a provocative weapon. He would relinquish the soiling only if his other needs—for support, for understanding, and for some personal achievement—could be met. Unfortunately, James had developed so unresponsive a personality that it would be difficult for anyone to fulfill his needs since James gave so little in return. The father did gratify some of these needs, and through therapy James was given encouragement to broaden his activities and venture out. The mother did also finally alter the superficial aspects of her behavior. With the accomplishment of these limited goals the soiling decreased, only to begin anew as the pressure of therapy to maintain changes was gone.

The Therapist as Surrogate Parent

Similar, although milder, difficulties were encountered in the therapy of Stephen, a seven-year-old boy who presented with a history of chronic encopresis interspersed with periods of continence. When seen, he was soiling daily and purposely avoiding the use of the toilet. His mother characterized him as "sneaky" in that he would empty his feces from his underwear into the toilet but that she was aware of this practice and punish him even if he denied soiling his pants. Actually, Stephen was a whiny, unhappy child who described himself as the helpless victim in his relationships with others. At the same time he proved himself to be stubborn and obstinate, with a malicious side to him. He was reported as never crying, regardless of what happened to him, as if by crying he would either show weakness or give satisfaction to others.

Stephen's mother was typically critical and outspoken. She openly berated him in the office with such comments as "he's like an animal" or "you can't trust him" while the child sat silently in his chair, apparently without emotion. This mother was a bitterly resentful and angry individual who blamed all of her discontent on her husband and her children. While describing herself as a martyr, she berated her husband as her social and intellectual inferior. As in other families with encopretic children, the father was a withdrawn, shy person who did not involve himself in family affairs and avoided the responsibilities of parenthood. In this case the father refused to come for therapy sessions and even opposed the whole idea of seeing a psychiatrist. The home atmosphere was gloomy and ungratifying except for occasional outbursts of anger by the father. The family rarely socialized or participated in any community or similar activities.

After a few weeks of therapy, the mother became angry with the therapist (who in this case was a female) and began openly to compete with her, reading and quoting books on child psychology. It seemed that the mother was disappointed that therapy was not going to transform her own unhappy life, and especially because the therapist was unable to magically change the father. Despite the mother's anger, or perhaps as a result of it, the mother became more active, less self-pitying, and less depressed. While feeling betrayed by the therapist, she continued to bring Stephen for sessions and to follow suggestions.

In the individual sessions, Stephen sat "like a lump" and refused to take any initiative. When he began any sort of activity, for example, drawing, he insisted that the therapist help him to an inappropriate degree. Rather than criticizing him for this feigned helplessness, as the mother often did, the therapist reacted in a supportive and cooperative manner, giving Stephen a great deal of praise and encouragement. He gradually responded and began to communicate his feelings of impotence and anger at his mother. Many sessions were spent in cooperative play without any great attempt at eliciting information or giving interpretations. Stephen looked forward to his sessions and enjoyed the attention and praise he was denied at home. It was also stressed that the sessions were his and that he could do as he wished with the time. As Stephen began to relate more warmly to the therapist and use the office as a sanctuary, he stopped soiling.

Therapy was continued beyond the cessation of encopresis in that Stephen still required help in the areas of self-assertion and socialization. These objectives were eventually accomplished without a recurrence of soiling. While the mother remained cool toward the therapist she was reported by Stephen as being less critical and generally happier. There was no discernible change in the father's behavior.

In Stephen's case an alteration of family relationships was not possible. Despite this obstacle, therapeutic results were obtained by supplying the child with a much needed relationship that was encouraging and empathic. The therapist took her cue by noting the child's needs and attempting to fulfill them as much as possible under the circumstances. Through becoming a surrogate parent, she was able to supply Stephen with enough satisfaction and freedom that he was willing to relinquish the soiling. Simultaneously the mother altered her own attitudes and decided to make a life of her own.

ENCOPRESIS RESULTING FROM A PERFECTIONISTIC, STERILE HOME ENVIRONMENT

Another child whose family again showed the pattern of an unempathic, critical mother and a withdrawn father was David, a four-and-a-half-year-old whose soiling was complicated by prolonged periods of constipation. In contrast to many other encopretic children, David demonstrated no evidence of any organic pathology. He was an attractive, bright, verbal child whose anger was readily provoked and openly expressed. History was relevant in that he was born with rectal stenosis which had required dilation from birth to three months of age. In addition, he was hospitalized during toilet training for an acute tonsillitis, after which time he reverted to daily soiling. Bladder training, on the other hand, was maintained.

David's parents were basically well-meaning individuals but were hampered in their relationships with their children by pathological attitudes and personality traits. Both were extremely compulsive and devoid of feeling, tending to intellectualize and view life in a logical, unemotional manner. They were very concerned with social appearances and conspicuous achievements. David's mother was meticulous in her housekeeping and dress, insisting that her children, who were immaculately dressed, remain spotless. She had little awareness of the usual exuberance of children or of their tendency to become dirty while playing. It was as if she expected her children to behave like little toy dolls. David's father was completely wrapped up in his own career, which involved his being away from home a great deal. When home he was often busy with work and became enraged if bothered. He also was a perfectionist, expecting model behavior from David and his sister. This family also did not socialize and had few extra-familial involvements.

David's mother was extremely upset by his soiling and had resorted to all kinds of remedies before seeking therapy. She had given him various purgatives during his periods of constipation and forced him to sit on the toilet for hours after he soiled. David's pediatrician had sensed the mother's unrealistic expectations toward her children and had suggested a nursery school as a means of breaking the power struggle between parent and child. The mother dutifully followed his advice but selected the most rigid, controlled school she could find. The selection of this school did not appear to be maliciously motivated but was rather an outcome of the mother's feelings about what was most proper for her children. In her everyday dealings with David and his sister, the mother was tied to a religiously kept schedule that superseded momentary feelings or desires. The entire home atmosphere had a mechanical, intellectual quality that was devoid of tolerance for feelings—which seemed to be viewed as human imperfections.

Both David and the parents (primarily the mother) were seen in therapy. David related openly and aggressively to the therapist. He would discuss his soiling, stating that it felt "good and warm." At the same time, he said he felt sad when he soiled because he felt he had failed his parents. David talked about his soiling and constipation as if these represented the one area of his life over which he had control. After a few sessions, David's initial "niceness" disappeared and he displayed an aggressive and controlling attitude toward the therapist. He would want to direct the sessions, insisting that he choose the activity for the day. Later he further tested the limits of his authority by refusing to come into the office, thus compelling the therapist to hold the session in the waiting room. On one occasion he was seen in the parking lot—he would not come out of the car. The mother was embarrassed by these incidents but she was reassured and David was allowed to have his own way. David was permitted to control the sessions but it was interpreted to him that he needed to boss other people around because he was so "bossed around" himself. He was also encouraged to verbalize how he felt instead of constantly having to prove he was boss.

Eventually David responded to the therapist's patient handling of his assertiveness and he became cooperative and productive in therapy. He began to make constructions out of blocks in the office, talking about his experience while he worked. He gradually was able to verbalize his anger at his mother and father for expecting so much from him. During these sessions, David was simply allowed to behave as a normal five-year-old child: he could make messes, he could get dirty, he could be silly if he wished, and the therapist participated in these activities.

The sessions with the parents centered on their lack of appreciation of childhood behavior. The parents seemed genuinely concerned for the children's welfare but had little ability to put themselves into the child's place or to experience within themselves the feelings that they aroused in others. However, they understood their lack of emotional responsiveness and trusted the therapist to set standards of behavior and to suggest ways of dealing with David and his sister. They relaxed their perfectionistic standards and stopped living by schedules although they remained somewhat mechanical and lacking in feeling. The children responded well to the looser family atmosphere and in sessions David appeared more relaxed and happy.

An interesting aspect of David's therapy was that after he had decided to cooperate in therapy, he began to construct complex winding "choo-choo" tracks which were always blocked by some sort of barrier. On one occasion, a tentative interpretation was made that the tracks might represent his intestines which were blocked and backed up. David did not acknowledge this suggestion but after he stopped withholding feces and soiling he constructed tracks without barriers.

After about a year of therapy David was free of bowel symptoms. He was appropriate in therapy and made a good adjustment in school. The parents remained cooperative and open to advice. Even after therapy was terminated, the mother continued to call for help in resolving momentary difficulties. In David's case, therapy was again directed at granting the child what he lacked in his home environment. David was allowed to be assertive in therapy, he was permitted to control something of his own, and, finally, to behave in a normal childish manner. At the same time the parents tried as much as they could to create a more human and satisfying life outside of therapy sessions.

Encopresis in Adolescence

In the cases just described the problems of the child could be directly ascribed to and were influenced by alterations in the familial mode of relating. Therapy consisted mainly of investigating the needs of the child and attempting to gratify them by restructuring family processes and by direct therapeutic intervention with the child. The prime objective of therapy was the eradication of those conditions which prompted the child to utilize soiling in lieu of a more appropriate mode of communicating.

While this approach has proved fairly successful with young children, its efficiency decreases as the child grows toward adolescence. When the soiling has continued beyond puberty, the symptom becomes more entrenched and seems to take on new meaning for the patient. By this time, the child's self-appraisals are only partially related to his immediate family and instead depend largely on relations with peers and achievement outside the home. At this time, an alteration of family attitudes may not be sufficient to eliminate the symptom.

Actually, encopresis in adolescence seems to be quite rare. It may be that most encopretic children stop soiling eventually even without treatment as a result of peer pressure, the inconvenience of the symptom, or possibly as a result of the greater independence from family pathology that accompanies increased maturation. On the other hand, some children may replace the soiling with more serious symptomatology as they are confronted with the developmental tasks of adolescence. Two young adolescent encopretic boys have been known to the author (one treated by a colleague and one currently in therapy), and their case histories are briefly presented here in order to demonstrate the difference of this symptom in childhood and in adolescence.

Daniel, age 13, was seen after he had been soiling for three years. The encopresis began insiduously after numerous protests that he was afraid to go to school because other children were teasing and bullying him. At first the mother occasionally allowed him to stay home, although criticizing him severely when he did, but finally insisted that he attend school regularly. It was later learned in therapy that Daniel had been given the job of "bathroom monitor," having to patrol bathrooms and report boys who were smoking or vandalizing school property. This job easily made him the target of other children's anger, and they often threatened him or even ganged up on him in the lavatories. It may be that these frightening experiences in bathrooms conditioned Daniel to avoid use of the toilet, or it may be that he experienced autonomous voiding during a moment of fear. In any case, Daniel consistently refused to mention his experiences at school beyond vaguely intimating that he was very frightened. He never mentioned his "job" or his experiences to his parents but instead refused to go to school—and when forced to go began soiling daily.

Daniel was an excellent student and scored in the very superior range on intelligence testing. However, he was extremely shy and fearful of social situations. He was somewhat obese and would sit or walk with his head bent. He appeared quite depressed and frightened during the initial interviews. On projective tests, the dominant themes were hopelessness, depression, poor self-image, and reactive anger. His responses were also indicative of a fear of losing control, of being overwhelmed by anger, and of suffering retaliation.

Past history revealed that Daniel had been repeatedly discouraged from individuation—his mother tied his shoe laces until he was nine years old—while at the same time he had been expected to meet exacting maternal demands. At the beginning of toilet training, at 18 months, Daniel had not complied quickly enough so that his mother concluded that he was being purposely spiteful and decided to "break" him by having him sit on the potty chair for hours at a time. Her rigid demands continued in many other areas, for example, if Daniel did not finish all the food on his plate, he had to sit at the table for one hour after dinner without talking.

The family situation was similar to others described previously. Daniel's father was a shy, isolated man who worked at night and either slept or retreated to his room during the day. The mother was critical, dissatisfied, and resentful. She also openly disparaged her husband for being a poor provider, for being socially inept, and for not measuring up to her own father whom she idolized but who had apparently paid her little attention. Her attitude toward Daniel was a mixture of criticism and infantilization. She demanded complete obedience and exceptional school performance while sabotaging any attempt at individualism or extra-familial activity. The family had no friends, did not socialize, and spent most of their leisure time watching television without communicating.

In therapy, Daniel expressed concern over perfectionistic demands which he felt unable to fulfill. He also demonstrated fear of others, a sense of disappointment toward his father and anger toward his mother. In the sessions with the parents, they became more resistant and unresponsive to suggestions, utilizing the time to complain about Daniel's lack of progress. They refused to see his soiling as part of a family process and were threatened by confrontations of their own problems. In the meantime Daniel still refused to attend school and continued soiling. It was therefore agreed to admit Daniel to a residential treatment center in order to remove him from his ungratifying and pathogenic environment.

On the ward, Daniel gradually lost his depressive demeanor and started socializing with other patients. He seemed less self-conscious, participated in group activities, and related well to the staff. Daniel's adjustment to the ward was hampered by his mother's frequent visits, during which she would criticize the staff and reassure Daniel that he would be home soon.

Despite Daniel's social improvement, he continued to soil daily and to avoid use of the toilet. His excuse was that he was afraid to sit on a toilet, but in therapy sessions he told his doctor that no one could make him give up his soiling because it was his "power." He alluded to obtaining some secret satisfaction from soiling and continued to resist urgings to give it up. Therapy was directed at showing him that his soiling was presently working against him in that it limited his efforts to do things on his own and to free himself from his mother. However, Daniel resisted these interpretations; although he relented somewhat by half heartedly using the toilet, his soiling continued despite efforts to conceal it from staff and patients. Daniel was discharged after three months on the insistence of his mother. While free from many of the personality problems that plagued him prior to admission, he continued to be sporadically encopretic. Follow-up therapy was declined by the family.

The significant aspect of Daniel's case appears to be the transformation of encopresis from a transpersonal mode of hostile communication to an intrapersonal source of gratification, independent of others. This perverse usage of soiling, as some sort of secret power, was also evident in the following case.

Jonathan was a 13-year-old boy who had been soiling for four years and had already been seen by two therapists without success. The soiling had begun at summer camp where, because of Jonathan's snobbish attitudes and lack of participation in camp activities, he was severely teased by his peers. One night his bunk mates held him down and pelted him with water bombs, threatening further punishment and generally terrifying him. It was on this occasion that Jonathan began soiling. He wrote his parents letters about wanting to come home but did not go into detail about what had happened. The parents ignored the letters, thinking that Jonathan was normally homesick and would eventually adjust. When they visited during parents' weekend, Jonathan spitefully refused to talk about his fears with his parents and insisted on sticking it out for the summer. His soiling stopped when he returned home only to recur the next spring when camp season approached. However, he decided to return to camp where he sarcastically insulted his peers and managed to become the counsellors' "helper" so as to avoid the embarrassment of having to fail in athletic events.

When Jonathan presented for therapy, he was a small, pale boy who looked younger than his age but acted like a little old man. He was extremely intelligent and very argumentative, excelling in logical analysis but lacking any emotion other than anger. He was contemptuous of most people, considering them his intellectual inferiors and unworthy of consideration. He seemed proud of having "defeated" two previous therapists. He was openly competitive with the therapist, trying to lay traps by which to trick him logically or making disparaging remarks about the therapy situation. After a few months this facade was dropped and Jonathan grudgingly admitted that he felt physically inferior and helpless in his interaction with peers. He also confessed that he was afraid to trust the therapist with his true feelings because he then would be vulnerable to ridicule. This defensiveness became more understandable as the parents were seen in therapy.

Briefly, the mother was the power in the household. She pursued her own ends and treated others with insensitivity, often humiliating them without awareness. The father passively withdrew from family affairs, returning home late from work and retiring to the television set. Both parents proved very responsive to therapy and in the course of about a year were able to markedly alter their mode of relating to each other and to their children. Despite extensive changes in the home situation and considerable improvements in Jonathan's character pathology, the soiling continued. Jonathan was able to verbalize many feelings about his soiling. Like Daniel he sometimes treated it as a semi-mystical act of power and freedom. At other times, he felt that if he continued to soil, he could reassure himself that he did not have to grow up. Throughout, he also bitterly disliked his soiling, recounting the inconvenience and the constant fear of discovery that it caused him. In one session, as he was describing how intensely he disliked having to limit his life because of his encopresis, he blurted out, "But I won't stop!" and then was startled at what he had said. His ambivalence about his soiling was evident, as was his current need of the symptom.

For Jonathan as for Daniel, what began as a reaction to fear, and later became a mode of punishing the parent, had finally taken on a personal meaning that was independent of others. As such, encopresis in adolescence resembles some cases of sexual perversion, where a childhood activity becomes a secret, somewhat ego-alien activity that is both hated and prized. These cases seem to indicate that after puberty separation from the family or a radical change in family relationships is no longer effective and that the symptom appears to become even more resistant to therapy.

CONCLUSION

In recent years, the model utilized for understanding and treating many childhood disorders has shifted from one which focuses on the child in isolation to one that stresses the child in his familial and social context. As has been described above, encopresis also appears to be best interpreted and treated in terms of complex interrelationships between the child and his environment.

While specific, and as yet unknown, predisposing factors are postulated as responsible for initial symptom choice, the eventual persistence of frequent soiling depends on particular types of family processes. Many families with encopretic children demonstrate a peculiar type of pattern which reinforces the prolongation of soiling for psychological motives. In young children, an alteration of this pathological family pattern may suffice to correct the symptom. In older children, individual therapy, in addition to work with parents, may be necessary to alter personality problems of the child as well as to allow him to learn more appropriate modes of communicating anger and disappointment. Finally, in the adolescent, changes in family dynamics are no longer sufficient to modify the encopretic pattern which by this time seems to have taken on a new meaning and significance for the patient.

At any age, chronic "neurotic" encopresis is difficult to treat successfully. The fact that such a disagreeable symptom is maintained by the child gives some evidence of the desperate situation in which he finds himself and the extent of prior damage that must be laboriously rectified in therapy.

REFERENCES

ANTHONY, E. J. An experimental approach to the psychopathology of childhood: Encopresis. *British Journal of Medical Psychology*, 1957, *30*, 146–175.

BAIRD, M. Characteristic interaction patterns in families of encopretic children. *Bulletin of the Menninger Clinic*, 1974, *38*, 144–153.

BEMPORAD, J. R., PFEIFER, C. M., GIBBS, L., CORTNER R. H., and BLOOM, W. Characteristics of encopretic patients and their families. *Journal of the American Academy of Child Psychiatrists*, 1971, *10*, 272–292.

FREUD, A. *Normality and pathology in childhood.* New York: International Universities Press, 1965.

FREUD, A., and BURLINGHAM, D. T. *War and children.* New York: Medical War Books, 1943.

HOAG, J. M., NORRISS, N. G., HIMENO, E. T., and JACOBS, J. The encopretic child and his family. *Journal of the American Academy of Child Psychiatrists*, 1971, *10*, 242–256.

KANNER, LEO. *Child psychiatry* (3rd ed.). Springfield, Ill.: Charles C. Thomas Publisher, 1966.

SHANE, M. Encopresis in a latency boy. *Psychoanalytic Study of the Child*, 1967, *22*, 296–314.

SHIRLEY, H. Encopresis in children. *Journal of Pediatrics*, 1938, *12*, 367–380.

ADDITIONAL SUGGESTED READINGS

BELLMAN, M. Studies on encopresis. *Acta Pediatrica Scandinaviea*, 1966, *170* (Supplement).

GARRARD, S. D., and RICHMOND, J. B. Psychogenic megocolon manifested by fecal soiling. *Pediatrics*, 1952, *10*, 474–483.

HUSCHKA, M. The child's responses to coercive bowel training. *Psychosomatic Medicine*, 1942, *4*, 301–308.

MINUCHIN, S., BAKER, L., ROSMAN, B. L., LIEBMAN, R., MILMAN, L. and TODD, T. C. A conceptual model of psychosomatic illness in children. *Archives of General Psychiatry*, 1975, *32*, 1031–1038.

NEALE, D. H. Behavior therapy and encopresis in children. *Behavioral Research Therapy*, 1963, *1*, 139–149.

PRUGH, P. G. Child experience and colonic disorders. *Annals of the New York Academy of Science*, 1954, *58*, 355–376.

WARSON, S. R., CALDWELL, M. R., WARINNER, A. KIRK, A. J., and, JENSEN R. A. The dynamics of encopresis: Workshop, 1953. *American Journal of Orthopsychiatry*, 1954, *24*,402–415.

12

ASTHMA: PSYCHOLOGICAL TREATMENT

James Egan

Asthma is a severe respiratory disease manifested by dysponea and wheezing that afflicts 5 to 7% of the population. The course is generally chronic and characterized by remissions and exacerbations. In approximately one-third of the cases there is a spontaneous recovery often at adolescence. Prior to adolescence boys are affected almost twice as frequently as girls. In 60% of the cases the onset is by 3 years of age.

It seems clear that constitutional factors play a prominent part in the etiology of asthma, and that chemical, infectious, allergic, physical, or psychological factors can precipitate attacks.

In general the earlier the onset, the more serious the asthma. This finding is illustrated by the observation that those with onset prior to 2 years of age have the highest mortality. Other unfavorable prognostic findings are infantile eczema and positive skin tests to egg whites in infancy. Favorable prognostic factors include asthma that is clearly allergic and discontinuous—i.e., with long symptom-free periods between attacks.

Early in the development of psychosomatic medicine the emphasis was on seeking specific personality traits that produced each disease. When this proved to be futile, an attempt was made to understand patients in terms of specific neurotic conflicts. This point of view is most clearly exemplified in the work of Franz Alexander and his followers.

RECENT TRENDS IN PSYCHOSOMATICS

More recently attention has shifted in two directions in the study of psychosomatic disorders. One is an increased emphasis on the effects on psychological functioning of a chronic illness. This has led to greater efforts in treating psychological symptoms, not so much in hopes of eradicating an etiologic factor, but rather in hopes of ameliorating the patient's response to the chronic disease.

The second direction has tended to emphasize the possibility that particular psychological configurations are the result of a chronic disease rather than the cause of it. This has most clearly been demonstrated in the case of peptic ulcers in children.

In cases of peptic ulcers one often finds gastric hypersecretions in association with dependent longings, and increased oral cravings and frustrations. Alexander (1950) suggested that peptic ulcers were the result of gastric hypersecretion owing to increased hypothalamic stimulation in response to unfulfilled oral needs.

It was shown by Mirsky (1958) that gastric hypersecretion is probably present as birth, at least in some peptic ulcer-prone individuals, and that this resulted in accelerated digestion and increased gastric emptying with a resultant relative enteroceptic sense of unfulfillment which could generate the intrapsychic configurations previously noted. To put it simply, this explanation accounts for the observed psychic reality of increased dependency needs but does not suggest that they are etiologic in the genesis of peptic ulcer disease. It is assumed nonetheless that these emotional needs may then perpetuate the disorder in accordance with Alexander's (1950) formulations.

It seems clear that a similar reformulation of our theories regarding asthma is called for, not just in order to achieve a harmony between current research and clinical findings but also to provide a rational basis for treatment. The argument has gone on for some time regarding the mind-body problem in asthma, between those who take strong positions that emotional factors are predominant, or insignificant in the etiology of asthma.

As with most disorders, there are probably many complex multifactorial issues involved, and in different persons, different factors predominate. I would agree completely with Knapp (1963) who states, "··· as in the case of the allergic predisposition, it seems less valuable to debate the existence of psychologic influences in asthma than to ask how they reinforce the asthmatic response, and to what extent."

It is this very issue that is crucial for the proper treatment of the asthmatic child. The lucky child who experiences the onset of asthma at seven, where it is seasonal and clearly related to a known allergin, and who functions well at other times, may need very little psychological help. He may only require reassurance and education to enable him to master his asthma and follow the required medical regimen.

There is evidence (Zealley, 1971) that such a patient will have considerably less psychopathology than the chronically ill asthmatic. There is also evidence that parents become more anxious and protective as the years pass, and they perceive the child as coping with a serious life-threatening disease.

A determination of the kinds of psychopathology present in the parents and child, and the effects on the asthmatic process will serve as a guide to psychological help. It is of interest that in 40% of asthmatic children, allergins cannot be documented by skin testing or history. Block and co-workers (1964) have demonstrated the reciprocal relationship between allergic and psychological precipitants. One can often document the triggering events from history, and when these are emotional then psychological help is warranted.

One of the most common emotional stimuli to an asthmatic attack is the threat of separation from the mother. It must be stressed that a threat of separation is fundamentally different from anxiety at being separated. It is these observations that led to "parentectomy" as a therapeutic maneuver.

PARENTECTOMY

Peskin treated asthmatic children at Mt. Sinai Hospital, New York City in the 1920s and 1930s. He noted that when the children were hospitalized many of them did well, only to relapse soon after returning home. It seemed clear to him that the allergic child was responding to allergins at home, and he thus concluded that removal from the allergic home—i.e., parentectomy—was in order.

For those children in whom fear of separation from the mother is the clinical precipitant, removal from the mother reduces that anxiety and consequently the asthma subsides. This phenomenon can often be seen when, after spending hours in an emergency room without breaking an asthmatic attack, the decision is made to hospitalize the child. It commonly happens that by the time the patient reaches the pediatric ward improvement is noted. The unsophisticated doctor might be led to believe that hospitalization could have been avoided if only he had waited a little bit longer. This response, often labeled the R-R (rapidly remitting) group in the pediatric literature, clearly points toward a psychologically based origin, in contradistinction to the steroid dependent group.

Purcell (1969) demonstrated an improvement in asthmatic children when they were kept in their own homes and the parents were removed. In this rather intricate experiment he controlled the environment, thereby preserving the allergic conditions. It confirmed the hypothesis that in the R-R group separation fears were the precipitants and not allergins.

The psychotherapeutic implications are clear. It is the task of the therapist to help the child and the parent(s) understand their feelings of helplessness, fear, and their conflicts over separation, autonomy, and independence. This task most often requires intensive psychotherapy.

PSYCHOTHERAPY

Sperling 1968 strongly advises working with the parents (generally just the mother alone) prior to treating the child psychologically. In her words, it is the "loosening of the asthmatic tie" by the mother that is necessary prior to helping the child overcome his conflicts over dependence-independence. In these instances the psychotherapeutic task is not unlike that of treating a child with school refusal syndromes in whom there are separation fears.

Sperling and others make the observation that, in many cases, the asthma develops during the anal-muscular stage of developing autonomy and mastery. The asthma is often used as a communication by these children, and part of the psychotherapeutic treatment will be to help them utilize words in place of somatic symptoms, to verbalize the infantile wishes for control and dominance, and the wished for yet feared separation from the mother.

In practice this is often a difficult not very exciting task, as many of our asthmatic patients and their mothers are not particularly insightful by any of the usual psychiatric standards.

RESIDENTIAL TREATMENT

Residential treatment is indicated only for the most serious, nonremitting cases of asthma. Vance and Taylor (1971) in studying the current status of residential homes for asthma in America note: "The following trends were observed: more intermediate stay facilities, family therapy, a reconsideration of minimum and maximum age limits, more readmissions, the absence of custodial care, the use of interdisciplinary teams, less emphasis on a favorable climate as therapy, and the creation of asthma units in existing multi-disease hospitals."

These trends reflect the increasing emphasis on holistically treating the child, and not just his asthma, as we increasingly understand the interrelationships between mind and body.

As advances are made in the out-patient treatment of asthmatic children, only the most seriously ill are referred for residential treatment. Thus, in a 15-year study of admissions and response to treatment at the Children's Asthma Research Institute and Hospital in Denver, there was a decrease from 98% to 12% of those who remitted rapidly after admission. This must be seen as a decrease in the rapidly remitting, psychologically triggered group. Hopefully it means that this group is receiving better psychological help and hence needs residential treatment less often.

INTERDISCIPLINARY TREATMENT

An interdisciplinary team approach is needed in treating the severely ill asthmatic child. The team often consists of the pediatrician, psychiatrist, social worker, teacher, allergists, parents, and clergyman.

Failure to participate in a multidisciplinary team approach usually reflects parental anxiety and a defensive bias about the etiology of the asthma. Obviously, the underlying familial forces that oppose change are likely to be revealed. This is clearly illustrated by the case of a 12-year-old boy with severe chronic asthma who required repeated hospitalization. Stabilization of his asthma occurred only when a diligent social worker recognized that the only time this child got to see his father, who lived apart from the family, was when the patient was hospitalized. The secondary gain of seeing his father was sufficient to help him "forget" to take his medicines.

BEHAVIOR MODIFICATION

Alteration of an asthmatic child's maladaptive behavior, including his asthma, is the number one priority for all. An understanding of the application of learning theory principles to the care of the asthmatic child will be of considerable importance. These treatment efforts can be both formal and informal.

An example of the latter is depicted in the vignette reported by Kluger (1969).

Patient: I can't go to school today because my asthma is worse.

Doctor: I know, but since it's not contagious, why can't you be in school?

Patient (irritated): Because I'm having trouble breathing!

Doctor: I can see that, but you will have trouble breathing whether you go to school or not. Remaining in bed won't help your breathing.

Patient (disgustedly): Boy, they don't even let you be sick in this hospital.

Here Kluger (1969) draws our attention to the ways in which we reinforce "sick" behavior in asthmatic children. Our efforts must be to discourage the child from becoming an unnecessary psychological cripple. Efforts must be made to help parents generalize these principles, and not respond to the child only when he wheezes, but equally so when discussing a good day at school or playing with a friend.

Alexander and co-workers (1972) report on the formal application of learning theory principles to the treatment of asthmatic children. They note an increased expiratory flow rate in those children who had been trained in systematic relaxation. Moore (1965) demonstrated subjective and objective improvement of bronchial asthma using relaxation with reciprocal inhibition in twelve patients.

SUMMARY

1. Asthma is a heterogeneous disease with multiple etiologic influences.
2. Treatment of the asthmatic child includes treatment of the child and his family.
3. Efforts must be made to distinguish those emotional disturbances secondary to asthma, from those that precipitate or perpetuate it.
4. Those children with strong psychological components often have less constitutional influences.
5. The predominate psychological conflicts tend to be around autonomy-independence, and helplessness-dependence.
6. The precipitant for asthma in the rapidly remitting patient is often fear of separation from the mother, and this requires psychotherapeutic intervention.
7. With more frequent team treatment of the child and his family there is a decreasing need for residential treatment.

REFERENCES

AAS, K., M. D. *The allergic child.* Springfield, Ill.: Charles C Thomas Publisher, 1971.

ALEXANDER, A. B., MIKLICH, D., and HERSHKOFF, H. The immediate effects of systematic relaxation training on peak expiratory flow rates in asthmatic children. *Psychosomatic Medicine*, 1972, *34*(5), 388–394.

ALEXANDER, F. *Psychosomatic Medicine*, New York: W. W. Norton & Co. Inc., 1950.

BLOCK, J., JENNINGS, P., HARVEY, E., and SIMPSON, E., Interaction between allergic potential and psychopathology in childhood. *Psychosomatic Medicine*, 1964, *26*, 307–320.

BLUMENTHAL, M. N., CUSHING, R. T., and FASHINGBAUER, T. J. A community program for the management of bronchial asthma. *Annals of Allergy*, 1972, *30*, 391–398.

BROWN, J. Asthma in childhood. *The Medical Journal of Australia*, March 31, 1973, 654–657.

Carmichael's manual of child psychology (3rd ed.) (Vol. II). Paul H. Mussen, Ed. New York: John Wiley, 1970.

COLLINS-WILLIAMS, C. *Paediatric allergy and clinical immunology (as applied to atopic disease*): *A manual for students and practitioners of medicine* (4th ed.). Toronto: University of Toronto Press, 1973.

ENGEL, G. L., M. D. *Psychological development in health and disease*. Philadelphia and London: W. B. Saunders, Co., 1962.

FALLIERS, C. J., M. D. Treatment of asthma in a residential center: A fifteen year study. *Annals of Allergy*, 1970, *28*, 513–521.

FEINGOLD, B. F. *Introduction to clinical allergy*. Springfield, Ill.: Charles C Thomas Publisher, 1973.

FINK, J. N., and SOSMAN, A. J. Therapy of bronchial asthma. *Medical Clinics of North America*, 1973, *57*(3), 801–808.

JESSNER, L., et al. Emotional impact of nearness and separation for the asthmatic child and his mother. *Psychoanalytic Study of The Child*, 1955, *10*.

JOHNSON, F. K., BAKER, G., and ALEXANDER, A. A. A psyche and soma reunited. A discussion of the need for an organized team approach when dealing with a child having a long term life-threatening illness. *Clinical Pediatrics*, 1971, *10*, 719–725.

KAUFMAN, W. Some aspects of psychotherapy in allergic practice. *Journal of Asthma Research*, 1972, *10*(2).

KLUGER, J., Childhood Asthma and the Social Milieu. *Journal of the American Academy of Child Psychiatry*, 1969, *9*, 360–361.

KNAPP, P. *The Asthmatic Child*. H. I. Schneer (Ed.), New York: Harper & Row, 1963.

MIRSKY, I. A., FUTTERMAN, P. and KAPLAN, S. Physiologic, psychologic, and social determinants in the etiology of duodenal ulcer. *American Journal of Digestive Diseases*, *3*: 285–314, 1958.

MITCHELL, R. G., and DAWSON, B. Educational and social characteristics of children with asthma. *Archives of Disorders of Childhood*, 1973, *48*, 467–471.

MOORE, N. Behavior therapy in bronchial asthma: A controlled study. *Journal of Psychosomatic Research*, 1965, *9*, 257–276.

PESHKIN, M. M. Asthma in children. *American Journal of Disorders of Children*, 1930, *39*, 774–781.

PINKERTON, P. The influence of sociopathology in childhood asthma. Recent Research in Psychosomatics, 8th European Conference on Psychosomatic Research, Knokke, Belgium, 1970. *Psychotherapeutic Psychosomatics*, 1970, *18*, 231–238.

PURCELL, K. Distinctions between subgroups of asthmatic children. Children's perceptions of events associated with asthma. *Pediatrics*, 1963, *31*, 486–494.

PURCELL, K., BRADY, K., CHAI, H., MASER, J., MOLK, L., GORDON, N., and MEANS, J. The effect on asthma in children of experimental separation from the family. *Psychosomatic Medicine*, 1969, *31*, 144–164.

REBUCK, A. S., and READ, J. Assessment and management of severe asthma. *American Journal of Medicine*, 1971, *51*, 788–798.

ROBINSON, G. The story of parentectomy. *Journal of Asthma Research*, 1972, *9*(4), 199–205.

SANERKIN, N. G., M. D. Terminology and classification of 'bronchial asthma' and 'chronic bronchitis': A reappraisal and redefinition. *Annals of Allergy*, 1971, *29*, 187–194.

SCHEER, M. S., M. D. Camp bronco junction: Second year of experience. *Annals of Allergy*, 1970, *28*, 423–433.

SCHNEER, H. I. (Ed.) The asthmatic child. New York: Harper & Row, 1963.

SPEER, F., M. D., and DOCKHORN, R. J., M. D. *Allergy and immunology in children*. Springfield, Ill.: Charles C. Thomas, Publisher, 1973.

SPERLING, MELITTA. Asthma in children. *Journal of the American Academy of Child Psychiatry*, 1968, *7*, 44–58.

STRAIN, J. J., and GROSSMAN, S. *Psychological care of the medically ill: A primer in liaison psychiatry*. New York: Appleton-Century-Crofts Div. of Prentice-Hall, Inc., 1975.

VANCE, V. J., and TAYLOR, W. F. Status and trends in residential asthma homes in the United States. *Annals of Allergy*, 1971, *29*, 428–437.

Vance, V. J., and Taylor, W. F. The financial cost of chronic childhood asthma. *Annals of Allergy*, 1971, *29*, 455–459.

Williams, J. S. Aspects of dependence-independence conflict in children with asthma. *Journal of Child Psychology and Psychiatry*, 1975, *16*, 199–218.

Wohl, T. H. Behavior modification: Its application to the study and treatment of childhood asthma. *Journal of Asthma Research*, 1971, *9*, 41–45.

Zealley, A. K. Bronchial asthma: A problem attributable to sampling when establishing its psychopathology. *Psychotherapeutic Psychosomatics*, 1971, *19*, 37–46.

13

SPEECH DISORDERS[1]

Clyde L. Rousey

Among out-patients and in-patients in psychological distress, the incidence of speech disorders is as high as 90% (Rousey & Toussieng, 1964; Green, 1962; Grimes, 1962; Page & Page, 1941). Such incidence is at least nine times greater than estimates made for the general population (Milisen, 1971). In such a context it is important to note that clinical studies (Kernberg & Rousey, 1970; Fleming & Rousey, 1974) suggest a reduction of speech disturbances coincident with improvement in psychological functioning. Thus, persons who practice psychotherapy have, without being consciously aware, been concurrently treating various forms of speech disorders.

Treatment of the various specific speech disorders closely mirrors the conglomerate of approaches used with other emotional disorders. Similarities probably exist because, in a broad sense, speech disorders and emotional problems both reflect a breakdown in communication. This chapter will focus on understanding and treating of speech disorders using some modifications of psychoanalytically oriented psychotherapy. Travis and Sutherland (1971), Backus and Beasley (1951), and Hejna (1960) provide a sample of what has been advocated so far in terms of various other types of psychotherapy for speech disorders. The more popular current treatment approaches for speech disorders emphasize operant procedures (Weston & Irwin, 1971), linguistic approaches (McReynolds & Engmann, 1975), or approaches assuming an organic substrata localized to some part of the central nervous system (Darley, Aronson & Brown, 1975). Diagnostic approaches of various authors are summarized in the volume edited by Travis (1971).

[1]The author is indebted to Carol G. Rousey, Ph. D. for her reading and helpful comments in the preparation of this manuscript.

A PSYCHOLOGICAL UNDERSTANDING OF SPEECH PRODUCTION

In the present context *speech* refers solely to the individual sounds which comprise the *spoken words* (i.e., verbal language) used by differing nationalities to express abstract and concrete thoughts. This differentiation is important since the writer proposes that speech and spoken words are independent forms of behavior and consequently are capable of expressing differing aspects of a person's psychological functioning. Specifically, speech is assumed to reflect primarily the affect life of individuals, while spoken language is one of the expressive modalities that reflect a person's cognitive functioning.

It is the cognitive aspects of language which allow feelings to be masked, subsequently complicating the work in psychotherapy, psychological testing, social work, and psychiatric examination. One limiting factor of spoken language for treatment is the necessity for obtaining as many corroborating expressions of thought as possible before making an interpretation. It is these connotative features of spoken language that account for the concept of overdetermination of symptoms.

The basis for thinking speech to be independent of language is threefold. In the only intensive longitudinal studies made of early infant sound development, Irwin (1947, 1948) was able to demonstrate the appearance of all the usual sounds heard in spoken language prior to the first year. This is significant since the onset of spoken language is generally placed sometime after the twelfth month. Further, there is little support for the old notion that it takes the first 6 to 8 years of life for speech sounds to appear correctly in a child's spoken language. Indeed, research data suggest there is, from a motoric standpoint, no developmental pattern in the speech of children (Hall, 1962; Healey, 1963). Finally, practicing speech pathologists know: (1) that one can have a speech disorder without a language disorder, a language disorder without a speech disorder, or both; and (2) that there is no known specific consonant sound which is related to a specific neurological state or condition.

In order to relate speech to emotional life, certain assumptions must be made. While these assumptions together with clinical and research data have been presented elsewhere in greater detail (Rousey, in press), it is necessary to summarize some of the more critical points before discussing the psychological treatment of speech disorders.

One basic assumption is that vowel sounds can be related to libidinal and aggressive drives, while consonants reflect developing object relationships over the varying periods of infantile sexuality. Relating speech in this manner to psychoanalytic concepts also requires knowledge of speech development.

To begin, research has shown that the majority of sounds made during the first 6 months of life are vowel sounds; during the next 6 months, however, the average child utters all of the consonant sounds that he will later use in spoken language. Now, if one assumes that drive discharge is the dominant theme during the infant's first 6 months while the anlage of object relationships is the dominant theme in the second 6 months of the first year, then the stage is set for relating vowels and consonants to these two dynamic factors.

There are additional similarities among vowels, consonants, and the previously mentioned psychological dimensions. For example, early drive discharge is usually conceived of as a grossly immodulated or an essentially unchecked and uncontrolled expression of feeling. This is strikingly similar to the nature of vowel production and utterance. Thus, although the tongue assumes differing shapes in vowel production, there is no major stoppage of sound as is the case with consonants. Further, in phonetic theory vowels are usually assumed to be energy carriers whereas consonants are seen as shaping and giving meaning to the vowel sounds. In a similar way, developing object relationships over the various periods of psychosexual development are assumed to give meaning and form to the various drives.

Elsewhere Rousey (1974, a) has postulated how the use of the various consonants is related to developmental struggles of the varying stages of psychosexual development.

> Utilizing Erikson's (1950) conceptualization of the development of infantile sexuality, the sounds *m*, *p*, *w*, *h*, *y* as in *y*ellow, *l*, *n*, and *t* are hypothesized as belonging to the oral respiratory-sensory stage, while *b*, *f*, *k*, *g*, and *d* are hypothesized as reflecting the oral-biting stage. The *ch* as in *ch*urch and the *j* as in *j*udge are felt associated with the anal-expulsive stage, while the *s*, *r*, *sh*, and *z* as in a*z*ure are theorized as reflecting the anal-retentive stage. The voiceless *th* as in *th*anks, the *v*, the voiced *th* as in *th*em, and the *z*

as in *zoo* are sounds believed associated with the phallic period.

In understanding how the above postulates are made, it is helpful to think of sounds as having what Werner (1957) has described as a physiognomic quality. For example, given a forced choice test, where individual sounds are to be placed in either an oral, an anal, or a phallic stage of psychosexual development, the majority of people will place such sounds as *m* or *f* in the oral period, *r* and *s* in the anal period, and either the voiced or unvoiced *th* sounds (e.g., *th*em [voiced] and *th*anks [unvoiced]) in the phallic period. Further help is available in understanding these postulates if one examines from a different perspective the data of Templin (1957), which were offered in support of the developmental notion of sound acquisition. Specifically, if one assumes that the pattern of sound acquisition she describes reflects a societal coping with psychological developmental issues, then the varying percentage of individual sound acquisition at varying ages can be interpreted as supporting the meanings which the present writer postulates for the various consonant sounds.

NORMAL SPEECH DEVELOPMENT

Normal speech development can also be described according to these assumptions. Thus, if there *were* appropriate mastery of areas expected to create developmental psychological stress, one would be surprised to find substitution of one sound for another (e.g., substituting *w* for *r*, as in *wed* for *red*) or distortions of sounds (e.g., sounds in a spoken word would be unintelligible) in the growing child. However, up until a mental age of approximately 5 years, it is not uncommon to find omissions of consonant sounds in words where two or three consonants occur in sequence (e.g., *bread* might be said as *bed* or *sprinkle* as *pinkle*). This one exception to the contention that sound production reflects affect life as opposed to cognition ability will be discussed in terms of treatment issues at a later point in this chapter.

In contrast to speech development, normal language development is assumed to follow and be related primarily to cognitive principles such as outlined by Brown (1973) and McNeill (1970). Lenneberg (1967) has outlined biological considerations.

In an otherwise asymptomatic child or adolescent, the appearance of sound deviations becomes an indicator that unusual stress is occurring in the person's emotional life. Such an indicator is analogous to the appearance of high fever as an early warning of a disturbance in normal physical functioning. As such, it provides the psychologist with a takeoff point for early intervention in emotional dysfunction.

SPEECH DISORDERS: AN OVERVIEW

Speech disorders are generally described in terms of delayed onset of talking, variations in articulation of sounds and in voice quality and production, stuttering, and speech and language variations secondary to neurological insult. Delayed onset of talking is often referred to as delayed onset of language. While this may be due to cognitive limitations, it is more often accurately thought of as a speech disorder as opposed to a language disorder since the locus of difficulty is principally on sound production. At a later age the phenomenon of elective mutism becomes a speech disorder which, while related to delayed onset of talking, is an entity all its own.

Examples of the customary articulation errors include (1) substitution of one sound (vowel or consonant) for another (here the person might say *wed* instead of *red*); (2) omission of a sound (here the person might say *ed* instead of *red*); or (3) distortions of sounds in words so that the average listener would not be able to understand the sounds which were present when the individual said the word *red*.

Variations in voice quality which might occur include such conditions as hoarseness (common to most readers who have ever become vocally excited at an athletic contest), breathiness (a condition where the speaker mixes an almost whisper with periods of standard phonation), harshness (where the sound produced is best described as hard, tight, and metallic), aphonia (where no phonation occurs), nasality (where all the sounds heard obviously resonate in the nasal cavities), and denasality (where nasal sounds such as *m*, *n*, or *ng*—as in com*ing*—do not resonate normally in the nasal cavities because of some obstruction). The phenomenon of too high or too low a pitch in terms of sex is also included under this general rubric. A related problem in voice production results when the larynx is removed or surgery is performed on the vocal folds. In addition to the obvious organic relationships, such an event has a profound psychological impact upon the person.

Problems in sound production are also found in the clinical entity known as stuttering. Little differentiation has been made between the presence of speech disorders and language disorders in persons whose expressive utterances earn them the designation as stutterers. However, it has been known for some time that persons who stutter do so on sounds, syllables, words or sentences. It is only the latter two forms of behavior which this writer includes under disturbances in language. Because stuttering is usually considered a speech disorder, treatment of all forms of the disorder will be discussed in the present essay while keeping in mind the distinction between speech and language.

Finally, the loss of capacity for understanding and expressing language (or a dysarthria affecting sound production, which is secondary to a trauma to the brain) is also found sometimes in children and adolescents. The trauma may result in regressive behavior and the onset of speech problems based on emotional reasons in addition to the language problems. Speech disorders which are a consequence of bona fide physical problems such as cerebral palsy, dysarthria, or cleft palate are infinitesimal in number. At least 95% of all speech disorders have no apparent or unequivocal neurological and organic basis. The following remarks about therapy for speech disorders are directed toward the large group of persons having talking problems seemingly unrelated to physical difficulties. Because of the psychological meanings associated with disordered speech production, the reader will be aware of the influence of Greenson's (1967) and Blanck and Blanck's (1974) works on treatment of varying psychopathologies.

GENERAL DISORDERS OF TALKING

Delayed Onset of Talking

Failure of the child to produce intelligible simple language or use sound to communicate by the age of 14 to 15 months must be considered an early warning of deviant development. The most appropriate step in treating such an event is a careful initial diagnosis. Clearly, profound bilateral peripheral deafness, central auditory integrating problems, and severe retardation are important factors to be considered when weighing the possibilities of any therapeutic intervention. Once these problems are corrected to the degree which is scientifically possible, treatment can proceed within the limits of the individual's potential. Failure to keep this elementary principle in mind has spawned false hopes and cruel disappointment in therapists, patients, and parents alike.

For example, a child who is congenitally and profoundly deaf will most likely never acquire usable verbal communication no matter how much teaching or therapy is provided. Similarly, a child born with a profound central auditory integrating difficulty will be limited in the development of verbal abilities. In contrast a child who reaches the mental age of at least 2 years should be able to develop some rudimentary form of verbal expression. The interaction among native capacity, parental and environmental reaction, and emotional response of the individual to these factors can artificially depress the potential level of communication ability. Such factors are best dealt with through parental counseling and/or casework procedures carried on in a process type interaction rather than in a single information-giving session.

While children with such difficulties constitute one subgroup of those who are delayed in the onset of talking, a much larger group of children exists who display no bona fide, clear neurological or organic reason for the symptom. Filippi and Rousey (1968) have described delayed onset of talking based on psychogenic factors. Specifically, they note that a high negative valence is often placed on sound production in young children who either are not yet talking or doing so in an unintelligible way. Often this is done by the mother as a displacement of her anger toward her husband. The resulting home environment is one in which sounds as would normally occur between mother and child are not only nonexistent—but even more importantly, sound making is actively discouraged. Seemingly, the child's sound productions remind the angry mother of all the worst aspects of her husband.

Treatment of this communication difficulty depends heavily on concepts pertaining to the development of early object relationships as proposed by Mahler, Pine, and Bergman (1975), Spitz (1965), and Kernberg (1975). Remembering that vowels are supposedly related to early drive discharge and object relationships, the therapist commences the communicative relationship on a one-to-one basis solely through the use of vowel sounds or noises. Such interaction is similar to the normally occurring reciprocal mother-child verbal interaction. Such vocal parameters as intensity, intonation, and pitch level are also an integral part of any verbalization of vowels or noises. These parameters allow communication of varying mixtures of libidinal and aggressive feelings. The nonverbal psychological acceptance and nurturance of the patient is an integral part of such interaction. In general, the closer the child is to the autistic phase as described by Mahler and co-workers (1975), the more physical contact is helpful. Such contact may take the form of rocking, holding the child on the therapist's lap, or just remaining physically close. Such closeness is, of course, discouraged if the child is in the symbiotic phase, for it is the therapist's intent in working with such a child to encourage separation from mother and father through the child's use of sound, and eventually to promote individuation through the tool of language. Standard playroom toys and arrangements for encouraging drive discharge to accompany vowel production and usage are helpful. As treatment progresses, the child will begin to use vowels and later consonants to form verbal language. With the advent of the use of consonants as well as vowels more complicated levels of object relations will become apparent in the play involved in therapy.

One immediate complication to successful treatment soon becomes apparent—that is, the response of the parents. For when the child begins to make more sounds (i.e., to express drives), the crux of the original problem, as noted earlier, must be faced by both parents. As a result, careful parent guidance and/or a casework process is necessary. The mother must begin to explore why the child's "incessant talking" bothers her and the conflict between the parents must be brought into focus so that the child will be free to make some progress. As the parents gradually become able to express their own feelings, they begin to permit the child the same freedom. The optimal form of treatment should be an intense one, with the child being seen at least three times a week and the parents being seen once a week. When no complications other than the psychological factors exist, two- to three-year-old children should begin talking and make considerable progress within a six-month time period. As such, this kind of intervention is immensely gratifying to the therapist, the patient, and the family.

Elective Mutism. A condition related to delayed onset of talking is the clinical phenomenon known as elective mutism. In such a condition the child or adolescent has begun talking but elects to talk to only certain people and remains silent in the presence of others. This problem has been approached therapeutically from rather traditional child guidance and psychoanalytic approaches as well as by recent operant conditioning procedures. Elective mutism is a disorder based on emotional charges attached to sound production as opposed to a cognitive or language disability. Brown, Wilson, and Laybourne (1963) describe the problem in ways similar to the dynamics proposed by Filippi and Rousey (1968) in their exposition on delayed onset of talking. Pustrom and Speers (1964) see elective mutism as a compromise expression of family conflict. Bradley and Sloman (1975) believe the problem to be more common in immigrant families. Halpern, Hammond, and Cohen (1971) and Shaw (1971) have described behavioral techniques for encouraging talking.

Chethik's (1973) case study of Amy presents the result of treatment of the disorder by a psychoanalytically oriented process.

In contrast to delayed onset of speaking or the later appearance of elective mutism are the problems with sound production in persons who are using sound and language freely. In the next part of this paper therapeutic considerations centering around such disturbances will be discussed.

Specific Deviations in Voice Quality

Variations in voice quality are reflected largely through vowels. As in the case of the other clinical problems, it is necessary to rule out any organic causes before treating these symptoms as being psychologically determined. Some of the more common voice problems with significant psychological components are hoarseness, breathiness, and nasality. In addition there is the relatively well-known problem of hysterical aphonia and the not so well-known secondary psychological complications to any surgery performed on the larynx.

Hoarseness. This condition generally can be simulated or provoked by an individual's phonating below his optimal pitch. Such an assumption does not rule out possible organic causes for hoarseness, such as cancer or vocal cord paralysis. However, if these physical conditions are not present, it is helpful to understand this voice deviation as a symptom of the person's trying to be more hypermasculine than is really appropriate. Such a symptom is a common bit of everyday psychopathology to many sports fans who become quite hoarse after prolonged cheering or correction of "erroneous officials' calls" at an athletic contest. The dynamic which seems apparent in such situations is that the fan is trying to be more aggressive than in reality is realistically possible. In boys around the oedipal period, hoarseness is often present without their ever going to or appearing in an athletic contest. The obvious dynamic involved is their assertion of a masculinity beyond their years in an effort to resolve their oedipal dilemma. Both parents contribute to this state of affairs in varying degrees. In some instances the child is identifying with the father's own style of coping with oedipal phenomena, and in others the child assumes the hypermasculine stance reflected in a hoarse voice upon the instigation of his mother. Quite often benign growths called "vocal nodules" subsequently appear on the child's vocal cords. Although a laryngologist can surgically remove these growths, they often reappear. A most effective way of treating this problem is by getting the child to phonate at a more appropriate pitch level. To do this requires psychotherapeutic help for the boy in coming to grips with his own family role and sexual identity. Vocal drills are notoriously ineffective by themselves.

In cases where the mother is unconsciously stimulating her son to be the father of the house, there is often a need for family therapy. This voice disorder is more easily treated in the younger child, since the psychological determinants have not yet become intertwined in the child's character patterns. Hoarseness does appear in adolescence and even adulthood on a reactive as well as chronic level. While hoarseness is most usually found in boys, the difficulty is sometimes seen in girls with essentially the same dynamics being operative.

Breathiness. This symptom is more common to adolescent girls than to adolescent boys. It seems related to suppression or reaction formation to the onrush of sexual feelings experienced by the developing adolescent girl which have no appropriate outlet. The adolescent girl whose sexual drives are ahead of boys her own age is caught in a predicament which she must deal with by (1) sublimating her sexual drives through extracurricular activities, (2) becoming promiscuous, or (3) somehow neutralizing her desires by invoking various psychological defenses. While the girl with a breathy voice is stereotypically thought of as extra-sexy, the present interpretation would be quite to the contrary. Indeed, the course of psychotherapy with females with breathy voices suggests they have significant problems with enjoyment of normal sexual feelings. With the above remarks in mind, the therapeutic task with these adolescent patients is to help them express their sexual drives in a sublimatory fashion as well as to deal with any secondary issues which may have developed as a result of the underlying conflict. The older the person, the more intensive and individual the psychotherapeutic process must become.

Hysterical Aphonia. A sudden and complete loss of voice, in the absence of organic factors, is a rare event. Two examples of representative comments about this problem can be found in works by Fenichel (1945) and Nemiah (1967). Freud's (1953) description of the circumstances surrounding Dora's loss of voice is an excellent clinical example of the psychological issues surrounding the onset of the problem. Specifically, her loss of voice seemingly was apparently related to being embraced by Herr K. "unexpectedly" and becoming aware of his simultaneously having an erection. Classical psychotherapeutic techniques are helpful in treatment of aphonia. The problem must be carefully assessed to make sure that it is not a symptom binding a psychotic process. While rare in children, hysterical aphonia is more "common" in adolescents.

Nasality and Denasality. These two voice symptoms represent opposites from both acoustic and psychopathological standpoints. In ordinary speech only the sounds *m* (as in *mom*), *n* (as in *no*) and *ng* (as in *going*) produce resonance in the nasal chamber. Assuming there is normal physiological functioning of the soft palate, the presence of nasality or denasality seems dynamically related to a conflict over the expression of aggression. In nasality (hyperresonance in the nasal chamber) aggression is likely to be expressed through indirect and passive means. In denasality (an atypical reduction of resonance in the nasal chamber) there is a more open and calculated expression of aggression without any real demonstration of feeling. Both of these voice variations are most likely present on a psychogenic basis in adolescence. Treatment along psychological lines must take into account characterological issues as opposed to neurotic conflicts.

Atypical Pitch Level and Control. The pitch level of males and females during childhood is not strikingly different. However, beginning in adolescence there is a definite perceptual and acoustic difference. Pitch change occurs in males in a gradual fashion. The breaks stereotypically associated with adolescent males occur less frequently than generally believed. At present, voice breaks at this age are seen as reflecting problems in mastery of impulse control. Assuming no organic laryngeal problems, ego strengthening measures are indicated in any treatment process. Inappropriately high-pitched voices in males, in the absence of organic or endocrine problems, suggest basic problems in sexual identification. The reverse is true in females. Early and intense psychotherapeutic intervention is indicated to allow the patient a chance to achieve what, for him or her, will be an appropriate sexual identity.

Psychological Reactions to Organic Trauma. Problems with voice production because of surgical removal of the larynx are fortunately a rare event in childhood and adolescence. Usually, this would be a result of some external trauma. In adults such surgery is often a consequence of cancer. Regardless of the etiology or the individual's age, removal of the larynx deprives the person of the ability to produce voiced sounds, a situation that can be responded to on many psychological levels. Obviously, the person will no longer sound the same and there will be a physical alteration of the body such as to challenge the self-concept of the most adjusted person. Successful teaching of esophageal speech or use of a prosthesis often requires concomitant psychotherapy. The required intensity and level of such treatment reflects the presurgical psychological adjustment of the person.

A more common surgical procedure on the child or adolescent is removal of vocal nodules. While many laryngologists will attempt some form of voice therapy first, occasions for surgery do arise. Quite often the nodules will reappear. Knowledge of the patient's presurgical psychological adjustment will help the treatment of the psychological response to any operation. The secondary gains of the surgery often further complicate any psychotherapy or voice reeducation procedures.

Specific Variations and Deviations in Vowel Production

Vowel Substitutions. Vowel difficulties in terms of substitution of one sound for another are rarely found. An example of a vowel substitution would be pronunciation of the word *sell* as *sail.* When present, such difficulties seem to herald a major fusion of aggressive and libidinal drives which are discharged indiscriminately and without modulation. In a teenager or an adult, one might well prognosticate extreme destructive behavior, while in a child the overt behavior might be contained, yet nonetheless environmentally disturbing. Clinically, the present writer has seen vowel substitutions occurring only in adolescent patients who have committed a major crime, such as murder or rape, and in children who are labeled as hyperactive. The therapeutic intervention for such a speech difficulty is obviously not to focus on correction of the sound but to provide the appropriate emotional and environmental support necessary to protect the individual and society.

"Foreign" Dialect. There are other variations in vowel production which are less pathognomonic yet still have important psychological meanings. Therapeutic intervention is not indicated where regional or "foreign" dialects are present. Thus, the distinctive Eastern pronunciation of the initial vowel found in the word *harbor*, the Southerner's pronunciation of the word *mother* as moth-*ah*, or the nasal twang of residents in the Bible belt represent vowel variations which, while suggestive of differences in drive discharge, do not represent pathological fusions of drives. Thus, the layman's perception of a "foreigner" in his midst probably represents some preconscious awareness of differences in expression of libidinal and aggressive drives as well as fear of the unknown way these drives will be expressed. It is thus more understandable why hearing a person talk like oneself is usually reassuring.

Another variation in vowel production which is not pathognomonic but important nonetheless for the therapist (in terms of understanding the psychological life of the person) is the variation seen in British speech patterns as compared to Latin American speech patterns. Stereotypically, it is common to describe British speech as being "clipped"; i.e., the vowels are shortened. Now, if vowels do reflect drive expression and if in England these are clipped, then we have a corollary in speech patterns of the general stereotype of the Englishman as inhibited in affect expression. In an opposite sense, if the stereotype of the Latin as being more free in affect expression is correct, one should expect, according to the present theory, to find vowel sounds more prolonged. This, of course, is what occurs in much of spoken Spanish where diphthongs are frequent. While these variations may be appropriate in given cultures, the appearance of such behavior in a native North American speaker would be justification for concluding that some changes in drive expression were occurring. Labov (1972) provides an example of this notion in describing how vowels change in the residents of Martha's Vineyard in Massachusetts in response to the unwelcome intrusion of summer tourists.

Mid-Central Vowel r and the Semivowel l. Whenever the vowel *r* becomes distorted so that, for example, the word *bird* is said in an accentuated fashion as *burrrd*, there is evidence (Decker and Rousey, 1974); (Filippi and Rousey, 1971) that the individual may have some other indications of minimal brain dysfunction. There are also associated problems with learning and impulsivity. Therapy focused on the sound will not in itself change the phonetic variation. Rather, some environmental, intrapsychic, or pharmacological controls are warranted to ameliorate the probable instability in ego functioning.

In contrast to the difficulties in production of the *r* are the problems with the *l* sound. When the *l* sound is said with an accompanying swallow, the specific product has been called a "dark *l*." This label refers to the fact that the sound is made in the back (dark) part of the mouth in contrast to the usual anterior movement of the tongue. Such a term probably originated in the days before electronic recording and thus was a convenient way to describe an acoustic production. The presence of the dark *l* is held to be related to psychological deprivation experiences sustained in interaction with the mother or mother figure. There are numerous ways individuals have of coping with such a psychological experience. Thus, a child or adolescent may become a voracious eater or be involved in drug or alcohol misuse. Another avenue of adjustment to this psychological deprivation would be for the child or adolescent to develop a significant degree of depression and inhibition of affect. A third avenue would be to develop a pathological degree of narcissism along the lines suggested by Kohut (1971). Each of these alternatives has its accompanying phonetic variations which in turn affect other consonants. These correlations will form the subject matter for the remainder of this chapter.

In the present context it becomes obvious that the treatment of choice for this sound variation is to intervene as early as possible when maternal deprivation is suspected. Environmental manipulation coupled with psychological work with both parents will usually facilitate the disappearance of the *l* difficulty. Depending on the severity of the deprivation, individual psychotherapy may be indicated. For one such child, play therapy focused for over a year on the repetitive act of feeding the therapist and being fed by the therapist. The most enduring act of play centered around activity at an ice cream store. Month after month, therapist and patient prepared and fed pretend ice cream cones to each other in a store that was open 24 hours a day. Finally, the patient was able to say that she was full and wanted to stop playing the "silly game." At that point trouble with the *l* sound had disappeared. As treatment progressed, the patient's mother was able to become more a part of the child's life as mother and daughter together baked foods of all sorts. Part of the clinical difficulty in treating this sound and its concomitant psychological state is the reluctance for society to think in terms of psychological maternal deprivation. Obviously, the kind of neglect discussed in the present context could occur in any socioeconomic or racial setting.

SPECIFIC DEVIATIONS AMONG CONSONANT SOUNDS

Earlier it was posited that consonant sounds reflect development of satisfactory object relationships. In the immediately preceding section discussion of the *l* sound and its relationship to maternal object relationships was noted. At this point we shall discuss only specific consonant deviations and their indicated treatment. It is not by accident that the *l* sound served as a bridge between the discussion of vowels and consonants, for in actuality the mother serves as the psychological bridge between drive expression and satisfaction and the child's interaction with the other objects in his or her world.

Substitution of w for l. In instances where the child substitutes the *w* for the *l* sound, there is a clearer clinical illustration of the interaction between need for drive fulfillment and object relationships. In such patients there is an inordinate demandingness which, despite all attention given, fails to satisfy. This kind of patient is still struggling to fill his need for nurturance. Because of the more open neurotic nature of the behavior, parent guidance is often helpful in letting the child attain some degree of satisfaction. This is not a speech symptom usually found in late childhood or adolescence, probably because if it is not resolved the child will either internalize the psychic dilemma (with the resultant development of a dark *l*) or begin displaying a pathological degree of narcissism.

Substitution of f for Voiceless th. The counterpart of disturbed maternal object relationships—i.e., disturbed object relationship with the father—is reflected in the substitution of *f* for the voiceless *th* sound (e.g., the word *both* becomes *bof*). Of interest is how this articulation pattern reflects both the area of conflict and the psychological solution selected. The conflict is around phallic issues (as reflected by the *th* sound) but the symptomatic solution is to use a sound (*f*) which represents an early stage of psychological development where phallic issues are secondary to oral needs. In some readers' minds the question may arise as to how the two-year-old who makes such an error can be dealing with phallic issues. It is by now commonly accepted that all stages of psychosexual development are present at all times except that at varying points certain psychological issues may predominate. Thus, the substitution and its inferred meaning are totally consistent with both psychoanalytic theory and with the dynamic meaning of psychological symptoms. In young children such speech problems can often be treated successfully by working with the parents. This sound variation is quite common among children of professional parents where the father is away in graduate school or in a residency program. Increasing the time spent between a father and his preschool child will often dramatically clear up the difficulty. Importantly, some therapeutic focus with the father on his feelings about this is a necessary accompaniment.

Continuation of this sound substitution into latency and adolescence is an indication of an increasing psychological toll being paid by the person for lack of father-child interaction. With the exception of Lynn's (1974) recent book, the role of the father in the child's psychological adjustment has been discussed relatively little. Isaacs (1948) notes that the father allows an infant to discover there are two different creatures in the world—male and female—a discovery that occurs when the child experiences the differences in smell, touch, sound, and bodily movement between men and women. As such, this interaction facilitates the separation-individuation process. Failure to engage in a process of differentiation between maleness and femaleness promotes a distorted sense of sexual identity, which has significant ramifications for self-differentiation in later childhood and adolescence.

In contrast to the inferences we have been making about relationships between specific misarticulations and their psychological correlates, many linguists see sound behavior as primarily culturally and environmentally determined. One evidence they present is the black person's substitution of *bof* for *both*. Yet clinical observation of both black and white speech patterns suggests that there is little hard evidence for such a conclusion, for it is not a given that every black says *bof* instead of *both* either within or among various subcultures. That some do cannot be denied. However, the same condition exists among white children. LaFon and Rousey (1970) and Rousey (1968) were able to show a significantly high incidence of this articulation error in children literally without a father as well as in situations where a "psychological absence" of fathering would be a reasonable hypothesis. A vignette of treatment of this speech difficulty within a psychotherapeutic context will further demonstrate the psychological issues.

The patient was a three-year-old white girl who was an only child. Her father had wished for a boy and was quite disappointed with the birth of a daughter. Complicating matters further was the fact that the child had a congenital hip dysplasia necessitating a cast from the first few months of life. The natural smells of elimination processes became attached to the cast and, although it was changed at appropriate times, the child literally was quite repelling from an odor standpoint. The father "managed" to leave all of the early care to the mother. There was, not surprisingly, a delay in onset of talking. Using the therapeutic guidelines discussed in the section on delayed onset of talking, it was possible to get her to talk intelligibly in a relatively short time. Of interest in the present context was the one remaining sound difficulty—a substitution of *f* for the voiceless *th*. At this point in time the child was close to four years of age. Play therapy was used as a treatment modality. After several months of work, the patient began to explore sexual differences through use of play dolls manufactured with appropriate sexual organs. As she was playing with these, she "accidentally" backed into a table and began complaining of the need for a band-aid to cover her buttocks. Since there was no real hurt, the therapist began to explore with her the fantasy behind such a request. It soon became apparent that she thought a penis would grow between her buttocks following removal of any band-aid. With this behavior it became possible to review some of her ideas about sexuality as well as to approach her feelings of not being valued by her father because she was a girl. There followed sometime after this a sequence of play which clearly illustrated her understanding of being a girl and her acceptance of this as well as the relationship between these factors and her speech problem. She drew for the therapist a picture of her dog complete with tail. As she looked at the picture, it appeared wrong to her. After some time she recognized it was because her real dog had had its tail bobbed. With the change in drawing completed, she was able to say "that's how little girl's dog should be." Recognizing the patient's knowledge of the basic difference between boys and girls as expressed in this action, the therapist recalled for her that she had difficulties saying words like *thank you*, *three*, and *both*. She was told the therapist thought she could now say those words like others and would have no further difficulty. She proceeded to confirm the therapist's remark. It is important to emphasize that at no time was direct work ever done in a teaching sense on her articulation difficulty.

In contrast to this child's psychological difficulties are those of an adolescent whose only articulation problem was a substitution of *f* for the voiceless *th*. This 14-year-old white boy had a psychiatric diagnosis of childhood schizophrenia. There were numerous indications of disorganization, including fear of being infected, backing into rooms with a coat over his head, and a conviction that it was better to be a girl than a boy. This patient could talk easily despite the massive amount of thought disorganization with which he contended. Early in the process of establishing a working alliance, the therapist's remarks took into account the crisis in sexual identity that was implied by this sound substitution. Other nonverbal cues revealing the patient's conflict over whether he was a boy or girl included such things as flirtatious actions, fantasies that the contents of a bean bag were testicles from bad boys, and talk about dressing up in women's clothes. As we focused on the conflict over sexual identity manifested not only through the obvious overt behavior but also by the appearance of the sound substitution of *f* for the voiceless *th*, the patient dropped his concerns about being infected by looking at other people and was able to enter the office easily. As the patient became more appropriate in his thoughts and actions and became more comfortable with being a boy, his articulation problem subsided. In this instance the disappearance of the speech problem and the correct articulation of words containing the voiceless *th* sound served as a basis for the therapist's making appropriate clarifying remarks about the improved psychological functioning. At no time was the patient's attention called to the specific speech error. This severely disturbed adolescent was able to progress in his emotional life to the point where he was discharged to a placement which would allow him to make maximal use of his cognitive potentials.

Substitution of w for r. Another quite common consonant problem is the substitution of *w* for *r*; thus the youngster might say *wabbit* instead of *rabbit*. Within the context of the present theory this error is felt related to object relationship disturbances associated with the anal period. Dynamically, there is a taking in, as reflected by use of the *w* sound (which is an oral sound in the present system), and problems in letting go, as reflected by the problem with the consonant *r*, an anal sound in the present system. Clinically, this sound variation is often seen in children who are struggling with mastery of toilet training. It is a sound difficulty often associated with obsessive thought styles and is not uncommon among underachieving students in the early grades of elementary school (Sehdev & Rousey, 1974). Parenthetically, a simple recording in baby books of letter difficulties experienced by children in their early talking could, under the present system, be of immense help to a therapist in any treatment process. Unfortunately, most baby books make no provision for such entries. A notable exception is the baby book by Hazen (1972).

In treating a child with this articulation error, the therapist often deals with behavior or fantasy material clearly related to anal issues. Thus, an extremely bright seven-year-old in treatment with this error found it hard to express his anger directly. He retained his feces and soiled a good deal. As this behavior became more focused in the therapy process, it was possible to anticipate a period of bowel retention by the "announcement" in his speech patterns of the *w* sound being substituted for the consonant *r*. The attendant problems with aggression produced some disorganization in thinking, a decidedly poor performance in motor activity, and a heavy use of obsessive and intellectual defenses. If all else failed, he would resort to reciting the alphabet, commenting on external events clearly beyond his years, or playing for months at a time at a task which could never be brought to fruition. As he progressed in therapy in this area, he finally got to the point where he was able to share the fantasy of having 10,000 bowel movements in the therapist's "wastebasket." In a related bit of play he was able to arrange some doll house furniture so that the toilet stool was upright rather than lying on its side. As this conflict was worked through in therapy, the articulation error of *w* for *r* disappeared.

An adolescent boy with the same sound difficulty displayed it most prominently whenever he would play Monopoly with the therapist and take his turn at being the banker. In this case not only the speech difficulty but also the overt hoarding behavior as banker and unwillingness to perform his duties clearly signaled his problems with open expression of aggression.

The therapeutic implications of a speech disorder can often be profitably brought to the attention of educators. Levy (1974) has discussed this possibility in detail. For the present, let us merely note that an elementary school teacher who insists on production of schoolwork in a child with a *w* for *r* substitution is likely to become involved in the kind of losing battle experienced by all parents who struggle with their children over toilet training. Alternative ways of letting the child share his schoolwork are indicated.

Whistle on s Sounds. Another speech symptom related to object relationship problems in the anal period is the presence of a whistling on sibilant sounds. Despite the seemingly logical assumption that such sound variations are related to missing teeth or interdental spacing, there is no evidence to believe this to be true. The presence of this sound variation seems intimately related to an unusual degree of anxiety. Its appearance is tied to anal issues surrounding the act of producing for parent figures and in later life to the threat of being "castrated" for failure to produce. Optimal treatment of this difficulty involves a reasonable mastery of both internal and external sources of anxiety. Since anxiety can be thought of as both reactive and chronic, analysis of this sound in the context of the other speech errors is necessary to make a satisfactory differentiation. In general, absence of other sound substitutions would lead one to think of a reactive anxiety state. Conversely, the presence of both the whistle on *s* sounds plus other sound errors would suggest chronic factors as predominating.

Lisping. The phenomenon of lisping, whether it be what is known as a lateral lisp or a frontal lisp, is unjustifiably associated in the layman's mind with missing teeth or interdental spaces. Clinically, it is most useful to think of the lateral lisp as being a symptom of the kind of pathological narcissism described by Kohut (1971). This sound variation is experienced by most listeners as if the person had a mouth full of saliva that cannot be contained and is being expelled from the sides of the mouth. Treatment of such persons is usually difficult, whether the approach is focused strictly on the speech difficulty or on the underlying psychopathology. Psychotherapeutic treatment that comes to grips with the psychological parameters is more successful with children than with older individuals, be they adolescents or adults. This sound deviation is a sequela to the earlier discussed speech disorder called a dark *l*. Thus, successful treatment of the lateral lisp in children usually temporarily produces a dark *l*. The countertransference problems of the therapist are usually marked because of the omnipotence of patients with such speech difficulties. In young children this omnipotence is often displayed by a good deal of messing in play, which seemingly illustrates their total disregard for others.

Frontal Lisp. The frontal lisp, in contrast to the lateral lisp, involves substitution of the voiceless *th* sound for the *s* sound; i.e., the word *sun* is pronounced *thun*, and *bus* becomes *buth*. In seeming disregard for the usual rules which govern symptoms (i.e., a regressive behavior is substituted for the age appropriate behavior), this symptom has an almost counterphobic quality about it. Thus, a phallic sound (the voiceless *th*) is substituted for an anal sound (the *s*). Of further significance is the observation that this sound difficulty is most often found in girls. The clinical behavior which accompanies the presence of this sound difficulty is a pseudo-level of maturity and assertiveness. While families, and especially fathers, often look with enjoyment at a daughter who is mature beyond her years, the front which the child displays through her behavior and speech reflects a headlong rush into the maturing process without a satisfactory resolution of childhood needs and relationships. Here the focus of therapy involves both work with the parents, who are accelerating the "growing-up" process in an inappropriate way, and helping the child relinquish the "adult" stance and consider the merits of childhood issues and feelings.

Substitution of v for Voiced th. The substitution of *v* for the voiced *th* involves strictly phallic sounds. When this substitution is heard, clinical examination will usually reveal hypersexual stimulation of the child. Such inappropriate sexual stimulation can happen in crowded, poverty level situations where sexual privacy is at a premium or it can happen in well-to-do situations where space is not an issue but intrusive handling can be. For example, the child who continues to be wiped after his or her toilet activities, sleeps with the parents of the opposite sex, or is actually the victim of a sexual attack may have such a substitution. Clinicians know that pure exposure to any or all of these sources of stimulation is not in and of itself always traumatic. Constitutional differences, accompanying affect, and the role played by the child all have an influence in the emotional response of the person involved. Such a traumatic experience is usually difficult to verify because of the various taboos and reluctance to talk about sex. This sound substitution does not develop in an adolescent or adult following a traumatic sexual encounter and seems largely related to childhood trauma. The trauma and resulting speech difficulty may and in fact often does carry over into adult life.

Substitution of b for v. A less serious, but nonetheless psychologically important, speech difficulty centers around the substitution of *b* for the *v* sound (i.e., *base* is said instead of *vase*). The difficulty is related to a failure to deal with the separation aspects of the oedipal struggle. This substitution is often seen in some native Spanish speakers who, when adopting English, always complain they can't say the *v* sound. The present author feels it not surprising in terms of the general tendency for Spanish families to be closely knit and for in-laws to continue living in closer than the usual proximity expected in families in the United States. Failure to master this substitution has grave implications for children in the United States when they are grown and wish to emancipate themselves from their own family and enter into marriage. Treatment of this speech disorder involves heavy focus on the family dynamics and attempts to deal with the derivatives of the oedipal struggle.

Substitution of d for Voiced th. The substitution of *d* for the voiced *th* (so that the word *those* is said *dose*) is clinically seen in the pseudo-verbally aggressive person. Such speech patterns fit into the stereotype associated with the tough kid who lashes out at the world in a verbal bullying sort of way more effectively than he would through action. Providing ways for the child to sublimate his problems with aggression will dramatically clear up this difficulty.

Sound Omissions. Another aspect of speech behavior is the presence of a sound omission. For example, the child might say *abbit* instead of *rabbit*, *pay* instead of *play*, or *pinkle* instead of *sprinkle*. While omission of sounds where two or more consonants occur in sequence is not unusual in the child up until around five years of age, omission of single consonants (e.g., the *r* sound in the word *r*un) in the three- or four-year-old would be one clinical indication of possible mental retardation. Capacity to include consonants in production of words seems related to cognitive development up to around 7 or 8. Between the mental age of 5 to 7 years, children freely articulate two and three consonant combinations. Articulation of two to three consonant combinations which involve sound substitutions or sound distortions is related to disturbances in affect rather than to limitations in cognitive ability.

One important variation to the above discussion occurs in the instance of a five- or six-year-old who has no omissions. Norris (1974), for example, presents a clinical case which illustrates how this absence of omissions led to the correct diagnosis of normal intellectual potential—despite results obtained on standard tests of intelligence that indicated a significant degree of retardation. Psychotherapeutic intervention produced a significant gain in intellectual functioning as measured by standard tests. A notable exception to the above premises occurs in the child of normal intelligence who is emotionally arrested. Here there may well be sound omissions in single, double, or triple consonant sequences. However, the child's use of expressive language plus other clinical data are useful in preventing an error in diagnosis. In the hands of a discerning therapist, speech data and formal psychological tests thus serve as a check and balance on each other in determining the appropriate therapeutic intervention.

Sound Distortions. At times the child may speak but do so in ways which are generally unintelligible. Again assuming no obvious and gross physical involvement of the tongue, lips, or soft palate, such behavior is clinically understood as reflecting overwhelming anxiety. Recommended treatment of this speech disorder follows traditional therapeutic practices for undue anxiety.

Other Speech Disorders

Stuttering. The speech disorder of stuttering presents a series of challenges in treatment. An adequate review of the disorder and its many facets, both from a diagnostic and treatment standpoint, has been completed by Van Riper (1971, 1973), Sheehan (1970), and Bloodstein (1969), to mention only a few. Part of the difficulty in treating this speech symptom has been the tendency to assume only one etiological factor. This way of approaching the problem collapses all symptoms and behavior so that differential treatment is impossible. In our experience, we feel that the symptom of stuttering can be grossly thought of as both a speech disorder and a language disorder. The behavior called stuttering consists basically of either a repetition or prolongation of sounds, syllables, words, phrases, or sentences. Sometimes there is some accompanying movement of the extremities or cognitive acts such as substituting silently a word which is synonymous with the feared word. The term stuttering is generally used in preference to stammering in the United States. In young children there is a tendency to call the same behavior dysfluency in an effort to avoid labeling.

From our own vantage point, we feel that the optimal treatment for this problem is primarily to concentrate along psychotherapeutic lines whenever the difficulty revolves around sounds or syllables. When the difficulty is on words, phrases, or sentences, a rather heavy dosage of prolonged spontaneous talking is indicated.

When stuttering occurs on sounds, it is helpful to note the specific sounds so that one can, using the previously presented material, infer the level of object relationship conflict. With this in mind plus other data from an appropriate psychological testing, the treatment of choice would follow the principles of traditional psychoanalytically oriented psychotherapy.

By contrast, where the problem is on words, phrases, or sentences, the present author has had success by encouraging a sort of verbal marathon for the patient (Rousey, 1958). Specifically, the person is asked to talk continuously and spontaneously ten hours a day for five consecutive days. No reading or singing is involved and the entire session is either monitored by a listener or is tape recorded so that content can be selectively studied at a later time. The hypothesis in this form of treatment is that some form of reorganization or transfer of function occurs in the brain. The exact process is at this point unclear.

In practice it is more common to see some combination of both of these clinical dimensions. Thus, in one adolescent whose stuttering on words and phrases was so severe that he could not be evaluated by a psychiatrist, treatment through the extensive talking method gave him quite fluent speech after only 5 days. At that point it became clear that a *w* for *r* sound substitution existed. Thus, the inference would be that not only was there some "internal restructuring of the speech circuits," which was accomplished through the talking, but there was also a major problem with aggression which had been obscured by a possible "neurological" factor.

Childhood Aphasia. Treatment of childhood aphasia represents more outright work with language than relief from speech symptoms. However, even here the reaction to an aphasia-producing trauma may produce a secondary affective response which inhibits use of sound. The clinician's primary task is carefully to evaluate the aphasic problems with the goal of determining if there is enough receptive language remaining to allow recovery of the expressive skills. Time of onset of the physical trauma as well as the extent of the problem becomes quite important in determining the prognosis. It is this therapist's opinion that almost any sort of language stimulation is helpful in facilitating whatever recovery is possible. So long as the verbal interaction between therapist and patient takes into account the psychological needs which are involved, then to the extent the brain is capable, there will be recovery of language. This point was demonstrated years ago in the work of Wepman (1951) and, inferentially, in the recent publications of Sarno, Silverman, and Sands (1970). No demonstrable relationship between specific language stimulation exercises and specific brain functioning seems logical at this point in our work in this area.

FINAL CLINICAL NOTE

Countertransference. A final therapeutic issue in dealing with speech disorders concerns the issue of countertransference in the therapist. If speech disorders are treated along the lines proposed in the present chapter, the therapist is liable to the same dynamics believed operative in any psychoanalytically oriented psychotherapy. Of interest at present is an additional form which countertransference can take. Specifically, the therapist who has enough observing ego to listen to himself as well as to the patient should be able to detect any personal emotional reactions displayed through sound variations during the treatment process. In so doing, another avenue is open to therapists for facilitating the growth of their patients. This concept is obviously applicable to patients in psychotherapy for presenting complaints other than speech disorders.

SUMMARY

This chapter has taken the position that speech disorders with the exception of gross and obvious neurological or physical handicaps reflect a person's affect state and object relationships. As such, recommended treatment adheres to conventional psychoanalytically oriented psychotherapy, modified slightly by an understanding of the psychological meanings of speech disorders. Most trained workers in the area of mental health have been practicing speech therapists for some time without knowing it.

A resumé of a theory of speech and personality was presented as a basis for treatment of the specific speech disorders along psychotherapeutic lines. This theory is in marked contrast to the usual cognitively based ways in which speech disorders are treated. Similarities between clinical and theoretical issues in psychotherapy in general, and speech disorders in particular, have also been discussed.

REFERENCES

BACKUS, O., and BEASLEY, J. *Speech therapy with children.* New York: Houghton Mifflin, 1951.

BLANCK, G., and BLANCK, R. *Ego psychology: Theory and practice.* New York: Columbia University Press, 1974.

BLOODSTEIN, O. *A handbook on stuttering.* Chicago: National Easter Seal Society for Crippled Children and Adults, 1969.

BRADLEY, S., and SLOMAN, L. Elective mutism in immigrant families. *Journal of the American Academy of Child Psychiatry*, 1975, 510–514.

BROWN, E., WILSON, V., and LAYBOURNE, P. Diagnosis and treatment of elective mutism in children. *Journal of the American Academy of Child Psychiatry*, 1963, 605–617.

BROWN, R. *A first language.* Cambridge, Massachusetts: Harvard University Press, 1973.

CHETHIK, M. Amy: The intensive treatment of an elective mute. *Journal of the American Academy of Child Psychiatry*, 1973, 482–498.

DARLEY, F., ARONSON, A., and BROWN, J. How motor speech is studied. In *Motor Speech Disorders.* Philadelphia, Pennsylvania: W. B. Saunders Company, 1975.

DECKER, L., and ROUSEY, C. Speech indicators of neurological dysfunction. In Clyde Rousey

(Ed.), *Psychiatric assessment by speech and hearing behavior*. Springfield, Ill.: Charles C. Thomas Publisher, 1974.

ERIKSON, E. *Childhood and society*. New York: Norton, 1950.

FENICHEL, O. *The psychoanalytic theory of neurosis*. New York: Norton, 1945.

FILIPPI, R., and ROUSEY, C. Delay in onset of talking: A symptom of interpersonal disturbance. *Journal of the American Academy of Child Psychiatry*, 1968, *17*, 316–319.

FILIPPI, R., and ROUSEY, C. Positive carriers of violence among children: Detection by speech deviations. *Mental Hygiene*, 1971, *55*, 157–161.

FLEMING, P., and ROUSEY, C. Quantification of psychotherapy change by study of speech and hearing patterns. In Clyde Rousey (Ed.), *Psychiatric Assessment by Speech and Hearing Behavior*. Springfield, Ill.: Charles C. Thomas Publisher, 1974.

FREUD, S. Fragments of an analysis of a case of hysteria. In *The standard edition of the complete psychological works of Sigmund Freud* (Vol. VII). London: Hogarth Press, 1953.

GREEN, A. *Speech of psychiatric patients: A hospital survey*. Unpublished M.S. Thesis, Purdue University, 1962.

GREENSON, R. *The technique and practice of psychoanalysis*. New York: International Universities Press, 1967.

GRIMES, J. *The status of speech and language of emotionally disturbed children*. Unpublished M.A. Thesis, Kansas University, 1962.

HALL, W. F. *A study of the articulation skills of children from three to six years of age*. Unpublished Doctoral Dissertation, University of Missouri, 1962.

HALPERN, W., HAMMOND, J., and COHEN, R. A therapeutic approach to speech phobia: Elective mutism reexamined. *Journal of the American Academy of Child Psychiatry*, 1971, *10*, 94–107.

HAZEN, B. *Baby's first six years*. New York: Golden Press, 1972.

HEALEY, W. C. *A study of the articulatory skills of children from six to nine years of age*. Unpublished Doctoral Dissertation, University of Missouri, 1963.

HEJNA, R. *Speech disorders and nondirective therapy*. New York: Ronald Press, 1960.

IRWIN, O. C. Infant speech: Consonantal sounds according to place of articulation. *Journal of Speech and Hearing Disorders*, 1947, *12*, 397–401.

IRWIN, O. C. Infant speech: Development of vowel sounds. *Journal of Speech and Hearing Disorders*, 1948, *13*, 31–34.

ISAACS, S. Fatherless children. In *Problems of Child Development*. London: New Education Fellowship Monographs, 1948.

KERNBERG, O. *Borderline Conditions and Pathological Narcissism*. New York: Jason Aronson, 1975.

KERNBERG, P., and ROUSEY, C. Variations in speech sounds during psychotherapy: An independent indicator of change. *Journal of the American Academy of Child Psychiatry*, 1970, *9*, 762–777.

KOHUT, H. *The analysis of the self*. New York: International Universities Press, 1971.

LABOV, W. *Sociolinguistic patterns*. Philadelphia: University of Pennsylvania Press, 1972.

LAFON, D., and ROUSEY, C. Residues of early father-child conflict. *Journal of Nervous and Mental Diseases*, 1970, *150*, 366–370.

LENNEBERG, E. *Biological foundations of language*. New York: John Wiley, 1967.

LEVY, N. Aspects of speech pathology and psychoanalysis for the educator. In Clyde Rousey (Ed.), *Psychiatric assessment by speech and hearing behavior*. Springfield, Ill.: Charles C Thomas Publisher, 1974.

LYNN, D. *The father: His role in child development*. Monterey, Calif.: Brooks/Cole, 1974.

MAHLER, M., PINE, F., and BERGMAN, A. *The psychological birth of the human infant*. New York: Basic Books, 1975.

MCNEILL, D. *The acquisition of language*. New York: Harper & Row, 1970.

MCREYNOLDS, L., and ENGMANN, D. *Distinctive feature analysis of misarticulation*. Baltimore, Md.: University Park Press, 1975.

MILISEN, R. The incidence of speech disorders. In L. E. Travis (Ed.), *Handbook of speech pathology and audiology*. New York: Appleton-Century-Crofts, 1971.

NEMIAH, J. Conversion reaction. In A. Freedman and H. Kaplan (Eds.), *Comprehensive textbook of psychiatry*. Baltimore, Md.: Williams & Wilkins, 1967.

NORRIS, V. Speech disturbance and the assessment of mental retardation in children. In Clyde Rousey (Ed.), *Psychiatric assessment by speech and hearing behavior*. Springfield, Ill.: Charles C Thomas Publisher, 1974.

PAGE, J., and PAGE, D. Criteria for mental hospitalization. *Journal of Abnormal Social Psychology*, 1941, *36*, 433–435.

PUSTROM, E., and SPEERS, R. Elective mutism in children. *Journal of the American Academy of Child Psychiatry*, 1964, *3*, 287–297.

ROUSEY, C. Stuttering severity during prolonged spontaneous speech. *Journal of Speech and Hearing Research*, *1*; 1958, 40–47.

ROUSEY, C. *Specific articulation difficulties of fatherless children*. Unpublished manuscript.

ROUSEY, C. The psychopathology of articulation and voice deviations. In L. E. Travis (Ed.), *Handbook of speech pathology and audiology*. New York: Appleton-Century-Crofts, 1971.

ROUSEY, C. (Ed.). *Psychiatric assessment by speech and hearing behavior*. Springfield, Ill.: Charles C Thomas Publisher, 1974. (a)

ROUSEY, C. *Slips of the tongue revisited*. Paper presented to Psychologists Interested in the Study of Psychoanalysis, American Psychological Association meeting, New Orleans, September 1974. (b)

ROUSEY, C. Disorders of speech in childhood and adolescence. In J. Nosphitz (Ed.). *Basic handbook of child psychiatry*. New York: Basic Books, in press.

ROUSEY, C. and TOUSSIENG, P. Contributions of a speech pathologist to the psychiatric examination of children. *Mental Hygiene*, 1964, *48*, 566–575.

SARNO, M., SILVERMAN, M., and SANDS, E. Speech therapy and language recovery in severe aphasia. *Journal of Speech and Hearing Research*, 1970, *13*, 607–623.

SEHDEV, H., and ROUSEY, C. Speech deviation: Indicator of underachievement. In Clyde Rousey (Ed.), *Psychiatric assessment by speech and hearing behavior*. Springfield, Ill.: Charles C. Thomas Publisher, 1974.

SHAW, W. Aversive control in the treatment of elective mutism. *Journal of the American Academy of Child Psychiatry*, 1971, *10*, 572–581.

SHEEHAN, J. *Stuttering: Research and therapy*. New York: Harper & Row, 1970.

SPITZ, R. *The first year of life*. New York: International Universities Press, 1965.

TEMPLIN, M. Certain language skills in children. *Institute of Child Welfare Monograph Series* (No. 26). Minneapolis: University of Minnesota Press, 1957.

TRAVIS, L. (Ed.). *Handbook of speech pathology and audiology*. New York: Appleton-Century-Crofts, 1971.

TRAVIS, L., and SUTHERLAND, L. Psychotherapy in public school speech correction. In L. Travis (Ed.), *Handbook of speech pathology and audiology*. New York: Appleton-Century-Crofts, 1971.

VAN RIPER, C. *The nature of stuttering*. Englewood Cliffs, N. J.: Prentice-Hall, 1971.

VAN RIPER, C. *The treatment of stuttering*. Englewood Cliffs, N. J.: Prentice-Hall, 1973.

WEPMAN, J. *Recovery from aphasia*. New York: Ronald Press, 1951.

WERNER, A. *Comparative psychology of mental development*. New York: International Universities Press, 1957.

WESTON, A., and IRWIN, J. Use of paired stimuli in modification of articulation. *Perceptual Motor Skills*, 1971, *32*, 947–957.

14

MENTAL RETARDATION: PSYCHOLOGICAL TREATMENT

Ruth LaVietes

In assessing psychotherapy for the mentally retarded, the wide variations subsumed in both the terms mentally retarded and psychotherapy should be considered.

The 6 million mentally retarded individuals in the United States comprise a spectrum that ranges from the most profoundly affected, with untestable intelligence and severe organic concomitants, to those who merge indistinguishably into the normal population. Those persons in the mildly retarded range of intelligence who comprise 85 to 90% of this broad classification are the group for which psychotherapy is usually considered. Greater degrees of retardation bring less struggle with reality. Mildly retarded individuals, with IQ's between 50 and 70, comprise the low end of the curve of intelligence distribution along with those whose normal or high genetic endowment has been lowered by somatic insult in pregnancy, birth, or post-natally. The former, usually labelled cultural-familial, undifferentiated, or "garden-variety," rarely show physical signs and are not suspected of retardation prior to entrance into school. The latter show minor somatic signs, differ from normal siblings, and are diagnosed in the preschool period. In both there is considerable variability in both symptoms and in degrees of impairment of the several mental functions, some of which are genetic-somatic and some of which are experientially determined.

Psychotherapy is also a diversely used term. Defined generally as a systematized, theoretically based psychological technique utilized by a professionally trained person for the purpose of effecting behavioral or personality change, psychotherapy varies in methodology, frequency, use of parameters, theoretical substrate, and skills and training of the therapist. The range is, in fact, so great as to make the term "psychotherapy" almost purportless unless further specified. It is necessary to describe psychotherapy precisely when considering its application to mental retardation because the multiple needs of the retardate can put him in contact with numerous interventions which resemble aspects of psychotherapy.

RISKS OF DEVELOPING PSYCHIATRIC DISORDER IN THE MENTALLY RETARDED

While most clinicians might not go so far as Webster (1963), whose opinion it is that "mental retardation is a clinical developmental syndrome that regularly includes an impairment in emotional as well as intellectual development," there is evidence that the incidence of psychiatric disorder in retarded children is high. In a study of 616 children, 30% had prominent psychiatric problems and only 10% were judged to be normal (Menolascino, 1965). In other studies (Chess & Hassibi, 1970; Philips & Williams, 1975) 40% and 87%, respectively, were found to be psychiatrically disturbed. The high risk for the development of psychiatric disorders can be ascribed to factors inherent in intellectual limitations, to the life experiences of such a child, and to the interaction between the two.

The potential for ego development can be limited from infancy in those whose adaptive capacities are constricted. Physiological difficulties, medical evaluations, and hospitalizations—more common in retardates—can predispose to higher anxiety, excessive emotional responsiveness, and difficulty in coping with change. Conceptualization of the self, dependent on encounters with the environment which separate self from non-self and give the external world a permanent existence, can be impaired by sensory handicaps (visual or auditory), motor impairment (poor motor control, awkwardness, hyperactivity), or integrative functions. Poor reality perception, as a form of perceptual or integrative problem, may lead to retaining primitive ways of thinking (maintenance of magical thinking, confusion of fantasy and reality, difficulty in directing aggression to the proper source of frustration) beyond the appropriate developmental stage. Slow development of language and speech delay appropriate expression of needs, investigation of the world, and conceptualization. Children who speak late tend to rely on earlier modes of expression, such as early sensory or motor patterns, as a life-long style. Object relations are delayed and may remain less differentiated, more dependent and need-filling. Delayed conceptualization slows comprehension of cause and effect. Fears are retained longer and defenses against them become more fixed, leading to rigidity. Fantasy is less available for problem solving, while thinking is concretistic and less used for coping with stress. If memory is poor, there are limits placed on the development of inner resources and less potential for planning. Poor control of attention contributes to difficulties in perception, memory, learning, and impulse control.

Low self-esteem is almost ubiquitous in mildly to moderately retarded children. They perceive their disappointment to others in some undefined way. Because he has failed the parent, the child feels in danger of losing parental love and support. He develops an increased need for praise and approval but has a decreased ability to elicit it. His low self-appraisal is aggravated by experiences within the family inasmuch as siblings, even younger ones, advance more rapidly and may resent the retardate's presence. Outside the family there are fewer environmental supports. He is excluded from social and community life. There is the stigma of attending a special school, and possibly of having a peculiar appearance. Other children may tease, avoid, ignore, or depreciate him. There are limits in social opportunities with peers, real difficulties in negotiating with the environment, and in mastering the ordinary tasks of childhood at appropriate developmental points. Encounters with the environment leave him feeling incompetent and ineffective. Yet he is overly dependent upon others for survival. In reaction to these chronic traumata, the retarded child reacts variously with distrust, withdrawal, inhibition, anxiety, fear of challenge, anger, and regressive or aggressive sources of satisfaction. Retarded children in institutions that are overly restrictive, controlled, and lacking the individualization and social structure of families, receive minimal stimulation for the development of appropriate interactive behaviors. Children become prone to excessive dependence, fears of the unfamiliar, rigidity, excess fantasy, and other maladaptive devices for coping with stress. On the other hand, certain behaviors which would be considered pathological in others might not be so in retardates. A certain amount of obsessional behavior, owing to limited inventiveness and anxiety about new situations, may serve a useful purpose in controlling anxiety and coping with the environment. Seeking of sensory or motor experience in excess of the average may be necessary at times to compensate for a paucity of inner resources.

Adolescence poses its special handicaps for the

retarded. Identification is complicated by a longer period of dependence on parents, social and vocational limitations, and interference with sexual experience by the need for realistic controls. Parental anxiety is heightened by fears of the adolescent's aggressive and sexual potential. The adolescent's future, a source of constant anxiety, may remain unmentioned as it makes others uncomfortable.

As the individual retardate passes through the developmental stages, each with its critical issues, without mastering the adaptational tasks required, his vulnerability to emotional disorder increases and his capacity to cope constructively is strained. Nonadaptive defenses—obsessional rigidity, identification with the aggressor, withdrawal, regression and projection—may serve to bind anxiety, although there can be breakthroughs in impulse control under stress. Poor judgment, which is often a concomitant of retardation, can aggravate these breakthroughs into episodes of acting out or other inappropriate reparative efforts to gain self-esteem. The risk factors which increase psychiatric vulnerability also lower intellectual potential.

The diagnostic range and symptoms in retarded children and adolescents do not differ from those found in the usual clinic population, but the incidence of psychosis is much higher (Philips & Williams, 1975). Thus, while there are no particular symptom clusters which are pathognomonic of emotionally disturbed retardates, their vulnerability to disorder is high and can be understood as the result of an interaction between their inherent limitations and the environmental stress which that engenders. Psychiatric disability among retardates presents more adaptive constriction than does the retardation itself. There is a place in society for those with intellectual restrictions but when these are combined with disorders of socialization, exclusion and segregation occur.

SUITABILITY OF PSYCHOTHERAPY FOR MENTAL RETARDATES

Many articles concerned with the value of psychotherapy for the retarded are polarized in one direction or another. Arguments which have been mentioned as contraindications to psychotherapy are:

1. Unawareness of problems and disinterest in seeking help; tendency to minimize psychogenic factors; inability to form a therapeutic relationship or understand the purpose of the individual offering it.
2. Inability to delay or control expression of impulses in the face of frustration.
3. Limitations in developing understanding and insights to modify behavior, in realizing the source and consequence of behavior and the cause-and-effect relationship.
4. Limitations in foresight and planning, in seeking and accepting socially appropriate substitute activities.
5. Poor ability to view others' behavior objectively and to adjust to needs of others; to understand interpersonal nature of problems.
6. Difficulty with verbal generalizations, with effecting a solution based on verbal understanding.
7. Limitations in developing self-reliance, in judging the self separate from others' behavior and standards, in internalizing rewards and punishments.
8. Difficulties in obtaining therapists because of (a) lack of understanding of mental retardation, (b) conflict of values between therapist and those of retardate, (c) therapeutic pessimism about treating retardation, (d) a view of retardates as uninteresting, unattractive, and repulsive, or (e) therapists inevitably assuming a parental role toward the patient.
9. Rigidity and nonadaptive nature of personality patterns.
10. Economic wastefulness of using limited professional resources on a group which would be least likely to benefit from them.

Those favoring treatment contend that obstacles can be overcome by modifying techniques, that the retarded are as much entitled to treatment as the non-retarded, and that results of treatment often prove that the retarded are treatable. Sternlicht (1965) points out the variability of intellectual function in the retardate, and the varieties of therapy capable of bypassing many of the obstacles. It is interesting to note that the first seven of the contraindications listed above apply more or less to psychotherapy with children and that if child therapists adhered to these criteria they would have few patients. The similarities between children and retardates as patients give clues as to the training and experience requirements for treating the mentally retarded.

TREATMENT TECHNIQUES

None of the techniques of treatment commonly used with children and adolescents is contraindicated in treating retardates, and all have been utilized. However, a therapist should be prepared to employ a wide variety of approaches in a manner flexible enough to shift with changing needs.

Establishing a therapeutic relationship in which there are positive expectations on both sides is the first task of therapy. The retarded youngster has had little experience of self-acceptance or acceptance by others. His individuality has received minimal attention from an environment which has emphasized adaptation to its behavioral norms. There has been slight encouragement for him to express his feelings or ideas, and scant personal time devoted to him in which he can determine the pace and type of communication. Thus, although the retardate may not fully understand the purpose of the therapeutic sessions, he usually is gratified by the opportunity to receive individual attention and close contact with a significant person. This by itself enhances his worth as a person despite his defects. His communications are valued, possibly for the first time and, as they are understood, he becomes more effective in this crucial area. The frequent difficulties in articulation and secondary process expression may make communications difficult to comprehend especially at the beginning of therapy, but it is preferable for the therapist to sacrifice precise understanding rather than constantly to request clarification. It is initially more important to promote freedom of expression than to introduce questions which may be seen by the patient as criticisms. In the unusual case in which the child or adolescent is disinterested in the therapy sessions, a preparatory period may be required to engender interest in and dependence on the therapist as a source of gratification. The use of rewards at first to make the child aware of and responsive to the therapist can initiate understanding of cause and effect and reality testing.

An obstacle to conducting therapy may be the poor impulse control exhibited within sessions and outside as a result of uncovering suppressed affects. A carefully defined structure may be necessary, whether in playroom or office, for some retardates. Acceptance is provided within the limits of time, space, safety, and preservation of property. The physical setting of the room, the type and quantity of materials available, and the number of distractions may have to be controlled. Even in verbal communication, direction may be required in the form of suggested topics or leading questions. Better control may be demonstrated by the conduct of the sessions themselves. Temper tantrums with poorly controlled aggression are common in the retarded individual in reaction to frustration, failure, disappointment, or jealousy. As there are limited ego resources to cope with tasks or strong feelings, the rage reactions are often out of proportion to the stimulus. Therapy is directed toward improving coping mechanisms and developing alternatives to explosive outbursts. Whether the episodes occur in the session or at other times they can be exploited therapeutically to demonstrate the difference between strong feelings along with verbal expression of them, both of which may be justified, and the behavioral expression, which is neither acceptable nor effective.

Since many mentally retarded children and adolescents have poorly developed language abstraction and verbal skills, psychotherapy must utilize alternatives to verbal communication to a greater degree than with the non-retarded patient. As with all children, however, considerable data concerning motivation, fantasy, relationships, and affects is gleaned from observation of facial expression, postural change, gestures, tone of voice, play activities, and attitudes toward the therapist and others. Play therapy is widely used even with adolescent patients (Maisner, 1950). Play allows the expression of emotions, the release of unacceptable feelings, escape from reality, discharge of energy, relief of tension, testing of competence at skills, desensitization of situations charged with strong emotions, role assumption, and rehearsal for future behavior. It permits closeness to feelings and persons without the risk of direct contact. Central themes of conflict can be expressed symbolically even when they are not fully understood in language. For example, a child suffering from separation anxiety can express this readily with toys while only minimally conscious of it in linguistic terms. The use of art materials and musical instruments as a form of play therapy can be utilized for emotional expression, role enactment, and tension release.

Relationship therapy, in which the patient learns about himself through a different kind of interaction with the therapist, underlies more specialized treatment interventions. The mentally retarded have characteristically been treated, advertently or not, as inferior, childish, and lacking in dignity and individuality. The therapeutic relationship counteracts this experience. Through his emotional control, patient search for solutions, human warmth, and respect for others, the therapist provides a model with whom the retardate can identify.

Strengthening of ego functions is a major aspect of therapy. Clarification of feeling states is helpful to the retarded individual. He may feel propelled to act without awareness of the provocation in reality or the emotion engendered. Nor does he have the word-abstraction, the label, for the feeling which will enable him to connect similar episodes. By attaching a feeling to a word and to a stimulus, the opportunity for control is enhanced, however slowly or repetitiously. The use of words rather than actions can be encouraged even without the development of an extensive vocabulary. Words which describe feelings are useful in freeing energy for more constructive purposes and for avoiding acting out behavior. Perception of reality is encouraged by the discussion of events in and out of therapy which are susceptible to varied interpretations. Correlations between events and reinforcement of memory is emphasized. Cause and effect can be demonstrated by attempts at alternative approaches to others. The patient has the opportunity to see himself reflected through the therapist's perceptions. The therapist also helps the patient to understand others through their words, expressions, and behavior. Reality support is given by reinforcement of workable attitudes and behavior. The postponement of gratification is encouraged by help with planning and decisions and by the use of reflection, fantasy, and play. The therapist may support the ego by encouraging defense mechanisms that work, for example, sublimation, by utilizing suggestion, advice, information, persuasion, and direction, by preventing destructive behavior, or by demonstrating the value of an alternative style. He may assume the role of an auxiliary superego with the use of prohibitions, commands, or expressions of accepted moral values.

Since the retardate has had an abundance of failure in his life, it is important that feelings of self-esteem be built into therapy by the use of corrective experiences of success within the sessions and as a result of the sessions. The content of the therapeutic hours themselves can be made ones of achievement for the child by the selection of activities for play and for discussion from which he will emerge with a sense of having performed well. The tangible products of a session, e.g., a simple airplane model completed or a drawing done with care, can be significant experiences, especially early in therapy. The object becomes a reminder of success as well as of therapy itself. Realistic praise and reassurance from the therapist gives support to the concepts of working toward achievement and delaying gratification.

Re-education plays a large part in therapy, particularly in the latter stages. First within therapy and later in the extratherapeutic environment, the mentally retarded child or adolescent needs to utilize what he has experienced and to rehearse various ways of managing stress. Initially, efforts to behave differently are made to please the therapist; subsequently they bring their own reward in the form of more effective functioning. The therapist suggests and teaches ways of resisting frustration, postponing gratification, substituting an activity for an earlier one that failed, controlling impulses, handling hostility, and gaining emotional control. Taking responsibility for one's own behavior is a constant theme. Discussion of forthcoming events, making decisions in advance, and outlining standards of acceptable conduct can be done within the shelter of therapy; subsequently they can be tried outside and reviewed in the sessions. Teaching the youngster when to seek help when he is faced with a problem is also rehearsed in therapy. It is especially important in the re-educative phase of therapy to enlist environmental support for the changes the child is attempting to consolidate. Social reinforcement in the form of praise, additional freedom, and greater responsibility in response to changed behavior will support therapeutic efforts.

The place of psychoanalytic techniques in the psychotherapy of retardates is questionable. In those cases reported in the literature where psychoanalysis has been successful, the children seem to have been either of borderline intelligence or incorrectly diagnosed as retarded. This is not to say that a trial of investigative therapy would not be warranted if the patient appeared capable of responding, but therapists should be prepared to work comfortably with other techniques. Interpretations to retardates must often be quite concrete and repeated frequently in many contexts. For example, if a child fears desertion the therapist may verbalize reassurance about this, get the mother to do so, have the mother doll seek out the child doll in play therapy, use the therapeutic appointments as a demonstration, etc. As all child therapists know, insight is not required for improvement.

Psychotherapy with retardates will generally take a longer time than with others because communication is slower, concepts are harder to grasp, repetition is neeessary, opportunities for corrective experiences are fewer, and real problems abound.

PLACE OF PSYCHOTHERAPY IN THE TOTAL TREATMENT PLAN FOR MENTAL RETARDATES

While the therapeutic session can be separated from the balance of the therapeutic interventions for purposes of discussion, in actuality psychotherapy for mentally retarded children must necessarily be only a part of a spectrum of therapeutic interventions. Mentally retarded individuals present considerable additional pathology. Susceptibility to infections, anomalous system development, convulsive states, motor disabilities, endocrine or enzyme abnormalities, and a plethora of somatic ailments are frequent, necessitating communication with pediatricians, neurologists, and various other medical specialists. Speech problems are common. Special educational, recreational, and vocational needs lead to contact with professionals in these areas. Families with retarded youngsters need help in adapting to the needs of the child while balancing these against the requirements of the rest of the family. A therapist treating a retarded child in any setting, whether in office, clinic, or institution, will find himself a part of a team of professionals and child-caring persons with whom he must coordinate his therapeutic efforts. They may look to him directly, e.g., parents, or indirectly, e.g., a social worker colleague treating the parents, for input into their role. In addition, the psychotherapist may utilize key persons in the child's environment to help in social reinforcement of the therapeutic process. The more consistent the life experience is with therapy, the more effective the latter will be.

The "team" necessitated for the mentally retarded child's needs is much more extensive and complex than the traditional child guidance team.[1] Coordination is more difficult. The child and his parents have multiple relationships either simultaneously or previously, inasmuch as the child has usually been evaluated or treated before by other professionals. The role of psychotherapy may be less influential in the child's life both as to importance and discreteness of function, since the therapist's identity is diffused by other helping persons in the environment. While the team factors are variable, depending upon the setting, those places in which psychotherapists are available are the most likely to have other professionals as well. In settings where there is a paucity of personnel, the more usual situation, it is unlikely that trained psychotherapists will be available.

[1] In the mental retardation institute where the author works, the following disciplines operate: endocrinology, cardiology, pediatrics, social work, special education, genetics, neurology, nutrition, radiology, psychiatry, nursing, physical medicine, dentistry, psychology, speech, audiology, occupational therapy, physical therapy, music and dance therapy, art therapy, opthalmology, and otorhinolaryngology.

TREATING PARENTS OF THE RETARDED CHILD

Most articles on psychotherapy with retarded children are based on work done within institutions, undoubtedly a result of the availability of patient groups and professional staff. Yet the great majority of retardates, and most of those for whom psychotherapy is feasible, are living with their families. Institutions are currently being reserved only for the more severely retarded or those with problems requiring specialized services. With trends moving away from separating retarded children from their homes, increasing numbers of families are facing the need to deal with the problems of living with a deviant child. As the nature of retardation brings with it high risk of psychiatric disorder, parent guidance early in the child's life can be helpful in the primary prevention of personality problems and in the maximization of the child's potential. There are numerous reality problems faced by parents of retarded children, such as deciding upon appropriate services, balancing the needs of the child versus those of the family, assessing the child's ability and the degree of autonomy to give him at various developmental stages, etc., all of which may require clinical help. Having a retarded child is a major stress for parents. Even the strongest family suffers under the strain of such an advent. Parents of retarded children, like all others, have vulnerable areas of potential psychopathology which can emerge in a characteristic manner under stress and interfere with the child's opportunity for maximizing his potential.

Guilt and depression are common reactions. The parent feels in some way responsible for the affliction, seeing it as a punishment for wrongdoing. Unconscious hostility to the child would not be unexpected in a situation in which a family's social, economic, and psychological well-being is adversely affected over a period of years or a lifetime. Compensation for guilt may take the form of overprotection, overdevotion to the child at the expense of spouse or siblings, or masochistic martyrdom. Siblings may have excessive demands placed on them for care-taking and supervision of the retardate, leading to angry reactions or to pathological personality development. Direct expression of hostility to the child from parents can break through when defenses are temporarily weakened. Ambivalence leads to the alternation of rejection and overprotection. The limitations inherent in mild retardation can be hard to comprehend and the child may be blamed for difficulties beyond his control. Denial is a parental defense which may be present in mild retardation with its absence of physical stigmata. This defense may lead to repetitive evaluations, inability to use special services effectively, or pressure on the child. Secrecy and avoidance of recognition of the retardation both with the child and among others may result in the child's unreal self-appraisal, suppression of meaningful affects and concerns, confusion, and isolation. A parent may exploit the retardation of the child to avoid social or sexual interaction, or to gratify a requirement for always being needed. Some parents who are overinvolved in working for the welfare of retardates are avoiding the personal aspects of the issue. Neglect of the child, in the form of underutilization of special programs, is often present in poor families because of their preoccupation with other survival issues and lack of sophistication about the nature of retardation and the services available.

Treating the parents may be of considerable benefit to the child even if he does not receive direct psychotherapy. A period of parent counseling prior to beginning sessions with the child or adolescent can set the stage for therapy. Unless contraindicated by the particular features of a case, the same person should treat child and parent, as this leads to the clearest and most economical comprehension of family interaction and capacity for effecting constructive change.

QUALITIES NECESSARY TO TREAT RETARDATES

Certain personality characteristics and attitudes appear to be important for therapists who treat retarded children. A conviction that the patient is worthwhile is essential. Optimism about the patient's possessing untapped capabilities and about the chosen treatment as a modality for realizing the patient's potential should be the underlying theme. It is helpful if the therapist finds something likeable in the patient and can convey this. While acceptance and relative permissiveness is desirable in encouraging the patient to express feelings and ideas, this should not be confused with passivity or the "watchful waiting" associated with traditional therapy. The therapist must be comfortable in taking an active role in defining treatment, its limits and structure. Discussion may need to be directed and problems delineated. An authoritative role may be necessary at times but punitiveness must be avoided. It may be difficult for the therapist to steer a course between whatever authority he exercises in decisions about the patient's life, particularly if treatment takes place within an institution, and distancing himself from decisions perceived negatively by the patient, e.g., whether or not to go home for a weekend. The therapist's flexibility is tested by the varied changes and approaches he makes as the patient fluctuates —to move from drawing the patient's ideas out at one point to directing the discussion at another. Countertherapeutic attitudes such as impatience, boredom, and hopelessness are almost inevitable from time to time. It is useful, as it is with other difficult patients, to build additional gratifications into the treatment process, such as research, supervision, or discussion with colleagues. Mental retardates may seduce therapists into assuming the role of protective approving parents because they appear so deprived and bereft of support. The experience of negativism with others may cause patients to provoke the therapist's rejection in order to test his constancy. The therapist may have difficulty in assessing the capabilities of the patient, either under- or overrating him. Ultimately the therapist must come to terms with his own feelings about being close to a person who must "settle" for a limited adaptation. He needs to remain optimistic in the face of realistic, significant limitations.

The training and experiential prerequisites for conducting psychotherapy with the retarded involve factors of skill, emphasis, cost, and availability. Previous training and experience with children is important not only in terms of the similarities in treatment technique between the child patient and the retardate but because the developmental viewpoint is helpful in understanding his behavior, ideation, and affects. Psychiatrists, psychologists, social workers, and teachers most often act as therapists. Each brings particular emphasis and strengths to the therapeutic endeavor. Because retarded children have ranked low on the scale of desirability as patients, they have often been assigned to the least experienced or least costly professional. This factor may be influential in evaluating results.

GOALS OF TREATMENT

Psychotherapy of mentally retarded children has as its general goal the alleviation of emotional and behavorial abnormalities which are inexplicable on the basis of mental retardation itself. As is true in the treatment of any group of individuals, a goal of therapy is the realization of maximum potential. For the retarded youngster the possibility that psychotherapy will raise intellectual function is of singular concern. To the degree that anxiety and avoidance interfere with maximum use of cognitive abilities, the retardate may also be limited by emotional conflicts. If psychotherapy can reduce the negative associations to learning, greater motivation and better intellectual functioning may result. Where the diagnosis of retardation is in doubt, a goal of therapy may be clarification of this question. However, there is little evidence that basic IQ will be affected by psychotherapy and the success of therapy cannot be judged by this standard.

A major goal is to help the retarded child to decrease his expectations in accordance with his capacities. He must learn the acceptance of limitations in the self while retaining self-esteem and adapting to the environment. Realistic self-appraisal is fundamental. Both child and family may have had expectations which were either too high or too low. Retarded children are puzzling to parents because their abilities can vary widely. This may cause parents to judge their totality by an area of good function. For example, "He can remember things that everyone else has forgotten," leads to heightened aspirations of intellectual function. Or if judgment is based on an area of poor function, e.g., "He can't seem to remember to look both ways when crossing the street no matter how many times I tell him," low aspirations for self-care can result. The psychotherapist who views the retarded youngster objectively can help him, and those in his environment, to sort out the complex of differing functions so that expectations from others and self can be based on sound individualized knowledge. The patient's maximum use of available intellectual capacity is facilitated by his ability to assess his strengths and weaknesses in the cognitive and interpersonal spheres.

While intrapersonal satisfactions are important in their own right, they are very much dependent upon social and vocational adaptation. Retardates want and need some measure of participation in normal society. No matter how benign or constructive their environment, dissatisfaction always results from segregation from the mainstream. Retardates should participate in whatever aspects of community life are feasible, and psychotherapy, along with other interventions, has as its goal the maximizing of abilities to achieve this. By developing ego capacities to assess reality, resist frustration, achieve emotional and behavorial control, and cope with disappointment, the retardate can be freed from unnecessary dependency on specialized programs. Even for those who cannot function outside an institution, hostel, special class, or workshop, maximum self-determination and emancipation from confines is the ultimate goal. An adjunct of greater freedom and independence for the retardate is the understanding of when and from whom to seek help at times of need.

RESULTS OF PSYCHOTHERAPY

The effectiveness of psychotherapy with retarded children and adolescents is as difficult to evaluate as with any other patient group. Population samples, type and amount of therapy, measures of change, and additional parameters of intervention are variable and uncontrolled in all reported studies. Many reports focus upon individual case studies, some of which turn out to have been misdiagnosed as retarded. Reports of real increase in IQ have been seriously questioned. Psychotherapists who undertake to work with the retarded are generally committed to their patients. This has the real advantage of maximizing the likelihood of success but may also influence estimation of outcome. Many therapists in this field have been novices and interventions were short term. Reports of the effectiveness of psychotherapy with retardates, dating from the 'thirties, have generally been favorable, although few studies have provided specific data in support of this impression. Improvement in the areas of adjustment to family and institutional life, discharge from institutions, greater independence, symptom relief, more adaptive defenses, development of constructive activity, and increase in tested intelligence have been mentioned. There are a few reports indicating no significant improvement. Patient factors which correlate with good results, according to various investigators, are presence of neurotic symptoms, mild degree of retardation, absence of organic brain damage, ability to verbalize, and awareness of problem. Therapist factors correlated with favorable outcome are warm and accepting attitude, use of relationship, directive, structured, or ego-supportive therapy, or use of a reality-oriented therapy with practical, limited, and immediate goals. Other parameters associated with good outcome are understanding and cooperative parents or institutional personnel, and the utilization of many disciplines working together.

The major thrust of reports of success in the psychotherapy of retardates has been to demonstrate that this form of treatment has a place in the total management of selected retardates, that it is feasible and justified.

CONCLUSION

Enough experience with retardates has been accumulated to indicate that a significant number of them are in need of psychotherapy and that they can benefit from it. Therapeutic technique needs to be modified to suit special requirements, and psychotherapy can only be a segment of the necessary professional services for the retardate.

The place of psychotherapy in the therapeutic package will be determined by the patient's requirement for this specialized treatment and alternative services which either duplicate crucial aspects of psychotherapy or accomplish its goals more rapidly, effectively, or economically.

REFERENCES

CHESS, S., and HASSIBI, M. Behavior deviations in mentally retarded children. *Journal of the American Academy of Child Psychiatry* 1970, *9*, 282–297.

CLARKE, A. M., and CLARKE, A. D. B. *Mental deficiency: The changing outlook* (3rd ed.). New York: Free Press, 1974.

LOTT, G. Psychotherapy of the mentally retarded. In F. Menolascino (Ed.), *Psychiatric aspects of the diagnosis and treatment of mental retardation.* Seattle, Wash.: Special Child Publications, 1971.

MAISNER, E. A. Contributions of play therapy techniques to total rehabilitative design in an institution for high-grade mentally deficient and borderline children. *American Journal of Mental Deficiency*, 1950, *55*, 235–250.

MENOLASCINO, F. Psychiatric aspects of mental retardation in children under eight. *American Journal of Ortho-psychiatry*, 1965, *5*, 852–861.

NEHAM, S. Psychotherapy in relation to mental deficiency. *American Journal of Mental Deficiency*, 1951, *55*, 557–572.

PHILIPS, I., and WILLIAMS, N. Psychopathology and mental retardation: a study of 100 mentally retarded children: Psychopathology. *American Journal of Psychiatry* 1975, *132*, 1265–1271.

ROBINSON H. B., and ROBINSON N. M. *The mentally retarded child.* New York: McGraw-Hill, 1965.

SARASON, S. *Psychological problems in mental deficiency* (3rd ed.). New York: Harper & Row, 1959.

STERNLICHT, M. Psychotherapeutic techniques useful with the mentally retarded: A review and critique. *Psychiatric Quarterly*, 1965, *39*, 84–90.

WEBSTER, T. G. Problems of the emotional development of young retarded children. *American Journal of Psychiatry*, 1963, *110*, 37–43.

15

LEARNING DISABILITIES: ASSESSMENT AND MANAGEMENT OF READING PROBLEMS

Carolyn S. Schroeder, Stephen R. Schroeder, & Melvyn A. Davine

Thousands of books and articles have been published on learning disabilities, many of which are of questionable utility to the practitioner. The purpose of this chapter is to equip the professional who is not an expert in the field with the necessary information to do consultation and selective referral of children with learning problems. The focus is on reading problems with a summary of the various theoretical approaches, the psychoeducational assessment instruments, and the management methods used with this specific learning disability.

Coinage of the Term *Learning Disabilities* (LD)

Notions of learning deficits in otherwise normal school children have origins before the turn of the century in the writings of Morgan (1896), and later Hinshelwood (1917) and Orton (1925, 1937). These were primarily speculations on possible neurological correlates of reading, e.g., "word blindness" and writing problems. This point of view gained impetus from the introduction of the term "minimal brain dysfunction" by Strauss and is seen in the works of his colleague, Werner, and their students, Kephart (Strauss & Kephart, 1955) and Cruikshank (Hallahan & Cruikshank, 1973). The psychoeducational approach, on the other hand, has its origins in Freudian psychodynamic psychology, the behaviorism of Skinner, and the psycholinguistic approach of Kirk (1972).

Samuel Kirk is generally credited with introducing the term "learning disability" in a talk given at the University of Illinois in 1963. That same year the study of learning disabilities was advanced greatly by the funding of three study groups by federal agencies within the Department of Health, Education and Welfare. Also in 1963 Congress passed PL88-164 which allotted funds for training and research in education. The Association of Children with Learning Disabilities, a vigorous parent-action group, was formed in 1964 and now numbers over 20,000 members. It has been instrumental in lobbying for government funding of programs and training institutes across the country specifically designed to advance the field of learning disabilities. Finally, with the passage of the Learning Disabilities Act of 1969, funds for service to the learning disabled became available.

Senf (1973) notes that the field of learning disabilities must be viewed in its sociocultural perspective. It grew out of the work of different professionals with different orientations, objectives, and points of view. In recent years the explosive growth has led to philosophical and professional disagreements that have resulted in anomalies which are puzzling to the outsider. There is little agreement among professionals in the field as to the differentiation of types of problems that fall within the definition of learning disabilities, the relative effectiveness of different approaches, of etiological correlates, or who should do the remediation. For example, two distinct professions, remedial reading specialists (Lerner, 1975) and learning disabilities teachers (Kirk, 1975), within the field of education are mandated to treat reading disabilities. They do not even agree as to how they differ in orientation and approach to remediation (Newcomer, 1975).

What then is a learning disability? Few professionals in the field would admit that they do not know the answer to this question, but they do seem to disagree substantially. In a questionnaire, Vaughan and Hodges (1973) asked 100 professionals active in the field of learning disabilities to rank 10 out of a list of 38 definitions (Table 1) of learning disability for their acceptability. Substantial accord was found among teachers, speech therapists, and directors of special education programs, but not among nurses, social workers, and psychologists. Acceptance patterns were similar for teachers and speech therapists but differed from program directors and other professionals. Their ranking of the five most preferred definitions was Baer, Kass and Myklebust, Chalfant, Colorado, Vail Conference, HEW Definition.

Apparently, formulating an acceptable definition of learning disabilities at this time does not matter and will not matter until more is known of the antecedents and consequents that underlie treatment of the various disabilities. In fact Bijou (1973) has argued against the use of the term because it is based upon a definition of learning as a hypothetical construct. "It is not useful to those whose responsibility it is to plan and carry out programs because in actuality there is not a specific treatment program for children in each of the diagnostic categories, . . . the remedial programs proposed for children in one category are *not* necessarily contraindicated for children in other categories." Thus, while there may be theoretical interest in the definition of learning disability, for practical purposes it is not very useful to know more than that the child is having difficulty in academic work at school and that his performance is below that which is expected on the basis of his IQ.

READING DISABILITY

The entire field of learning disabilities began originally with professional concern over children's reading problems. Reading remains a central issue in the field of learning disabilities. It is estimated that two-thirds of all children referred for learning disabilities have reading difficulties. It also is estimated that at least 15% of elementary school children in the United States have reading skills one year or more below expected grade placement and the same percentage are one and a half years behind in the later grades (HEW Report, 1969). Since the analysis of reading disabilities is characteristic of the broader field of learning disabilities, for the sake of brevity we will restrict our subsequent discussion to reading problems.

The analysis of reading disability has occurred under many rubrics: reading retardation, reading disorders, word blindness, strephosymbolia (twisted symbols), receptive written language disorders, and, perhaps the most controversial of all, dyslexia. Each of these reflects a different etiological view but in terms of current functioning, all suggest a dysfunction. The diagnosis of reading disability, whether medical or psychoeducational in orientation, implies an underlying substrate which is causing the child to perform below his expected level. Furthermore, the implication is that this impairment must be removed before suitable progress in reading can be realized.

It is important to note that the prevalent definitions of reading disability rest on the phrase "expected performance level." The assumption is that we know what should be age-appropriate levels of functioning for reading. While we do have some information on age-appropriate reading, it is also true that our expectancies have been strongly influenced by sociocultural variables.

Table 15-1 DEFINITIONS AND SOURCES

A	A child with a learning disability is any child who demonstrates a significant discrepancy in acquiring the academic and social skills in accordance with his assessed capacity to obtain these skills. In general, these discrepancies are associated with specific disabilities such as: gross motor, visual memory, visual discrimination, and other language related disabilities.	Baer (McDonald)
B	An identifiable perceptual or communicative handicap is an impediment in one or more of the basic learning processes involved in the understanding or reception, organization or expression of written or spoken language. This includes a condition referred to as a specific learning disorder, rather than a learning problem which is primarily due to speech, visual, hearing, or motor handicaps, limited intellectual functioning; emotional disturbance; or to environmental disadvantages.	State Advisory Comm. on Spec. Ed. 1972
C	The term is used as a generic one which covers any difficulties in acquiring knowledge possessed by children (or adults) with average (or above) intelligence. (IQs approx. over 75.)	Bannatyne (McDonald)
D	It is synonymous with marked underachievement. It is not seen as a population of children or another discrete category of handicapped children. Rather it is a new way of looking at children who have difficulties in school. It is part of a school based classification system which includes "behavior disorders." It thus cuts across traditional categories of handicapped children and represents a departure from the medical model to a more appropriate school based model.	Trippe (McDonald)
E	Learning disability refers to one or more significant deficits in essential learning processes requiring special education techniques for remediation. Children with learning disability generally demonstrate a discrepancy between expected and actual achievement in one or more areas, such as spoken, read, or written language, mathematics, and spatial orientation.	Kass and Myklebust 1969
F	The term "children with specific learning disabilities" means those children who have a disorder in one or more of the basic psychological processes involved in understanding or in using language, spoken or written, which disorder may manifest itself in imperfect ability to listen, think, speak, read, write, spell, or do mathematical calculations. Such disorders include such conditions as perceptual handicaps, brain injury, minimal brain dysfunction, dyslexia, and developmental aphasia. Such terms do not include children who have learning problems which are primarily the result of visual, hearing or motor handicaps, of mental retardation of emotional disturbance or of environmental disadvantage.	HEW 1970
G	Learning disabilities are the presumptive product of disturbances in the normal time-table of development. Uneven levels of functioning, with performance in some areas within or above age level expectancy and in others below, are characteristic of such disruption.	Gateway School (McDonald)
H	Children whose behavior is characterized by disorganization and difficulty in the development of generalization to a degree which interferes with their education progress. Because of their failure to generalize, special educational presentations and special learning situations are required.	Kephart (McDonald)
I	A learning disability refers to an educationally significant discrepancy between estimated intellectual potential and actual level of performance in one or more of the processes of speech, language, perception, behavior, reading, spelling or arithmetic.	Chalfant (McDonald)
J	A learning disability is an impediment to the learning process and exists, to a varying degree, when conditions in the educational process and/or specific functioning of the child are such that a child's normal progress toward stated objectives of the school district's general educational program cannot be maintained without intervention by specialized personnel, materials, educational strategies, and/or modifications of the educational process.	Colo. Vail Conference 1972

From "A Statistical Survey into a Definition: A Search for Acceptance" by R. Vaughan and L. Hodges, *Journal of Learning Disabilities*, 1973, *6*, No. 10, 69–73. Copyright 1973 by The Professional Press, Inc. Reprinted by special permission of Professional Press, Inc.

For instance, Thorndike (1973) in an extensive cross-cultural study of reading performance in 15 countries found that in some developing countries, e.g., India or Chile, where the literacy rate is low, learning disability is not recognized as an educational problem. In the Scandinavian countries with their extremely high literacy rate, the term is simply inapplicable, because the national programs are individualized and each student learns to read at his own rate. In the United States 75% of the student population attends high school, whereas only 20% does so in England. Whether or not we choose to attend to reading disabilities is primarily culturally determined.

The most common term used to denote reading disability is dyslexia, which currently refers to all types of reading disabilities. Originally, however, dyslexia was used by Hinshelwood (1917) to distinguish mild reading problems from "true congenital word-blindness." Recent neuropsychological views (Money, 1962; Schain, 1972) are that it should be reserved for reading problems with a known neurological correlate. These would be post-traumatic dyslexia, i.e., reading difficulties resulting from insult to the brain; and developmental dyslexia or specific dyslexia, i.e., selective disturbance in maturation of higher neurological functions—those responsible for the acquisition of reading and writing skills and constitutional in origin.

While the term *dyslexia* has had heuristic value in promoting research into specific neurological dysfunction related to reading, this research has yet to benefit the teacher. Owen, Adams, Forrest, Stolz, and Fisher (1971) found that, of the 304 dyslexic children in their study, only four could be diagnosed as definitely neurologically impaired. For practical purposes, therefore, "reading difficulties" seems a suitably neutral term if it refers to failure to read at the age-appropriate norm in schools. Theoretical controversy over the meaning of the term *dyslexia* is beyond the scope of this paper.

Theoretical Approaches to Reading Difficulties

There are a host of putative symptoms presumed to be "pathognomic signs" of reading difficulty. Only major trends will be examined and evaluated briefly.

Minimal Brain Dysfunction (*MBD*). This term refers to dysfunctions of the nervous system resulting in behavioral and learning disabilities which are not due to social and cultural provocations (Clements, 1966). In medical practice, this becomes synonymous with learning disorders among children not manifesting gross neurological impairment or mental retardation (Schain, 1972). Essentially, it is the neurological equivalent of learning disability.

Over 100 "soft" neurological signs have been associated at one time or another with the diffuse MBD syndrome (Wender, 1971). Some motor symptoms most frequently mentioned are clumsiness in fine motor tasks, choreiform movements, disturbed muscle tonus, reflex asymmetries, and dysdiodochokinesia (poor rapid alternating movements). Sensory signs frequently mentioned are poor stereognosis, poor graphesthesia, and finger agnosia. Associated miscellaneous symptoms are poor attention span, mixed laterality, hyperactivity. Each list encountered differs and there is little agreement among neurologists as to whether symptoms cluster reliably and what their clinical significance is (Schain, 1972; Adams, Kocsis, & Estes, 1974; Barlow, 1974).

Perhaps the most thorough normative study of MBD symptoms in learning disabled children is by Peters, Romine, and Dykman (1975). This was a well-controlled study of 82 boys, age 8 to 11 years, referred to the University of Arkansas Medical Center Child Guidance Clinic and 45 normal, equal chronological age (CA), control boys from similar socioeconomic backgrounds. IQ's of the LD sample were 90 or above; those for the control sample are not reported. Of the LD sample 73% had a significant reading disability. All were rated on a scale of 0 – 4 on a special set of 80 items considered soft neurological signs. LD children differed significantly from the control group on 44 symptoms. Further it was found that there was a significant negative relationship between age and the incidence of specific neurological signs in LD children. Younger LD children showed more discriminatory signs in motor development and showed first signs of improvement in gross motor functions and body orientation. These delays were assumed to be related to delays in neurological maturation.

Present research seems to point toward significantly more delays in maturation of LD children. The authors are careful to note, however, that these signs have no established anatomical specificity. The strategy of this research has been correlational. At present it is not possible to infer these maturational lags as causes of reading disability. Senf's (1973) and Keogh's (1971) cautions are pertinent here. Studies on LD children are difficult to compare because of the populations from which subjects are drawn (clinic versus classroom).

Knowledge of Right-Left Body Orientation. This view was based on the findings of Harris (1957) and Money (1962) that dyslexic children show inferior right-left orientation compared to normal readers. These differences are also negatively related to age. The notion was very popular in visual-motor training programs of the 1960s that maturation of orientation in space and consistent directional habits were necessary prerequisites for reading. In a review of the existing evidence, Benton (1968) notes that right-left discrimination is a complex concept involving both somatosensory components and a linguistic component that correlates highly with intelligence. When intelligence level was controlled in comparisons of normal and dyslexic children, no difference in right-left orientation was found between the two groups (Benton & Kemble, 1960; Balow, 1963; Coleman & Deutsch, 1964). Right-left impairment seems primarily symbolic and not perceptual and is a reflection rather than a cause of a basic language disability.

Reversals of Letters and Words. Orton (1924, 1937) proposed that poor readers fail because they tend to reverse letters and words. This "sin of reversal," as Kinsbourne (1973a) calls it, was thought to be due to failure of cerebral dominance to develop adequately. In fact mirror image reversals of letters are a common error in the development of graphic discrimination by at least half of all kindergarten children (Calfee, Chapman, & Venezky, 1972). Shankweiler and Liberman (1972) found that letter reversals accounted for only 10% of the errors of poor readers in the third grade. Word reversal was very infrequent, but there was a tendency to transpose letters within words. Ilg and Ames (1950) reported letter reversal in normal children until 9 years of age.

Children could be reversing letters for a variety of reasons, e.g., failure in serial ordering and temporal sequencing (Gibson & Levin, 1975), or failure to comply with orthographic rules in learning to write. Kinsbourne (1973) notes that most frequently reversed symbols have clearly distinguishable forms, but that both form and *orientation* are required for their correct identification. Orientation, however, both develops more slowly than form discrimination in children and is more difficult to remember. Number of reversals increases with the difficulty of items being remembered, and their hierarchical pattern is invariant. From age 4 to age 8 the most common errors are mirror-image reversals, next are inversions, then inverted reversals, and finally rotations. Reversals in the reading process can, however, be eliminated by carefully sequenced teaching.

Again, reversals, rather than being the cause, are more likely to be a reflection of perceptual processes occurring in learning to read.

Poor Perceptual-Motor Integration. There are a number of perceptual-motor curricula in existence today which are based upon what Gibson (1969) calls motor copy theories of development. The thesis of each of these is that reading disability is the result of poor perceptual, perceptual-motor, or sensory-motor development and that remediation can be brought about by training exercises to overcome the various deficits that resulted at specific maturational stages. There is little research to substantiate the theories underlying these programs which grew out of speculations on minimal brain dysfunction. It is only recently that adequately controlled research on the effectiveness of these remedial programs for different learning disabilities has been performed. These will be treated in a subsequent section on remediation.

The motor copy theories of development have nonetheless spurred some thought about the causes of reading difficulties. One hypothesis is that progress through the stages of early motor development is the main influence in determining later cognitive development and, therefore, reading ability (Dunsing & Kephart, 1965). Perhaps, this is best illustrated by the statement by Getman (1964), "Thoughts which do not get into the muscles never fully possess the mind."

This is the rationale for visual training exercises related to beginning reading. Research on poor readers, however, has not borne out this contention (Keogh, 1974). Lawson (1968), in a factor analytic study of children, found that visual problems were not significantly related to specific reading disorders. That motor development is closely correlated with intelligence at an early age is undoubtedly the case. Bayley (1968) in her factorial study of the development of mental abilities found at least six perceptual-motor attributes differentiated by age 6 months. However, early motor responsiveness was not predictive of IQ at the age of eight years. Also the common observation of the development of reading skills in paraplegics, cerebral palsy victims, and the blind makes Getman's assumption dubious.

Another concept which persists as a result of motor copy theories of development is that of reading readiness. It has been held by Getman (1965) that training reading at too early an age leads to reading difficulty because the necessary sensory-motor integration is not adequately developed. That the development of prereading skills is important for good reading habits can hardly be doubted. Gibson and Levin (1975) note that prereading skills include analysis of speech sounds, early production and discrimination of writing, intermodal relations, and a variety of cognitive factors, i.e., serial ordering, selecting discriminative features of stimuli, phonetic analysis of graphic displays. It is equally true that most children below age 4 have not developed these skills. But the inference that this is simply a result of poor perceptual-motor coordination is unwarranted. Kinsbourne (1973) notes that there are so many cognitive processes involved that each child displays his own pattern of difficulties in learning to read.

A final concept which grew out of early neurological speculation on reading disorders and culminated in the Doman-Delacato Theory of Neurological Organization (1966) is that reading difficulties are a result of mixed dominance. Delacato's theory of organization of neural function has been unanimously rejected by neurologists because it lacks support from neuroanatomical research (Rabinovitch, 1965; Whitsell, 1967).

Functional asymmetry is, however, characteristic of most mobile organisms. Hand preference in humans develops somewhat irregularly until stabilizing at about age 10 (Hecaen & Ajuriaguerra, 1964). Both hand and eye preference tendencies are probably inherited (Merrell, 1957), but are also influenced by environmental events (Hildreth, 1948). Hand-foot preferences are more closely associated than hand-eye preferences (Merrell, 1957). Asymmetry develops for different organs at different rates. Thus ocular control develops almost fully by age two, much earlier than handedness.

The fact that mixed asymmetry occurs more often among children with reading difficulties than among normals (Peters et al., 1975) suggests a relationship. However, the clinical significance of dominance is unclear. Sperry (1970), from a review of the literature and from evidence collected from patients with congenital and surgical absence of the corpus callosum, has suggested that the minor hemisphere mediates configurational, spatial, synthetic, and geometric activity, while the major hemisphere is specialized for sequential, verbal, logical, and analytic activity. These two sets of functions "compete for brain space" and may be related to the evolution of cerebral dominance and laterality. If so, lateral asymmetry noted in poor readers may be a sign of abnormal development of cerebral dominance. Such speculation would support recent neuropsychological research by Rourke (1975) that brain-behavior relationships involved in reading difficulties are primarily at the cortical level.

Cognitive Models of the Reading Process. Gibson and Levin (1975) note that there are over 30 models of the reading process in existence. One set of models, the information-processing models, stresses a paradigm of successive mental transformations that must occur in a synchronized fashion for reading to be successfully accomplished. The other set of models, the "analysis by synthesis" models, stresses how the reader constructs meaning for himself as he reads, forms hypotheses as to what is to follow, and confirms predictions by reading (Goodman, 1967). Such components analyses (Posner, Lewis, & Conrad, 1972) allow generalizations about what good readers do when they read.

Cognitive models have yet to yield significant benefits to the professional concerned with reading difficulties, but they do suggest some fruitful lines of research into the causes of and possibly the remediation of reading disorders. A few examples follow.

Intermodal Integration. Since reading is a multimodal task involving extraction of patterned information from the printed page, integration of visual-symbolic and auditory-verbal information this is likely to be a stumbling block for some poor readers. Vellutino has compared this skill in normal and poor readers in two studies (Vellutino, Steger, & Kandel, 1972; Vellutino, Smith, Steger, & Kaman, 1975) in subjects ranging in age from 6 to 15 years. Subjects were presented tachistoscopic exposures of both verbal and nonverbal stimuli and were asked to identify and/or reproduce them both orally and graphically. Poor readers were similar to normals on visual reproduction but not on verbal encoding. Vellutino's conclusion was that the perceptual inaccuracies often observed in reading and written language of deficient readers are due primarily to poor verbal identification and not to misperception of their visual features.

Birch and Belmont (1964) found that retarded readers matched for age and IQ with normal readers were inferior on auditory-visual matching. However, Jones (1974) showed that, when auditory-visual matching is compared with relevant intramodal and visual-auditory matching tasks, retarded readers make fewer correct responses than normals only when an auditory pattern is the initial stimulus. Together with the Vellutino studies, Jones' study suggests that a significant factor in reading difficulty involves problems of auditory analysis, storage, and reproduction rather than visual processing. Such research tends to support the findings cited by Hammill and Larsen (1974) that little relationship exists between auditory-visual integration skills as currently measured and general reading ability.

Serial Ordering. Immaturity in development of serial ordering is likely to be related to difficulties in spelling and calculating (Kinsbourne, 1973). McLeod (1965) and Bannatyne (1967, 1971) noted that poor readers do poorly on WISC digit span and sequencing scores. That such skills are likely to be related to analysis of phrases and syntactic structure is obvious. However, as yet there is not much research in this area.

Language Analysis. Belmont and Birch (1966) examined in detail the WISC profiles of 150 retarded and 50 normal 9- and 10-year-old readers. Some of their findings were that retarded readers differed from normals more in their verbal than in their performance scales. They suggested that this was due to poorer use of symbolic language. Johnson and Myklebust (1967) suggested that poor readers do poorly at segmentation of language, especially differentiation of phonemes. However, Liberman (1971) points out that such problems may be more closely related to the physical rather than to the semantic or communicative properties of language. Stanley and Hall (1973) found that poor readers require longer interstimulus intervals than normals to identify letters in masking experiments. While the research in this area is sparse, it does appear promising.

Learning and Retention Rate

Camp (1973) reported on a tutoring program for severely retarded readers, ages 8 to 18. Her results show that learning and retention rates of retarded readers differed quantitatively but not qualitatively from those of normals. The implications of her work are that improvement of poor reading and retention depend more on amount of training rather than on any deficit in the perceptual or motor equipment the reader brings to the task. This is a point that is rarely made in reading research. Most of it is aimed at finding out what is wrong with the reader's performance rather than what can be done to remedy it.

Genetic Factors in Reading Difficulty

A number of studies tend to implicate genetic factors in reading difficulties. Bakwin (1973) found that, in 338 pairs of twins, reading performances were alike in 84% of the identical twins but in only 29% of the fraternal twins. Lenneberg (1967) documented several studies indicating that speech disorders and reading disorders tend to run in families. Owen and co-workers (1971) found that dyslexic children who had discrepancies between their verbal and performance scores on the WISC also had siblings and mothers with similar reading problems. While the evidence to consider the role of genetic factors in reading difficulties is compelling, it is likely that such methods will encounter the same resistance as those examining the heretibility of intelligence.

Extrinsic Factors in Reading Difficulty

As might be expected, a variety of cultural factors affects the development of poor reading—for example, lack of reading and writing materials, lack of good reading models, lack of verbal stimulation by parents and peers (Durkin, 1966). Bannatyne (1971), in studying case histories of dyslexics, found lack of verbal communication between mother and child, lack of reference to logical relationships, and variations in dialect to be factors. In the United States, there is a high ratio of boys to girls among poor readers. However, this is not true in many other countries (Thorndike, 1973).

There is also a variety of other childhood disorders which may be related to reading difficulties. The most common of these are hyperactivity (Kinsbourne, 1973), emotional disturbances, short attention span, and severe failure set. Since poor readers often exhibit many of these behaviors, it is frequently difficult to evaluate each factor's potential importance. In addition, all of these factors may be antecedent conditions for the development of reading difficulty and must be dealt with on a per case basis. These are discussed in depth in other chapters of this book. The present review will focus on the academic aspects of reading difficulties.

PSYCHOEDUCATIONAL ASSESSMENT OF READING PROBLEMS

The problems inherent in diagnosing a reading difficulty reflect on a smaller scale the problems of the entire field. As we pointed out in our opening remarks, there is no general systematic approach to definition, diagnosis, remediation, or research. Part of this problem can be explained by the newness of the field as well as the development of a label, learning disability, that is more acceptable to parents and teachers than labels such as slow, dumb, delinquent, aggressive or whatever you like (Divoky, 1974). As Divoky points out, learning disabled children are whomever the diagnostician wants them to be.

There is no standard battery of psychological or educational tests used in the diagnosis of reading problems. The assessment procedures used vary with the training of the examiner as well as with the current approach being taken by the school or clinic in which he works. Some educators and psychologists have become so disenchanted with the traditional testing approach that they have instead opted for remediation on an individual basis rather than diagnostic categorization. Diagnostic-prescriptive generating methods, a task analysis, and a functional analysis of the child's behavior and his learning environment are among the most systematic of these approaches. A survey of the various diagnostic tests with their strengths and weaknesses should give the reader some insight into which tests a psychologist might use with nonachieving children.

Problems in the Diagnosis of Individual Cases

Assessment generally involves a survey of performance skills designed to reveal what a child can and cannot do and then a prescription of the remedial steps necessary to help him acquire the needed skills. Traditionally, psychologists approached diagnosis of the child by giving him standardized psychological and educational test batteries which compare his performance to that of other children his age. The processes which they are assessing are assumed to be involved in the referral problem. The child's strengths and weaknesses should give clues to the specific problem, and thus the appropriate remediation. Unfortunately, many of the tests used to diagnose reading disabilities focus on processes that have little or no relationship to reading achievement. With the "induced birth" of the learning disabilities field came a proliferation of tests with little or no supportive research. For example, reading disabilities have not been shown to be significantly related to visual-motor problems. Yet tests such as the Developmental Test of Visual Motor Integration (Beery & Buktenica, 1967) and the Frostig Developmental Test of Visual Perception (Frostig, 1961) are often used to diagnose or predict reading difficulties.

Another problem with standardized tests is that they are not designed to ferret out specific deficits, which often affect a child's performance on all of the tasks. For example, if a child is required to read instructions in order to demonstrate a skill which does not involve reading, it is likely that the child with a reading disability will be scored as failing the task. Standardized tests do serve a function, however, in revealing where the child stands in relationship to his age group and whether or not he is performing specific tasks at the rate one would predict from his performance in other areas. The weakness of such tests, however, is that they fall short of telling *why* a child fails a task. They tell you only that he fails. Consequently, the difficulties diagnosticians have in translating their findings from standardized tests into remedial programs can easily be understood. Most diagnosticians who rely primarily on standardized tests do not even try to give specific programming suggestions, but rather rely upon the classroom teacher to translate the findings and recommendations into appropriate programs. However, it is not enough to agree with the teacher that a child cannot read or to discuss his vocal encoding skills when the teacher is primarily asking how she can help the child to read.

Psychological Tests

Intelligence Tests. Intelligence tests such as the Stanford-Binet and Wechsler Intelligence Scale for Children (WISC) are used to determine whether a child is retarded, average, or superior in relation to the general population. General intelligence for children whose IQ is 70 or above has not been found to be a primary cause of reading disabilities (Kline, 1969; Bush & Mattson, 1973; Black, 1971). The scatter of subtest scores on the WISC, as well as the existence of a discrepancy between the Verbal Scale (VS) and Performance Scale (PS), has been frequently used to diagnose learning disabilities as well as to plan remedial programs (Keogh, Wetter, McGinty, & Donlon, 1973; Barnwell & Denison, 1975). Children with reading problems do better on the Performance Scales than on the Verbal Scales, with a usual discrepancy of 15 points or higher (Black, 1973; Rourke, Dietrich, & Young, 1973; Belmont & Birch, 1966). Current literature does, however, leave some doubt about the validity of attributing this pattern of functioning exclusively to learning disordered youngsters. Barnwell and Denison (1975) recently compared VS-PS discrepancies of 15 or more points and subtest scatter on the WISC in three groups of children from a pediatric clinic population: (1) children having learning problems without behavioral problems; (2) children having behavioral problems; and (3) children with learning and behavioral problems. All three groups were found to have similar VS-PS discrepancies and subtest scatter.

A study worth remembering on subtest scores was done by Rugel (1974). He reviewed 25 studies reporting WISC subtest scores of disabled readers. He used a category system similar to Bannatyne's (1968) that clustered the subtests into three categories—sequential, conceptual, and spatial. Although most studies, including this one, do not differentiate types of disabled readers, it appears that disabled readers as a group score significantly lower than normals on sequential subtests such as Digit Span, Coding, and Arithmetic but score higher than normal readers on the spatial subtests of Block Design, Picture Completion, and Object Assembly. He found that the disabled readers had a less severe deficit in conceptual categories, e.g., Vocabulary and Similarities, with no differences on Comprehension. This pattern of deficits would suggest problems in short-term memory and attentional processes rather than in visual-spatial skills (Rugel, 1974). Belmont and Birch (1966) found markedly lower vocabulary scores for their problem 9- and 10-year-old readers and suggested that the problem was more one of language and its usage than perceptual or manipulative skills. At the present time one cannot say that the individual disabled reader would conform to these patterns or that there is a clear relationship between learning disabilities and subtest scatter, but they do give a logical framework in which to analyze the various subtests beyond the overall verbal and performance scaled scores.

To conclude, the WISC alone is not a good diagnostic tool to predict or assess reading problems. It does, however, give the diagnostician information on general intellectual level and on specific strengths and weaknesses. These are at least clues for further investigation in planning the individual child's remedial reading program.

McCarthy Scales of Children's Abilities (*MSCA*). This is an individually administered test that measures mental and motor abilities of children ages 2½ to 8½ (McCarthy, 1972). There are 18 tests from which are derived six scales: Verbal, Perceptual-Performance, Quantitative, General-Cognitive Index (GCI), Memory, and Motor. The GCI is composed of the Verbal, Quantitative, and Perceptual-Performance Scales and gives a standard score with a mean of 100 and a standard deviation of 16. In a sample of 35 normal children the GCI and Stanford-Binet were found to correlate, .81 (McCarthy, 1972).

Research on the MSCA has been scarce, but what has been done is promising. Kaufman and Kaufman (1974) found the GCI to be approximately 20 points lower than IQ scores for MBD diagnosed children who were not achieving in school. These underachieving children scored significantly lower than their IQ-matched control group on the Quantitative and Perceptual Scales as well as on the Memory tests which required sequencing. While further research is needed, the design of the MSCA subtests and the six scales seem more related to performance of academic skills than to IQ per se and should therefore be more helpful in planning remedial programs.

Illinois Test of Psycholinguistic Abilities (*ITPA*). This battery, devised by Kirk, McCarthy, and Kirk (1968), has grown in popularity among psychologists and educators as a tool both for diagnosing children with language problems and for planning remedial programs (Kirk & Kirk, 1971; Ferinden, Jacobson, & Kovalinsky, 1970; Bush & Giles, 1969). The ITPA consists of 12 subtests that reportedly measure discrete psycholinguistic abilities as outlined in Osgood's Model of Language Behavior (1957). The 12 subtests are combinations of three psycholinguistic dimensions: (1) channel of communication (auditory, vocal, visual, and motor); (2) level of organization (representational and automatic); and (3) process (reception, association or expression). Remediation programs based on the ITPA assume that the subtests measure distinct abilities necessary to language development and that these abilities are important to academic achievement. Research on the ITPA, and in particular with children having difficulty in reading, gives little support for these assumptions (Sedlock & Weener, 1973; Burns & Watson, 1973). The ITPA measurement of language skills is not basically relevant to how a child is able to handle meaningful communication and language structure (Blackley & Stern, 1975). Consequently, reading programs based on the ITPA are of minimal utility. As O'Connor (1975) suggests, it would be more logical and beneficial simply to use specific criterion measures of concept formation and language skills. For example, if a child is confusing prepositions, then he should be tested on a task that actually assesses his use of prepositions.

Perceptual Motor Tests. Perceptual motor functioning has long been felt to play a significant role in learning problems. Tests such as the Frostig Developmental Test of Visual Perception (Frostig, 1961), the Bender-Gestalt Visual-Motor Test, and the Beery-Buktenica Developmental Test of Visual Motor Integration (VMI) (Beery & Buktenica, 1967) have been used both to identify problems in this area and to lay the groundwork for remedial programs (Frostig & Horne, 1964). Getman's (1965) and Kephart's (1960) approaches to learning disabilities have also focused on the perceptual-motor processes. What bearing these processes have on reading proficiency has been the subject of many research studies, the bulk of which are poorly controlled, do not clearly define the experimental population, or lack reliable measures of what constitutes improvement in learning (Silverman & O'Bryan, 1972; Hammill, Goodman, & Wiederholt, 1974).

It is fair to say that, in their haste to remediate, professionals have taken what seemed like a plausible approach to learning problems and turned it into an accepted fact without first empirically determining its validity. The ease with which tests in the perceptual-motor area are administered and the backing they have received from disciplines as varied as neurology, optometry, psychology, and education seem to have made them impervious to the ever increasing evidence against them as predictors of reading problems and the basis for remedial programs. Let it be enough to say that tests linking perceptual-motor processes to reading problems are suspect and at present should not be used for that purpose. This is not to say that perceptual-motor processes may not be important to learning reading, but we are currently not in a position to specify a precise enough relationship. For a more detailed discussion of these issues see Olson, 1968; Smith and Marx, 1972; Silverman and O'Bryan, 1972; Ackerman, Peters, and Dykman, 1971; Hammill et al., 1974; Goodman and Hammill, 1973.

Educational Tests

When a child with a history of reading failure is referred to a mental health clinic, the psychologist or learning disabilities specialist responsible for his evaluation may initially administer a battery of tests designed to assess his level of intellectual functioning or learning aptitude. If the outcome of testing is to have any implication for treatment, however, it is essential that the teacher or remedial specialist working with the child eventually receive some information about his current level of academic functioning. It is thus important for the professional evaluator to focus directly on the child's level of reading skills development (or his lack of skill development).

Although there are literally hundreds of diagnostic instruments currently being used to assess children's reading difficulties, the majority of these fall into two categories: (1) formal testing instruments such as standardized diagnostic reading tests and other tests of academic achievement in which it is possible to judge the child's performance objectively without examiner bias (Guthrie, 1973), and (2) informal tests ranging from individual reading inventories (Johnson & Kress, 1971) to task-analysis-derived criterion-referenced tests in which the child's reading deficiencies are carefully monitored so as to allow rational educational instruction or remediation. Each of these approaches to the assessment of children's reading difficulties is outlined below.

Achievement Tests. Tests of general academic achievement typically contain reading subtests. Two of the most widely used achievement tests are the Wide Range Achievement Test (WRAT; Jastak & Jastak, 1965) and the Peabody Individual Achievement Test (PIAT; Dunn & Markwardt, 1970). Both the WRAT and PIAT are standardized, norm-referenced testing instruments which enable the examiner objectively to judge each child's level of reading achievement in relation to other children in his grade or age group. For example, both tests provide information about each child's relative standing in terms of grade-level equivalents and percentiles.

Although the reading subtests of the WRAT and PIAT have been found to correlate highly (Soethe, 1972), there is at least one reason why the PIAT may be regarded as the preferred test. The Wide Range Achievement Test in reading is solely a test of word recognition, while the PIAT contains measures of both reading recognition and comprehension.

Diagnostic Reading Tests. A diagnostic reading test is usually given to a child who has done poorly on the reading subtests of an achievement test battery in order to more accurately determine reading strengths and weaknesses in various word recognition and comprehension skills (Miller, 1974). Probably the most popular diagnostic reading test currently in use is the Durrell Analysis of Reading Difficulty (Durrell, 1955). The Durrell contains subtests of oral reading, silent reading, listening comprehension, word recognition and analysis, and phonetic analysis.

Although the Durrell, like the achievement tests outlined above, is a standardized testing instrument, the grade-norms provided for the test are not considered to be as important as the examiner's observation of individual reading errors. Guthrie (1973) has commented on the need to provide the teacher with specific diagnostic information:

> The description of the results of tests usually includes the areas which were tested and the grade levels of the children who were examined. Accuracy in describing the areas which were tested is important. It is seldom useful to say the child is [performing] at the fourth grade level. ... [For example], if a child was observed to have a 4.5 score in spelling, it could be assumed that this meant the child was performing at the middle of fourth grade in this area of academic work. It should be emphasized that the educational remediation of children depends on the criterion-referenced characteristics of the test. That is, the teacher who will ultimately work with the child must know specifically what the child was capable of doing at the point when he was tested (p. 98).

Informal Reading Inventories. The individual informal reading inventory is a clinical technique devised by reading specialists to provide extensive information about a child's reading performance. The technique is an informal one in that specific methods are not standardized, and no norms have been established to evaluate individual performance. For this reason, the results obtained from administering an individual reading inventory are only as good as the examiner's observations (Johnson & Kress, 1971).

Although the individual reading inventory may vary somewhat in format according to the examiner, it is usually composed of a series of graded word lists (the sight-word knowledge inventory) and a series of graded oral reading paragraphs. A number of specially constructed phonetic analysis and structured analysis word lists may also be used to assess the child's word attack skills (Miller, 1974). According to Miller (1974), the examiners either construct their own word lists and reading passages by consulting the child's basal reader series (primer to grade six) or else rely on commercially available materials, such as the Dolch Basic Sight Word Test, the Kucera-Frances Corpus (1967), Fry's Instant Words (1972), and the Gray Oral Reading Tests (1963).

In administering the individual reading inventory, the child's reading errors and word recognition skills are meticulously recorded. For example, the child may exhibit an inability to use word "parts" (i.e., root words, prefixes, suffixes, etc.) to decode unknown sight words (structural analysis). However, since a reading specialist will typically administer such an inventory, this information may be readily translated into an effective remedial program.

Criterion-Referenced Testing. Within the field of learning disabilities, the primary goal of educational testing is to facilitate instructional decisions. However, even after a "decision" has been made and an educational prescription has been posited on the basis of the test data collected, it is still necessary to monitor the child's progress in an objective manner. This monitoring activity lies at the heart of a relatively new area of measurement technology known as criterion-referenced testing (Proger & Mann, 1973).

In contrast to the norm-referenced psychometric model, in which a child's test score is basically measured against test scores obtained by other children, criterion-referenced measurement is concerned with comparing a child's test score with a criterion test score defining an absolute standard of task mastery (Shoemaker, 1972). For example, a child is tested by a reading specialist and is found to be grossly deficient in the word recognition skill of structural analysis (as defined above). Lacking access to a formal "criterion-referenced" instructional program, the examiner decides to analyze this reading skill into its component parts (i.e., a hierarchy of subskills needed to achieve proficiency in the task). In the examiner's informal program each component skill represents a discrete educational objective, and the ability of the child to progress from one level to the next within the hierarchy is contingent on his exhibiting an absolute level of task mastery (e.g., 19/20 items correct or 95%). Thus, initially the child may be required to identify only the "roots" of compound words spoken by the examiner (e.g., earth-worm, rail-road, etc.). Eventually, however, he will be expected to identify and locate not only small "root" words, but also prefixes, suffixes, and syllables when stimulus words are presented in their written from. By testing the child each day and monitoring his progress within the "sequenced curriculum of instructional units," the teacher will be able to determine which objectives the child has mastered and which ones are still troublesome. While this example admittedly represents a gross oversimplification of the criterion-referenced measurement systems currently in use, it serves to demonstrate how the adoption of a criterion-referenced approach to educational assessment may "individualize goals, monitor progress, and provide a base for instruction improvement" (Hofmeister, 1975, p. 87).

MANAGEMENT OF READING DIFFICULTIES

Professionals from many disciplines are currently developing methods for helping children with learning problems. One result of this multidisciplinary effort has been a proliferation of treatment approaches encompassing "such diverse activities as psychotherapy, drugs, phonic drills, speech correction, tracing, crawling, bead stringing, trampoline exercises, orthoptic training, auditory discrimination skills, and controlled diet" (Bateman, 1965). To the confused parent of a learning-disabled child, and to the concerned professional faced with the task of matching treatments to children, the existence of such diverse activities elicits an obvious question: Which treatment or remedial approach works best?

The present state of the art, however, permits no better than a disappointing "all of them and none of them." Many practitioners seem to have profited not at all from the great debate over beginning reading instruction, in which research findings that ran counter to the mainstream of educational thought were either curiously misinterpreted or even blatantly ignored (Chall, 1967). Similarly a good number of learning disabilities specialists have continued to espouse specific treatment approaches despite empirical evidence to the contrary. There are, of course, numerous reasons for the continued survival of controversial paradigms within each scientific discipline (Kuhn, 1962). Probably the most important one within the present context is that many professionals, being more concerned with answering practical, timely questions than with accumulating tested knowledge, have inundated the research literature with a large number of small, poorly controlled studies that invariably both support and refute any treatment approach one might advocate. Indeed, some investigators, alarmed at the contradictory findings that abound, have gone so far as to argue that any remedial program which includes individual attention, sympathetic understanding and parental involvement—in short, a caring person—will help (Bettman, Stern, Whitsell, & Gofmann, 1967).

While the identification of learning disability "types" and remedial treatments may currently prove too superficial to permit definitive research (Senf, 1973), let alone prescriptive management, the fact still remains that about 10% of any school population are annually referred to speech educators, psychologists, and pediatricians with learning problems that require immediate attention. For this reason, it is important for professionals who work with these children, either directly or indirectly, to be aware of the remedial programs currently in practice and the assumptions underlying their use, if only to be able to offer parents proper guidance (Silver, 1975).

In general, approaches to treating the child with learning disabilities fall into two major categories: (1) task-oriented approaches and (2) process-oriented approaches. To those educators who advocate a task-oriented approach to remediation, conventional wisdom will dictate focusing on the child's performance of the *academic task*—i.e., the subject matter to be learned. In process-oriented approaches, on the other hand, attention is centered on the cognitive abilities or *mental processes* presumed to underlie task performance.

The following discussion is divided into four

parts. First, the current status of visual-motor training programs will be outlined, including the developmental approaches of Frostig and Horne (1964) and Kephart (1960) and the controversial optometric visual training programs (Flax, 1972; McGrady and McCarthy, 1971; Keogh, 1974). Second, the traditional psychoeducational approach to remediation, diagnostic-prescriptive teaching, will be described, and the validity of the basic assumptions underlying its use will be examined. These two sections effectively represent the most prevalent process-oriented approaches to remediation. This is followed by a consideration of the more traditional academic approach to remediation as advocated by specialists in (remedial) reading. Finally, on the basis of the remedial approaches initially reviewed, an argument will be made for adopting a behavioral analysis approach to educational management. Both the academic and behavioral approaches represent task-oriented treatment models.

PROCESS-ORIENTED APPROACHES TO REMEDIATION

Developmental Approaches. Treatment programs such as those suggested by Kephart (1960) and Frostig and Horne (1964) are based on the assumption that incompetence in beginning reading (and other academic tasks) is a function of perceptual immaturity or maldevelopment and that a remedial course of "perceptual-motor" training is essential to both preventing and correcting initial school failure. Inherent in this approach is the belief that the ability of the child to acquire proficiency in a higher-order "cognitive" skill such as reading is dependent upon the prior development of more primitive "sensory-motor" and "perceptual" skills (Frostig, 1968). According to Frostig and Maslow (1968):

> Education which focuses solely on academics will hardly influence the *developmental abilities* which underlie the ability to learn. Education must focus on each of these abilities directly in order to modify them optimally (p. 107, emphasis added).

Although the relatively high incidence of visual-perceptual and perceptual-motor dysfunction reputedly found within samples of learning-disabled children has undoubtedly contributed to the continued popularity of "perceptual-motor" training within some educational circles, there is little evidence to support this approach. Hammill (1972) made an in-depth review of the research literature for the purposes of (a) investigating the relationship between visual-perceptual functioning, as measured, and reading comprehension, and (b) determining the effects of visual-perceptual training, not only on reading, but on visual-perceptual functioning itself. On the basis of the empirical data examined, Hammill concluded that little correlation currently exists between measures of visual perception and tests of reading comprehension, that training visual perception does not facilitate school learning "and that, in the final analysis, visual perception processes may not even be trainable, at least not by existing programs" (pp. 552, 557). The results of studies conducted since Hammill's cogent review have confirmed these conclusions: not only do research findings continue to suggest a lack of clear equivalency between reading disability and disturbances of visual perception (Black, 1974), but there is still no reason to believe that visual-perceptual training programs are more efficient than traditional academic approaches to remediation (Belmont, Flegenheimer, & Birch, 1973).

Psychologists and educators, however, have not been the only professionals involved in "visual-training." According to Carlson and Greenspoon (1968), there are currently many optometrists in private practice who employ a wide variety of educational and sensory-motor-perceptual training techniques in an attempt to correct educational problems in children. A detailed account of the controversy surrounding developmental optometric training programs is beyond the scope of this chapter; however, Paragraph 3 of a joint organizational statement issued by the American Academy of Pediatrics, the Division for Children with Learning Disabilities of the Council for Exceptional Children, and the American Academy of Ophthalmology and Otolaryngology delineates rather well the current status of the art in the eyes of its critics:

> 3. No known scientific evidence supports claims for improving the academic abilities of learning disabled or dyslexic children with treatment based solely on: (a) visual training (muscle exercises, ocular pursuit, glasses), (b) neurologic organizational training (laterality training, balance board, perceptual training). Furthermore, such training has frequently resulted in unwarranted expense and has delayed proper instruction for the child (McGrady & McCarthy, 1971).

The Psychoeducational Approach: The diagnostic-prescriptive teaching model. Traditional psychoeducational evaluation of children with learning disorders has attempted to isolate specific characteristics of the child—typically, deficits or weaknesses in auditory and visual information-processing skills presumed to underlie the learning problem (Keogh, 1971). Such information, it is postulated, not only facilitates a diagnosis of the problem, it also guides the plan for treatment. Lerner (1975) has summarized the major educational strategies based upon differential diagnosis of individual strengths and weaknesses of children:

> Within the LD framework some authors suggest that to diagnose and thereby treat problems in children it is important first to assess specific and discrete underlying psychological functions and then to build up those that are found to be deficit areas.... Other authorities suggest that, following assessment of areas of deficits and strengths in mental processing, treatment procedures utilize the areas of strength in teaching. Still other authorities suggest that treatment should both teach through the assets while building up deficits (p. 121).

Implicit in this approach to remediation are two closely related assumptions: (1) that central processing dysfunctions, as currently measured, are responsible for learning problems; and (2) that, once identified, modality strengths (or other personological variables) form an effective base for differential educational programming.

Although there continues to be increased interest among learning disabilities specialists in diagnostic-prescriptive teaching, the validity of this approach has been questioned by a number of educators. According to Newcomer (1975), not only have empirical studies failed to support the construct validity of several of the most popular measures of psychological processes used in education (e.g., ITPA, Frostig, etc.), but there is little evidence to suggest that these "processes," as currently measured, relate to academic tasks such as reading in a practically significant manner (predictive validity) (p. 147).

To underscore this latter point, Hammill and Larsen (1974) recently reviewed studies that adopted correlational statistical procedures to examine the relationship of reading ability to measures of several auditory perceptual skills (e.g., auditory discrimination, sound blending, auditory memory, etc.). The authors failed to find any evidence to suggest that particular auditory skills, as measured, are essential to the reading process or that children who fail to read proficiently do so because of auditory-perceptual deficits.

Another area of learning research which has served to undermine the diagnostic-prescriptive model has been aptitude-treatment interaction research (Bracht, 1970; Ysseldyke, 1972). According to Ysseldyke (1972), the goal of aptitude-treatment interaction research within the field of learning disabilities is to identify significant disordinal interactions between modality strengths and individualized instructional programs. Thus far, however, the premise that certain LD children have a preferred modality that facilitates their learning has received little empirical support (Sabatino & Streissguth, 1972; Ringler & Smith, 1973; Waugh, 1973; Newcomer & Goodman, 1975). In the majority of these experiments, children identified as either "auditory (or visual) learners" who were taught by a method that corresponded to their modality preference did not significantly outperform those who were taught by a method different from their modality preference.

Task-Oriented Approaches

Academic Approaches: Remedial Reading. Individual tutoring in reading, remedial reading specialists, and remedial educational procedures for children deficient in the skill, all existed long before the field of learning disabilities emerged as an independent subspecialty in the 1950s. In contrast to the psychoeducational (diagnostic-prescriptive) approach to remediation espoused by some learning disabilities specialists, the "reading specialist" has traditionally adopted a more strictly "academic approach" to treatment (Senf, 1973). Lerner (1975) describes this approach as one that focuses on the reading task itself rather than on processing abilities presumed to underlie the task. In general, this involves adopting a criterion-referenced system approach to reading in which (1) the reading task is analyzed in terms of its component skills and (2) the child's reading skill development is carefully charted. Remediation would then focus on those components of the reading act not yet mastered.

A large number of remedial reading methods are currently available (Frierson & Barbe, 1970; Myers & Hammill, 1969; Money, 1966). Based largely on the pioneering work of Monroe (1932), Orton (1937), and Gillingham and Stellman (1936) in the United States and Schonell (1938) in Great Britain, most of these remedial techniques differ from one another in their choice of a specific sensory modality (e.g., auditory-phonics approach, visual word-form configuration training, etc.) or in their emphasis within a multisensory approach. For example, in Grace Fernald's "hand-kinesthetic" technique, the child is presented with a word written in crayon in blackboard-sized print and is instructed to trace the word while saying each part of the word as he traces it. Unfortunately, each of these methods lacks an adequate research base that would establish a reliable connection to improved reading performance. Moreover, the few longitudinal studies undertaken to show the effects of remedial reading instruction on school performance have indicated that (1) no one method is superior to any other and (2) while there is typically an increase in measured reading level at the end of intervention, this improvement is only transitory (Silberberg, Iverson, & Goins, 1973).

Behavioral Techniques Applied to Reading Difficulties. Behavioral analysis and modification of learning difficulties has its origins in the writings of Skinner (1968), Bijou (1970, 1973), and Lindsley (1971). More recent applications to remediation of reading difficulties are found in the work of Lovitt (1975), Bradfield (1974), and others. Behavior analysis is often placed in opposition to traditional teaching approaches by the educational community. But, as Lindsley (1971) insists, behavior analysis is not an approach, i.e., a panacea or cure, meant to supplant whatever ails the teaching profession. Good teachers are good behaviorists but the reverse is not necessarily true. The tools of behavioral analysis comprise a technology which the teacher can add to his/her arsenal of skills to improve the acquisition and performance of any behavior of any pupil.

Behavioral analysis remains neutral to the previously discussed hypotheses on reading success and failure. When antecedent conditions, however, can be specified or their relevance determined empirically, they are relevant to remediation of reading difficulties. Behavior analysis provides the technology for reaching such decisions. It is based on the evaluation and changing of specific observable behaviors only. In this respect it does not deal with hypothesized underlying causes of behavior but only with its antecedents and consequences.

The teacher arranges the conditions most conducive to the individual child's learning, so that these become permanent methods which the child uses for future study tasks. The programming steps involve the following (Bijou, 1970): (1) statement in precise, objective terms of the desired terminal or goal behavior; (2) assessment of the pupil's repertoire which is relevant to the task; (3) arrangement of the sequence of materials and criteria for success; (4) determination of an entry point where the student can start with a high success rate; (5) management of the contingencies that lead to improvement on the task; (6) keeping accurate records of performance which can be used to make decisions about program changes.

It can be seen that the major assumption underlying behavior analysis is that the rules governing the change and maintenance of performance are the same for all students. Thus, while certain diagnostic variables, e.g., blindness, deafness, etc., might affect functional assessment, point of entry into a program, and training materials to be used, the basic steps in programming would remain the same regardless of the original cause of the difficulty.

There are probably as many good behavioral teaching technologies as there are good teachers; however, a few technologies for teaching reading have been more formalized and, therefore, are more amenable to evaluations. They are precision teaching (Lindsley, 1964), performance-determined instruction (Gray, 1974), programmed instruction (Silberman, 1965), and computer-assisted instruction (Atkinson, 1968). Although there is a voluminous literature on the latter two technologies, few of these findings have been translated into usable knowledge for the teacher. At present the instrumentation is too costly to implement on a large scale. Therefore, these topics will not be reviewed in this paper although their future potential is great.

Precision teaching was originally developed by O. R. Lindsley (1971) at the University of Kansas and is currently implemented in two major experimental programs: the Therapeutic Education Center in the San Francisco Unified School District (Bradfield & Criner, 1974) and the Experimental Education Units at the University of Washington (Kunzelman, Cohen, Hulten, & Mingo, 1970). Basically, it involves breaking down all of the components of the reading act into small steps called "movements." These programs are taught sequentially, one at a time. Progress through the program is dictated by performance carefully charted by the student himself and arranged by the teacher. Precision teaching has been used very successfully with poor readers (Bradfield & Criner, 1974; Haring & Krug, 1975), but its utility relative to other programmatic systems remains to be determined.

Performance Determined Instruction (PDI) is a reading program developed at the Monterey Speech and Hearing Institute (Gray, Baker, & Stancyk, 1969). Behavior principles are used in teaching reading, and the program decision-making strategy is the Test-Operate-Test-Execute (TOTE) system from Miller, Galanter, and Pribram (1960). Although the results of the PDI reading system have been positive, as with precision teaching, its relative effectiveness has not been compared to that of other systems. Both precision teaching and performance-determined instruction are stylized versions of the principles discussed earlier (Bijou, 1970). Many teachers who are effectively using their own behavioral system of remedial reading will probably not switch to the more formal systems until there is more evidence of their superiority. In any case, as Lovitt (1975) points out, applied behavior analysis is a method and not an answer to remediation. With respect to reading, little research has been done as yet on setting realistic criteria for performance of students with different reading difficulties or in programming generalization and maintenance of reading skills learned during training. Nevertheless, behavioral technology provides a means to answering such questions in a systematic way.

CONSULTATION TO THE SCHOOLS[1]

In the final analysis the fate of the child with reading problems rests with the teacher. As Bijou (1970) so aptly put it, the teacher is "the Lone Arranger." Regardless of a researcher's or specialist's approach to reading problems, it will be of little value unless it can be transmitted to the teacher.

The consultant's relationship with the school should be established from the start of the assessment process. Since the classroom is the place where the child is failing, the teacher can bring much useful information to bear on the assessment problem. The consultant should establish a working relationship with the school to judge what can and cannot be done to help the teacher. The remediation program should be developed out of observations which take into account the teacher, the child, and his school.

DEFINING THE PROBLEM

The point of entry into consultation is usually with the relevant concerns of the teacher. The consultant can assist in defining concerns and

[1]Thanks are due to Dr. Ann P. Turnbull and the Special Education section of the Division for Disorders of Development and Learning, Child Development Institute for many of the ideas in this section.

translating them into observable behaviors. As with the child, so with the teacher, the best approach is an individualized one which analyzes concerns, strengths, and weaknesses. Only after the relationships between teacher and pupil are assessed, can an appropriate and practicable remedial approach be chosen. Although teachers are often self-deprecating when they confer with the consultant, they are usually the most knowledgeable and critical people in the pupil's program (Constanza & Klapman, 1970).

Observation

Observing the child via diagnostic tests and standard examination procedures is a natural part of problem assessment. Even more important is observing the child in the setting in which he fails, for it is the school that will have to change to meet his needs. How and when material is presented, under what conditions, and how the child is reinforced for reading will determine his progress. Observing the contraints under which the teacher is working (25 or 40 pupils), the physical environment (open versus closed classroom), the support staff (guidance counselors, resource teachers, teacher consultants, teacher aides), the socioeconomic level of the school, and administrative support for the teacher are all vital to the success of a program. For example, poor readers in lower socioeconomic neighborhoods are often mixed with the mentally retarded, whereas schools in higher socioeconomic areas will refer to them as learning disabled. These conditions will certainly affect the type of program the school provides for the child with reading problems. Such considerations do not necessarily define program limitations, but they indicate a starting point to bring about desired changes. Any program that does not take the school's limitations into account is doomed to failure.

Making simple suggestions during the observation phase is a useful way to get a baseline on how much of the final program the school can carry out. It also should indicate to the consultant whether or not his/her suggestions are concrete and explicit enough to be followed.

Intervention

This is the point where most consultants start to work with the school. Their work is usually in the form of a report of their findings and recommendations. Constraints on time and distance from the school must be considered. At the very least, however, telephone conversations with teachers, questionnaires asking for specific information, and work samples should be carefully processed before the consultant suggests a remedial program. The facts are that professional consultant reports are rarely utilized by teachers. As Waugh (1970) pointed out, no business would continue to function if only 38% of its finished product were ever used.

School consultants must find more effective ways of reaching consumers. Pope and Haklay (1974) suggest the use of teacher-consultants as intermediaries between the professional and the teacher. Constanza and Klapman (1970) offer suggestions regarding the nature of the report that is sent to the school. The solution to these problems can only come from a clearer understanding by teachers and consultants of what both parties have to offer.

There are some simple but important guidelines that one should keep in mind when consulting with a school:

1. The use of jargon in written or verbal communications should be avoided. In the field of learning disabilities there is not so much a communication gap but a communication gorge. Terms such as MBD, P-M problems, LD problems, remedial reading, etc. are not even agreed upon by experts. Yet teachers are expected to understand them and translate them into remedial programs. The more concrete and precise the information, the greater will be its utilization.
2. Start out with simple recommendations that can be implemented easily. Turnbull and Rosenthal (1974) found that teachers readily implemented suggestions such as cutting down length of assignments, using rulers for the child to keep his place while reading, providing special work spaces with fewer distractions, giving more precise and shorter directions, rewarding for small improvements, decreasing length of work periods, and breaking tasks into smaller steps.
3. Be aware of the range of alternatives open to the child, e.g., resource room, tutors, self-contained

classes, etc. In suggesting the use of volunteer tutors, list possible resources from which such people could be drawn. Peers can also be excellent tutors, but it is important for the teacher to allow the tutored pupil to give tutoring help in other subjects.

4. The child with school problems is usually under a great deal of stress. His/her self-concept is affected by failure. It is important to include programs for reinforcing positive feelings about one's self in any remedial program. What does the child do best? What other roles can he or she play in the classroom? These are important factors which affect feelings of worth that can easily be overlooked. Recently a student teacher reported visiting a classroom that had three reading groups: the Jet Planes, the Freight Trains, and the Dump Trucks.

5. In suggesting materials and specific programs, include advice on where these can be purchased, the price, etc. Hammill and Bartel (1970) give an excellent list of resources for this purpose.

6. The relevance of the recommendations to the particular child should always be kept in mind. For example, if a child is fourteen years old and not reading, then it would be better to focus on teaching everyday words found on safety signs, in want ads and maps than to focus on a phonetic approach to reading.

This list of recommendations for consulting with the teacher is limited. However, it is important to specify the behaviors necessary for successful consultation. The next step is to determine empirically the importance of each behavior. Otherwise, the consultation is likely to be a waste of time.

SUMMARY

The purpose of this chapter has been to equip the professional with the necessary information to do consultation and selective referral of children with learning problems. An attempt was made to summarize the theoretical underpinnings of reading problems since this is the problem for which children are referred most often.

Our introductory remarks illustrate that there is no single comprehensive approach to the study of reading difficulties. This is not surprising since there is not at present a generally acknowledged model of the reading process. Nor is there a generally accepted definition of reading. Gibson and Levin (1975) offer the following definition: "Reading is extracting information from text." However, according to Elkonin (1973), "Reading is a creation of the sound form of the word on the basis of its graphic representation." Such widely disparate notions reflect our current lack of understanding of the complexities of reading.

An examination of the presumed causes of reading disability yields a variety of hypotheses, mostly unsubstantiated. Their relation to acquiring reading skills and their relative importance for diagnosis and remediation are highly problematic. It is important to know in general which factors are likely to be related to reading difficulty. But Kinsbourne's (1973) caution still holds—each poor reader presents a unique set of problems to the clinician and should be treated accordingly.

The status of diagnostic approaches to reading problems is also in flux. The proportion of dyslexics for whom there is a known neurological correlate is small. The psychoeducational approaches to diagnosis can be divided into two classes. The process-oriented approaches, usually consisting of standardized tests (WISC, ITPA, and VMI), are falling into disfavor because their hypothesized underlying causes for reading problems have not successfully differentiated remediation approaches. Psychologists and educators have moved more toward functional analyses of reading problems, using criterion-referenced instruments, diagnostic reading tests, informal reading inventories, task analysis, work samples, educational tests, and achievement tests. The utility of process-oriented approaches awaits the results of future research.

The situation in management and remediation is similar to that in diagnosis. Remedial reading programs based on process-oriented approaches have been disappointingly unsuccessful when subjected to careful scrutiny in controlled research. Recent remedial programs based on behavioral technology, which address directly the behaviors to be taught rather than attempt to eliminate the underlying causes of reading problems, have been more successful. But research in this area is still very limited in extent and scope.

Future efforts in the field of diagnosis and remediation must avoid discussing learning disability in generalities but focus on careful observation of the specific behaviors in question, a more precise taxonomy of the behaviors which compose the problems labeled learning disability, and more effective research on the basic components which define learning.

REFERENCES

ACKERMAN, P. T., PETERS, J. E., and DYKMAN, R. A. Children with specific learning disabilities: Bender Gestalt test findings and other signs. *Journal of Learning Disabilities*, 1971, *4*, 35–44.

ADAMS, R., KOCSIS, J., and ESTES, R. Soft neurological signs in learning-disabled children and controls. *American Journal of Disabilities in Childhood*, 1974, *128*, 614–618.

ATKINSON, R. C. Computerized instruction and the learning process. *American Psychologist*, 1968, *23*, 225–239.

BAKWIN, H. Reading disability in twins. *Developmental Medicine and Child Neurology*, 1973, *15*, 184–187.

BALOW, I. Lateral dominance characteristics and reading achievement in the first grade. *Journal of Psychology*, 1963, *55*, 323–330.

BANNATYNE, A. The etiology of dyslexia and the Color Phonics System. In *Proceedings of the Third Annual Conference for Children with Learning Disabilities, Tulsa, Oklahoma*. San Rafael, Calif.: Academic Therapy Press, 1967.

BANNATYNE, A. Diagnosing learning disabilities and writing remedial prescriptions. *Journal of Learning Disabilities*, 1968, *1*, 28–35.

BANNATYNE, A. *Language, reading, and learning disabilities*. Springfield, Ill.: Charles C Thomas Publisher, 1971.

BARLOW, C. "Soft signs" in children with learning disorders. *American Journal of Diseases in Childhood*, 1974, *128*, 605–606.

BARNWELL, A., and DENISON, H. WISC Scale discrepancies: Are they diagnostically significant for learning disabilities? *Pediatric Psychology*, 1975, *3*, 9–11.

BATEMAN, B. Learning disabilities—yesterday, today, and tomorrow. *Exceptional Children*, 1965, *31*, 166–177.

BAYLEY, N. Behavioral correlates of growth-birth to thirty-six years. *American Psychologist*, 1968, *5*, 1–17.

BEERY, K., and BUKTENICA, N. A. *Developmental tests of visual-motor integration*. Chicago: Follett Publishing Co., 1967.

BELMONT, L., and BIRCH, H. An intellectual profile of retarded readers. *Perceptual and Motor Skills*, 1966, *22*, 787–816.

BELMONT, I., FLEGENHEIMER, H., and BIRCH, H. G. Comparison of perceptual training and remedial instruction for poor beginning readers. *Journal of Learning Disabilities*, 1973, *6*, 230–235.

BENDER, L. A. A visual-motor gestalt test and its clinical use. *American Orthopsychiatric Association*, Research Monograph, No. 3, 1938.

BENTON, A. Right-left discrimination. In S. Grossman (Ed.), *Pediatric Clinics of North America*, 1968, *15*, 747–758.

BENTON, A., and KEMBLE, J. Right-left orientation and reading disability. *Psychiatric Neurology*, 1960, *139*, 49–56.

BETTMAN, J. W., JR., STERN, E. L., WHITSELL, L. J., and GOFMANN, H. F. Cerebral dominance in developmental dyslexia: Role of opthalmologist. *Archives of Opthalmology*, 1967, *78*, 722–729. (Cited by P. Gardiner, The eye and learning disability. *Developmental Medicine and Child Neurology*, 1974, *16*, 95–96.)

BIJOU, S. What psychology has to offer education—now. *Journal of Applied Behavior Analysis*, 1970, *3*, 63–71.

BIJOU, S. Helping children develop their full potential. In S. Grossman (Ed.), *Pediatric Clinics of North America*, 1973, *20*, 579–585.

BIRCH, H., and BELMONT, L. Auditory-visual integration in normal and retarded readers. *American Journal of Orthopsychiatry*, 1964, *34*, 852–861.

BLACK, F. W. An investigation of intelligence as a causal factor in reading problems. *Journal of Learning Disabilities*, 1971, *4*, 139–142.

BLACK, F. W. WISC verbal performance discrepancies as indicators of neurological dysfunction in pediatric patients. *Journal of Clinical Psychology*, 1973, *30*, 165–167.

BLACK, F. W. Achievement test performance of high and low perceiving learning disabled children. *Journal of Learning Disabilities*, 1974, *7*, 178–182.

BLACKLEY, S., and STERN, B. Personal communications, University of North Carolina, Chapel Hill, N.C., 27514, 1975.

BRACHT, G. H. Experimental factors related to aptitude-treatment interactions. *Review of Educational Research*, 1970, *40*, 627–645.

BRADFIELD, R. *Behavior modification of learning disabilities*. San Rafael, Calif.: Academic Therapy Publications, 1974.

BRADFIELD, R., and CRINER, J. Precision-teaching the learning disabled child. In R. Bradfield (Ed.), *Behavior modification of learning disabilities*. San Rafael, Calif.: Academic Therapy Publications, 1974.

BURNS, G. W., and WATSON, B. L. Factor analysis of the revised ITPA with underachieving children. *Journal of Learning Disabilities*, 1973, *6*, 371–376.

BUSH, W. J., and GILES, M. T. *Aids to psycholinguistic teaching*. Columbus, Ohio: Charles E. Merrill, 1969.

BUSH, W. J., and MATTSON, B. D. WISC test patterns and underachievers. *Journal of Learning Disabilities*, 1973, *6*, 251–256.

CALFEE, R., CHAPMAN, R., and VENEZKY, R. How a child needs to think to learn to read. In L. W. Gregg (Ed.), *Cognition in learning and memory*. New York: John Wiley, 1972.

CAMP, B. Learning rate and retention in retarded readers. *Journal of Learning Disabilities*, 1973, *6*, 11–17.

CARLSON, P. V., and GREENSPOON, N. K. The uses and abuses of visual training for children with perceptual-motor learning problems. *American Journal of Optometry*, March, 1968, 161–169.

CAY, M. N. The Bender Visual-Motor Gestalt Test as a predictor of academic achievement. *Journal of Learning Disabilities*, 1974, *7*, 59–61.

CHALL, J. *Learning to read: The great debate*. New York: McGraw-Hill, 1967.

CLEMENTS, S. *Minimal brain dysfunction in children*. (Monograph No. 3, U.S. Public Health Service Publication No. 1415). Washington, D.C.: U.S. Government Printing Office, 1966.

COLEMAN, R., and DEUTSCH, C. Lateral dominance and right-left discriminations: A comparison of normal and retarded readers. *Perceptual and Motor Skills*, 1964, *19*, 43–53.

CONSTANZA, V., and KLAPMAN, H. Developing direct classroom consultation. *Journal of Learning Disabilities*, 1970, *3*, 351–354.

DELACATO, C. *Neurological organization and reading*. Springfield, Ill.: Charles C. Thomas Publisher, 1966.

DIVOKY, D. Education's latest victim: The "LD" kid. *Learning*, October, 1974, 20–25.

DUNN, L. M., and MARKWARDT, F. C. *Peabody Individual Achievement Test: Manual*. Circle Pines, Minn.: American Guidance Service, 1970.

DUNSING, J., and KEPHART, N. Motor generalizations in space and time. In J. Hellmuth (Ed.), *Learning disorders* (*Vol. 2*). Seattle, Wash.: Special Child Publications, 1965.

DURKIN, D. *Children who read early*. New York: Teacher's College Press, 1966.

DURRELL, D. D. *Durrell Analysis of Reading Difficulty*. New York: Harcourt, Brace, Jovanovich, 1955.

ELKONIN, D. In J. Downing (Ed.), *Comparative reading*. New York: Macmillan, 1973, 551–579.

FERINDEN, W. E., JACOBSON, S. and KOVALINSKY, T. *Educational interpretation of the Stanford-*

Binet Intelligence Scale, Form L-M and the Illinois Test of Psycholinguistic Abilities. Linden, N.J.: Remediation Associates, 1970.

FLAX, N. Comment—The eye and learning disabilities. *Journal of the American Optometric Association*, 1972, *43*, 26.

FRIERSON, E. C., and BARBE, W. S. *Educating children with learning disabilities*. New York: Appleton-Century-Crofts, 1970.

FROSTIG, M. *The Marianne Frostig Developmental Test of Visual Perception*. Palo Alto, Calif.: Consulting Psychologists Press, 1961.

FROSTIG, M. Education of children with learning disabilities. In H.R. Myklebust (Ed.), *Progress in learning disabilities* (Vol. 1). New York: Grune and Stratton, 1968.

FROSTIG, M., and HORNE, D. *The Frostig Program for the development of visual perception*. Chicago: Follett Publishing Company, 1964.

FROSTIG, M., and MASLOW, P. Language training: A form of ability training. *Journal of Learning Disabilities*, 1968, *1*, 105–115.

FRY, E. B. *Reading instruction for classroom and clinic*. New York: McGraw-Hill, 1972.

GETMAN, G. *The physiology of readiness experiment*. Minneapolis: P.A.S.S., Inc., 1964.

GETMAN, G. The visuomotor complex in the acquisition of learning skills. In J. Hellmuth (Ed.), *Learning disorders* (Vol. 1). Seattle: Special Child Publications, 1965.

GIBSON, E. J. *Principles of perceptual learning and development*. Englewood Cliffs, N.J.: Prentice-Hall, 1969.

GIBSON, E., and LEVIN, H. *The psychology of reading*. Cambridge, Mass.: MIT Press, 1975.

GILLINGHAM, A. B., and STELLMAN, B. L. *Remedial work for reading, spelling, and penmanship*. New York: Hackett and Wilhelms, 1936.

GOODMAN, K. Reading: A psycholinguistic guessing game. *Journal of the Reading Specialist*, 1967, *6*, 126–135.

GOODMAN, L., and HAMMILL, D. The effectiveness of Kephart-Getman activities in developing perceptual-motor and cognitive skills. *Focus on Exceptional Children*, 1973, *4*, 1–9.

GRAY, B. A behavioral strategy for reading training. In R. Bradfield (Ed.), *Behavior modification of learning disabilities*. San Rafael, Calif.: Academic Therapy Publications, 1974.

GRAY, B., BAKER, K., and STANCYK, S. Performance determined instruction for training in remedial reading. *Journal of Applied Behavior Analysis*, 1969, *2*, 255–263.

GRAY, W. S. *Gray Oral Reading Tests*. Indianapolis, Ind.: Bobbs-Merrill, 1963.

GUTHRIE, J. T. Educational Assessment of the handicapped child. In S. Grossman (Ed.), *Pediatric Clinics of North America*, 1973, *20*, 89–103.

HALLAHAN, D., and CRUIKSHANK, W. *Psychoeducational foundations of learning disabilities*. Englewood Cliffs, N.J.: Prentice-Hall, 1973.

HAMMILL, D. D. Training visual perceptual processes. *Journal of Learning Disabilities*, 1972, *5*, 552–559.

HAMMILL, D. D., and BARTEL, N. R. *Teaching children with learning and behavior problems*. Boston: Allyn-Bacon, 1975.

HAMMILL, D. D., GOODMAN, L., and WIEDERHOLT, J. L. Visual-motor processes: What success have we had in training them? *The Reading Teacher*, 1974, *27*, 469–478.

HAMMILL, D. D., and LARSEN, S. C. The relationship of selected auditory perceptual skills and reading ability. *Journal of Learning Disabilities*, 1974, *7*, 429–435.

HARING, N., and KRUG, D. Evaluation of a program of systematic instruction procedures for extremely poor retarded children. *American Journal of Mental Deficiency*, 1975, *79*, 627–631.

HARRIS, A. J. Lateral dominance, directional confusion and reading disability. *Journal of Psychology*, 1957, *44*, 283–287.

HECAEN, H., and AJURICAGUERRA, J. *Left-handedness: Manual superiority and cerebral dominance*. New York: Grune and Stratton, 1964.

HEW report, Reading disorders in the United States. Arleigh B. Templeton (Chairman).

Report of the Secretary's (HEW) National Advisory Committee on Dyslexia and Related Reading Disorders, August, 1969.

HILDRETH, G. Manual dominance in nursery school children. *Journal of Genetic Psychology*, 1948, *72*, 25–45.

HINSHELWOOD, J. *Congenital word-blindness*. London: Lewis, 1917.

HOFMEISTER, A. Integrating criterion-referenced testing and instruction. In W. Hively and M. C. Reynolds (Eds.), *Domain-referenced testing in special education*. Minneapolis: Leadership Training Institute/Special Education, University of Minnesota, 1975.

ILG. F., and AMES, L. Developmental trends in reading behavior. *Journal of Genetic Psychology*, 1950, *76*, 291–312.

JASTAK, J. F., and JASTAK, S. R. *Wide Range Achievement Test: Manual*. Wilmington, Del.: Guidance Associates, 1965.

JOHNSON, D., and MYKLEBUST, H. *Learning disabilities*. New York: Grune and Stratton, 1967.

JOHNSON, M. S., and KRESS, R. A. Individual reading inventories. In D. D. Hammill and N. R. Bartel (Eds.), *Educational perspectives in learning disabilities*. New York: John Wiley, 1971.

JONES, B. Cross-modal matching by retarded and normal readers. *Bulletin of the Psychonomic Society*, 1974, *3*, 163–165.

KASS, C., and MYKLEBUST, H. Learning disability: An educational definition. *Journal of Learning Disabilities*, 1969, *2*, 377–379.

KAUFMAN, N. L., and KAUFMAN, A. S. Comparison of normal and minimally brain dysfunctioned children on the McCarthy Scales of Children's Abilities. *Journal of Clinical Psychology*, 1974, *30*, 69–72.

KEOGH, B. K. Hyperactivity and learning disorders: Review and speculation. *Exceptional Children*, 1971, *37*, 101–109, a.

KEOGH, B. K. A compensatory model for psychoeducational evaluation of children with learning disorders. *Journal of Learning Disabilities*, 1971, *4*, 544–548, b.

KEOGH, B. K. Optometric vision training programs for children with learning disabilities: Review of issues and research. *Journal of Learning Disabilities*, 1974, *7*, 219–231.

KEOGH, B. K., WETTER, J., MCGINTY, A., and DONLON, G. Functional analysis of WISC performance of learning-disordered, hyperactive and mentally retarded boys. *Psychology in the Schools*, 1973, *10*, 178–181.

KEPHART, N. C. *The slow learner in the classroom*. Columbus, Ohio: Charles E. Merrill, 1960.

KINSBOURNE, M. School problems. *Pediatrics*, 1973, *52*(5), 3–17, (a).

KINSBOURNE, M. *Perceptual learning determines beginning reading*. Washington, D.C.; Paper presented at Society for Research in Child Development, 1973, (b).

KIRK, S. *Educating exceptional children*. Boston: Houghton Mifflin, 1972.

KIRK, S. A., and KIRK, W. *Psycholinguistic learning disabilities: Diagnosis and remediation*. Urbana, Ill.: University of Illinois Press, 1971.

KIRK, S. A., MCCARTHY, J. J., and KIRK, W. *The Illinois Test of Psycholinguistic Abilities: Examiner's Manual*. (Rev. ed.) Urbana, Ill.: University of Illinois Press, 1968.

KIRK, W. The relationship of reading disabilities to learning disabilities. *The Journal of Special Education*, 1975, *2*, 133–137.

KLINE, C. Rebuttal. *Journal of Learning Disabilities*, 1969, *2*, 57.

KUCERA, H., and FRANCIS, W. N. *Computational analysis of present-day American English*. Providence, R.I.: Brown University Press, 1967.

KUHN, T.S. *The structure of scientific revolutions*. Chicago: University of Chicago Press, 1962.

KUNZELMAN, H., COHEN, M., HULTEN, M. G., and MINGO, A. *Precision teaching*. Seattle, Wash.: Special Child Publications, 1970.

LAWSON, L. Ophthalmological factors in learning disabilities. In H. Myklebust (Ed.), *Progress in learning disabilities* (Vol. 1). New York: Grune and Stratton, 1968.

Lenneberg, E. H. *Biological foundations of language*. New York: John Wiley, 1967.

Lerner, J. Remedial reading and learning disabilities: Are they the same or different? *Journal of Special Education*, 1975, *2*, 119–131.

Liberman, I. Basic research in speech and lateralization of language: Some implications for reading disability. *Status Report on Speech Research*, Haskins Laboratories, Storrs, Conn. January-June, 1971.

Lindsley, O. Direct measurement and prosthesis of retarded behavior. *Journal of Education*, 1964, *143*, 62–81.

Lindsley, O. Precision teaching in perspective: An interview with Ogden R. Lindsley. *Teaching Exceptional Children*, 1971, *3*, 114–119.

Lovitt, T. Characteristics of ABA, general recommendations, and methodological limitations. *Journal of Learning Disabilities*, 1975, *8*, 432–443.

McCarthy, D. *Manual for the McCarthy scales of children's abilities*. New York: The Psychological Corporation, 1972.

McGrady, H. J., and McCarthy, J. M. The eye and learning disabilities. *Division for Children with Learning Disabilities Newsletter*, *2*(1), 1971.

McLeod, J. A comparison of WISC sub-test scores of pre-adolescent successful and unsuccessful readers. *Australian Journal of Psychology*, 1965, *17*, 220–228.

Merrell, D. Dominance of eye and hand. *Human Biology*, 1957, *29*, 314–328.

Miller, G., Galanter, E., and Pribram, K. *Plans and the structure of behavior*. New York: Holt, Rinehart & Winston, 1960.

Miller, W. H. *Reading diagnosis kit*. New York: The Center for Applied Research in Education, 1974.

Money, J. (Ed.). *Progress and research needs in dyslexia*. Baltimore: Johns Hopkins, 1962.

Money, J. *The disabled reader: Education of the dyslexic child*. Baltimore: Johns Hopkins, 1966.

Monroe, M. *Children who cannot read*. Chicago: University of Chicago Press, 1932.

Morgan, W. A case of congenital word blindness. *British Medical Journal*, 1896, *2*, 1378.

Myers, P. I., and Hammill, D. D. *Methods for learning disorders*. New York: John Wiley, 1969.

Newcomer, P. L. Learning disabilities: An educator's perspective. *Journal of Special Education*, 1975, *9*, 145–149.

Newcomer, P. L., and Goodman, L. Effect of modality of instruction on the learning of meaningful and nonmeaningful material by auditory and visual learners. *Journal of Special Education*, 1975, *9*, 261–269.

O'Connor, P. Whether or whither the school psychologist? Unpublished manuscript, Department of Special Education, University of North Carolina, Chapel Hill, North Carolina, 1975.

Olson, A. V. Factor analytic studies of the Frostig Developmental Test of Visual Perception. *Journal of Special Education*, 1968, *2*, 429–433.

Orton, S. "Word blindness" in school children. *Archives of Neurology and Psychiatry*, 1924, *14*, 581–615.

Orton, S. *Reading, writing and special problems in children*. New York: Norton, 1937.

Osgood, C. E. Motivational dynamics of language behavior. In M. R. Jones (Ed.), *Nebraska Symposium on Motivation* Vol. V. Lincoln, Neb.: University of Nebraska, 1957.

Owen, F., Adams, P., Forrest, T., Stolz, L., and Fisher, S. Learning disorders in children: Sibling studies. *Monographs of the SRCD*, 1971, *36*, No. 4.

Peters, J., Romine, J., and Dykman, R. A special neurological examination of children with learning disabilities. *Developmental Medicine and Child Neurology*, 1975, *17*, 63–78.

Pope, L., and Haklay, A. A followup study of psychoeducational evaluations sent to schools. *Journal of Learning Disabilities*, 1974, *7*, 239–244.

POSNER, M. I., LEWIS, J. L., and CONRAD, C. Component processes in reading: A performance analysis. In J. F. Kavanagh and I. G. Mattingly (Eds.), *Language by ear and eye*. Cambridge, Mass.: MIT Press, 1972.

PROGER, B. B., and MANN, L. Criterion-referenced measurement: The world of gray versus black and white. *Journal of Learning Disabilities*, 1973, *6*, 73–85.

RABINOVITCH, R. Neuropsychiatric factors. Paper read at the annual meeting of the International Reading Association, Detroit, 1965.

RINGLER, L. H., and SMITH, I. L. Learning modality and word recognition of first-grade children. *Journal of Learning Disabilities*, 1973, *6*, 307–312.

ROURKE, B. Brain-behavior relationships in children with learning disabilities. *American Psychologist*, 1975, *30*, 911–919.

ROURKE, B. P., DIETRICH, M., and YOUNG, I. C. Significance of WISC verbal-performance discrepancies for younger children with learning disabilities. *Perceptual and Motor Skills*, 1973, *36*, 275–282.

RUGEL, R. P. WISC subtest scores of disabled readers: A review with respect to Bannatyne's recategorization. *Journal of Learning Disabilities*, 1974, *7*, 48–56.

SABATINO, D. A., and STREISSGUTH, W. O. Word form configuration training of visual perceptual strengths with learning disabled children. *Journal of Learning Disabilities*, 1972, *5*, 435–441.

SCHAIN, R. (Ed.). *Neurology of childhood learning disorders*. Baltimore: Williams & Wilkins, 1972.

SCHONELL, F. J. *Backwardness in the basic subjects*. Edinburgh and London: Oliver and Boyd, 1938.

SEDLOCK, R. A., and WEENER, P. Review of research on the Illinois Test of Psycholinguistic Abilities. In L. Mann and D. A. Sabatino (Eds.), *The first review of special education* (Vol. I). Philadelphia: J.S.E. Press, Bottomwood Farms, Inc., 1973.

SENF, G. Learning disabilities. In S. Grossman (Ed.), *Pediatric Clinics of North America*, 1973, *20*, 607–640.

SHANKWEILER, D., and LIBERMAN, I. Misreading: A search for causes. In J. F. Kavanagh and I. G. Mattingly (Eds.), *Language by ear and eye*. Cambridge, Mass.: MIT Press, 1972.

SHOEMAKER, D. M. Improving criterion-referenced measurement. *Journal of Special Education*, 1972, *6*, 315–324.

SILBERBERG, N. E., IVERSEN, I. A., and GOINS, J. T. Which remedial reading method works best? *Journal of Learning Disabilities*, 1973, *6*, 547–556.

SILBERMAN, H. Reading and related verbal learning. In R. Glaser (Ed.), *Teaching machines and programmed learning* (Vol. II). Washington, D.C.: National Education Association, 1965.

SILVER, L. B. Acceptable and controversial approaches to treating the child with learning disabilities. *Pediatrics*, 1975, *55*, 406–415.

SILVERMAN, H., and O'BRYAN, K. G. Learning disabilities: Implications of research for the classroom. Paper presented at the First Annual International Symposium on Learning Problems, Toronto, Canada, February 23–25, 1972.

SKINNER, B. F. *The technology of teaching*. New York: Appleton-Century-Crofts, 1968.

SMITH, P. A., and MARX, R. W. Some cautions on the use of the Frostig test: A factor analytic study. *Journal of Learning Disabilities*, 1972, *5*, 359–362.

SOETHE, J. W. Concurrent validity of the Peabody Individual Achievement Test. *Journal of Learning Disabilities*, 1972, *5*, 560–562.

SPERRY, R. Cerebral dominance in perception. In F. Young and D. Lindsley (Eds.), *Early-experience and visual information processing in perceptual and reading disorders*. Washington, D.C.: National Academy of Sciences, 1970.

STANLEY, G., and HALL, R. Short-term visual information processing in dyslexics. *Child Development*, 1973, *44*, 841–844.

STRAUSS, A., and KEPHART, N. *Psychopathology and education of the brain-injured child* (Vol. II). New York: Grune and Stratton, 1955.

THORNDIKE, R. *Reading comprehension: Education in fifteen countries.* New York: John Wiley, 1973.

TURNBULL, A., and ROSENTHAL, S. *A model of special education services at the Division for Disorders of Development and Learning.* Unpublished manuscript, Department of Special Education, University of North Carolina, Chapel Hill, N.C., 1974.

VAUGHAN, R., and HODGES, L. A statistical survey into a definition: A search for acceptance. *Journal of Learning Disabilities*, 1973, *6*, 69–73.

VELLUTINO, F., SMITH, H., STEGER, J., and KAMAN, M. Reading disability: Age differences and the perceptual-deficit hypothesis. *Child Development*, 1975, *46*, 487–493.

VELLUTINO, F., STEGER, J., and KANDEL, G. Reading disability: An investigation of the perceptual deficit hypothesis. *Cortex*, 1972, *8*, 106–118.

WAUGH, R. On reporting the findings of a diagnostic center. *Journal of Learning Disabilities*, 1970, *3*, 630–634.

WAUGH, R. P. The relationship between individual modality preference and performance after four instructional procedures. *Exceptional Children*, 1973, *39*, 465–469.

WENDER, P. *Minimal brain dysfunction in children.* New York: Wiley-Interscience, 1971.

WHITSELL, L. Delacato's "Neural Organization": A medical appraisal. *California School Health*, 1967, *3*, 1–13.

YSSELDYKE, J. E. Diagnostic-prescriptive teaching: The search for aptitude-treatment interactions. In L. Mann and D. Sabatino (Eds.), *The First Review of Special Education.* New York: Grune and Stratton, 1972.

16

DRUG AND ALCOHOL ABUSE[1]

Robert B. Millman

During the past decade, there has been an explosive increase in the incidence of psychoactive drug taking in youthful populations in the United States. In some areas over 80% of high-school-age children have used one or more drugs for nonmedical purposes. There is frequently no sharp line that distinguishes appropriate use from misuse of any drug. Drug abuse may therefore be defined as the use of any substance in a manner that deviates from the accepted medical, social, or legal patterns within a given society. It is behavior that results from the complex interaction of an adolescent, his social and cultural environment, and the pharmacology and availability of particular drugs.

No single factor is the basis of all drug-taking experience and no person's drug taking has a single etiology. Initially, psychoactive drugs may be taken merely to feel differently. People have always tried to alter their state of consciousness. Little children will spin around in place or hold their breath until they get dizzy; the smell of gasoline or glue is felt to be pleasurable for similar reasons. Drugs are taken to reduce tension and anxiety, to decrease fatigue and boredom, to facilitate social interaction, to change activity levels, to improve mood, to heighten sensation and awareness, to satisfy curiosity, and for many other reasons. If caffeine, nicotine, prescription and over-the-counter depressants and stimulants are included, few people in this country would be found who take no psychoactive drugs. Some young people experiment with drugs that are considered dangerous from a medical or legal point of view and do not repeat the experience. Others use them intermittently and do not harm themselves. Still others persist in drug-abuse behavior patterns that lead to physical or psychosocial deterioration for a variety of reasons.

In some cases an adolescent may become dependent on drugs or their behavioral concomitants in order to function at what he perceives to be a satisfactory level. This *psychological dependence* or *habituation* varies in intensity and may culminate in *compulsive drug abuse*, where the supply and use of particular drugs become primary con-

[1]This work was supported in part by DHEW PHS Career-Teacher Grant in Drug and Alcohol Abuse 6 T01 AA07005-02.

The author gratefully acknowledges permission to use portions of this material which first appeared in the section entitled "Drug Abuse, Addiction, and Intoxication" in the TEXTBOOK OF MEDICINE edited by Beeson and McDermott, Philadelphia, Saunders, 1975. He also acknowledges the assistance of Elizabeth T. Khuri, M.D., Berniece B. Hess, R. N., and the staff and patients of the Adolescent Development Program.

cerns of living. In addition, certain drugs have the capacity to produce *physical dependence*. This is an altered physiological state induced by the repeated administration of a drug that requires the continued administration of the drug to prevent the appearance of a syndrome characteristic for each drug, the *withdrawal*, or *abstinence*, syndrome. The term *addiction* has been used in the literature to refer to either behavioral or pharmacologic events. As used herein, it refers to a pattern of compulsive drug use that includes both physical dependence and an overwhelming involvement with the supply and use of a drug. Neither a diabetic on insulin nor a compulsive user of marijuana—nor a well-adjusted patient in methadone-maintenance treatment—is an addict in this sense of the term.

In order to provide effective treatment, it is necessary to appreciate the patterns of abuse, the psychological factors that determine drug-abuse behavior, and the adverse effects that occur incident to this behavior. The drugs that will be considered in some detail may be grouped into six major classes: (1) opiates; (2) central nervous system depressants, including alcohol, hypnotics, and tranquilizers; (3) central nervous system stimulants, including the amphetamine group and cocaine; (4) cannabis; (5) psychedelics; and (6) miscellaneous inhalants.

Patterns of Abuse

People have used substances that induce alterations in mood, perception, and behavior for medical, religious, or recreational purposes since ancient times. It is instructive to recognize that the patterns and prevalence have been an integral part of the sociocultural milieu of many societies. It is during the adolescent years that people often have begun experimenting with and using drugs.

Adolescent drug-abuse patterns and prevalence continue to change rapidly in response to a variety of factors, which include the cultural and economic climate, media emphasis, the availability of particular drugs, the impact of treatment programs, and legal sanctions. Accurate assessment of the character and extent of emerging drug-abuse patterns is difficult given the rapidity of change, great geographical and cultural variation, and the illegal or otherwise stigmatized nature of the phenomena. It is also likely that some surveys exaggerate the prevalence or severity of the problem in order to demonstrate or dramatize the need for public funding and expansion of treatment programs.

Despite the limitations of attempting to generalize some summary statements might be useful. Young people often begin their drug use with beer and wine, though the initial alcohol exposure may also be hard liquor. During this initial period, the use of nicotine and, somewhat later, marijuana may begin. Use of depressants, excitants, or LSD may then occur, in large part depending on sociocultural factors; opiates are often the last drug in this decidedly nonlinear and complex progression. In some areas, however, opiates are used early, just after the initial alcohol exposures.

Many people stop at particular points in this sequence, depending on a variety of factors. Some young people will use only one drug or group of drugs during a particular period. More often, youthful drug abusers will use a variety of drugs, depending on their assessment of the situation, their needs, and the availability of drugs. This so-called *polydrug abuse* varies in severity from the benign use of alcohol and marijuana in preparation for a concert, to the disorganized, dangerous multiple-abuse patterns of severely disturbed young people. It is interesting to note that as young people give up more dangerous abuse patterns, they often return to the drugs they used earlier.

Psychobiological Factors

Personality characteristics influence the choice of drugs and patterns of abuse of individual users and in part determine the psychoactive effects drugs will elicit in a given situation. Controversy exists as to whether drug abuse implies a personality disturbance that antedates drug use and also whether specific patterns of abuse correlate with certain personality types. Most authorities agree that the experimental or intermittent use of drugs is not necessarily an indication of psychopathology. At the same time, compulsive drug use is frequently associated with serious psychopathology. Present evidence suggests that personality characteristics vary considerably in drug-abusing populations and that psychological factors play a markedly variable role in the etiology of drug abuse. The problem is that none of these characteristics and no predictive test will determine whether or not a person will become a compulsive user nor which people will use which drug. There is no good evidence for the existence of a well-defined addictive or alcoholic personality type or other specific psychodyanamic constellation. Whereas premorbid personality disturbances are crucial in the etiology of some cases of compulsive drug use, the psychopathology noted in other cases may be a reaction to the behavioral patterns of compulsive abuse in a society that condemns the drug-dependent life.

Conditioned learning is an integral part of the development and maintenance of compulsive drug-abuse patterns. The feelings of dysphoria that the drug taking behavior allayed or some of the situations attendant to the behavior become, in time, the conditioned stimulus to the experience of drug craving and the persistence of drug-seeking behavior. This may occur in the presence or absence of physical dependence. The drug craving and withdrawal syndrome that long-abstinent ex-addicts experience when they return to a site of former drug use is in part a reflection of this conditioning process. Learning also influences the effects drugs have on individual users. Marijuana or alcohol will elicit different and sometimes contrary responses depending on group expectations or pressure, particularly in these youthful users. Marijuana is used in some cultures as a work stimulant or appetite depressant, in contrast to its well-publicized but poorly documented effects on American adolescents of decreased motivation or increased appetite.

In some adolescents compulsive drug use may be an attempt at self-treatment of painful affects of shame, rage, loneliness, guilt, and depression. Others may be seeking to satisfy or control unacceptable drives, particularly sexual longings, security needs, or primitive sadistic and aggressive impulses. It has been postulated that there may be an impairment in affect or drive defense such that these feelings and desires are experienced as overwhelming. Pathological narcissism is a frequent finding. Denial, splitting, and externalization are commonly employed defenses against these overwhelming affects. Other elements may include pathologic dependency, sadomasochistic impulses, and an inability to identify and articulate feelings such that painful emotions may be experienced as somatic complaints. There may be superego pathology based on faulty ego-ideal formation or value systems; or the superego may consist of an idealized, overly demanding aspect coexisting with more primitive superego functioning.

It has also been postulated that drugs fill needs that were left unresolved during the process of attachment to the mother. They may serve as a loved or loving object of symbiotic attachment for the compulsive user—or as a replacement for a defect in the psychological structure. These children are unable to pursue needs for admiration and for love. They do not build up a system of activity, interests, and relationships that could serve as a buffer against depression, boredom, and narcissistic withdrawal.

Some of these children have neurotic, personality, or psychotic disorders. Borderline or psychotic youngsters use heroin and other drugs in an attempt to cope with intolerable paranoid and angry feelings. Compulsive users of amphetamines may be seeking a feeling of power and competence and relief from feelings of depression or loss. Alcohol use may facilitate the denial of feelings of vulnerability and loneliness and allow the expression of long-suppressed anger.

Not only does the choice of drugs reflect personality characteristics (as it does various social factors), so also do abuse patterns reflect ego-structure pathology. A depressed obsessive character may use heroin compulsively, but in a structured, organized fashion. Most young people will use a variety of drugs as they become available or as they develop a taste for them, the so-called *polydrug-abuse* pattern. This includes a spectrum of use and users from well-organized, reasonably healthy young people using marijuana and occasional "ups" and "downs" to the chaotic use pattern of borderline or psychotic patients who take many different drugs in diverse combinations and suffer frequent adverse reactions and overdoses.

It should be evident that withdrawal of some of these severely disturbed people from the drug may result in a deterioration of their psychological function. It is not unusual for a reasonably well-compensated young heroin addict to deteriorate into a psychotic state when he is detoxified or when he is stabilized on methadone. In other cases the psychopathology is a result of the drug use or its concomitants, and symptoms will abate after withdrawal.

FAMILIAL FACTORS

Adolescent drug-abuse behavior is influenced by family dynamics and drug-use patterns, though no particular familial patterns are predictive for drug abuse. Often families will lack consistency in the setting and enforcing of limits. There may at the same time be a gratification of all material needs coupled with inappropriately stringent parental demands. A self-centered concern with success and prestige is often seen with little real caring for the subjective experience of the child. Some of these patterns occur in both wealthy and disadvantaged families. The reaction of the family to the drug-using behavior may provide covert reinforcement for continuing similar behavior. In some families the drug use is a shared behavior that is sanctioned, and children are supplied with drugs by parents or siblings. This is particularly true in some inner-city families with several heroin- or alcohol-dependent members.

Some parents violently condemn the controlled and occasional use of marijuana, even when they themselves engage in alcohol abuse. Children may be made to feel that they have severe psychological or social problems and that they are morally inadequate. They often feel they might just as well identify strongly with the "sick" group and take more drugs. Alternatively, adolescents have been convinced that alcohol is the drug of choice for mature adults. Some have been weaned off marijuana and onto alcohol after much anger, cajoling, and prayer.

It has long been known that the children of alcoholics and other drug abusers have a markedly increased chance of becoming drug abusers. Recent studies suggest that the influence of genetic factors in the development of alcoholism may be more important than the quality of nurturing. Children of alcoholic biologic parents who were raised by nonalcoholic parents were more likely to become alcoholic than were children of nonalcoholic biologic parents raised by alcoholics. It has been postulated that a genetic disturbance could produce an impairment of certain central nervous system functions during infancy, which might result in an impairment in object relations. That a child does not receive the necessary "good enough mothering" might be as much a function of the child's innate inability to relate as it is of the mother's.

Sexual problems are frequent in this population. Often these precede the drug-abuse experience and may be a predisposing factor. In other cases the inability to perform satisfactorily may be a result of drug taking. Many young people find that they are able to suppress their feelings of anxiety and sexual inadequacy through the use of depressants or opiates. Some males are able to sustain an erection only when they are "stoned." Low doses of sedatives and alcohol increase desire, relieve inhibitions, and improve performance. The great vogue that Quāālude and similar sedatives had in recent years relates to this phenomenon. When young people become dependent on these drugs to perform sexually, they may increase the dose and find themselves unable to perform at the higher level. The effects of low doses of opiates are similar in increasing desire and improving performance; males report that ejaculation is delayed significantly. At higher doses there is decreased interest and patients often report an inability to reach orgasm. Cannabis in its various forms has increased sexual desire and sensitivity in some people; in others it has been associated with a marked disinterest in sex. Stimulants also have been reported as having markedly variable influence on sexual interest and performance. It should be remembered that the compulsive use of *most* drugs is associated with decreased sexual interest and performance.

Sociologic Factors

Adolescence as we know it is a recent historical phenomenon dependent upon unique cultural, economic, and psychological realities. Drug-abuse behavior in the young should be considered in the context of these complex psychosocial determinants. Adolescence is a time when an individual is confronted with his own powerlessness in an alien world and his lack of an adult identity. Youth are told that this is a crucial period of preparation that should not be lived for its own sake. Testing and experimentation are an integral part of the young person's search to discover himself and his society and the progression from the dependence of childhood to the independence of maturity. Yet during the entire period, the rules of behavior remain those of the adult world, with enthusiasm, curiosity, and spontaneity distrusted and initiative frequently mistaken for aggressiveness.

The societal institutions with which the adolescent comes into contact may be hostile or unresponsive, including the family and particularly the educational system. Insecurity and fear are common to most youngsters; few are sure that they will measure up to the demands of society. Many can't wait to grow up. Others have a pervasive and realistic dread of the future. The frequently reported inability of some adolescents to focus on long-range goals, their desire for immediate gratification, and their lack of appreciation for the possible consequencs of behavior might be anticipated in light of these pressures.

Peer affiliation and acceptance are crucial for adolescents' sense of self; they need to compare what they appear to be in the eyes of others with what they feel they are. Many of them do not have the necessary experience or confidence to develop productive relationships, and there are often few avenues of expression open to them aside from drugs and sex. Early sexual activity is frequently unsatisfactory and may be a source of intense anxiety for some young people.

If the problem of being young is compounded by poverty, minority ethnic-group status, or physical and/or intellectual disability, little pleasure, sense of dignity, or uniqueness, and almost no power remain for the adolescent in the "straight" world. Many families are in disarray and a pervasive sense of helplessness or resentment communicates itself to children trying to make their way. Successful role models in adult legitimate society are often unknown or distant.

Some youngsters, particularly those who live in urban ghettos, acquire an enormous and sophisticated range of survival skills on the street. They may be perceptive judges of people and situations. At the same time, they are often unprepared for the educational system and find classes boring, irrelevant, and frequently mortifying. Failure is almost inevitable. In this context, the self-administration of psychoactive substances remains one of the few pleasurable options for many adolescents; it may be a predictable, reliable method by which to punctuate their lives.

Young people are most often introduced or "turned on" to the various drugs by a close friend or relative. Initially, the intent may be to share an exciting experience or to diffuse some of the shame or guilt associated with drug taking, which then becomes a focus for group identification and activity. Most of these youngsters believe themselves able to control their drug taking so that it will not be personally destructive—this despite the exhortations of parents, media, etc., as to the dangers of drug use, and occasionally despite their own familiarity with victims of this behavior. Interestingly, in most cases they are right; the drugs are less destructive to them than they have been led to believe.

The more aberrant an adolescent's drug-abuse behavior pattern is for his particular social milieu, the more likelihood there is a significant degree of psychopathology. White middle-class heroin addicts tend to show more psychopathology than black heroin addicts from the inner city. Jewish alcoholics tend to have more psychopathology than do Irish alcoholics. This has significant bearing on treatment approaches.

Some aspects of drug taking in young women are distinct from abuse patterns in males. Often a boyfriend or lover will have been involved initially, and then "turned her on." He is responsible for the constant and formidable task of supplying both of their drug needs. In the inner city it is not unusual for a young girl to be prostituting herself so as to provide her lover with sufficient drug money. When the male leaves or is taken away, perhaps to jail or a hospital, it is not unusual for these women to "clean up" or at least significantly decrease their drug use. In contrast to this situation, young girls' use of alcohol, depressants, and opiates may in some circles receive fewer sanctions and be more stigmatized than similar behavior in young boys. The girls in these situations appear to be more emotionally disabled and the drug taking more a means of self-medication.

PHARMACOLOGIC FACTORS

The nature of the psychophysiologic effects of any given drug influences its initial abuse potential for particular youngsters as well as the subsequent patterns of abuse. Then, too, the dose and route of administration of particular drugs influence the psychoactive effects. All too often, treatment strategies betray an ignorance or lack of concern for the clinical pharmacology of these drugs, an attitude which then renders the strategy ineffective. A child who is addicted to opiates and in withdrawal, though his objective symptoms be mild, is a poor candidate for any kind of insight therapy. He will agree or acquiesce to anything if there is a possibility of obtaining medication to allay his severe subjective discomfort and craving.

Tolerance refers to the necessity for increasing the dose or, conversely, to the decreased effect a given dose of a drug will elicit upon repeated administration. This phenomenon may be either *pharmacodynamic* (cellular) in type, which means that central nervous system cells adapt to drug concentrations or *drug disposition* (metabolic), in which there is more rapid inactivation or excretion of a drug. Both types occur with the same drugs, though the former is more important in determining clinical tolerance. With opiates, alcohol, and general depressants, physical dependence develops concurrently to tolerance and, though poorly understood, may be related to pharmacodynamic tolerance mechanisms. *Cross-tolerance* refers to the ability of one drug to induce tolerance to another. *Cross-dependence* refers to the ability of one drug to suppress the abstinence syndrome produced by withdrawal of another. Cross-tolerance and cross-dependence may be complete or partial as in the case of alcohol and the barbiturates.

DIAGNOSIS

If adequate treatment is to be provided, it is necessary to characterize the specific problems of drug abuse and dependence, the individual psychopathology of the user, and the social set within which he is using the psychoactive substances. In all cases, the nature and degree of drug-induced psychoactive effects and the presence of any abstinence symptoms should be assessed. This requires careful history taking, when possible, and a complete psychiatric and physical examination. Drug abusers are often poor historians and may minimize or exaggerate the extent of their drug use, depending on their perception of the situation, their needs, and the attitudes of the examiners. It is likely that an opiate user will exaggerate the extent of his use so as to obtain more opiates during the detoxification process and perhaps suffer decreased abstinence symptoms. At the same time, a college student may neglect to tell his psychiatrist that he is using 30 or 40 mg diazepam in order to keep himself functioning, since this might be considered to be evidence of weakness or serious psychopathology. These difficulties may be minimized if the patient perceives the examiner as acting in his behalf, as not unduly moralistic, and as genuinely interested in his particular situation.

Evaluation of the mode of administration of the abused drugs is important in establishing a diagnosis. Signs of repeated intravenous injections ("tracks") suggest heroin, amphetamine, or cocaine abuse. These drugs are also sniffed, whereby the material is inhaled and absorbed through the mucous membrances of the nasopharynx and respiratory tract. Chronic sinusitis or perforation of the nasal septum may suggest this mode of administration. Personal hygiene and patterns of dress may further define the clinical picture.

It is sometimes difficult to distinguish drug effects, particularly those of acute anxiety, paranoid ideation, and even hallucinations and delusions, from the various psychiatric disorders. Often the picture is a mixed one, with elements of several drug effects and a severe psychological disorder presenting concurrently. In some cases supportive care and even protective custody may be called for until such time as a more coherent picture emerges. More precise diagnostic impressions will emerge as drug effects, abstinence syndromes, and the resistance of the patient wane with continued treatment and development of a therapeutic alliance.

Pressing social or legal needs should be identified with a view toward providing realistic, often necessarily short-term solutions. The characteristics of the family relationships should be obtained, with particular care taken to determine the drug-abuse patterns of all family members. Often the youngster's drug-abuse pattern reflects that of his father, older sibling, or other important family member.

Routine qualitative procedures for the detection in urine, of morphine (the major metabolite of heroin), methadone, amphetamines, cocaine, and the most frequently abused general depressants, are currently available in many laboratories. Results will generally be positive if a dose sufficient to produce pharmacologic effects has been taken within 24 hours prior to the urine sample. Since results ordinarily are not immediately available and false positives do occur, these tests should be used to confirm the clinical impression. They are most useful as an adjunct to the long-term evaluation of patients already in treatment. In emergency situations, blood levels of suspected drugs can usually be obtained immediately.

Diagnosis and Treatment of Acute Drug Poisoning

Drug poisoning, or *overdose*, most often occurs incident to an adolescent's attempt to get as "high" or "stoned" as possible. Only the opiates and sedatives create any appreciable risk of death due to direct drug effects. Often a boy or girl will take a variety of drugs, perhaps several hypnotics such as methaqualone (Quāālude) or secobarbital (Seconal), a large quantity of alcohol, and marijuana. After waiting for half an hour, the youngster may not feel high enough and will "take another hit" of whatever is available, and overdose. Accidental overdoses may be due in some cases to "drug automatism," where individuals become confused, forget the drugs they took, and ingest more. Opiates—particularly methadone, with its slow onset and long duration of action alone or in combination with other depressants—are especially dangerous. Controversy exists as to whether many of these so-called "accidental" overdoses are suicide attempts. Other cases are frank suicide attempts. Very young children who gain access to improperly stored depressant medication form another distinct group. Acute care remains the same whatever the motivation; long-term care should vary depending on the particular circumstances.

Table 16-1, adapted from the *Textbook of Medicine*, summarizes the signs of toxicity and treatment of some common drug poisonings. Additional information is presented as part of the discussion of specific pharmacological agents. Clinical appraisal must be used to diagnose the agent or combination responsible for the overdose picture and to assess its severity. Blood levels of particular drugs or amounts taken are less useful as indicators of potential danger since individuals who have developed tolerance will react differently to similar doses. Often it may be necessary to institute rapid treatment on a presumptive basis when a definitive diagnosis cannot be made, particularly in those situations where there is a possibility of an opiate or sedative-hypnotic overdose. Emergency hospitalization is indicated in all cases of severe depressant overdose. If possible, when an opiate overdose is suspected, a narcotic antagonist might be administered on site or in an office, though hospitalization is still indicated. Failure to respond suggests an overdose of another drug.

General Treatment Considerations

As distinct from most other patients, drug abusers frequently know more about the behavior

Table 16-1 COMMON DRUG POISONINGS, SIGNS OF TOXICITY, AND TREATMENT

DRUG	MILD TOXIC SIGNS	TISSUE FOR DIAGNOSIS	TREATMENT	SEVERE OVERDOSE SIGNS	TREATMENT
Opiates: Heroin, Morphine, Demerol, Methadone	"Nodding" drowsiness, small pupils, urinary retention, slow and shallow breathing; skin scars and subcutaneous abscesses; duration 4–6 hrs; with methadone, duration to 24 hrs	Blood, Urine	Naloxone (Narcan) 0.01 mg/kg iv, nalorphine (Nalline) 0.1 mg/kg iv, levallorphan (Lorfan) 0.02 mg/kg; repeat in 10–15 min if necessary; then repeat in 3 hrs if necessary	Coma; pinpoint pupils, slow irregular respiration or apnea, hypotension, hypothermia, pulmonary edema	Naloxone, nalorphine, levallorphan; if no response by second dose, suspect another cause; treat shock; find and detect infection
Depressants: Alcohol	Confusion, rousable drowsiness, delirium, ataxia, nystagmus, dysarthria, analgesia to stimuli	Blood, urine, breath	Alcohol excitement: diazepam or chlorpromazine	Stupor to coma; pupils reactive, usually constricted; oculovestibular response absent; motor tonus initially briefly hyperactive, then flaccid; respiration and blood pressure depressed; hypothermia; with glutethimide, pupils moderately dilated, can be fixed; with meprobamate, withdrawal seizures common; with methaqualone, coma, occasional convulsions, tachycardia, cardiac failure, bleeding tendency	Intubate, ventilate, gavage; drainage position; antimicrobials; keep mean blood pressure above 90 mm Hg and urine output 300 ml/hr; avoid analeptics; hemodialyze severe phenobarbital poisoning
Barbiturates		Blood	None needed for acute toxicity; withdraw drug under supervision if patient is a chronic user		
Glutethimide (Doriden)		Blood			
Meprobamate (Equanil)		Blood			
Methaqualone (Quaālude, Sopor, Mandrax)	Hallucinations, agitation, motor hyperactivity, myoclonus, tonic spasms	Blood, Urine			As above; diuresis of little help
Chlordiazepoxide (Librium)	Usually taken with another sedative if poisoning the attempt	Blood, Urine			
Diazepam (Valium)					
Stimulants: Amphetamines, Methylphenidate	Hyperactive, aggressive, sometimes paranoid, repetitive behavior; dilated pupils, tremor, hyperactive reflexes; hyperthermia, tachycardia, arrhythmia. Acute torsion dystonia	Blood, Urine	Reassurance if mild; Chlorpromazine if intense	Agitated, assaultive and paranoid excitement; occasionally convulsions; hypothermia; circulatory collapse	Chlorpromazine
Cocaine	Similar but less prominent than above; less paranoid, often euphoric	Blood clinical appraisal	Reassurance; Chlorpromazine	Twitching, irregular breathing, tachycardia	Sedation

Table 16-1 (CONTINUED)

DRUG	MILD TOXIC SIGNS	TISSUE FOR DIAGNOSIS	TREATMENT	SEVERE OVERDOSE SIGNS	TREATMENT
Psychedelics (LSD, mescaline, psilocybin, STP)	Confused, disoriented, perceptual distortions, distractable, withdrawn or eruptive, leading to accidents or violence; wide-eyed, dilated pupils; restless, hyperreflexic; less often, hypertension or tachycardia		Reassure; "talk down"; do not leave alone Diazepam	Panic	Reassure; diazepam satisfactory; avoid phenothiazines
Atropine-scopolamine (Sominex)	Agitated or confused, visual hallucinations, dilated pupils, flushed and dry skin		Reassure	Toxic disoriented delirium, visual hallucination; later, amnesia, fever, dilated fixed pupils, hot flushed dry skin, urinary retention	Reassure; sedate lightly; (1) avoid phenothiazines; (2) do not leave alone
Antidepressants:					
Imipramine (Tofranil), amitriptyline (Elavil)	Restlessness, drowsiness, tachycardia, ataxia, sweating	Clinical Blood		Agitation, vomiting, hyperpyrexia, sweating, muscle dystonia, convulsions, tachycardia or arrhythmia	Symptomatic; gastric lavage
MAO inhibitors: tranylcypromine (Parnate), phenelzine (Nardil), pargyline (Eutonyl)	Hypertensive crises, agitation, drowsiness, ataxia	Clinical Blood	Withdrawal	Hypotension; headache; chest pain; agitation; coma, seizures and shock	Symptomatic; gastric lavage
Phenothiazines	Acute dystonia, somnolence, hypotension	Clinical Blood	Benadryl 0.50; withdrawal	Coma; convulsions (rare); arrhythmias; hypotension	Symptomatic; gastric lavage

Source: *Textbook of Medicine*, eds. Beeson and McDermott (Philadelphia: W. B. Saunders Company, 1975). Used by permission.

and disability incident to drug taking than do their physicians. Serving to further complicate therapeutic efforts, drug abusers are often faced with prejudice and hostility on the part of treatment personnel that are revealed in statements such as, "He did it to himself." Since many drug takers' personality characteristics and behavior patterns occur in response to the attitudes of society, an inquiring, compassionate attitude is crucial in the treatment of this group of patients. The chronic use of most drugs may be associated with a subculture that rejects conventional values and orientation. To be effective, therapists should be sensitive to these value systems.

These patients commonly do not show consistent progress. Some will resume the use of drugs after withdrawal or will alter their drug-using patterns. Others tend not to stop the drug use. Still others will drop out of treatment incident to their continued drug use, or perhaps seek a "magical" solution. Many of these adolescents frustrate the efforts of a well-meaning treatment team, who may be provoked to give up on a particular boy or girl. A major fallacy on the part of the helping persons is a conceptual one; physicians often regard substance abuse as an acute illness, not unlike pneumonia, and amenable to complete cure. In general, this is an unrealistic assumption. Most psychological and social difficulties tend by nature to be chronic; then, too, the character of pharmacological dependence may also be more protracted than previously imagined. Since the clinical course in some of these patients may be reminiscent of diabetes or schizophrenia, with remissions and exacerbations, the need for patience and continuing enthusiasm is important. At the same time, the adolescent patient continues to change in relation to his society. His self-image may improve and his sense of power and dignity may increase given adequate opportunity and support. In contrast to adult patients, the youthful are more likely to develop the necessary skills and tastes to live reasonably contented with themselves and in society without drugs. Treatment may therefore be considered a holding action with particular patients.

Patients will often minimize or exaggerate the extent of their drug use or in other ways distort data so as to create a desired effect. Direct confrontation of these failures to tell the truth, particularly at the outset of treatment, may lead to increased resistance and power struggles. At the same time, if the therapist accepts the information without reservation, he may further increase the patient's sense of guilt and undermine the therapeutic alliance. This is a difficult problem with all patients, but particularly in drug-abusing adolescents. If possible, the therapist must adopt the stance of an accepting, interested ally, such that the responsibility for behavior and improvement rests squarely on the patient. An attitude of gentle but persistent curiosity is more effective than approach as an adversary. When distortions are suspected, it may be useful to listen carefully but neutrally. Some experienced therapists find it useful to gloss over questionable issues, at different treatment stages, to consider in more depth other confirmed problems and behavior.

Upon entering treatment the adolescent should, if possible, be withdrawn from his drug or drugs of abuse. If dependence on depressants or alcohol is suspected, hospitalization or close observation in a therapeutic setting is indicated. In-patient or out-patient detoxification from opiates is also indicated immediately. Withdrawal from the other drugs of abuse may require hospitalization or simply close observation, depending on the extent of psychological dependence, the psychopathology, and the availability of social supports.

Those patients who continue to use drugs, whether they admit or deny this behavior, present difficult problems for the therapist. Clearly, psychotherapeutic and social progress are significantly retarded when patients are able to "act out" through continued drug taking. In these cases, it may be useful to reinforce the positive aspects of a nondrug-dominated life rather than talk about the dangers of drug use once again. At the same time, the therapist should clearly support the idea that there is no point in a therapy or counseling session while a patient is "stoned." The patient will get little out of it and the therapist will waste his time. Antisocial or aggressive behavior may be considered in a similar vein. Many of these young people have been living in a violent world, where this sort of behavior is necessary for survival and dignity and also serves as a defense against painful affects, particularly shame and rage. The therapist or treatment team should work to prevent the unacceptable behavior by means of rules and regulations that are firmly but nonpunitively enforced. Every attempt should be made to keep these patients in treatment; these behaviors are an integral part of the disease. On occasion when the drug-taking or antisocial behavior is disruptive to a group situation or has not improved over a period of time, it may be necessary to transfer a patient to another, perhaps more structured setting or discharge him.

After withdrawal from a drug or control of its use is accomplished, underlying psychopathology and character disturbances may be better identified. Often these disturbances increase in severity when the controlling influence of the drug is no longer present. Psychotic episodes have been precipitated by withdrawal from all drugs. Similarly, psychotic behavior has developed soon after patients are stabilized on methadone.

Whenever possible, patients should be treated within the family group. Modes of familial interaction that provoke drug-abuse behavior should be identified and altered. It may be necessary to provide care for other family members who are abusing drugs, or to provide support for nondrug-using members. Families must sometimes be advised to protect themselves from the abuses of a drug-using adolescent who steals to support his habit or engages in other disruptive acts. It is occasionally necessary to suggest that a family turn a compulsive drug user out so that he will be forced to seek treatment. On other occasions, it is necessary to encourage the separation of the patient from a family situation that is destructive, particularly one in which there are other compulsive drug users present.

Treatment of the psychopathology that led to, or resulted from, the drug-abuse behavior will obviously depend on the individual personality patterns. This is discussed in detail elsewhere in this book. Certain general considerations deserve emphasis. These youngsters have generally been unable to get adequate satisfaction from any phase of their lives save the intermittent drug "high" and perhaps the attendant life style. Drug usage has substituted for defenses, relationships, and other satisfactions. These young men and women are disappointed in themselves; they feel inadequate and helpless in the face of the real problems of living. The therapist must be sensitive to this profound lack of self-esteem as well as to the various modes of denial they employ. It is useful to work in the context of providing realistic alternatives to drug-use behavior. Patients should be encouraged to identify the extremes of emotion that they have been unable to recognize. The pattern of self-indulgence in regard to some aspects of life and self-denial in relation to other relationships and desires should be gently clarified. The patient's inability to adequately assess the risks of particular behaviors requires careful work and often firm intervention. The overwhelming guilt that many of these youngsters feel should be recognized and to some degree assuaged.

These youngsters need help in developing relationships that do not depend on drugs; they often trust no one. This requires very practical, concrete training in understanding others and living with them. Group techniques are useful in this regard, though with some populations it may be necessary to keep the groups informal and loose rather than structured. Sex education and counseling should be an integral part of most drug-abuse treatment programs. These patients will often deny the existence or minimize the extent of a severe sexual problem. Very practical kinds of help should be gently offered.

Most adolescent drug abusers should be treated without medication, particularly those agents that are liable to abuse. The ease of prescribing and the power of the medication often lead to a situation where the therapists overmedicate inappropriately. This may serve to further rigidify the previous coping patterns even if the new drugs are medically sanctioned. On the other hand, many compulsive drug users are medicating themselves in order to function, and it is unrealistic to expect to be able to treat some of this significant pathology through psychotherapeutic means alone. In these cases, despite the risk of abuse or noncompliance, psychotropic drugs should be considered an integral part of the therapeutic regimen. The particular medications employed will depend on the specific diagnosis and precise identification of target symptoms and affectual states.

The use of depressants or minor tranquilizers should be minimal since these are subject to abuse. If a tranquilizer is necessary, chlordiazepoxide hydrochloride (Librium) is less sedating and seems to be subject to less abuse than diazepam (Valium). Major tranquilizers are usually not abused and should be used when indicated. If a tricyclic antidepressant is indicated, imipramine hydrochloride (Tofranil) would be the drug of choice since it causes less sedation and is less subject to abuse than amitriptyline hydrochloride (Elavil). Lithium is useful in certain circumstances. The use of methadone and disulfiram (Antabuse) is indicated in the treatment of some adolescents. This will be discussed in later sections.

Behavior-modification techniques have been increasingly used in the treatment of this population. There is little evidence that aversive techniques are useful, though positive-reinforcement operant conditioning has been used effectively as an integral part of other treatments. A form of this is the staff approval and respect a young boy or girl might be rewarded with for abstinent or mature behavior. Systematic desensitization utilizes relaxation techniques or hypnosis to reduce the anxiety or other dysphoric feelings which may be a factor in drug abuse. Emphasis is placed on recognition of these feelings as conditioned stimuli for the experience of drug craving or drug use. Techniques related to this include yoga, meditation, biofeedback, and dance therapy. These are attractive to youthful populations and may be particularly valuable.

When the drug-abuse behavior is primarily determined by social factors, as is often the case in inner-city, ethnic minority youngsters or the rural poor, the focus of treatment should be on providing realistic, attractive alternatives to drug abuse. Some need a place to live or legal representation. Many of these youngsters need help in returning to school or preparing for their High School Equivalency Diploma. They may have lost a good deal of time and confidence and require encouragement to return to an academic milieu. Others need practical vocational training and job placement so that they can support themselves in "straight" society. Many of them will benefit from exposure to pleasurable options such as sports events, cultural exhibitions, and hobbies. A surprising number of these youngsters will benefit from exercises and procedures designed to improve their ability to relate to each other in a context other than drugs or criminal behavior. Group or milieu therapy is particularly useful with this group of adolescents, particularly with therapists who have shared similar cultural experiences. The general focus should be on common problems, sexual difficulties, methods of coping, and the establishment of trusting relationships with each other. The generation of a sense of identity and dignity within a group may be a crucial aspect of this approach.

The therapeutic-community model has recently been adopted widely in the treatment of adolescents. Originally established to treat heroin addiction, many have begun to treat other categories of drug abusers as well. These are generally communities that are self-regulatory in nature and staffed with a varying mix of former drug users and professional therapists. The youngster remains in the closed, drug-free environment for prolonged periods of time, frequently one to two years. He is encouraged to develop a new set of living skills and confidence that will enable him to remain drug free upon completion of the program. A variety of therapeutic techniques are employed to aid *residents* to recognize their deficiencies and change them. The sense of isolation that many young people feel may be reduced through this experience. Role models for responsible behavior are provided by the program staff and graduates. These communities vary considerably in the nature of the therapeutic milieu created and in the complex system of rewards and punishments the residents live with. These facilities may be an important resource in the treatment of severely disturbed youngsters who are unable to function in society.

A useful model that provides the diverse treatment capability necessary for adolescent drug abusers combines an in-patient and out-patient therapeutic-community structure with extensive medical and psychiatric backup. Individual treatment plans may be formulated within this organization. Clients are encouraged to identify strongly with the program. Professional and paraprofessional counselors, some with drug-abuse histories of their own, provide social, educational, legal, and recreational help, depending on the individual need. Medical care is provided for all clients and individual psychotherapy is available for a limited number. Patients may move from the in-patient to the out-patient, or day-care-center, phase to a more limited involvement as they develop ties to the larger society and have less need for program support. Individual patients begin at the appropriate phase of the program. If difficulties arise with any patient on any level, more supportive care is available.

Many youthful drug abusers are admitted to psychiatric or general hospitals for acute care. Liaison should be established between these traditional medical facilities and the longer-term institutions and treatment programs so that effective referrals can be made.

The lack of good comparative data makes it difficult to evaluate the efficacy of various treatment approaches. Particular therapeutic communities may be poorly run or in other ways may be unsuitable for patient referral. It is useful to have an appreciation for these different approaches and some notion of their applicability for particular patients. At the same time, it is important to remember that it may be necessary to try several modalities, either individually or often in appropriate combination.

An important aspect of the treatment program is the follow-up of those who have completed treatment or dropped out prematurely. Drug use tends to be chronic, and adolescents are often too proud to admit slippage. It is best to build into the program provision for revisits at intervals. The primary goal is to encourage these young people to reenter treatment if this is necessary. Continued contact, however infrequent, with the treatment program may also be necessary as a source of support, relationships, and validation. It is also useful to evaluate the effectiveness of any therapeutic program on a continuing basis. Optimally, a counselor or other skilled professional should be responsible for the follow-up of a panel of patients. Home visits or, in the inner city, extensive tracking may be necessary to secure the necessary contact.

Many of the young people referred to psychiatric facilities or treatment programs are not in need of intensive care. While their drug use may appear to be incomprehensible and dangerous to their parents, it may be a reasonably normal behavior pattern within their social milieu. At the same time, they often have serious concerns about their abilities, potential, and even sanity. There is a real danger of overtreatment here. All too often the relatively benign drug use becomes a cause of great concern and a focus for treatment. Their great need may be some validation of their own experience, e.g., telling them that smoking marijuana occasionally or experimenting with sedatives is "no big deal." It is not easy to be young, and on occasion, warm support and encouragement in a few informal sessions may be useful.

Prevention

Since the causes of drug abuse are complex and varied, approaches to prevention of this behavior should not be oversimplified. The provision of reasonable, rewarding emotional, educational, vocational, and recreational alternatives to drug use should be of prime concern. This is a difficult task. Educational programs that provide accurate information on the various drugs and their adverse effects should be available. The stringency of legal sanctions is controversial, and a great deal has been written on this topic with little resolution. It seems clear that the users of these drugs who have not been major dealers are victims and have committed only victimless crimes. As such, they should be treated and not punished. Physicians must be extremely prudent in their prescribing practices with respect to abusable drugs.

OPIATES (NARCOTIC ANALGESICS)

People have used derivatives of opium for medical, religious, or recreational purposes since the beginning of recorded time. Opium is derived from the poppy plant, *Papaver somniferum*, and contains more than 20 alkaloids, including morphine and codeine. Heroin, the most frequently abused opiate in the United States, is chemically converted from morphine in illegal laboratories. Demerol and methadone are synthetic narcotic analgesics which are pharmacologically similar to the opiates.

In this country the incidence of heroin use rose precipitously during the 1950s and 1960s, particularly in urban youthful populations; in New York City in 1971, for example, heroin addiction was the major cause of death in males aged 15 to 35 years. There were an estimated 200,000 to 300,000 heroin addicts in the country at that time. There appears to have been a decline in use of heroin and an increase in abuse of street methadone since that time. Most recently, heroin and methadone abuse appear to be increasing, as indicated by rising morbidity and mortality rates, arrest records, and requests for treatment.

PATTERNS OF ABUSE

Young people are generally introduced to heroin ("turned on") by a friend or relative already using the drug. Most often they have experience with other drug use, particularly alcohol and marijuana, and are aware of the dangers of becoming addicted to heroin, either through exposure to intensive educational or media campaigns or through personal contact with victims of the heroin life style. At the same time, few believe that they will be unable to control the drug use such that it will be personally destructive. On the contrary, in some inner-city areas the use of heroin represents an exciting, demanding goal-oriented life that may be more attractive than the life they know. Every user is a real or potential dealer of drugs and many fantasize about the wealth and power they will have when they become "heavier" dealers.

The drug is first taken by "sniffing," in which the white or brown powder is inhaled and absorption occurs through the mucous membrances of the nasopharynx and respiratory tract. Street heroin ("smack," "scag," "junk," "dope") is adulterated ("cut") with quinine or lactose as it passes from the importer through successive levels of dealers to the street user. The amount of heroin in a street package is highly variable and may vary from 3 to 30 mg and cost anywhere from three to ten dollars.

Nausea and vomiting are often associated with the initial drug experiences; these symptoms abate with continued use. Opiates produce a feeling of relaxation and contentment, with relief of the dysphoric effects of anxiety and pain. Use may be intermittent at the outset, separated by days or weeks. Some young people experiment with the drug and do not continue its use. Those who do continue, develop tolerance to its euphoric effects such that they either increase the dose or begin to use it more efficiently by injecting the drug subcutaneously ("skin-popping") or eventually intravenously ("mainlining"). Intravenous injection produces a "rush" warm flushing of the skin, and intensely pleasurable feelings in the entire body that are often compared to sexual orgasm. Many years of continued intravenous use of opiates or other drugs leads to obliteration of patent, available veins so that addicts must return to the subcutaneous mode of injection.

As tolerance increases and people become aware of their physical dependence ("habit," "Jones"), more drug must be used more often. Young people, especially the urban, minority-group poor with little access to legitimate sources of money, must devote all their time and energy to the acquisition of heroin. Strong identification with the "junkie" subculture provides them with an ideology that makes the life style palatable as well as a source for the transmission of skills and information for securing the drug. Any source of money is acceptable, and food, clothing, dignity, sexual desire, and aspirations become subordinate to the constant need for heroin. Some middle-class or wealthy adolescents are able to support their habits with parental subsidies; this may necessitate using their allowances or often stealing from their parents.

During the past five years, when heroin was not available or in poor supply, many adolescent addicts used methadone to allay their withdrawal symptoms. It is longer acting and less expensive than heroin though it is usually available in oral form only and provides less of a "high" than heroin. Some young people have relatively short experiences with heroin before they turn exclusively to methadone, and a few are primary methadone addicts. Most adolescent heroin users will use other drugs as they are available. Mixed addictions and dangerous polydrug abuse are often seen. Some of these young men and women attempt to "kick the habit" at intervals; many are repeatedly arrested, hospitalized for the complications of heroin use, or are periodically unable to get any drug. These abstinent periods are a part of the disease and also serve to lower tolerance for short periods, thus making the "habit" easier to bear.

Youthful opiate addicts are a heterogeneous group. The incidence of preexisting psychopathology appears to depend on how deviant the behavior is relative to a given social milieu and how difficult it is to get the drugs. Inner-city, minority-group adolescents are often remarkably stable considering their difficult living situations; a high degree of personality integration and intelligence is necessary to survive as a street addict. Middle-class adolescents, on the other hand, are often severely disturbed, and the drug use represents an attempt at self-medication for borderline or psychotic personality disorders. A number of these people are able to function as street addicts, but decompensate acutely when the opiate is withdrawn. The relief of anxiety afforded by the opiates as well as the very structured existence heroin addiction demands, may have been important in maintaining psychological homeostasis.

Pharmacology

Opiates administered to a nontolerant individual induce analgesia through a decreased perception of the painful nature of stimuli and a resultant decrease in anxiety and tension. Somnolence and an inability to concentrate also occur. Opiates cause pupillary constriction, stimulation of central nervous system centers to produce nausea and vomiting and respiratory depression. All opiates are absorbed after subcutaneous or intravenous use. Morphine and heroin lose much of their analgesic potency when taken orally, codeine and demerol remain quite active, and methadone retains most of its activity after oral administration. After subcutaneous administration, methadone and morphine exert approximately equal analgesic effects, heroin is three times stronger and more rapid acting, and demerol and codeine are approximately one-tenth as potent. After intravenous injection, morphine and heroin are effective almost immediately; duration of action is 3 to 6 hours. Oral administration prolongs the effects of all opiates, particularly that of methadone, where effects occur in 30 minutes and persist in nontolerant people for 4 to 10 hours.

Addiction and Withdrawal Process

A marked degree of tolerance develops to most acute narcotic effects after repeated use of any opiate, and the lethal dose increases significantly. Whereas a 10-mg dose will produce euphoria in a nontolerant individual, addicts may use 5 gm daily. Tolerance does not occur equally to all opiate effects since addicts will continue to demonstrate pupillary constriction and constipation. Cross-tolerance occurs with all narcotic analgesics.

Physical dependence, marked by the development of an abstinence syndrome ("cold turkey") upon withdrawal of narcotics, develops in association with tolerance. The syndrome is quite variable in severity and depends on the particular drug, the magnitude and duration of the opiate use, as well as the personality and situation of the addict. It has developed in some people after only a few exposures on succeeding days. With heroin, 4 to 6 hours after the last dose, the first withdrawal signs seen are purposive in nature and include drug craving, anxiety, restlessness, and irritability. Running eyes and nose, yawning, and perspiration occur 8 to 12 hours after the last dose. A restless sleep, the so-called "yen sleep," may occur, from which the addict awakens with dilated pupils, sneezing, coughing, nausea, vomiting, diarrhea, abdominal cramps, "bone" pains, goose flesh, and very rarely, convulsions and cardiovascular collapse. With heroin, most withdrawal symptoms peak at 2 to 3 days and are dissipated in 7 to 10 days. With methadone, the onset is more gradual and the severity is generally less, though symptoms may persist for several weeks. Under some circumstances, addicts will experience the abstinence syndrome as life threatening and excruciatingly painful, even when the magnitude of their habit was small and their pharmacological dependence minimal. The intense psychological dependence on the drug may contribute to the severity of their symptoms. These should be taken seriously and treated vigorously.

Most addicts experience a return of drug craving after being withdrawn from opiates, however gradually, and usually resume their use of narcotics. The traditional psychologic theory of relapse suggests that after detoxification, the psychologic causes of drug dependence have been removed, but that addicts have an "addictive personality" disorder that causes them to continue to take drugs. Evidence is accumulating that metabolic and neurophysiologic changes persist long after the detoxification process has been completed, as does some tolerance. This protracted abstinence syndrome, may be associated with the commonly reported experience of drug hunger and the high incidence of relapse. A similar protracted abstinence syndrome may exist with general depressants and alcohol. Conditioned associations are also involved in the experience of recurrent drug craving. Narcotic addiction with its implicit relapses after abstinent periods should be viewed as a disease of complex etiology in which profound neurochemical, psychological, and social factors determine the drug-seeking behavior.

ADVERSE REACTIONS

When a known dose of an opiate is taken under aseptic conditions, medical complications are almost unknown. The patterns of use, including unknown and markedly variable doses, nonsterile needles, syringes, and drug, the variety of adulterants used to dilute the opiate, and the often violent life style are responsible for the extensive morbidity and mortality (estimated to be about 1 to 2% per year) associated with opiate abuse.

More than three-quarters of all narcotics deaths are caused by acute heroin reactions. The syndrome is marked by the acute onset of cyanosis, pulmonary edema, respiratory distress, and coma. Whereas a portion of these reactions may be attributable to true pharmacologic overdoses, others may be a result of opiate-induced cardiac arrhythmias or hypoxia, acute reactions to adulterants, and allergic reactions. Most other adverse effects are due to infections in various organ systems, including skin abscesses and cellulitis, bacterial endocarditis, and viral hepatitis. These are covered in detail in textbooks of medicine.

TREATMENT

Narcotic Dependence. Every attempt should be made to reach young people early before they have severed their community and educational-system ties and while it is still possible for them to develop the skills and tastes necessary to succeed in the "straight" world. Then, too, the impact of pharmacological and conditioning factors will be far less significant than in "hard-core" addicts with a history of 10 or 20 years of heroin addiction. However, many adolescents are still enjoying the excitement of the narcotic-dependent life; they have not yet experienced the almost inevitable associated pain and degradation. It is often difficult to get these people into treatment, and once in, it is very difficult to hold them. If possible, patients should be withdrawn from narcotics at the outset of treatment. In some cases, particularly those with a long history of opiate use and repeated treatment failures, it may be necessary to provide methadone maintenance for varying periods of time.

Narcotic Withdrawal Syndrome. Detoxification with decreasing doses of oral methadone is the most effective, humane method of withdrawing people from narcotics. This should be done on an in-patient basis if the patient's condition necessitates close medical or psychological supervision. Out-patient detoxification is indicated in well-motivated people who are already involved in a treatment program. Doses ranging from 20 to 40 mg daily are instituted, followed by a gradual reduction of dosage to zero over the course of 2 weeks, or longer if possible. Since the disease tends to be chronic and the relapse rate after detoxification is extremely high, provisions must be made for referral of all patients to an appropriate long-term treatment program.

Patients who are dependent on a sedative hypnotic in addition to an opiate should be withdrawn in an in-patient setting. Optimally, the patient should be withdrawn from the depressant initially, while the methadone dose is maintained at a level sufficient to allay any abstinence symptoms yet low enough to prevent excessive sedation (20 to 40 mg). When the depressant withdrawal is completed, the opiate detoxification might proceed. Under some circumstances, e.g., incarceration in correctional institutions, it is necessary to detoxify patients from both classes of drugs simultaneously.

Long-term Treatment. Since addiction has psychological, physiological, and social determinants, treatment is most effectively provided by a well-organized team approach rather than by individual practitioners.

Psychosocial Approaches—Abstinence Programs. A multitude of programs exists, of varying philosophies and competence, that emphasize abstinence from opiates as a primary form of treatment. If an adolescent is willing, he should probably be admitted to one of these inpatient therapeutic communities for protracted periods of time, perhaps 1 to 2 years. These have been discussed in a previous section. The particular community selected should have enthusiastic leadership, strong professional backup, provide extensive rehabilitative services, and be culturally appropriate for a particular youngster. Psychologically disabled, polydrug-abusing patients require this extensive supportive system. Patients often leave prematurely ("split") or refuse to enter because they are loath to leave their friends or family to enter so narrow a world. Some young addicts are unable to cope with the stringent rules of the community, and others want to return to the street life. Provisions must be made for prolonged follow-up of these people, with alternate referral attempts. In selected cases, out-patient treatment programs have met with a measure of success. Therapeutic communities are valuable for many people, though the relapse rates on return to society are high and follow-up studies are presently inadequate.

Since many young people are arrested because of drug abuse, many states have developed alternatives to jail which involve the nonpunitive incarceration of drug-dependent people for the purposes of rehabilitation (civil commitment). These programs generally include a period in a locked facility, followed by close supervision of the individual in the community. If renewed drug abuse or other antisocial behavior is noted, the addict is reinstitutionalized. These programs have been hampered by a lack of rehabilitative services, unskilled treatment personnel, and poor leadership.

As noted earlier, traditional out-patient psychotherapeutic techniques alone have not been effective for the majority of adolescent opiate abusers, particularly when a patient's drug use continues. Psychotherapy is useful in encouraging a patient to enter a therapeutic community or methadone program. It is also indicated in the treatment of well-motivated people once abstinence is achieved or the drug dependence is controlled as in a methadone program. Group therapy, behavioral techniques, and medication in combination are effective in certain circumstances, as we have outlined previously.

Methadone Treatment. Treatment with methadone is being developed for "hard-core" adolescent addicts who had a long history of addiction, repeated treatment failures, and who refuse other forms of treatment. Methadone treatment derives from the two major properties that distinguish methadone from the other narcotics: good oral efficacy and long duration of action. Oral methadone is administered daily in doses sufficient to allay abstinence symptoms and stabilized such that patients will be tolerant to the euphoric effects of the drug and experience no drug craving. In adolescent patients, the "maintenance" dose should be kept as low as possible (30–50 mg). Optimally, medication should be dispensed in a clinic situation that provides medical care and extensive rehabilitative services so as to facilitate reentry into society. To these ends, close ties might be maintained with vocational-training programs and schools. Long-term methadone maintenance has been shown to be medically safe, with minimal side effects when properly administered. Performance and learning are normal in methadone-maintained subjects.

Programs utilizing methadone maintenance for varying periods of time (6 months to 2 years) followed by a slow detoxification process, have shown promise in the treatment of adolescent addicts. The model of a day hospital or out-patient therapeutic community utilizing methadone may be useful in this population as well. A variable percentage of patients in methadone treatment will abuse other drugs and may become dependent on sedative-hypnotics or alcohol or both. These patients often require an in-patient detoxification and intensive psychotherapy if these are available. Referral to a therapeutic community may be necessary after detoxification.

ALCOHOL

Just as their parents, adolescents use and abuse alcohol more than any of the other psychoactive drugs. Similarly, it is often difficult to distinguish between social and/or normal drinking and patterns of alcohol consumption that could be termed abuse. It is useful to define alcohol abuse as drinking that adversely affects an individual's physical or psychosocial functioning. The term "alcoholism" is ambiguous and has been used to refer to a wide range of drinking patterns ranging from alcohol use that is considered deviant for a given social group to alcohol addiction characterized by compulsive use and physical dependence.

Patterns of Abuse

The vast majority of young people begin drinking in association with friends at social functions. They also often have parents who drink. Most will continue to drink in a manner acceptable to their cultural milieu. As noted, there are no predictive psychological or social variables to determine which of the great number of adolescents who experiment with alcohol will develop into problem drinkers.

Inner-city youths begin drinking early, sometimes at 10 to 12 years of age, and often in association with drug-taking of other kinds. Middle-class and suburban young men and women may begin drinking at an older age. Alcohol is legal, relatively inexpensive, and therefore accessible to most young people. Some youngsters will drink and take other drugs to get as "stoned" as possible to be able to fully enjoy particular events or gatherings. A few of these will come to depend on the alcohol for satisfactory functioning and will begin drinking daily, perhaps alone, to ward off depression and often to enable them to fall asleep. The depression, anxiety, and inability to sleep that follow a day of heavy alcohol intake may be a strong reinforcement of drinking behavior the next day. This combination of psychic dependence and early physical dependence may lead to an addictive pattern, where the use of alcohol and other drugs dominate the user's life.

The normal or neurotic adolescent who develops an alcohol problem may be reacting to an acute or chronic stressful situation such as loss of a loved one or the fear of sexual inadequacy based on several threatening experiences. Often the drug and alcohol use lead to a deterioration of the life situation. The psychopathology noted may be in large part a reaction to the alcohol use rather than an etiological factor.

Alcohol is used as a disinhibiting "social lubricant" in withdrawn, alienated, schizoid personalities. For the "borderline" it provides an escape from reality; for the passive, dependent personality it may produce infantile passivity and narcissism. There is some evidence that alcohol may act as an antipsychotic tranquilizer, though in other patients it may allow a latent psychotic to act out his psychosis without concomitant anxiety.

Pharmacology

In general, psychoactive effects are similar to those of other general depressants or tranquilizers. At low doses, anxiety is reduced and individuals may perform better in social situations. Low doses may also enhance sexual competence and pleasure. Moderate dosage impairs visual-motor coordination, though auditory and tactile sensations are unchanged. Sustained attention to stimuli becomes difficult and judgment is impaired. Sexual performance is generally impaired, also. The degree of intoxication in nontolerant social drinkers depends on the amount of alcohol consumed and correlates roughly with blood alcohol levels. Absorption of alcohol is delayed by the ingestion of food or congeners in beverage alcohol. The consumption of 180 ml of distilled spirits on an empty stomach will produce a blood-alcohol level of 100 mg per 100 ml, which is associated with a state of mild inebriation. At blood levels above 200 mg per 100 ml, gross intoxication and sedation occur. Continued, frequent drinking leads to the development of tolerance such that chronic alcohol abusers are able to function effectively and appear sober even at high blood alcohol levels. The range of tolerance is narrow compared to that for the depressants or the opiates. Whereas opiate addicts may use amounts 100 times in excess of their initial intake, blood alcohol exceeding 450 mg per 100 ml would generally be seen only in association with severe somnolence and coma. The lethal level of alcohol in alcohol-dependent adolescents is similar to that of normal drinkers and is in the range of 500 to 600 mg per 100 ml.

Cross-tolerance between alcohol and the general depressants occurs, though not between the opiates and alcohol. When alcohol and depressants are taken together, synergism and/or potentiation of psychoactive effects may occur. Some synergism or potentiation may also occur with opiates. The combination of alcohol with various depressants has proven to be lethal as a result of these additive effects.

Psychoactive effects also depend on the personality of the user and the setting. If a youngster consumes alcohol at a rock concert or party where inebriation is expected, it is likely that he will get drunk. At the same time, individuals who fear the consequences of drunkenness, may occasionally be able to maintain a sober demeanor despite high consumption.

Addiction and Withdrawal Process

After acute intoxication, the generalized discomfort, headache, nausea, diarrhea, agitation, mild tremulousness, depression, and inability to sleep, termed the "hangover," may be the equivalent of the first signs and symptoms of a withdrawal syndrome. Continued drinking in high concentrations for prolonged periods will increase the severity of this syndrome, which is now characterized by the development of tremulousness as early as 6 hours after cessation of drinking, and usually remits or is significantly diminished by the third day. Auditory and visual hallucinations may occur in association with the tremulous state. Seizures may occur from 12 to 24 hours after termination of drinking, are grand mal in type, and generally are followed by a postictal state. Youthful alcohol addicts usually have not been drinking long enough to develop frank delirium tremens, though this does occur. It is marked by confusion, disorientation, delusions, hallucinations, psychomotor agitation, and autonomic dysfunction. This syndrome, which peaks from 72 to 96 hours after cessation of drinking, is a potentially lethal illness that requires hospitalization and intensive care.

The acute withdrawal syndrome is followed by persistent withdrawal symptomatology characterized by tremulousness, anxiety, depression, and insomnia lasting up to 6 months after the cessation of drinking. This symptom complex may act as a physical and psychological reinforcement to the inital causative pathology.

Adverse Reactions

The chronic abuse of alcohol may lead to a variety of medical disorders including gastritis, pancreatitis, and liver disease, The combination of alcohol abuse and poor dietary intake may rarely result in peripheral neuropathies marked by motor and sensory impairment in the upper and lower extremities, pain, paresthesias, and even paralysis.

Alcohol abuse is a significant factor in accidents of all kinds as well as in situations which result from violent and aggressive behavior. More than half of all highway and nonhighway fatalities involve individuals who have been drinking, and evidence suggests that the majority of alcohol-related automobile fatalities may result not from episodic acute intoxication but from chronic intoxication or addiction. Homicide, assault, and other violent crimes occur frequently in settings where the perpetrator, the victim, or both are intoxicated. Alcohol abuse is considered to be a factor in adolescent suicide as well.

Treatment

It is often difficult to obtain an accurate drinking history even when an adolescent is willing to discuss other drug use. Dependence on alcohol suggests weakness and may not convey the sense of romance that is implicit in some other drug-use patterns. A realistic, encouraging, non-judgmental attitude on the part of the examiner will facilitate the history taking and prepare the way for therapeutic intervention.

Alcohol Withdrawal Syndrome. It is necessary to attempt to interrupt the drinking pattern as quickly as possible. Controversy exists as to whether effective psychotherapy may be accomplished when a patient is drinking; at any rate, patients should be maintained in treatment though they continue to drink, and a variety of means should be attempted to change this behavior pattern. If compulsive use and physical dependence are suspected, it may be necessary to hospitalize or otherwise remove the youngster from his drinking milieu.

All patients should be observed for mild withdrawal signs and symptoms for a period of several hours, to determine whether the syndrome is abating or beginning to develop. If the symptoms abate, it may be possible to treat the patient in an office or clinic setting. If possible, an in-patient milieu should be sought for the initial stages of treatment, lasting several weeks to many months. Facilities vary, although alternatives to traditional psychiatric and medical facilities in the form of nonmedical detoxification centers or therapeutic communities have become available. If the patient presents with severe delirium tremens or the development of that syndrome appears likely, hospitalization in an intensive care setup is indicated on an emergency basis. In general, patients get better care and the incidence of complications is less in a facility that focuses on alcoholic or other drug-abusing patients.

Treatment should begin with a careful search for associated surgical and medical illnesses, particularly cerebral trauma, subdural hematoma, pneumonia, meningitis, and liver disease. The patient may be suffering from malnutrition, hypovitaminosis, and fluid and electorlyte disturbances. The severe degree of agitation and the profuse perspiration which characterize the fully developed form of the disease may require the use of 6000 ml of fluid and appropriate electrolyte replacement. It is good practice to give B vitamins in all cases, particularly thiamine intramuscularly, to prevent or treat Wernicke's encephalopathy.

Benzodiazepine derivatives, particularly diazepam and chlordiazepoxide, are indicated in doses sufficient to blunt the patient's agitation and to prevent exhaustion, yet not compromise the patient's ability to tolerate oral food and fluids or to take part in his environment. The absolute suppression of agitation and tremor often requires an amount of drug that could seriously depress respiration. Many centers use diazepam 10 mg p o Q I D and reduce the dosage to zero in 5 to 7 days. In extreme cases with intense agitation, intravenous medication might be used to induce a calm state, followed by 5 to 10 mg diazepam IM orally every 2 to 4 hours. The dosage should be adequate and continuous. The use of medication *as necessary* depending on signs or symptoms often leads to power struggles and/or complications.

It has been suggested that an element in severe delirium tremens is sensory deprivation. It is known that the hallucinations and agitation occur more frequently at night and often respond to reassurance of a personal nature. Patients should therefore be encouraged to be as active as possible, eating regularly and taking part in group activities. If possible, an authority figure, perhaps a nurse, aide, or specially trained counselor, should be in frequent attendance reassuring the patient when he hallucinates and continually providing cues to reality.

Long-term Treatment. As for other compulsive drug-abuse syndromes, individual group and family therapy, therapeutic communities, behavior-modification techniques, and drug therapy of psychopathology may be successful long-term approaches. Alcoholics Anonymous, so valuable for some adult alcoholics, has not heretofore been particularly useful in the treatment of the adolescent abuser or polydrug abuser, though adolescent groups are now being setablished.

Disulfiram (Antabuse) may be a valuable adjunct to other forms of treatment. As a potent aldehyde dehydrogenase inhibitor, it causes a build-up of acetaldehyde leading to the clinical picture of an alcohol-disulfiram reaction: nausea, vomiting, cramps, flushing, vasomotor collapse. It should not be used in patients with a history of psychosis, severe medical illness, or those taking an MAO inhibitor or isonicotinic acid hydrazide (Isoniazid). After a patient has abstained from alcohol for at least 12 hours, he should be given 250 mg in a single dose. Subsequently, he may be given 125 to 250 mg daily, preferably at night, since the sedation that some patients experience facilitates sleep. Therapy should be continued for many months, and in some cases for years.

CENTRAL NERVOUS SYSTEM DEPRESSANTS

Abuse of depressants by young people has increased significantly over the past decade. These drugs are manufactured in massive quantities by pharmaceutical companies and become available for abuse purposes through illicit diversion. Physicians' prescriptions also represent a drug source for some adolescents, either directly or indirectly via theft or sale from adults. All drugs in this class are subject to abuse. The most commonly used "downs" for "nonmedical" purposes are the short-acting barbiturates, secobarbital (Seconal, "reds"), pentobarbital (Nembutal, "yellows"), and secobarbital and amobarbital (Tuinal, "double trouble"), and assorted other hypnotics such as glutethimide (Doriden), methaqualone (Quāālude, "sopers"). Recently, diazepam (Valium) and amitriptyline (Elavil) have been increasingly abused for their depressant properties.

Patterns of Abuse

Many young people occasionally use low doses of these drugs, in combination with alcohol or marijuana, to get "high" for a concert or a party or to enhance their sexual performance. Other youngsters use large quantities of these drugs on a daily basis in order to function and may be compulsive users of alcohol and opiates as well. In this milieu the acquisition and use of drugs becomes a primary focus of living. In many of these disturbed youngsters, the drug use may represent self-medication for intolerable internal or external experience.

The "high" that depressant users describe may be compared to the sense of peace or numbness that occurs just prior to sleep in normal individuals. Anxiety and inhibitions are blunted and the world is limited to the immediate. There may be a feeling of freedom or aggressiveness that sometimes leads to antisocial or violent behavior. At low doses some individuals experience enhanced sexual pleasure and ability, but high doses impair sexual performance. Some users seem to be seeking an obtundation that is close to unconsciousness, in an attempt to cope with anxiety or pain.

Pharmacology

Central nervous system effects vary from mild sedation to coma depending on the drug, the dose, the route of administration, the excitability of the nervous system, and tolerance. Small doses may produce an initial stimulation similar to that derived from alcohol. Duration of action varies with the particular drug. After-effects, including impairment of performance and judgment, depression, drowsiness, and irritability, may persist for many hours.

Tolerance develops rapidly to all central nervous system depressants. The lethal dose of depressants varies, though in distinction to the opiates, the range between this dose for tolerant and nontolerant individuals is significantly narrower. When more than ten times the hypnotic dose is taken at one time, overdose may occur. Acute poisoning therefore occurs in a setting of chronic intoxication. The combination of sublethal doses of depressants, alcohol, or opiates may also result in overdose. Cross-tolerance occurs between all depressants. Partial cross-tolerance occurs between alcohol and the depressants.

Adverse Effects

Acute depressant poisoning (overdose) varies in severity from mild intoxication to coma and occurs both accidentally and incident to suicide attempts in adolescent and preadolescent populations. The signs and symptoms of intoxication resemble those of alcohol intoxication, with individuals showing sluggishness, slurred speech, slowness of thinking and movement, narrowed attention span, and emotional lability. Neurologic examination demonstrates nystagmus, diplopia, strabismus, vertigo, ataxia, positive Romberg's sign, hypotonia, dysmetria, and decreased superficial reflexes.

ADDICTION AND WITHDRAWAL PROCESS

Physical dependence as indicated by withdrawal signs and symptoms develops to all the general depressants and is similar to the symptoms of the alcohol withdrawal syndrome. It varies in severity depending on the drug, dose, and frequency of use, though in contrast to the opiate abstinence syndrome, it may be life threatening. The withdrawal syndrome produced when short-acting sedatives are withdrawn is more abrupt in onset and more severe than with the longer-acting sedatives and tranquilizers.

After discontinuation of only therapeutic doses of sedatives, the first manifestation of the withdrawal syndrome may be the rebound increase in rapid-eye-movement sleep that is associated with a sense of having slept badly and vivid nightmares. After 0.6 gm per day of pentobarbital or its equivalent for 1 or 2 months, approximately half of the patients experience insomnia, tremors, anorexia, and irritability, and 10% may have a seizure. Higher doses lead to an increased incidence of seizures and the development of a delirium that is characterized by disorientation to time and place, auditory and visual hallucinations, and sensorial clouding. Increased irritability and seizures usually occur within the first 3 days after withdrawal, and the delirium usually occurs between the fourth and seventh days and may be associated with hyperthermia, tachycardia, agitation, and cardiovascular collapse. The syndrome generally clears by about the eighth day, though with long-acting barbiturates and the benzodiazepines, seizures may not occur until the seventh or eighth day. Persistent psychotic symptoms over many months probably relate to preexisting psychopathology.

TREATMENT

Mild depressant intoxication or poisoning requires only supportive reassurance. If severe poisoning is suspected, emergency hospitalization and intensive care is indicated. If physical dependence is suspected, close observation or hospitalization is mandatory. When the diagnosis is confirmed, a suitable general depressant should be administered after the intoxication clears but before major withdrawal symptoms have begun. Phenobarbital orally is suitable substitution therapy for most of the sedatives, though Diazepam or pentobarbital may also be used. Patients who are taking lesser known sedatives should probably be withdrawn from the original drug of abuse if it is known. Sufficient doses of the depressant should be given to produce a mild but manageable level of intoxication marked by ataxia, dysarthria, and lateral nystagmus. Phenobarbital withdrawal usually requires approximately one sedative dose (30 mg) for each hypnotic dose of the sedative that the patient has been using, given in divided doses 3–4 times daily. A test dose may be necessary but in no case should the initial daily dose exceed 600 mg. Patients may be stabilized at this level for 1 to 2 days, after which the dose should be reduced by 30 mg or less daily. The patient should be closely observed for signs of increased withdrawal, such as tremulousness and insomnia, at which time the withdrawal regimen should be suspended for 1 to 2 days. If symptoms are severe, additional phenobarbital may be given. Delirium and fever should be treated vigorously, but once established, the delirium may persist for several days. Phenothiazines or butyrophenones, may lower the seizure threshold and are not indicated nor is diphenylhydantoin. In general, the pentobarbital substitution technique may take from 10 days to 3 weeks. It should not be hurried but may be concurrent. In combined addictions, if possible, the withdrawal of the depressant should precede that of the opiates.

Compulsive abusers of depressants, alone or in combination with other drugs, are considered more difficult to treat than any other class of adolescent drug abuser. The incidence of severe psychopathology is higher in this group; they are frequently withdrawn, depressed, and may be suicidal. The course is characteristically marked by frequent relapses, use of a wide variety of drugs, and antisocial or intoxicated behavior while in treatment. It is often necessary to secure long-term hospitalization or residence in a therapeutic community for many of these young people, since they are unable to function in society without strong supports.

STIMULANTS

The most frequently abused drugs in this category ("ups," "speed") include the amphetamine group made up of amphetamine, dextroamphetamine, and methamphetamine, all synthetic derivatives of ephedrine, and cocaine, an alkaloid of the coca plant, which grows in the Andes. Other stimulants that are subject to abuse are methylphenidate (Ritalin), phenmetrazine (Preludin), and diethylpropion (Tepanil).

Patterns of Abuse

Stimulant use by hard-driving students, athletes, and musicians who want to increase their efficiency or productivity is common. Most often the drugs are taken orally, used intermittently, and produce virtually no dependence. Rarely, individuals find they must continue to take the drugs at ever-increasing doses in order to perform satisfactorily. Depressants are often used to ensure sleep, and concurrent dependence on both drugs may occur.

A distinctly different pattern of abuse occurs in polydrug-abusing adolescents when the stimulants are used primarily for their mood-elevating properties ("the high"). Methamphetamine ("crystal," "meth") is the preferred agent since it has the most powerful central effects. The drugs are most often sniffed or injected intramuscularly or intravenously, though they are also taken orally. The "rush" that occurs after sniffing or injection is described as a feeling of great well-being, physical power, and intelligence. There is little need for food and sleep, and users often plan and discuss ambitious projects for many hours. The drug effects are dissipated after 4 to 6 hours and may be experienced as an unpleasant sense of depression ("coming down," "crashing"). Chronic users ("speed freaks") of stimulants often have severe personality or affective disorders. The drug use decreases their depression and anxiety, improves their general level of functioning, and may even enhance their ability to eat and sleep. Use of these drugs may become compulsive and result in "runs" of days or even weeks, to maintain the good feeling or, more importantly, to stave off the "crash." The development of tolerance requires the use of increasing doses at ever more frequent intervals so that 1 gm might be injected every 2 to 4 hours. At this stage, the compulsive user may be irritable and paranoid and characteristically involves himself in complicated, often unnecessary tasks such as reorganizing or painting a room or taking a television set apart. When the drug supply ends or the user becomes too disorganized to continue, the "run" ends. Depressants or alcohol, sometimes in large quantities, are often used to minimize the duration and intensity of the "crashing" phase and induce sleep. Following a stimulant "run," there is generally a period of prolonged sleep, from which the user will emerge feeling depressed and apathetic. All other drugs may be used in combination with the stimulants; the combination of heroin and either amphetamines or cocaine is termed a "speed ball."

Patterns of abuse of cocaine, like those for amphetamines, run the gamut from intermittent sniffing of the much-adulterated white powder by well-functioning youngsters to compulsive intravenous use by severely disturbed people. Psychoactive effects include improvement of mood, increased energy, and decreased need for food or sleep, but cocaine is much shorter acting and much more expensive than the amphetamines. It is used in "runs" such that from 1 to 10 gms might be taken in a single day. Recently the use of the drug by affluent and middle-class adolescents has increased explosively; it is regarded as luxurious punctuation for a variety of occasions, to be used in conjunction with alcohol and marijuana.

Pharmacology

In low doses, stimulants increase alertness, physical and cognitive ability, particularly when these have been compromised by lack of sleep. Tolerance develops to all of the amphetamine effects but apparently not to cocaine, except for a narrow degree of psychologic tolerance to the drug's euphoric properties, which dissipates rapidly. Cross-tolerance exists between the amphetamines, but not between the amphetamines and cocaine. Abrupt cessation of stimulant use does not produce major physiological symptoms. However, some workers feel that the depression, apathy, and prolonged sleep characterized by an increased percentage of rapid-eye-movement electroencephalographic patterns and the experience of nightmares might be considered an abstinence syndrome.

Adverse Effects

The intravenous use of these drugs involves the same complications of nonsterile conditions previously discussed in the section on opiates. Irritation or, rarely, perforation of the nasal septum is a complication of sniffing stimulants. Chronic users describe a sensation of something crawling under their skin ("cocaine bugs") and may have excoriations and open sores from constant scratching. Severe overdose reactions or death from these drugs is rare. Extensions of the sympathomimetic effects with possible convulsions and cerebrovascular accidents is a rare complication. Inflammation of the blood vessels or hepatitis resulting from direct toxic effects of methamphetamine has been reported but requires clarification. Large intravenous dosages of cocaine may act directly on heart muscle to cause cardiac arrhythmias. The lethal dose of amphetamines is varied depending on tolerance; that of cocaine is estimated to be about 1.2 gms.

There is often considerable preexisting psychopathology in compulsive stimulant abusers, and the abuse itself engenders severe psychological complications. The most frequent adverse effects are paranoid ideation and stereotyped, compulsive behavior. Experienced users are often aware of these reactions and will not act on paranoid ideas or delusions. When this insight is lost, antisocial or irrational behavior results. Continued use may lead to an amphetamine or cocaine psychosis that may be clinically indistinguishable from acute paranoid schizophrenia. Psychotic episodes may be inevitable in all people if the stimulant dose and frequency of use are continually increased or high doses maintained. The preexisting personality structure may determine the ease with which these ego disruptions occur; psychotic breaks have been precipitated in some individuals after only one small dose of amphetamine. The etiology of these pathological states may be related to the ability of the amphetamines and cocaine to inhibit the re-uptake inactivation of the catecholamines, dopamine, and norepinephrine, and thereby potentiate their synaptic effects. The psychotic reactions appear while the individual is drug influenced and most often abate within a few days to several weeks after drug use ceases. Prolonged psychotic episodes have been precipitated and probably relate to the premorbid personality structure.

Treatment

Treatment will depend on the pattern of abuse and the individual personality characteristics of the user. Many adolescents using varying quantities of these drugs require no treatment at all. Others using these drugs intermittently may benefit from advice as to the actual dangers, and encouragement to the effect that they can perform satisfactorily without the drugs. Compulsive users of stimulants should be helped to terminate their use as quickly as possible. It may be necessary to hospitalize some adolescents or, if possible, confine them in a safe, supportive environment to attempt to alleviate some of the anxiety of withdrawal. Short-term hospitalization and appropriate psychotropic medication is indicated for the treatment of severe paranoid ideation or overt psychotic episodes. Following stimulant withdrawal, depressive symptoms should be sought and the possibility of suicide considered. Compulsive or polydrug abusers will require long-term supportive care as described in previous sections.

Physicians should prescribe these drugs with great caution. Some authorities suggest that narcolepsy and the childhood hyperkinetic disorders are the only medical indications for the amphetamines.

CANNABIS (MARIJUANA AND HASHISH)

Cannabis in its various forms has become an integral part of the youth culture in this country; estimates suggest that between 30 and 40 million Americans have used the drug and that more than 70% of some adolescent populations report its use. Both marijuana and hashish are derived from the hemp plant, *cannabis sativa*, which contains varying amounts of the major psychoactive compound, delta-9-tetrahydrocannabinal. Marijuana refers to the dried mixture of leaves, flowering tops, seeds, and stems of the plant; hashish is the compressed resin secreted by the flowering tops and is four to eight times more potent than marijuana.

Patterns of Abuse

Geographical, social, and cultural considerations are important in determining whether an adolescent will use cannabis and at what age. Personality characteristics influence the frequency and patterns of abuse. In some inner-city areas as well as some affluent suburbs, young people begin smoking at 10 to 14 years of age. In other situations, the first exposure may not be until high school. Some use of alcohol often precedes marijuana use, though other drugs do not generally come into the picture until later. Many young people experiment with the drug and do not continue its use; others use it intermittently, often in groups where the ritual of preparing and smoking a "joint" may be a major focus of social interaction. A few adolescents develop a compulsive use pattern, where the acquisition, use, and discussion of cannabis become the primary life concerns. Other drugs are often used in conjunction with large quantities of marijuana. These are often severely disturbed people who function poorly and in whom the drugs represent an attempt at self-medication. Many youngsters of borderline or psychotic personality organizations present as "heads," or compulsive users.

Marijuana is usually smoked in homemade cigarettes, "joints." Hashish is smoked in a variety of small pipes. Both preparations may be ingested in combination with a variety of foods and drinks. The potency of the material varies markedly, though they are three to four times more potent when smoked than when taken orally.

Pharmacology

After inhalation, effects begin within minutes, peak within 1 hour, and are dissipated within 3 hours. Oral ingestion delays the onset and prolongs the effects. The acute physiologic effects are dose-related and include conjunctival vascular congestion, an increased heart rate, dryness of mouth and throat, fine tremors of fingers, and altered sleep patterns. Orthostatic hypotension and loss of consciousness occur rarely.

Psychoactive effects are highly variable and depend on the dose, the route of administration, the personality of the user, his prior experience with the drug, his personal expectations and those of his group, and the social setting in which the drug is used. Users describe an altered and often enhanced perception of visual, auditory, tactile, and gustatory stimuli. Mood changes are complex and labile. A sense of relaxed well-being is frequently reported, though anxiety and depression may also be precipitated. Drowsiness or hilarious hyperactivity may occur. Time seems to pass slowly and short-term memory may be impaired. Motor performance, particularly of complex tasks such as driving in traffic, is impaired as is reaction time. Although heightened attention may be responsible for the enhanced sensory perception, alterations in attention span are probably responsible for the reported decrements in performance and cognitive function.

A variable degree of tolerance develops to the psychologic and physiologic effects of the drug such that naive users demonstrate greater decrements in performance and increased physical effects as compared with chronic users. At the same time, a learning process appears to be involved since inexperienced users of cannabis report fewer subjective effects and get less "high."

Adverse Effects

Adverse physical effects of acute or chronic cannabis use have been of little clinical significance and no deaths have been reported. Interference with DNA and RNA synthesis, interference with pituitary function and, in turn, testosterone production, and disruption of the immunological system are possible toxic effects under current investigation.

Adverse effects are generally psychologic in nature, infrequent, and similar to those seen with psychedelic drugs. The acute panic reaction, transient paranoid ideation, and depression are the most common and usually abate in several hours. Prolonged psychotic reactions have been precipitated by cannabis though it is probable that significant psychopathology was present prior to the drug use. Higher doses are associated with an increase in these reactions. The cannabis-induced lability of affect and altered perceptions may be sufficiently disordering for the individual of borderline personality adjustments to precipitate an acute psychotic break. An acute brain syndrome, or toxic delirium, has also been reported with cannabis use. "Flashback" phenomena similar to those seen with psychedelic use, occur infrequently.

An "amotivational syndrome" has been described, in which chronic heavy users of cannabis demonstrate impaired goal-directed activity, apathy, inability to master new problems, and magical thinking. This has not been documented by extensive field studies here or abroad. Although no evidence of psychological deterioration from chronic use has been documented, it is nonetheless likely that preexisting psychopathology may be aggravated so that users become less able to function effectively.

Many people who derive enjoyment from the use of cannabis do, in fact, then experiment with other drugs. If one took no drugs, including alcohol and nicotine, obviously there could be no progression to harder drugs. However, it is clear that the psychobiological and social predisposition of a youngster is more important in the development of severe drug problems than whether he or she has ever used marijuana or alcohol.

Treatment

Treatment of the frequently seen acute reactions is firm, supportive reassurance. The patient should be continually reminded that he is feeling this way because of the drug that he took and that the effects will wear off shortly ("talking down"). Tranquilizers may be indicated in aggressive or violent states.

PSYCHEDELICS

In this country, the most frequently abused drugs comprising this category are related to the indolealkylamines, such as synthetic lysergic acid diethylamide (LSD, "acid"), psilocybin ("magic mushrooms"), psilocin, dimethyltryptamine (DMT), and diethyltryptamine (DET), or to the phenylethylamines, such as mescaline, which is derived from the peyote cactus, and the substituted amphetamines, such as 2,5-dimethoxy-4-methylamphetamine (DOM, "STP"). Phencyclidine ("angel dust"), actually an anesthetic agent, has been abused for its psychedelic effects. These drugs produce bizarre alterations in perception, thought, feeling, and behavior, and are sometimes classified as hallucinogens or psychotomimetics.

Patterns of Abuse

Psychedelic use has primarily been among middle-class, white, educated youth in this country who are seeking a mystical, enriching experience. Use peaked to an estimated 500,000 to 1 million range in the 1967–69 period, when the media-popularized youth culture developed complex metaphysical and religious beliefs as well as a social style that supported the search for altered states of consciousness. The pervasive feelings of boredom, emptiness, and lack of meaning in many young people's experience contributed to the popularity of psychedelic drugs. The apparent recent decline in use may be related primarily to a disillusionment with this class of drugs as any kind of answer to life's problems, though fear of adverse effects of the drugs and of increasingly stringent legal penalties also may play a role.

Most of the psychedelic drugs available through illicit channels, whatever they were claimed to be, have actually consisted of LSD in differing doses. It is usually synthesized in illegal laboratories and made available in liquid, impregnated sugar cubes or paper, capsules, and tablets, that are orally ingested. Users are ordinarily unaware of the dose they ingest. Use is generally intermittent, varying from one "trip" weekly, monthly, or yearly. The drug is usually taken in groups so that support is available in the event of an acute panic reaction or "bad trip." Naive users will often be attended by a guide experienced with the drug effects. It is well recognized that a supportive, safe environment facilitates an enriching experience ("good trip"). Rarely, some adolescents take the drug more often ("acid heads"), such that they may remain intoxicated for prolonged periods. These people often have psychotic or borderline personality disorders and the drug use becomes an integral part of a delusional system.

Pharmacology

LSD is more than 100 times more potent than psilocybin and 4,000 times more potent than mescaline in producing psychoactive effects. The usual street dose varies from 100–400 μg and produces central sympathomimetic stimulation within 20 minutes after ingestion, characterized by mydriasis, hyperthermia, tachycardia, hypertension, piloerection, increased alertness, and facilitation of reflexes. Nausea and vomiting occasionally occur.

Psychoactive effects are fully manifest within 1 to 2 hours, though they vary markedly depending on the personality and expectations of the user, the setting, and the dose. Perceptions are heightened, distorted, and may be experienced as overwhelming. Afterimages are prolonged and overlap with ongoing perceptions. Objects may seem to waver or melt. Illusions and synesthesias, the overflow of one sense modality into another, are common. Thoughts may assume extraordinary importance or clarity, and body distortions are commonly perceived. Time may seem to pass very slowly. The self may be experienced as mystically boundless and the world as possessed of unlimited and profound meaning. True hallucinations with loss of insight rarely occur, though some apparently susceptible people have them repeatedly. Mood is labile, remarkably variable, and may range from euphoric grandiosity to paranoid reactions marked by depression and panic. The syndrome generally begins to clear after 10 to 12 hours, and distorted perceptions, tension, or fatigue may persist for an additional 24 hours. Tolerance to LSD develops rapidly, such that repeated daily doses become ineffective in 3 to 4 days. Cross-tolerance has been demonstrated between most of the psychedelics, implying some common mechanism of action. Physical dependence does not occur to any of the psychedelics.

Adverse Effects

Acute physical toxicity is minimal at doses of the psychedelic drugs that produce marked psychological effects, and no toxic deaths have been reported. Increased chromosome breakage and an increased incidence of congenital defects in children born to LSD users has been reported, though the evidence is controversial. LSD may also disrupt the body's normal immunological system, but this has not been clinically significant. Phencyclidine toxicity, characterized by hypertension, hyperreflexia, seizures, and very rarely coma and death, has been reported.

The acute panic reaction ("bad trip," "freakout") is the most frequent complication of psychedelic use. This takes the classical forms of hysteria and paranoia, with sensations of breathlessness and fears of bodily harm, paralysis, and insanity most common. These symptoms abate in most instances as the drug effect is dissipated. Infrequently prolonged psychotic episodes may be precipitated. These are characterized by paranoid ideation, grandiosity, bizarre delusions and hallucinations, affectual disturbances, and may be clinically indistinguishable from the functional psychoses, but generally abate more rapidly or respond more readily to treatment. Depressive reactions have been triggered by the drug experience as well. "Flashback" phenomena, the recurrence of some aspect of a previous "trip" when the individual is not under the influence of the drug, occur. In general, these episodes are mild, though severe episodes with associated psychotic behavior have been reported. The relationship of the psychedelics to the functional psychoses requires further study. It is clear that adverse reactions and psychotic episodes occur more often in a setting of high doses of the drugs taken by emotionally disturbed young men and women in unstable or frightening situations. It is not clear whether the psychedelics can precipitate prolonged psychotic reactions in reasonably healthy young people. It is not surprising that polydrug abusers with psychopathology usually steer clear of this group of drugs after one or more bad experiences.

TREATMENT

Treatment of the acute panic reaction requires the provision of a warm, supportive environment, a well-lighted room, and someone in constant attendance. The youngster should be continually reminded that he has taken a psychedelic drug and that the strange things he is experiencing are part of the drug effect, happen to many people, and will pass in time. The consensual reality should be repeatedly and gently affirmed. Experienced users of the psychedelic drugs often provide the best treatment for these "bad trips." In particularly agitated patients, chlorpromazine 50–100 mg or diazepam 20–40 mg orally or intramuscularly may be used. "Flashbacks" are treated with reassurance, psychotherapy, or medication when they are severe. In general, these decrease with time if psychedelic use ceases. Treatment of prolonged psychotic episodes is similar to treatment of the functional psychoses and is discussed elsewhere in this volume.

MISCELLANEOUS INHALANTS

AMYL NITRITE

The inhalation of amyl nitrite ("poppers," "amies") is a widespread phenomenon in adolescent populations. Use is intermittent and characterized by an instantaneous feeling ("rush") of flushing, dizziness, hilarity, and rapid heart rate. Effects last for a few minutes. Adverse effects are rare, but may include postural hypotension with loss of consciousness.

ORGANIC SOLVENTS

"Sniffing" a wide range of organic solvents, particularly the toluene in glue, has received considerable attention from the mass media and law-enforcement agencies. It is likely that this publicity has contributed significantly to the incidence of this practice. The material is usually squeezed or sprayed into a plastic bag and the vapors inhaled. Psychoactive effects are short-lived and resemble the intoxication produced by alcohol. Adverse effects are rare though suffocation due to the plastic bag has occurred. Chronic exposure as in the case of industrial workers may have serious adverse effects. Aerosol sprays containing fluorocarbon propellants have been inhaled as a means to get "high." Adverse effects are not known as yet though cardiac arrhythmias are a potentially serious complication.

NITROUS OXIDE

Some youthful populations obtain cannisters of this gas for recreational purposes. Inhalation produces a short-lived experience of intoxication and hilarity. Adverse effects are rare; forced inhalation of nitrous oxide could produce respiratory depression.

TREATMENT

Treatment of young people who use these inhalants will depend on the individual personality characteristics. Chronic glue sniffers, though rarely seen, are often reported to be severely disturbed. On the other hand, the intermittent use of amyl nitrite or nitrous oxide may occur in normal adolescents.

REFERENCES

BERNSTEIN, B., and SHKUDA, A. N. The young drug user: Attitudes and obstacles to treatment. New York: Center for New York City Affairs, New School for Social Research, June 1974.

BIHARI, B. Drug dependency: Some etiological considerations. *The American Journal of Drug and Alcohol Abuse*, 1976, *3*(3), 409.

BRECHER, E. M., and Editors of Consumer Reports. *Licit and illicit drugs. The Consumers Union Report on narcotics, stimulants, depressants, inhalants, hallucinogens, and marijuana, including caffeine, nicotine, and alcohol.* Mount Vernon, N. Y.: Consumers Union, 1972.

CHERUBIN, C. E. A review of the medical complications of narcotic addiction. *International Journal of the Addiction*, 1968, *3*, 167.

DISHOTSKY N. I., LOUGHMAN, W. D., MOGAR, R. E., and LIPSCOMB, W. R. LSD and genetic damage. *Science*, 1971, *172*, 431.

DOLE, V. P. Narcotic addiction, physical dependence and relapse. *New England Journal of Medicine*, 1972, *206*, 988.

DOLE, V. P., and NYSWANDER, M. A medical treatment for diacetylmorphine (heroin) addiction. *Journal of the American Medical Association*, 1965, *193*, 646.

ERIKSON E. H. *Childhood and society* (2nd ed.). New York: Norton, 1963.

FENICHEL, O. *The psychoanalytic theory of neurosis*. New York: Norton, 1945.

ISBELL, H., ALTSCHUL, S., KORNETSKY, C. H., EISENMAN, A. J., FLANARY, H. G., and FRASER, H. F. Chronic barbiturate intoxication. An experimental study. *Archives of Neurological Psychiatry*, 1950, *64*, 1.

JAFFE, J. Narcotic analgesics and Drug addiction and drug abuse. In L. S. Goodman and A. Gilman (Eds.), *The pharmacological basis of therapeutics* (5th ed.). New York: Macmillan, 1975.

KALANT, H., LEBLANC, A. E., and GIBBINS, R. J. Tolerance to, and dependence on, some nonopiate psychotropic drugs. *Pharmacological Review*, 1971, *23*, 135.

KANDEL, D., SINGLE, E., and KESSLER, R. C. The epidemiology of drug use among New York State high school students: Distribution, trends and change in rates of use. *American Journal of Public Health*, 1976, *66*(1), 43–53.

KAUFMAN, E. The psychodynamics of opiate dependence: a new look. *American Journal of Drug and Alcohol Abuse*, 1974, *1*(3), 349–370.

KERNBERG, O. F. *Borderline conditions and pathological narcissism*. New York: Jason Aronson, 1975.

KHANTZIAN, E. J. Opiate addiction: A critique to theory and some implications for treatment. *American Journal of Psychotherapy*, 1974, *28*, 59–70.

KHANTZIAN, E. J., MACK, J. E., and SCHATZBERG, A. F. Heroin use as an attempt to cope: Clinical observations. *American Journal of Psychiatry*, 1974, *131*, 160–164.

KISSIN, B., and BLANE, H. T. *Medical and psychological treatment of alcoholism*. New York: Plenum Press, 1977.

MENDELSON, J. Alcohol abuse and alcohol related illness. In P. B. Beeson and W. McDermott (Eds.), *Textbook of medicine*. Philadelphia: W. B. Saunders Co., 1975.

MILKMAN, H., and FROSCH, W. A. On the preferential abuse of heroin and amphetamine. *Journal of Nervous and Mental Disease*, 1973, *156*(4), 242–248.

MILLMAN, R. B. Drug abuse in adolescence: Current issues. In E. Senay and V. Shorty (Eds.), *Developments in the field of drug abuse*. Proceedings of the First National Drug Abuse Conference, 1974. New York: National Association for the Prevention of Addiction to Narcotics, 1974.

MILLMAN, R. B. Drug abuse addiction and intoxication. In P. B. Beeson and W. McDermott (Eds.), *Textbook of medicine*. Philadelphia: W. B. Saunders Co., 1975.

MILLMAN, R. B., and KHURI, E. T. Drug abuse and the need for alternatives. In J. Schoolar

(Ed.), *Current issues in adolescent psychiatry*. New York: Brunner/Mazel, 1973.

OAKLEY, S. R. *Drugs, society and human behavior*. St. Louis: C. V. Mosby, 1972.

PLUM, F. Acute drug poisoning. In P. B. Beeson and W. McDermott (Eds.), *Textbook of medicine*. Philadelphia. W. B. Saunders Co., 1975.

PREBLE, E., and CASEY, J. Taking care of business —the heroin user's life on the street. *International Journal of The Addictions*, 1969, *4*(1), 1–24.

RUBIN, V., and COMITAS, L. *Ganja in Jamaica*. The Hague and Paris: Mouton and Company, 1975.

SCHUCKIT, M. A., GOODWIN, D. A., and WINOKUR, G. A study of alcoholism in half-siblings. *American Journal of Psychiatry*, 1972, *128*, 1132–1136.

SNYDER, S. H. Catecholamines in the brain as mediators of amphetamine psychosis. *Archives of General Psychology*, 1972, *27*, 169.

A survey of substance use among junior and senior high school students in New York State. Report No. 1: Prevalence of Drug and Alcohol Use, Winter 1974/75. New York: New York State Office of Drug Abuse Services, 1975.

WURMSER, L. Psychoanalytic considerations of the etiology of compulsive drug use. *Journal of the American Psychoanalytic Association*, 1974, *22*, 820–843.

ZINBERG, N. E. Addiction and ego function. In R. S. Eissler, A. Freud, Marianne Kris, and A. J. Solnit (Eds.), *The psychoanalytic study of the child*. New Haven: Yale Univ. Press, 1975.

17

SEXUAL PROBLEMS: BEHAVIOR MODIFICATION[1]

George A. Rekers

A wide variety of sexual problems come to the attention of clinicians treating children and adolescents. Only a subset of these problems has been treated with behavior modification techniques, as reported in uncontrolled case studies. Even fewer of these sexual problems have been treated behaviorally in experimental studies using intrasubject replication or group designs to identify the treatment variables. Although behavioral intervention techniques for sex-related problems hold considerable promise, the area remains ripe for more systematic treatment research.

THE RANGE OF TARGET BEHAVIORS

The diagnostic term *sexual deviation* has been applied to "individuals whose sexual interests are directed primarily toward objects other than people of the opposite sex, toward sexual acts not usually associated with coitus, or toward coitus performed under bizarre circumstances as in necrophilia, pedophilia, sexual sadism, and fetishism. Even though many find their practices distasteful, they remain unable to substitute normal sexual behavior for them" (American Psychiatric Association, 1968, p. 44). It is beyond the scope and purpose of this chapter to review the complex diagnostic considerations involved in evaluating sexual adjustment of children. A competent clinical evaluation of a potential sexual problem requires familiarity with the literature on normal psychosexual development as well as the literature on deviant patterns. Treatment may be required for sexual behavior problems in childhood or adolescence before a firm diagnosis of "sexual deviation" is warranted. The wide range of target behaviors for intervention is suggested by the literature on normal and deviant sexual development cited in the "Additional Readings" section at the end of this chapter.

Virtually all child and adolescent sexual problems may be operationally defined in terms of target behaviors that may be amenable to behav-

[1]The writing of this chapter was supported, in part, by United States Public Health Service Research Grants MH21803 and MH28240, awarded to the author by the National Institute of Mental Health. The author conducted a major portion of this literature review at the library of the Institute for Sex Research at Indiana University, Bloomington, Indiana, and the helpful cooperation of the Institute is gratefully acknowledged. Appreciation is expressed to Kathy McCormick for her competent assistance in the bibliographic and editorial preparation of this manuscript.

ioral intervention. However, it appears that the behavior modification literature on sexual problems has been limited to the treatment of excessive masturbation and gender disturbances in childhood, and to fetishism, transvestism, sadism, exhibitionism, transsexualism, homosexuality, promiscuous sex behavior, and dating behavior deficits in adolescence. The main behavior modification studies are few enough to allow for a review of each one with enough detail on the treatment procedures to give the experienced behavior therapist a full grasp of the clinical intervention techniques that were applied.

SEXUAL PROBLEMS IN CHILDHOOD

Excessive Masturbation

Relatively little has been published on the treatment of "compulsive" public masturbation in children, although there have been several theoretical articles on the problem (e.g., Mertz, 1955; Hammerman, 1961). In 1932, Dunlap reported a case of compulsive masturbation successfully alleviated through the use of negative practice (Dunlap, 1932/1972; Lehner, 1960). There appears to be no empirical research on the behavioral treatment of inappropriate forms of masturbation in children, but an uncontrolled case report was published by Wagner (1968), who successfully trained a teacher to behaviorally treat the public masturbation of an 11-year-old girl in her classroom. The child masturbated almost constantly, frequently achieving obvious orgasm. With continuous, fixed interval and periodic reinforcement schedules, a variety of positive social reinforcements was used to shape and strengthen the incompatible responses of attending to academic assignments and participating in classroom activities. An aversive verbal contingency was applied to the occurrence of the masturbatory response. After 74 school days, the public masturbation had ceased entirely, the treatment effect persisting to the end of the first school year (the 129th day). A 4-month follow-up found no recurrence of the behavior.

Child Gender Identity and Gender Behavior Disturbances

Although major questions remain regarding the etiological variables in a deviant sex-role development (Bentler, 1976; Green, 1975; Money & Ehrhardt, 1972; A. C. Rosen, 1969; Rosen & Teague, 1974; Zuger, 1970a, 1970b), the available longitudinal data indicate that boyhood effeminate behavior is predictive of male homosexuality (Bakwin, 1968; Green, 1974; Lebovitz, 1972; Zuger, 1966, 1970a; Zuger & Taylor, 1969) and is retrospectively reported by adult male homosexuals (Bieber et al., 1962; R. B. Evans, 1969; Holemon & Winokur, 1965), adult male transvestites (Prince & Bentler, 1972), and adult male transsexuals (Benjamin, 1966; Bentler, 1976; Green & Money, 1969). Adult gender identity problems are generally accompanied by social and emotional maladjustments (Hoenig, Kenna, & Youd, 1970; Pauly, 1965, 1969; Walinder, 1967) and have been completely resistant to all forms of psychological treatment (Baker, 1969; Benjamin, 1969; Pauly, 1969) with the single exception of an adolescent transsexual treated behaviorally by Barlow, Reynolds, and Agras (1973).

The treatment of gender identity and gender behavior disturbances should, therefore, be instituted in early childhood to prevent adult sexual orientation disturbance and its associated psychological adjustment problems (Green, 1974; Rekers, Bentler, Rosen, & Lovaas, in press; Stoller, 1970). Pioneering work on the treatment of boyhood gender disturbances (Greenson, 1966, 1968) indicated the need for modifying specific feminine sex-typed behaviors which unfortunately have been quite resistant to therapeutic interventions (Stoller, 1968; Zuger, 1966). Although ethical issues are raised in the behavioral treatment of childhood gender disturbances (Franks & Wilson, 1975, p. 528; Rekers, 1975a; Rosen & Rekers, 1975), a careful consideration of the clinical issues reveals that intervention at the earliest age possible is the most humane and appropriate approach to the needs of these troubled individuals (Rekers, in press; Rekers, Bentler, Rosen, and Lovaas, in press; Rekers & Lovaas, 1974; Rosen, Rekers, & Bentler, 1977).

In a brief, uncontrolled case study, Dupont (1968) described a social learning theory approach to the treatment of an 8-year-old boy who had dressed in his mother's clothes two or three times weekly over several months' time. Without seeing the boy or the mother, the therapist met only once with the father who agreed to terminate the spankings and other negative attention given to the deviant behavior (which appeared to reinforce the behavior), and to explain to the boy that positive attention and affection would be contingent upon his normal behavior. Although no systematic data were obtained, Dupont reported that after one week of this intervention, no further transvestite behavior was observed by the parents for the next twelve years. This appears to be the first report of a behavioral treatment for mild transvestic behavior in a child.

Research on Extrinsic Reinforcement Control Techniques. The first systematic experimental investigation of the behavioral treatment of more pronounced childhood gender disturbances was initiated by Rekers and Lovaas (1971). The preadolescent boys in this behavioral treatment research program were independently evaluated by a clinical psychologist or psychiatrist as manifesting serious, chronic gender disturbances. The inappropriate gender behaviors included not only dressing in female attire and improvised cross-dressing, but other cross-gender behaviors as well: actual or imagined use of cosmetic articles; stereotypic feminine behavior mannerisms, gestures and gait; aversion to masculine activities, coupled with preference for girl playmates and feminine activities; preference for assuming a female role in play and social interaction; and feminine voice inflection and a predominantly feminine content in speech (Rekers, 1975b; Rekers, Amaro-Plotkin, & Low, 1977; Rekers & Yates, 1976; Rosen, Rekers, & Friar, 1977). All children evaluated by Rekers and his colleagues were screened by the UCLA Department of Pediatrics with a medical history, physical examination, including examination of external genitalia, chromosome analysis including two cells karyotyped and 15 counted, and sex chromatin studies. Baseline endocrinological studies are considered unnecessary unless abnormalities are detected in the physical exam. (For example, see Rekers, Yates, Willis, Rosen, & Taubman, 1976).

The first experimental demonstration of reinforcement control over sex-typed behavior in a gender behavior disturbed child was presented by Rekers (1972), who described the treatment of a 7-year-old black boy, Wayne. After obtaining a baseline of sex-typed play behavior with a set of masculine and feminine toys, a paraprofessional therapist shaped masculine behavior with contingent positive social reinforcement and extinguished feminine behavior by the contingent withdrawal of social attention. The experimental procedure followed the *ABABABA* reversal, intrasubject replication design where *A* represented the baseline and reversal conditions in which there were no differential reinforcement contingencies and the *B* condition represented the treatment sessions. During the pre-treatment baseline sessions, Wayne's behavior was consistently feminine both when alone and in the presence of adults. Three sets of five 10-minute therapy sessions were introduced, separated by sets of reversal sessions. Each time the therapy sessions were introduced, the feminine behavior sharply decreased and the masculine behavior increased. When the contingencies were withdrawn early in treatment, however, Wayne reverted to predominantly feminine behavior. During the course of treatment, the female therapist, male strangers, and female strangers became discriminative for masculine play with the baseline toys, indicating stimulus generalization of the treatment effects. Finally, after the third set of therapy sessions, Wayne's acquired masculine behavior in the presence of the therapist appeared to be resistant to extinction. The treatment effects did not generalize to playing alone with the baseline toys, however. Recently, a 3-year follow-up of this boy in his natural environment found predominantly masculine play behavior, and an independent clinical psychological evaluation of the boy and an interview with the mother yielded no evidence for a gender disturbance.

Rekers (1972) also reported on the intrasubject treatment studies of two other, more seriously gender-disturbed boys. In addition to the same gender *behavior* disturbance manifested by children like Wayne, these boys were independently diagnosed as manifesting a "cross-gender (feminine) *identity*," which was evidenced by a long-standing developmental history of making verbal statements about the desire or preference to be a girl, to grow up to become a "mommy," to deliver children, and to breast-feed infants. The first of these cross-gender identified boys to be behaviorally treated was Kraig, a 4-year 11-month old boy found to be physically normal, with the exception of having one undescended testicle. Kraig had a 3-year history of frequent cross-dressing and other feminine behaviors characteristic of gender disturbance. Before treatment, Kraig had been described by a psychiatric authority on gender identity problems as one of the most severe cases he had assessed, and his clinical history clearly paralleled the retrospective reports of adult transsexuals.

Kraig was treated sequentially in the clinic and home environments by his mother who was trained to be his behavior therapist. An intrasubject replication study was conducted employing a multiple baseline design across behaviors and environmental settings and a reversal design in the clinic setting (see Rekers & Lovaas, 1974, for detailed procedures and data). After obtaining baseline observational measures of sex-typed play and verbal behavior in the clinic, the mother was trained to reinforce masculine behaviors socially by using the procedures described above for Wayne. The investigator shaped the mother's therapeutic behavior by prompting her and reinforcing her over an earphone while observing the mother-child interaction from behind a one-way mirror. She smiled, attended to, and verbally reinforced Kraig's masculine play, and ignored feminine behavior by picking up a book on her lap to "read." The *ABABABA* reversal design demonstrated that Kraig's sex-typed behaviors were strongly controlled by his mother's attention, and she was successfully trained to increase masculine behavior and in effect to eliminate most feminine responding during only three sets of 10-minute therapy sessions spaced over several weeks' time. Through the course of treatment, the data indicated strong generalization of the treatment effects to play with the baseline toys in the presence of adult figures. Generalization to Kraig's play when he was alone in the playroom progressed more slowly, but by the end of the clinic treatment he played in a predominantly masculine mode in all situations, including the alone condition.

Before and during treatment in the clinic, Kraig's feminine behaviors had been reliably recorded in the home with a time-sampling procedure using a daily behavior checklist. These measures indicated that the clinic effects did not generalize to the home setting, even though the mother had been trained as therapist in the clinic. The mother was then trained to mediate a token reinforcement system for nongender and subsequently for gender behaviors in the home. Blue tokens served as secondary positive reinforcers (S^{r+}) and could be exchanged for the back-up reinforcers of certain candies, treats, and rewarding activities. Red tokens served as secondary negative reinforcers (S^{r-}) and were discriminative for (a) a response-cost condition (i.e., each red token received resulted in the loss of one blue token), (b) a time-out from reinforcement procedure (i.e., each red token resulted in a loss of five minutes of a rewarding activity such as watching television), or (c) a mild swat from the father. The token system successfully increased Kraig's helpful, appropriate nongender behaviors and suppressed several undesired nongender behaviors. Red tokens were then delivered for the single feminine behavior of "playing with dolls," which immediately decreased entirely and did not reoccur during the next 29 weeks that the contingency remained in effect. Following a multiple baseline replication design, "feminine gestures" were then successfully treated in the same manner, followed by intervention for "play with girls."

At the end of this formal 10-month behavioral treatment program, Kraig was indistinguishable from any other boy in terms of gender-related behaviors, according to reports from his parents, neighbors, school teacher, and two assistants sent to make systematic observations in the home and school environments. Kraig now referred to himself as a boy and assumed male roles in play. A follow-up psychological evaluation 26 months after termination of treatment revealed durability of the treatment effects with no resumption of cross-gender identification. He was found to be relatively less skilled in some desired masculine play behaviors, however. Subsequent to the initial report of these data, a research assistant made weekly visits to the home for several months to train Kraig and his father in playing ball together. An additional follow-up evaluation was conducted 3½ years after treatment by an independent clinical psychologist who interviewed the boy and family members and administered a complete battery of psychological tests. The boy was found to have normal male gender identity and a normal emotional, social, and academic adjustment. The permanence of the treatment effects appeared to be a function of the mother's acquired skills in behavior modification, which extended the treatment program indefinitely on an informal basis in Kraig's home setting.

Similar treatment techniques were employed by Rekers (1972) to treat an 8-year-old cross-gender identified boy in the clinic, school, and home environments. Carl had been previously treated in psychoanalytic, individual and family therapy for a period of 8 months in a largely unsuccessful attempt to alleviate his transsexual problem and difficulties in social relationships. Carl's feminine behavior was increasingly leading him to social isolation, ridicule, and chronic unhappiness. His mother requested behavioral treatment to relieve his social isolation and to lessen the emotional depression and anxiety associated with his sex role deviance.

With a multiple-baseline intrasubject design across stimulus environments and across behaviors, Carl was treated in one setting at a time in order to assess the generalization of treatment effects (Rekers, Lovaas & Low, 1974). The major portion of Carl's treatment took place in the home and school settings since (1) Carl felt overly self-conscious in the clinic with its one-way mirrors, and (2) previous investigations with Kraig found no generalization of treatment effects from the clinic to the natural environment. Since Carl enjoyed telling elaborate fantasized stories while drawing pictures on a chalkboard, the clinic treatment procedure was designed to obtain reinforcement control over the sex-typed verbal behavior during the boy's story telling. After obtaining a baseline measure of masculine and feminine speech content, the therapist introduced a differential social reinforcement contingency in which Carl's questions regarding masculine or neutral topics were answered by giving short, nonleading, direct answers, expressing positive interest. If Carl referred to a feminine topic, the therapist immediately withdrew social attention by looking away and reading a magazine. If Carl persisted with direct questions on feminine topics, the therapist expressed disinterest. An *ABA* reversal design demonstrated reinforcement control over sex-typed speech; the therapeutic contingency resulted in a sharp decrease in feminine speech and an increase in masculine content. The data suggested a generalized suppression effect to feminine voice inflection as well, even though that behavior was not specifically treated.

Carl's mother was trained to administer a token and point economy reinforcement procedure in the home which increased Carl's masculine play with his brother and decreased his feminine gestures, feminine speech content, feminine voice inflection, and predominant play with his sister. Since Carl's treatment in the clinic had not generalized to the home or to the school setting, his teacher was trained to apply a response-cost procedure to his disobedient "brat" behaviors and to his feminine gesture mannerisms. When the contingency was applied to the brat behaviors, they decreased immediately. The contingency for feminine gestures resulted in a gradual suppression of both gestures and feminine speech. These effects were stimulus-specific to the classroom setting, necessitating a reintroduction of the contingencies into Carl's new classroom when he was promoted to the next grade level.

The contingencies in this formal behavior modification program were discontinued after a 15-month period. Reports from individuals in Carl's natural environments and from psychologists who conducted diagnostic testing and interviews all concurred that Carl's previous feminine behaviors had been markedly reduced to only rare occurrences and there was no evidence for a cross-gender identification after treatment. Major improvements were also found in Carl's overall social and emotional adjustment. Since Carl was inept at most games and sports played by his male peers and was receiving only minimal encouragement from a new stepfather, he was treated for an additional 15 months with a specific set of behavior-shaping procedures to overcome his deficits in throwing a ball, socking a playground ball, and in playing kickball. This training was combined with a companionship relationship established between Carl and a psychology student who modeled appropriate masculine behaviors and took Carl on numerous trips to the park, beach, etc. A 12-month follow-up after this additional treatment provided evidence of continued stability of the therapeutic gains. The data suggest that Carl's sex-role development has become normalized.

The intrasubject replication data obtained in these three gender-disturbed children treated by Rekers (1972) demonstrated a direct functional relationship between the reinforcement contingencies and the sex-typed behavior. Since the treatment effects were relatively response-specific and setting-specific, it appears necessary to treat all feminine behaviors in the major settings in which they occur. It is thus more reasonable to train the parents and teachers to serve as the behavior therapists for a gender-disturbed child; it then becomes imperative, however, to obtain reliable observational data on the child's sex-typed behavior in order to monitor his progress under this paraprofessional treatment. This became especially apparent in Green's (1974) attempt to informally replicate Rekers' (1972) procedures for three child patients. Green provided parents with instructions to administer similar point economy reinforcement procedures, including response-cost contingencies. However, he did not obtain or report any systematic, reliable observational data by which to evaluate the intervention outcome but instead provided an informal clinical discussion of the difficulties encountered in training the parent to discriminate specific feminine behaviors and to carry out the reinforcement procedures. His three treatment failures point out the necessity of training the parent accurately to observe sex-typed behavior in the clinic and at home, and also of pre-training the parent carefully in the clinic setting. By omitting these two components, Green's partial replication unfortunately did not succeed. Green concluded that his behaviorally-based treatment program was essentially unable to evaluate whether or not sex-typed behavior is amenable to change by reinforcement schedules since experimental control procedures are necessary and closer attention must be given to parental cooperation and ability to mediate the contingencies in the home.

In contrast to Green (1974), Bates, Skilbeck, Smith, and Bentler (1975) gave careful attention to parental involvement in administering behavioral treatment procedures for gender-disturbed boys. Unlike the treatment strategy of Rekers and his colleagues, these investigators did not focus on attempting to decrease the boys' effeminate mannerisms and play interests, but focused instead on the acquisition of masculine behaviors and social skills. Several of the boys received individual social reinforcement from a therapist for masculine behavior and athletic play, in conjunction with teaching their parents to apply social and material reinforcers and token systems with behavior charting. Bates and co-workers then developed behavior modification groups of gender-disturbed boys for the purpose of systematically reinforcing masculine and pro-social behaviors with structured point-economy systems and individual behavioral charting. These boys' groups were conducted concurrently with parents' groups, the aims of which were to increase the parents' cooperative behavior, to foster their successful use of reinforcement strategies in the home, and to instruct them in systematic behavioral charting of their child's behavior. The major emphasis throughout this entire research program was to develop and validate new assessment techniques for boyhood gender disturbances (Bates & Bentler, 1973; Bates, Bentler, & Thompson; 1973 Bates et al., 1974). Consequently these kinds of rigorous empirical measures were nonexistent at the time of the pre-intervention evaluation of their subjects. Unfortunately, therefore, this treatment could not be evaluated by controlled comparisons with objective outcome measures. Bates and colleagues' pioneering research in the field has, however, provided the necessary assessment techniques for future research, and their clinical report of behavioral treatment success corroborates the results of the earlier single-subject research of Rekers.

More recently, Rekers and his colleagues have

reported on the results of other behavior modification techniques in the treatment of gender-disturbed boys. Intrasubject replication data were obtained in a study by Rekers, Yates, Willis, Rosen, and Taubman (1976) in which a series of reinforcement procedures were programmed in differing stimulus environments (i.e., in alone, mother-present and father-present conditions, and in different therapy rooms) in order effectively to eliminate the kind of stimulus-specific behavioral treatment effects reported in the earlier studies. The simultaneous introduction of the treatment procedures for sex-typed play in the clinic and home environments was also designed to minimize the probability of stimulus-specificity of the intervention, although *stimulus* generalization was found to the cross-gender behavior mannerisms. Response-cost and verbal prompt procedures were then applied to modify the child's "flexed elbow" feminine mannerism. At the follow-up 25 months after treatment terminated, evaluation by an independent clinical psychologist indicated the therapeutic change to a male gender identity. This appears to be the first published study documenting a successful change of childhood gender identity by pre- and post-diagnostic assessment procedures.

In Rekers' previous studies, response-cost contingencies had been successfully applied to cross-gender mannerisms but the children appeared to have had initial difficulties in discriminating those target behaviors. Consequently, another study (Rekers, Willis, Yates, Rosen & Low, in press) was designed in which reliable observational measures were obtained for eight sub-types of cross-gender behavior mannerisms. A discrimination training was provided for an 8-year-old boy in which he successfully learned to self-observe his cross-gender mannerisms by means of a videotape feedback procedure coupled with a S^{r+} contingency. However, this procedure alone did not reduce the frequency of the child's *in vivo* performance of mannerisms. Consequently, a combined response-cost and verbal prompt contingency was applied in the clinic and home settings to a single-target mannerism: limping the wrist. Marked decreases resulted in the target mannerism and response generalization of the treatment effect occurred on all other types of cross-gender mannerisms in both the clinic and home environments. The same response-cost and verbal prompt procedure was then successfully applied to suppress the boy's high-pitched feminine-like voice inflections. As in earlier studies, token economy procedures were applied in the home to suppress doll-play and predominant play with girls, and to increase masculine play. These treatment effects were replicated in a multiple baseline intrasubject design across behaviors and across the clinic and home settings. The 2-year follow-up psychological assessment by an independent clinician found a marked shift to an essentially normal gender-role adjustment.

Research On Behavioral Self-Control Techniques. In order to treat childhood gender disturbance successfully, intervention on multiple sex-role behaviors in multiple environments is necessary. Research findings indicate that the behavior therapist needs to supplement the traditional office-visit model of mental health service delivery with staff visits to the home, play, and school environments of the child. This has required more professional staff time than is normally available for an individual child client. Even where parents and teachers are trained to take on therapeutic roles for the child, considerable professional time is required for the adequate supervision of those co-therapists. In terms of cost-efficiency and the available financial resources, most parents would not be able to afford the investment in professional time required for the only treatment intervention which has been experimentally demonstrated to be effective in normalizing the child's gender-role behavior.

To increase cost-efficiency and minimize potential stimulus specificity of extrinsic reinforcement effects, self-control strategies have been successfully introduced to these cases (Rekers & Varni, in press; Varni & Rekers, 1975). In an initial study, an *ABA* reversal design demonstrated the successful but stimulus-specific effects of parent-mediated extrinsic social reinforcement. In a clinic setting, a 6-year-old boy was successfully trained to use a wrist-counter to self-monitor his masculine play. A "bug-in-the-ear" device was used for training the self-monitoring response in a behavioral cueing procedure that was gradually phased out over time. An *ABA* reversal replication demonstrated the reactive effect of self-monitoring, but the effect extinguished over time. The boy was then trained to give himself a small piece of candy for each point recorded on his wrist-counter. When this self-reinforcement procedure was superimposed upon the self-monitoring instruction, it produced exclusively masculine play, replicated in a *BAB* design. A subsequent study extended this approach to investigate the possibility that self-regulation strategies would result in greater stimulus generalization and response generalization to the treatment effects for child gender disturbance, as compared to the results of externally mediated social reinforcement procedures. Again, no generalization of the social reinforcement effect was found using a parent behavior therapist. A self-monitoring procedure applied in the clinic eliminated all the variability in the data and produced nearly exclusive masculine play, and generalization of this effect was found with another set of sex-typed toys. In the school setting, an initial reactive effect was found with a self-monitoring procedure, but it was extinguished over time. When a self-reinforcement procedure was superimposed upon the self-monitoring of cross-dress-up play, that behavior substantially decreased and response generalization of that effect was recorded to feminine role play, which also decreased. Play with girls was not similarly influenced in this boy.

Similar positive outcomes have been obtained with a number of gender-disturbed boys, and we may look forward with some confidence to replication of these behavioral treatment effects in other young boys. It has not yet been determined whether these treatment procedures will produce changes in future preference for sex mates. Perhaps sexual preference is a response that is independent of the child behaviors that have been treated so far. At the present time one can only speculate that a preventive treatment for transvestism, transsexualism, and homosexual orientation disturbance has indeed been isolated. This could be determined by comparing the long-term outcome of these children to that of non-treated gender-disturbed children such as those followed by Green (1974).

SEXUAL PROBLEMS IN ADOLESCENCE

The problem of homosexual behavior has received the greatest amount of research attention from behavior therapists, while other adolescent sexual problems have received relatively scant attention. Although some of the other adolescent problems are closely related in terms of the target behavior treated (e.g., fetishism for female garments and transvestism), they will be reviewed here under separate headings for the sake of convenience.

HOMOSEXUALITY

Homosexual orientation and behavior in adolescents has been treated in approximately two dozen reported cases with aversion therapy and/or non-aversive behavioral techniques.

Aversion Therapy Approaches. MacCulloch and Feldman (1967) reported the treatment of 43 homosexuals by a technique of anticipatory avoidance learning using an electrical aversive stimulus. Two of these patients were 18-year-old lesbian girls and three were adolescent males between 15 and 20 years of age. The patient views a homosexual slide projected on a screen "for as long as he finds it attractive" and receives a shock if he/she does not switch it off in 8 seconds. To assist in delaying extinction, a mixture of trials was presented with one-third reinforced, one-third delayed, and one-third non-reinforced schedules. Although the authors did not present data for the adolescents separately, an inspection of the tables and text reveals that the two lesbian adolescents made significant improvement—all homosexual fantasy, interest, and practice was eliminated, and one began heterosexual intercourse while the other developed a heterosexual dating relationship. Unfortunately, it is impossible to determine from the published report any details regarding the three male adolescents except that only one of them improved. These results persisted at the 12-month follow-up.

Larson (1970) reported a somewhat simplified adaptation of the MacCulloch and Feldman technique of anticipatory avoidance aversion therapy to the treatment of three male homosexuals, one of whom was an 18-year-old male. He reported success for all three patients when they were taught to associate anxiety with the habit of thinking about or gazing at male partners and to associate anxiety relief with a female image. The 18-year-old boy had had 30 to 40 homosexual experiences from the age of 14, and had had no heterosexual experience. After 10 treatment sessions over a 5-week period, a 4-month follow-up found that he had ceased homosexual activity, had minimal homosexual fantasy, and had developed heterosexual masturbatory fantasies and behavior.

A set of monozygotic twins discordant for homosexuality were studied by Davison, Brierly, & Smith (1971). The 18½-year-old homosexual boy was treated by aversion therapy in which electric shock was paired with male projected pictures with intermittent and varying delayed reinforcement schedules. Eight months of out-patient treatment resulted in his verbal report of a loss of homosexual desires. He was followed over a 2-year period, during which time he reported that his sexual orientation remained heterosexual, matching the adjustment of his identical twin brother. No systematic or replicated treatment data were presented in this case study, but the results paralleled those of other experimental studies.

McConaghy (1969, 1970) also reported a series of 40 homosexual patients who were randomly assigned to apomorphine aversion therapy or to aversion-relief therapy. These patients included both adolescents (from age 17 years) and adults (up to 56 years), but unfortunately results for the adolescent boys were not separately reported. Subsequent research by McConaghy and Barr (1973) investigated the relative efficacy of three forms of aversive therapy for homosexual impulses based on classical, avoidance, and backward conditioning paradigms. The patients ranged from adolescence (age 15 years) through adulthood (age 59 years). Again, the adolescent patients were not separated from the adults for data analysis, but the study is mentioned here for its successful treatment of homosexual adolescents, as measured by decreases in penile volume to male pictures. The number of booster treatments was positively correlated to the degree of treatment success. The findings were of theoretical significance, since backward conditioning was no less effective than the other two forms. The investigators suggested that these results support the contention that these aversive therapies do not act by setting up conditioned reflexes, and that an alternative mechanism is operative which is compatible with their findings that pretreatment measures of general conditionability in the aversion procedure correlate with treatment response.

In another group designed study, McConaghy (1975) randomly allocated 31 male homosexual patients (aged 15 to 45 years) to receive either electric shock aversive therapy or positive conditioning, in which pictures of nude women were associated with pictures of nude men and later with pictures of heterosexual relationships. Penile volume responses were measured in all experimental conditions. Aversive therapy was followed by a significant reduction in homosexual feelings and behavior, but the positive conditioning technique proved ineffective. McConaghy suggested that aversive therapy reduces the secondary reinforcement properties of stimuli associated with homosexual behavior.

> . . . This both limits and defines the type of patient most likely to be helped. Clearly this therapy will not be of use if the patient is almost exclusively homosexual and seeks treatment to become more heterosexual. It will be of more value to such patients if they consider they are excessively preoccupied by homosexual fantasies or compelled to become involved in behavior they find guilt-provoking, distasteful, dangerous, or excessively time-consuming. (1975, p. 319)

One of the several male sexual deviates treated by Callahan and Leitenberg (1973) was a 19-year-old male with a 6-year history of overt homosexual experience with various partners, a regular pattern of masturbation with male fantasy, and a complete lack of heterosexual dating experience. In the first phase of treatment, homosexually oriented and heterosexually oriented slides were presented and changes in penile circumference were recorded by plethysmography. If penile circumference increase exceeded 15% of full erection, electric shock was administered to the first and third fingers of the patient's hand. Absence of erection avoided the shock. Erection to homosexual stimuli was partially suppressed during 10 sessions, but homosexual urges outside the treatment setting reportedly increased. The second phase consisted of covert sensitization sessions in which the therapist presented verbal descriptions of homosexual acts coupled with descriptions of aversive consequences such as nausea, vomiting, discovery by family, etc. Seven such sessions effectively suppressed erection to slides depicting homosexual content and reduced subjective reports of deviant sexual arousal. An 8-month follow-up evaluation indicated durability of the therapeutic gains and a pattern of heterosexual dating. Although these investigators had major difficulties in conducting controlled intrasubject experimental comparisons with their patient population, their overall results across several subjects suggested that subjective measures of sexual deviation were more substantially reduced by covert sensitization than by contingent shock procedures.

Canton-Dutari (1974) reported a combined method to teach 54 active male homosexuals, aged 13 to 25 years (mean age 17), to control sexual arousal in the presence of a homosexual stimulus. During the first 3 weeks of treatment, the patients were taught to combine full body relaxation with a special contraction-breathing procedure in order to inhibit orgasm during masturbation. Then the patient was given 3 weeks of aversive therapy in which mild shock was given for reported sexual arousal to homosexual stimuli and was maintained until the contraction-breathing took place. For the next 4 weeks, the patient was instructed to allow orgasm only in the presence of a heterosexual photo, substituting heterosexual for homosexual mental images. Individual psychotherapy sessions were then commenced which focused on heterosexual dream content and the therapist-patient (male-male) relationship. After 16 weeks of treatment, 91% of the patients reported control of their sexual arousal to homosexual stimuli, and erection to female stimuli took place in 78% of the patients. Of the 49 successfully treated patients, only one had returned to homosexual behavior at the 11-week follow-up. Twenty-two of the patients were followed for 3½ years and 11 (50%) remained exclusively heterosexual. Unfortunately, this study presented only a clinical summary of cases without objective assessment data. The absence of experimental control procedures in such clinical reports renders the evidence inconclusive with regard to the variables potentially producing therapeutic behavior changes.

Non-Aversive Behavioral Techniques. Many clinicians consider the use of physically unpleasant sensations in psychological therapy to be practically, ethically, and/or aesthetically unacceptable. Others have pointed out the theoretical limitations of aversion therapy for homosexual behavior and recommend the use of techniques to increase appropriate heterosexual responsiveness and social dating skills. While some clinicians have assumed that alternate patterns of sexual arousal will occur if deviant arousal is eliminated by aversion therapy (e.g., Bond & Evans, 1967), this has not been conclusively demonstrated (Herman, Barlow, & Agras, 1974). Even supplementary techniques designed to increase heterosexual arousal such as aversion-relief (Feldman & MacCulloch, 1965) are of questionable effectiveness (Barlow, 1972). Homosexual individuals with little pretreatment heterosexual interest have a very poor prognosis with aversion therapy (Feldman & MacCulloch, 1971)—a finding that indicates a therapeutic need for developing or strengthening heterosexual patterns of arousal (Herman et al., 1974). Since adolescent patients with homosexual problems have had a relatively shorter conditioning history of deviant fantasies and sexual behavior (as compared to the more frequently studied adult patients), the acquisition of appropriate social dating skills and of heterosexual responsiveness may be relatively more important than the direct elimination of deviant sexual patterns, which perhaps are not yet irreversibly entrenched. However, relatively few procedures have been found effective in developing heterosexual arousal (Barlow, 1973; McConaghy, 1975), although investigations have indicated that this is therapeutically necessary (Bancroft, 1970; Barlow, 1974; Feldman & MacCulloch, 1971). Various behavioral techniques hold potential for shaping heterosexual fantasies, desensitizing the individual to anxiety associated with sexual stimuli, instructing in sexual technique, shaping social and assertive behavior, and developing specific dating behaviors in adult and adolescent homosexuals (Salter & Melville, 1972).

Gold and Neufeld (1965) treated a 16-year-old boy who reported chronic difficulties in his relationships with other boys and regarded himself as a rather unsuccessful individual in all spheres. At age 12, he had been homosexually seduced by a young man and had indulged in homosexual fantasies, usually associated with masturbation, from that time onward. He gradually became active in homosexual practices and had appeared in juvenile court for soliciting men in restrooms. The initial nonspecific treatment consisted of six sessions of desensitization to reduce interpersonal anxiety and the fear of failure in diverse social situations such as school examinations and sports involvement. After the neurotic disturbances were successfully treated, two types of covert sensitization procedures were applied to the homosexual problem. Sessions of "imaginary" aversive deconditioning consisted of suggesting and reinforcing images in which increasingly attractive males were rejected sexually, first in situations of great danger and gradually in the absence of external prohibitions. Subsequently, a discrimination learning task was conducted, in which the boy visualized a choice situation between an attractive young man and an attractive young woman. The male image choices were paired with prohibitions and punishing consequences, whereas the fantasized female choices were paired with pleasant consequences. After 10 treatment sessions over a 3-week period, the boy reported improvement in overall feelings of well-being and had ceased homosexual practice and fantasies, although he retained mild attraction to males. Three booster sessions were conducted over the next 3 months. At the 12-month follow-up, the boy was found to be succeeding academically, socially and vocationally, and he was dating a girl regularly. The homosexual behavior had not recurred.

Using neither physical nor imagined aversive contingencies, Bentler (1968b) presented treatment case studies of three homosexual boys, age 14, 16, and 20 years, respectively. In individual therapy sessions, Bentler socially reinforced the traditional heterosexual dating sequence in focused discussions regarding relationships with girls. Behavior rehearsals of heterosexual social interaction were conducted. To provide fantasy material for masturbation, Bentler encouraged the boys to focus on the sexual features of girls' bodies and to engage in petting between therapy sessions. This was accompanied by instructions to reinforce such heterosexual fantasy with the orgasm of masturbation instead of doing so with homosexual fantasies. The youngest boy was seen weekly for 7 months and by the end of the therapy he had increased his heterosexual behaviors from zero to three on the Bentler scale (1968a). His homosexual fantasies ceased and he enjoyed fantasizing sexually with pictures of nude women. The 16-year-old was seen weekly for 11 months during which time his score on the Bentler scale increased from zero to ten (up to heterosexual intercourse). His extensive repertoire of pretreatment homosexual fantasies was reduced substantially to minor levels. The 20-year-old was treated with behavior rehearsal to eliminate occasional effeminate gesturing, in addition to the other procedures. During 2 months of treatment his heterosexual behavior increased to four on the Bentler scale, and treatment was abruptly terminated with his induction into the army. These procedures were reportedly successful in changing fantasies associated with masturbation, in eliminating homosexual behavior, and in increasing the amount of heterosexually oriented social behavior.

Taking a somewhat different approach, Huff (1970) presented the case study of a 19-year-old adolescent boy who complained of stage fright and homosexuality. Following the theoretical formulation of Ramsay and vanVelzen (1968), Huff reasoned that the boy's homosexual adjustment was necessitated, in great part, by an irrational fear of the opposite sex. The treatment of choice was assumed to be the desensitization of this phobia rather than aversion therapy. The pretreatment administration of the MMPI and Leary Interpersonal Checklist revealed the boy to be very complaining and disturbed, thinking of himself as shy, passive, and weak. In the initial two sessions, deep muscle relaxation was taught, and an anxiety hierarchy to physical intimacy with women was set up. Desensitization procedures proceeded over the next 18 sessions from the lowest to highest anxiety-provoking situations in the hierarchy. The boy's daily records of sexual behavior and fantasies before, during, and after treatment revealed a sharp decrease in homosexual fantasy and behavior, and a substantial increase in heterosexual fantasy and behavior as therapy progressed. At the end of treatment and at 6-month follow-up, the boy's heterosexual interests predominated over infrequent homosexual interests. Heterosexual dating began and the boy found himself sexually aroused by girls. The post-treatment of the MMPI and Leary Checklist found substantially less distress, a self-concept closer to his ideal self-concept, and a positive change in his conceptualization of his mother. As an apparent result of the desensitization procedure, he had achieved a more positive feeling toward women as sexual partners and as people from whom he might obtain nurturance. Huff conceptualized the boy's therapy as the resolution of an approach-avoidance conflict:

> When the approach value of women became greater than their avoidance value, Mr. J. reported he felt less homosexual and began to be sexually aroused to scenes presented in the desensitization session. It was as if homosexuality represented a compromise sexual adjustment rather than a free choice of equally available sex objects. When the approach gradient was raised above the avoidance gradient then this compromise was no longer necessary and the selection of women as sexual objects was made. (Huff, 1970, p. 102)

More recently, Herman et al. (1974) used classical conditioning procedures directly to increase heterosexual responsiveness in a 16-year-old boy. Using an intrasubject experimental design and a backward presentation phase to control for sensitization, investigators demonstrated that the classical conditioning paradigm was effective in increasing heterosexual arousal in this adolescent and in one adult (the procedures failed for a second adult). The pattern of increased penile response to the female slide (the CS) generalized to other female slides and was also paralleled by increases in the other heterosexual measures of subjective attitudinal assessment of arousal, reports of fantasies outside the laboratory, and records of masturbatory fantasy. It should be noted that major procedural difficulties were encountered in the implementation of the classical conditioning technique. Critical attention had to be given to the habituation to the UCS slide, the intensity of the UCR and to the temporal relationship between the CS, UCS, and UCR. With this classical conditioning procedure, sexual responsiveness to the male slides did not show a decrease when responses to female stimuli increased. This indicates that simple acquisition of heterosexual arousal may be insufficient to treat adolescent homosexuality and that physical aversion therapy or covert sensitization may be required to decrease homosexual arousal. Finally, Herman and his colleagues noted that this adolescent boy had considerable difficulty in implementing new social-sexual behaviors in the natural environment after heterosexual responsiveness had been increased. Although they did not report additional behavior shaping, they recommended teaching the patient sufficient hetero-social skills to implement his new arousal. Bentler's (1968b) social learning therapy techniques could be useful at this very point.

Single-case experimental design methodology was used to evaluate the separate effects of feedback and reinforcement to increase heterosexual arousal in three males (two of them 15 years and one 21 years of age) who had extensive histories of homosexual behavior throughout their adolescent years (Barlow, Agras, Abel, Blanchard, & Young, 1975). Penile circumference changes were recorded by mechanical strain gauge (Barlow, Becker, Leitenberg, & Agras, 1970), and analogue feedback was provided to the subjects visually by means of a voltmeter which was adjusted so that the positions of the needle on the scale represented amount of penile erection. No-feedback sessions provided a control condition for the effects of exposure to erotic homosexual stimuli. Some experimental treatment conditions included contingent verbal and contingent monetary reinforcement for criterion responding (with appropriate control conditions). The data failed to confirm the effectiveness of biofeedback to increase heterosexual arousal. The effects of the reinforcement contingencies were weak and clinically insignificant in view of the lack of generalization to probe sessions. The results also pointed out the difficulties in relying on the patient's self-report as an indicator of treatment progress, since the subjective reports by the patients and relatives were discrepant with the objective measures of sexual arousal patterns.

These findings of Barlow and his colleagues underscore the need for caution in drawing inferences regarding the mechanisms of therapeutic change from uncontrolled case reports which lack experimental replication procedures to isolate the effective therapeutic variables. An "exposure" effect or other undefined source of change may be responsible for the positive results obtained in the uncontrolled case studies.

Transvestism

Bentler (1968b) presented the successful treatment case studies of three adolescent boys, aged 11, 13, and 16 years old. The youngest boy had been encouraged to be sexually effeminate by his mother. He had stereotypic feminine gestures, limp wrists, played with dolls, and avoided boys' games. The major therapeutic goal was to enhance socially appropriate, sex-typed behavior by social reinforcement and modeling by the therapist. The therapist systematically expressed disapproval following effeminate behavior. Four months of weekly behavior shaping sessions resulted in cessation of cross-dressing behavior, reduction of effeminate behavior, and an increase in masculine interests.

The other two transvestites were similar in that they had a fetishistic sexual involvement with women's clothes and their sexual fantasies were clearly heterosexual in nature. The boys rarely masturbated, but when they did it was not by manual manipulation but by rolling on the bed with feminine clothes. In individual sessions, the therapist socially reinforced verbalizations about heterosexual dating, conducted behavior rehearsals of heterosexual social interaction, encouraged heterosexual encounters, and encouraged frequency of masturbation with heterosexual fantasy rather than transvestic fantasy. With 7 and 12 months, respectively, of weekly therapy sessions cross-dressing ceased, masturbation with heterosexual fantasy increased, and social dating behavior reportedly increased. No follow-up evaluation was reported.

Transsexualism

There appears to be only one successful attempt to change gender identity in a diagnosed transsexual—a case of a 17-year-old boy systematically treated with behavioral procedures by Barlow, Reynolds, and Agras (1973). This published report was a significant contribution to the literature in light of the fact that all other treatment approaches for transsexualism had failed, and because, unlike many other reports of behavior modification of adolescent sex problems, specific procedures were experimentally demonstrated to be responsible for the therapeutic changes.

This adolescent patient had every major component previously described as contributing to the diagnosis of transsexualism: (1) a validated history of spontaneous cross-dressing before age 5 persisting into adolescence; (2) early development and continuity of feminine interests, coupled with avoidance of masculine activities; (3) reports of early cross-gender fantasies and identification that persisted into adolescence; (4) extremely effeminate behavior from childhood into adolescence; (5) gender inappropriate vocational interests; (6) reported cross-gender sexual fantasies from age 12 to time of referral, and (7) requests for physical change of sex.

During pretreatment baseline three measures were administered: (1) a score of 32 out of a possible 40 was obtained on a "transsexual attitude scale" based on a card sort procedure using statements such as "I want to have female genitals"; (2) daily records in a notebook revealed the patient to have an average of 7 homosexual and no heterosexual urges and fantasies each day; (3) daily measures of penile circumference found sexual arousal to male nude slides to average around 50% of a full erection, but virtually no arousal to female nude slides.

Barlow and co-workers attempted to alter the deviant patterns of sexual arousal first by increasing heterosexual arousal through techniques of "fading," and second by decreasing arousal to transsexual fantasies and to male stimuli by electric shock aversion therapy. Although treatment was administered daily for 2 months, no changes were found in the patterns of sexual arousal, reports of sexual urges and fantasies, nor the transsexual attitude scale scores. This failure to change sexual arousal patterns led the investigators to attempt direct modification of sex-role behaviors. Modeling, videotape feedback, and social reinforcement were used to alter gender-specific motor behaviors (sitting, standing, and walking) from predominantly feminine to predominantly masculine. A multiple baseline design across behaviors demonstrated that the treatment procedures resulted in a change to masculine motor behaviors, as reliably recorded by trained behind-the-scene observers. This treatment phase extended over a 2-month period and also included modeling and reinforced practice in male role behavior, e.g., discussing sports and dates with other males and rehearsing dating behavior. Daily voice re-training for 3 weeks, with the use of prompting and feedback methods, successfully eliminated his high pitch and feminine voice inflections. The boy reported liking these newly acquired masculine behaviors, but all other aspects of gender identity and sexual arousal remained at baseline levels at this point.

A direct attempt to modify transsexual thoughts and fantasies was then initiated by developing competing gender-appropriate fantasies in which the patient visualized himself as a boy having intercourse with a girl. Successively longer and more detailed heterosexual fantasies were prompted and socially reinforced by the female therapist. An *ABA* reversal design demonstrated that the praise (rather than the practice alone, or expectancy effects) was responsible for the increasing ability to fantasize in the gender-appropriate manner. Transsexual attitudes as measured by the card sort procedure also decreased dramatically with this therapy. The boy's continuing notebook recordings indicated a transfer of these newly developed heterosexual fantasies to the natural environment. At the end of this 2-month phase of 34 sessions the patient behaved, thought, and felt like a boy but his sexual arousal patterns remained deviant.

The boy was now diagnostically a homosexual after nearly one year of treatment. A classical conditioning procedure was administered to increase heterosexual arousal. Slides of nude females were used as the CS followed by slides of nude males (the UCS). *ABA* reversal replication demonstrated that the classical conditioning procedure was responsible for the increased sexual arousal to females as measured by penile circumference changes. Reports of sexual attraction to girls in the natural environment increased at this time. Since homosexual attraction was still present, the investigators applied a combined aversion therapy procedure, incorporating electrical aversion and covert sensitization techniques. Unlike the first attempt, the 20 aversion therapy sessions administered over a 2-month period resulted in a gradual reduction of homosexual arousal. Masculine components of sitting, standing, and walking showed sharp increases at this point in time, although no direct therapeutic attempts had been made to alter them.

After treatment, the boy's parents reported overall improvement in his social, academic, and emotional adjustment. He was seen in supportive, individual sessions over the next year at weekly, then monthly, and finally 3-month intervals. The transsexual card sort remained at zero, masculine behavior continued stable at high levels, heterosexual arousal continued to predominate, heterosexual fantasies continued to increase, and the boy began appropriately dating a steady girlfriend. Gender-relevant motor behaviors, sex-typed social behavior, vocal characteristics, sexual fantasies and attitudes, and patterns of sexual arousal had been changed one by one, resulting in a total change from transsexual to normal adjustment. In most instances, procedures were experimentally demonstrated to be responsible for the therapeutic changes in intrasubject replication designs. The adolescent boy's gender identity and total sexual adjustment was changed through behavior modification procedures, and he no longer requested that his body be changed through medical and surgical sex-reassignment procedures.

Fetishism

It has been hypothesized that sexual deviations are learned in a gradual process occurring during "masturbation to a memory," that the memory need not have been sexually stimulating at the initial time of experience, and that the memory may be altered by psychological processes of recall.

McGuire, Carlisle, and Young (1965) advanced this etiological theory and illustrated it with seven case histories including that of an adolescent with a fetish for female underwear. At age 14, a boy was sexually stimulated by the sight of a girl dressed only in her underwear. With the passage of time, his memory of the actual girl became vague but store displays continually reminded him of the stimulus details of underwear which he used as a cue in his fantasy. By age 17, he no longer had any sexual interest in girls but was sexually stimulated by the female underwear he collected.

> Perhaps more important than the *initiation* of deviant interests is the process by which they change, or develop from more normal interests during regular masturbation to fantasy. This is because fantasies, based on memory, are subject to their usual psychological processes of recall with the result that distortion and selection of cues take place. In addition, a particular cue initially given the slightest emphasis becomes more and more dominant because of the positive feedback involved in the conditioning process; the more sexually stimulating it becomes, the more emphasis it is given in a masturbatory fantasy and consequently, by conditioning it becomes still more stimulating. Other sexual stimuli are, in the meanwhile, being deconditioned so that sexual interest becomes more and more specific (McGuire et al., 1965, p. 186).

Strzyewsky and Zierhoffer (1967) presented a case report of an 18-year-old boy who was successfully treated by a drug-induced aversion conditioning for fetishism with superimposed transvestism. At age 12, this boy began masturbating while secretly observing his mother undress. He then began masturbating while touching his mother's clothes which he took from the wardrobe. By age 14, he began to dress in his mother's clothes and observe himself in the mirror while masturbating. His fetishistic-transvestic practices continued to age 18 at the frequency of 2 or 3 times a week. He sought treatment on his own and was treated as a hospital in-patient. Three times daily for 5 days, he was given an injection of 4 – 5 mg. apomorphine and as its effects of nausea and vomiting occurred, the patient was shown colored slides of himself holding lingerie and cross-dressing which were accompanied by his own tape-recorded descriptions of the slides. Follow-up observations were made over a year's time during which the patient reported only a few isolated instances of milder fetishistic behavior, which gradually extinguished altogether.

The majority of the earlier attempts to treat adult fetishism by avoidance therapy also involved the pairing of the fetishistic object with the noxious drug effect. The general consensus now, however, is that electric shock is preferable as the avoidance stimulus since (1) the temporal contiguity between the deviant response and aversive stimulus is more easily controlled; (2) shock eliminates the medical risks attendant with apomorphine administration; (3) shock procedures do not require the expense and inconvenience of hospitalization; and (4) shock is comparatively less personally offensive to the patient and administering staff (Rachman & Teasdale, 1969).

Electric shock was used as the aversive stimulus by Bond and Evans (1967), who reported an instrumental, anticipatory avoidance conditioning approach to the treatment of underwear fetishism in two adolescent boys. One boy, aged 16, had begun fetishistic activities at the age of 11 and since then had had a history of approximately two incidents monthly, in which he stole brassieres and panties. The fetishism of the other boy had begun at age 17 and consisted of stealing panties and slips to fondle during masturbation. He was treated after a 2-year history of this deviance. Unpleasant electric shock was administered to the boy's fingers contingent upon picking up an item of female underwear. Neutral objects were never associated with shock and the fetishistic objects were related with delayed shock on a 70% partial reinforcement schedule. Shock was terminated as soon as the object was placed in a box. Each boy received eight 30-minute sessions, one per week. The fetishistic behaviors were reportedly suppressed entirely, and booster sessions were projected. Although these treatment case histories were not experimental studies, the therapeutic effect appeared to be replicated in two similar adolescent cases.

SADISTIC SEXUAL FANTASIES

Mees (1966) presented a case study of an adolescent boy who, from the age of 12, regularly masturbated with fantasies about physically binding and injuring women and about being injured while dressing as a woman. He read sadistic pulp magazins and occasionally cross-dressed. At age 17, he assaulted a woman with the intention of carrying out a sadistic fantasy. Two years later, he was committed as mentally ill to a state hospital where examination found him to be developing a paranoid schizophrenic reaction. On an in-patient basis, the boy was taught to keep detailed records of his fantasies and sexual behavior for a 25-week baseline period. During the subsequent 14 weeks of daily aversion treatment, the patient was instructed to visualize selected parts of his deviant fantasy and to signal when the imagery was clear, at which point he was administered an uncomfortable electric shock to a finger. Since no change in the rate of either normal or sadistic fantasy or masturbation was observed during the initial 3½ weeks of aversive conditioning, the boy was instructed to write a "normal seduction" fantasy for substitution. During the eighth week of treatment, the sadistic fantasy weakened and normal heterosexual fantasy occurred before climax with increasing frequency. During the 11 post-treatment weeks, two abortive sadistic fantasies occurred and normal fantasy regularly accompanied masturbation. The substitution of sadistic by normal fantasies was gradual, and treatment consisted of a total of over 6000 shocks in 65 sessions over a 14-week period. Although replication data are lacking, the finding of an extended, stable pretreatment baseline tends to minimize the probability of adventitious influences (such as reactive effects of the self-observation) accounting for the therapeutic gains.

EXHIBITIONISM

Adult exhibitionists have been successfully treated by a variety of conditioning techniques, including reciprocal inhibition (Bond & Hutchinson, 1960), partial reinforcement schedule with imaginal stimuli (Kushner & Sandler, 1966), and by an anticipatory avoidance technique (D. R. Evans, 1968). Several successful treatments of adolescents have also been reported in the behavior modification literature.

MacCulloch, Williams, and Birtles (1971) described the treatment of a 12-year-old boy who had a compulsion to undress and expose his erect penis to older women. Not only was he shy and socially unskilled with girls his own age, but his exhibitionistic behavior was occurring so frequently that court action was likely. Therefore, a preliminary trial of conventional psychotherapy was abandoned in favor of a conditioning approach to achieve a more rapid resolution. The patient and his mother consented to a method of anticipatory avoidance aversion therapy designed to reduce the age of the boy's heterosexual approach objects. Slides of women over 25 years of age were the stimuli (CS_1) associated with shock onset (and hence anxiety) and slides of girls his own age were the stimuli (CS_2) associated with shock avoidance (anxiety relief) in a modified form of faradic anticipatory avoidance conditioning as described by Feldman, MacCulloch, Orford, and Mellor (1969). The technique thereby combined aversion to older females and desensitization to young girls within a single treatment program. The procedure included reinforced, delayed, and non-reinforced avoidance trials and presentation of the CS_2 on a partial schedule in order to reduce the generalization decrement to the real-life situation. The boy was given 18 20-minute sessions of therapy using six CS_1 and six CS_2 slides. A modified Sexual Orientation Measure questionnaire resulted in the maximum score for both "older women" and "girls my age" prior to treatment and during the first two treatment sessions, but by the fifth session, his score for older women had begun to drop, reaching the minimum score by the eighth session where it remained through follow-up. At the completion of treatment, 25% of the boy's masturbatory fantasy still concerned older women, but he was able to control the start of the cognitive chain which had previously led to the exhibitory behavior. At the 6-week and 5-month follow-ups, he reported that his masturbatory fantasy exclusively concerned girls his age and the compulsive ideas about exposing himself were absent.

Callahan and Leitenberg (1973) treated a 15-year-old boy with a 4-year history of exposure which had resulted in police action, expulsion from high school, and two institutional commitments. By replicated, counterbalanced intrasubject presentations, two different aversion therapy approaches were compared: (1) 4 sets of 6 treatment sessions of covert sensitization in which an imagined aversive event was followed by the imagined exhibitionistic behavior, and (2) 3 sets of 6 sessions in which shock was made contingent on erection to slides during exposure fantasy. The data did not reveal any difference in the relative effectiveness of one treatment over the other, but by the end of treatment and at the 18-month follow-up, overall improvement was found. Penile plethysmography indicated that the boy's erectile response to slides of nude females under instructions to fantasize intercourse was 83% of maximum, while instructions to think of exposure resulted in only 14% erection. Mean daily urges to expose decreased from a baseline of 4 to 5 daily to less than one daily at follow-up, and incidents of reported exposure decreased to zero from a baseline of once every other day. Appropriate dating behavior was reported subsequent to treatment as well.

There appears to be only one case in the literature in which an adolescent exhibitionist was treated by positive rather than aversive conditioning. Lowenstein (1973) proceeded on the assumption that fantasy plays a causal role in creating and perpetuating sexual deviations and that orgasm can be made contingent upon infrequent fantasies in order to reinforce acceptable social behavior. A 17-year-old boy was referred for treatment by a probation officer prior to his court appearance for exhibitionism. He exposed himself to adolescent girls several times weekly in a wooded area. He sought their surprised reaction, and he traced this behavior back to age 10. He rarely masturbated, considering it "dirty," and he was judged to be essentially male identified. The boy was instructed to use a running diary to record a baseline of daily events, sexual stimulation, and drive to expose himself. After the one-week baseline, the boy was trained through counter-conditioning and reciprocal inhibition techniques to masturbate every day while fantasizing about sexual intercourse with a female. Competing behavior was encouraged by instructing him to associate with people in busy activity as much as possible, since exposure was less frequent under these conditions in his history. He continued to record his thoughts of exposure and rated the strength of the need to expose on a 1 – 10 scale. After the 20-day treatment period, the drive to expose himself reportedly decreased, to reappear only on occasions of experienced anxiety. Overt instances of exposure reportedly ceased entirely and no instances were reported by the boy at the 12-month follow-up. Lowenstein speculated that the increase in masturbation reduced sexual drive and its deviant expression.

Promiscuous Sex Behavior

Anant (1968) reported the use of a verbal aversion technique to treat the long-standing promiscuous sex behavior of a 20-year-old girl institutionalized for mental retardation (WAIS IQ of 59). Her promiscuous heterosexual behavior had occurred all through her adolescent years and she had had an illegitimate child at age 15. She was unable to hold down a simple job because of her indiscriminate sexual advances toward all male customers. The treatment consisted of training in relaxation, the imagination of aversive consequences paired with imagined sexual behavior with strangers, and the practice of these scenes twice daily on her own time. In 10 one-hour sessions over a 2-week period, the therapist asked her to visualize scenes based on three dangers of indiscriminate sex with strangers: risking unwanted and embarrassing pregnancy, contracting venereal disease, and risking being murdered by a sex-criminal. After treatment, the girl was able to accept a new job and maintained it satisfactorily without inappropriate sexual behavior for the duration of the 8 months of follow-up.

Shaping Appropriate Heterosexual Dating Behavior

Very little attention has been given to the problem of treating the individual who manifests simple learning deficits in appropriate social behavior with members of the opposite sex. M. Rosen (1970) has discussed the need for programming appropriate boy-girl relationships in mentally retarded individuals, particularly among those educable, mildly retarded persons with potential for independent functioning in the community. Specifically he proposes desensitization where social fears exist, reinforced practice and role-play to initiate dating behavior, and instructions in masturbation as an alternative to deviant sexual behavior.

In a controlled group design study, Melnick (1973) demonstrated that minimal dating behavior in older adolescents is amenable to modification based on the social learning procedures of vicarious learning, behavioral rehearsal, response feedback, and direct reinforcement. Groups which received higher amounts of feedback benefited more from treatment. The combination of videotape feedback and participant modeling produced significant behavioral change—participant modeling alone did not. This appears to be the only study that demonstrates specific behavior modification techniques for increasing boy-girl dating behavior.

CONCLUDING COMMENT

Insufficient data exist presently to substantiate any particular learning theory formulation of child and adolescent sexual development, although plausible theories exist and are apparently supported by some evidence. This chapter has been limited to a brief review of the behavior modification techniques that have been applied to child and adolescent sexual problems; it has not been possible to present a theoretical discussion of the learning principles involved in the etiology, maintenance, and modification of sexual deviance (See Bandura & Walters, 1963; Bentler, 1968b; Clark, 1965; D. R. Evans, 1968; Feldman & MacCulloch, 1965; Fensterheim, 1974; Franks, 1967; McGuire, Carlisle, & Young, 1965; Rachman, 1966; Rachman & Hodgson, 1968; Thorpe, 1972; Thorpe, Schmidt, & Castell, 1963).

Instead this chapter has reviewed the relatively few behavior modification studies that have employed innovative behavioral treatment approaches to child and adolescent sexual problems. Many of these studies were uncontrolled case reports and only a few used either intrasubject replication designs or group comparisons. The application of behavior modification to these problems is still in its infancy, and consequently this review has revealed areas in which future research is required to provide the replication that is necessary before a definitive statement can be made regarding the efficacy of many of these behavioral intervention techniques.

REFERENCES

AMERICAN PSYCHIATRIC ASSOCIATION. *Diagnostic and Statistical Manual of Mental Disorders* (2nd ed.). Washington, D. C.: Author, 1968.

ANANT, S. S. Verbal aversion therapy with a promiscuous girl: Case report. *Psychological Reports*, 1968, *22*, 795–796.

BAKER, H. Transsexualism: Problems in treatment. *American Journal of Psychiatry*, 1969, *125*, 1412–1418.

BAKWIN, H. Deviant gender-role behavior in children: Relation to homosexuality. *Pediatrics*, 1968, *41*, 620–629.

BANCROFT, J. H. J. A comparative study of aversion and desensitization in the treatment of homosexuality. In L. E. Burns and J. L. Worsley (Eds.), *Behavior therapy in the 1970's*. Bristol: Wright, 1970.

BANDURA, A., and WALTERS, R. H. *Social learning and personality development*. New York: Holt, Rinehart, and Winston, 1963.

BARLOW, D. H. Aversive procedures. In W. S. Agras (Ed.), *Behavior modification: Principles and clinical applications*. Boston: Little, Brown, & Co., 1972.

BARLOW, D.H. Increasing heterosexual responsiveness in the treatment of sexual deviation: A review of the clinical and experimental evidence. *Behavior Therapy*, 1973, *4*, 655–761.

BARLOW, D. H. The treatment of sexual deviation: Towards a comprehensive approach. In K. S. Calhoun, H. E. Adams, and K. M. Mitchell (Eds.), *Innovative treatment methods in psychopathology*. New York: John Wiley, 1974.

BARLOW, D. H., AGRAS, W. S., ABEL, G. G., BLANCHARD, E. B., and YOUNG, L. D. Biofeedback and reinforcement to increase heterosexual arousal in homosexuals. *Behavior Research and Therapy*, 1975, *13*, 45–50.

BARLOW, D. H., BECKER, R., LEITENBERG, H., and AGRAS, W. S. A mechanical strain gauge for recording penile circumference change. *Journal of Applied Behavior Analysis*, 1970, *3*, 73–76.

BARLOW, D. H., REYNOLDS, E. J., and AGRAS, W. S. Gender identity change in a transsexual. *Archives of General Psychiatry*, 1973, *28*, 569–576.

BATES, J. E., and BENTLER, P. M. Play activities of normal and effeminate boys. *Developmental Psychology*, 1973, *9*(1), 20–27.

BATES, J. E., BENTLER, P. M., and THOMPSON, S. K. Measurement of deviant gender development in boys. *Child Development*, 1973, *44*, 591–598.

BATES, J. E., SKILBECK, W. M., SMITH, K. V. R., and BENTLER, P. M. Gender role abnormalities in boys: An analysis of clinical ratings. *Journal of Abnormal Child Psychology*, 1974, *2*, 1–16.

BATES, J. E., SKILBECK, W. M., SMITH, K. V. R., and BENTLER, P. M. Intervention with families of gender-disturbed boys. *American Journal of Orthopsychiatry*, 1975, *45*, 150–157.

BENJAMIN, H. *The transsexual phenomenon*. New York: Julian, 1966.

BENJAMIN, H. Introduction. In R. Green and J. Money (Eds.), *Transsexualism and sex reassignment*. Baltimore: Johns Hopkins, 1969.

BENTLER, P. M. Heterosexual behavior assessment. I. Males. *Behaviour Research and Therapy*, 1968, *6*, 21–25. (a)

BENTLER, P. M. A note on the treatment of adolescent sex problems. *Journal of Child Psychology and Psychiatry*, 1968, *9*, 125–129. (b)

BENTLER, P. M. A typology of transsexualism: Gender identity theory and data. *Archives of Sexual Behavior*, 1976, *5*, 567–584.

BIEBER, I., DAIN, H. J., DINCE, P. R., DRELLICH, M. G., GRAND, H. G., GUNDLACH, R. H., KREMER, M. W., RIFKIN, A. H., WILBER, C. B., and BIEBER, T. B. *Homosexuality: A psychoanalytic study*. New York: Basic Books, 1962.

BOND, I., and EVANS, D. Avoidance therapy: Its uses in two cases of underwear fetishism. *Canadian Medical Association Journal*, 1967, *96*, 1160–1162.

BOND, I. K., and HUTCHINSON, H. C. Application of reciprocal inhibition therapy to exhibitionism. *Canadian Medical Association Journal*, 1960, *83*, 23–25.

CALLAHAN, E. J., and LEITENBERG, H. Aversion therapy for sexual deviation: Contingent shock and covert sensitization. *Journal of Abnormal Psychology*, 1973, *81*, 60–73.

CANTON-DUTARI, A. Combined intervention for controlling unwanted homosexual behavior. *Archives of Sexual Behavior*, 1974, *3*, 367–371.

CLARK, D. F. A note on avoidance conditioning techniques in sexual disorders. *Behaviour Research and Therapy*, 1965, *3*, 203–206.

DAVISON, K., BRIERLEY, H., and SMITH, C. A male monozygotic twinship discordant for homosexuality. *British Journal of Psychiatry*, 1971, *118*, 675–682.

DUNLAP, K. *Habits: Their making and unmaking*. New York: Liveright, 1972. (Originally published, 1932).

DUPONT, H. Social learning theory and the treatment of transvestite behavior in an eight-year-old boy. *Psychotherapy: Theory, Research and Practice*, 1968, *5*, 44–45.

EVANS, D. R. Masturbatory fantasies and sexual deviation. *Behaviour Research and Therapy*, 1968, *6*, 17–19.

EVANS, R. B. Childhood parental relationships of homosexual men. *Journal of Consulting and Clinical Psychology*, 1969, *33*, 129–135.

FELDMAN, M. P., and MACCULLOCH, M. J. Application of anticipatory avoidance learning to the treatment of homosexuality. I. Theory, technique, and preliminary results. *Behavior Research and Therapy*, 1965, *2*, 165–183.

Feldman, M. P., and MacCulloch, M. J. *Homosexual behavior: Theory and assessment.* Oxford: Pergamon, 1971.

Feldman, M. P., MacCulloch, M. J., Orford, J. F., and Mellor, V. The application of anticipatory avoidance learning to the treatment of homosexuality: Developments in treatment technique and response recording. *Acta Psychiatrica Neurologica Scandinavica*, 1969, *45*, 109–117.

Fensterheim, H. Behavior therapy of the sexual variations. *Journal of Sex and Marital Therapy*, 1974, *1*, 16–28.

Franks, C. M. Reflections upon the treatment of sexual disorders by the behavioral clinician: An historical comparison with the treatment of the alcoholic. *Journal of Sex Research*, 1967, *3*, 212–222.

Franks, C. M., & Wilson, G. T. *Annual review of behavior therapy theory and practice: 1975.* New York: Brunner/Mazel, 1975.

Gold, S., and Neufeld, L. A learning approach to the treatment of homosexuality. *Behaviour Research and Therapy*, 1965, *2*, 201–204.

Green, R. *Sexual identity conflict in children and adults.* New York: Basic Books, 1974.

Green, R. Sexual identity: Research strategies. *Archives of Sexual Behavior*, 1975, *4*, 337–352.

Green, R., and Money, J. *Transsexualism and sex reassignment.* Baltimore: Johns Hopkins, 1969.

Greenson, R. R. A transvestite boy and a hypothesis. *International Journal of Psychoanalysis*, 1966, *47*, 396–403.

Greenson, R. R. Dis-identifying from mother: Its special importance for the boy. *International Journal of Psychoanalysis*, 1968, *49*, 370–374.

Hammerman, S. Masturbation and character. *Journal of American Psychoanalytic Association*, 1961, *9*, 287–311.

Herman, S. H., Barlow, D. H., and Agras, W. S. An experimental analysis of classical conditioning as a method of increasing heterosexual arousal in homosexuals. *Behavior Therapy*, 1974, *5*, 33–47.

Hoenig, J., Kenna, J., and Youd, A. Social and economic aspects of transsexualism. *British Journal of Psychiatry*, 1970, *117*, 163–172.

Holemon, E., and Winokur, G. Effeminate homosexuality: A disease of childhood. *American Journal of Orthopsychiatry*, 1965, *35*, 48–56.

Huff, F. W. The desensitization of a homosexual. *Behaviour Research and Therapy*, 1970, *8*, 99–102.

Kushner, M., and Sandler, J. Aversion therapy and the concept of punishment. *Behaviour Research and Therapy*, 1966, *5*, 179–186.

Larson, D. E. An adaptation of the Feldman and MacCulloch approach to treatment of homosexuality and the application of anticipatory avoidance learning. *Behaviour Research and Therapy*, 1970, *8*, 209–210.

Lebovitz, P. S. Feminine behavior in boys: Aspects of its outcome. *American Journal of Psychiatry*, 1972, *128*, 1283–1289.

Lehner, F. J. Negative practice as a psychotherapeutic technique. In H. J. Eysenck (Ed.), *Behavior therapy and the neuroses.* Oxford: Pergamon, 1960.

Lowenstein, L. F. A case of exhibitionism treated by counter-conditioning. *Adolescence*, 1973, *8*, 213–218.

MacCulloch, M. J., and Feldman, M. P. Aversion therapy in management of 43 homosexuals. *British Medical Journal*, 1967, *2*, 594–597.

MacCulloch, M. J., Williams, C., and Birtles, C. J. The successful application of aversion therapy to an adolescent exhibitionist. *Journal of Behavior Therapy and Experimental Psychiatry*, 1971, *2*, 61–66.

McConaghy, N. Subjective and penile plethysmograph responses following aversion-relief and apomorphine aversion therapy for homosexual impulses. *British Journal of Psychiatry*, 1969, *115*, 723–730.

McConaghy, N. Penile response conditioning and

its relationship to aversion therapy in homosexuals. *Behavior Therapy*, 1970, *1*, 213–221.

McConaghy, N. Aversive and positive conditioning treatments of homosexuality. *Behaviour Research and Therapy*, 1975, *13*, 309–319.

McConaghy, N., and Barr, R. F. Classical, avoidance and backward conditioning treatments of homosexuality. *British Journal of Psychiatry*, 1973, *122*, 151–162.

McGuire, R. J., Carlisle, J. M., and Young, B. G. Sexual deviations as conditioned behavior: A hypothesis. *Behaviour Research and Therapy*, 1965, *2*, 185–190.

Mees, H. L. Sadistic fantasies modified by aversive conditioning and substitution: A case study. *Behaviour Research and Therapy*, 1966, *4*, 317–320.

Melnick, J. A comparison of replication techniques in the modification of minimal dating behavior. *Journal of Abnormal Psychology*, 1973, *81*, 51–59.

Mertz, P. Therapeutic considerations in masturbation. *American Journal of Psychotherapy*, 1955, *9*, 630–639.

Money, J., and Ehrhardt, A. A. *Man and woman, boy and girl: The differentiation and dimorphism of gender identity from conception to maturity.* Baltimore: Johns Hopkins, 1972.

Pauly, I. Male psychosexual inversion. Transsexualism: A review of 100 cases. *Archives of General Psychiatry*, 1965, *13*, 172–181.

Pauly, I. Adult manifestations of male transsexualism. In R. Green and J. Money (Eds.), *Transsexualism and sex reassignment.* Baltimore: Johns Hopkins, 1969.

Prince, C. V., and Bentler, P. M. A survey of 504 cases of transvestism. *Psychological Reports*, 1972, *31*, 903–917.

Rachman, S. Sexual fetishism: An experimental analogue. *Psychological Record*, 1966, *16*, 293–296.

Rachman, S., and Hodgson, R. J. Experimentally-induced "sexual fetishism": Replication and development. *Psychological Record*, 1968, *18*, 25–27.

Rachman, S., and Teasdale, J. *Aversion therapy and behavior disorder: An analysis.* Coral Gables, Fla.: University of Miami Press, 1969.

Ramsey, R. W., and vanVelzen, V. Behavior therapy for sexual perversions. *Behaviour Research and Therapy*, 1968, *6*, 233.

Rekers, G. A. Pathological sex-role development in boys: Behavioral treatment and assessment. *Dissertation Abstracts International*, 1972, *33*, 3321B. (University Microfilms No. 72–33, 978.)

Rekers, G. A. *Experimental treatment of sex-role behaviors in a transsexual boy: An intrasubject study with ethical implications.* Paper presented to the meeting of the Western Association of Christians for Psychological Studies, Santa Barbara, Cal., May 1975. (a)

Rekers, G. A. Stimulus control over sex-typed play in cross-gender identified boys. *Journal of Experimental Child Psychology*, 1975, *20*, 136–148. (b)

Rekers, G. A. Atypical gender development and psychosocial adjustment. *Journal of Applied Behavior Analysis*, in press.

Rekers, G. A., Amaro-Plotkin, H., and Low, B. P. Feminine sex-typed mannerisms in normal boys and girls as a function of sex and age. *Child Development*, 1977, *48*, in press.

Rekers, G. A., Bentler, P. M., Rosen, A. C., and Lovaas, O. I. Child gender disturbances: A clinical rationale for intervention. *Psychotherapy: Theory, Research, & Practice*, in press.

Rekers, G. A., and Lovaas, O. I. Experimental analysis of cross-sex behavior in male children. *Research relating to children: ERIC Clearinghouse on Early Childhood Education*, 1971, *28*, 68. (Abstract)

Rekers, G. A., and Lovaas, O. I. Behavioral treatment of deviant sex-role behaviors in a male child. *Journal of Applied Behavior Analysis*, 1974, *7*, 173–190.

Rekers, G. A., Lovaas, O. I., and Low, B. P. The behavioral treatment of a "transsexual" preadolescent boy. *Journal of Abnormal Child Psychology*, 1974, *2*, 99–116.

Rekers, G. A., and Varni, J. W. Self-monitoring and self-reinforcement processes in a pre-transsexual boy. *Behaviour Research and Therapy*, in press.

Rekers, G. A., Willis, T. J., Yates, C. E., Rosen, A. C., and Low, B. P. Assessment of childhood gender behavior change. *Journal of Child Psychology and Psychiatry*, 1977, *18*, 53–65.

Rekers, G. A., and Yates, C. E. Sex-typed play in feminoid boys vs. normal boys and girls. *Journal of Abnormal Child Psychology*, 1976, *4*, 1–8.

Rekers, G. A., Yates, C. E., Willis, T. J., Rosen, A. C., and Taubman, M. Childhood gender identity change: Operant control over sex-typed play and mannerisms. *Journal of Behavior Therapy and Experimental Psychiatry*, 1976, *7*, 51–57.

Rosen, A. C. The intersex: Gender identity, genetics, and mental health. In S. Plog & R. Edgerton, *Changing perspectives in mental illness*. New York: Holt, 1969.

Rosen, A. C., and Rekers, G. A. *Ethical issues in the treatment of childhood gender-role disturbances*. Paper presented at the meeting of the California State Psychological Association, Anaheim, Cal., March 1975.

Rosen, A. C., Rekers, G. A., and Bentler, P. M. Ethical issues in the treatment of children. *Journal of Social Issues*, 1977, in press.

Rosen, A. C., Rekers, G. A., and Friar, L. R. Theroretical and diagnostic issues in child gender disturbances. *Journal of Sex Research*, 1977, *13*.

Rosen, A. C., and Teague, J. Case studies in development of masculinity and femininity in male children. *Psychological Reports*, 1974, *34*, 971–983.

Rosen, M. Conditioning appropriate heterosexual behavior in mentally and socially handicapped populations. *Training School Bulletin*, 1970, *66*, 172–177.

Salter, L. G., and Melville, C. H. A re-educative approach to homosexual behavior: A case study and treatment recommendations. *Psychotherapy: Theory, Research and Practice*, 1972, *9*, 166–167.

Stoller, R. J. Male childhood transsexualism. *Journal of the American Academy of Child Psychiatry*, 1968, *7*, 193–209.

Stoller, R. J. Psychotherapy of extremely feminine boys. *International Journal of Psychiatry*, 1970–1971, *9*, 278–280.

Strzyewsky, J., and Zierhoffer, M. Aversion therapy in a case of fetishism with transvestistic component. *The Journal of Sex Research*, 1967, *3*, 163–167.

Thorpe, G. L. Learning paradigms in the anticipatory avoidance technique: A comment on the controversy between MacDonough and Feldman. *Behavior Therapy*, 1972, *3*, 614–618.

Thorpe, J. G., Schmidt, E., and Castell, D. A comparison of positive and negative (aversive) conditioning in the treatment of homosexuality. *Behaviour Research and Therapy*, 1963, *1*, 357–362.

Varni, J. W., and Rekers, G. A. *Behavioral self-control treatment of "cross-gender identity" behaviors*. Paper presented at the 9th Annual Convention of the Association for Advancement of Behavior Therapy, San Francisco, December 1975.

Wagner, M. K. A case of public masturbation treated by operant conditioning. *Journal of Child Psychology and Psychiatry*, 1968, *9*, 61–65.

Walinder, J. *Transsexualism: A study of forty-three cases*. Goteborg: Scandinavian University Books, 1967.

Zuger, B. Effeminate behavior present in boys from early childhood I. The clinical syndrome and follow-up studies. *Journal of Pediatrics*, 1966, *69*, 1098–1107.

Zuger, B. Gender role determination: A critical review of the evidence from hermaphroditism. *Psychosomatic Medicine*, 1970, *32*, 449–467. (a)

Zuger, B. The role of familial factors in persistent effeminate behavior in boys. *American Journal of Psychiatry*, 1970, *126*, 1167–1170. (b)

ZUGER, B., and TAYLOR, P. Effeminate behavior present in boys from early childhood. II. Comparison with similar symptoms in non-effeminate boys. *Pediatrics*, 1969, *44*, 375–380.

ADDITIONAL READINGS

NORMATIVE DATA ON SEXUAL DEVELOPMENT

ANGERILLI, A. F. The psychosexual identification of preschool boys. *Journal of Genetic Psychology*, 1960, *97*, 329–340.

ASAYAMA, S. *Adolescent sex development and adult sex behavior in Japan*. Tokyo: Japanese Association for Sex Education, 1974.

BAKWIN, H. Erotic feelings in children. *Indian Journal of Pediatrics*, 1971, *38*, 135–137.

BELL, A. P. Adolescent sexuality and the schools. *North Central Association Quarterly*, 1969, *43*, 342–347.

BRODERICK, C. B. Preadolescent sexual behavior. *Medical Aspects of Human Sexuality*, 1968, *2*(1), 20–29.

CAPES, M. Sexual development in childhood and its problems. *British Medical Journal*, 1972, *5831*, 38–39.

CONN, J. H. Factors influencing development of sexual attitudes and sexual awareness in children. *American Journal of Diseases of Children*, 1939, *58*, 738–745. (a)

CONN, J. H. Sex attitudes and sex awareness in young children. *Child Study*, 1939, *16*, 86–87. (b)

CONN, J. H. Children's reactions to the discovery of genital differences. *American Journal of Orthopsychiatry*, 1940, *10*, 747–754. (a)

CONN, J. H. Sexual curiosity of children. *American Journal of Diseases of Children*, 1940, *60*, 1110–1119. (b)

CONN, J. H. Children's awareness of the origins of babies. *Journal of Child Psychiatry*, 1948, *1*, 140–176.

CONN, J. H. Children's awareness of sex differences. II. Play attitudes and game preferences. *Journal of Child Psychiatry*, 1951, *2*, 82–99.

CONN, J. H., and KANNER, L. Children's awareness of sex differences. I. *Journal of Child Psychiatry*, 1947, *1*, 3–57.

DIAMOND, M. A critical evaluation of the ontogeny of human sexual behavior. *Quarterly Review of Biology*, 1965, *40*, 147–175.

ELIAS, J., and GEBHARD, P. Sexuality and sexual learning in childhood. *Phi Delta Kappan*, 1969, *50*, 401–405.

GAGNON, J. H. Sexuality and sexual learning in the child. *Psychiatry*, 1965, *28*, 212–228.

HALVERSON, H. M. Genital and sphincter behavior of the male infant. *Journal of Genetic Psychology*, 1940, *56*, 95–136.

HAMPSON, J. G., MONEY, J., and HAMPSON, J. L. Hermaphrodism: Recommendations concerning case management. *Journal of Clinical Endocrinology and Metabolism*, 1956, *16*, 547–556.

JOHNSON, W. R. Awakening sexuality of girls. *Sexual Behavior*, 1973, *3*(3), 3–6.

KANNER, L. Infantile sexuality. *Journal of Pediatrics*, 1939, *4*, 583–608.

KATCHER, A. The discrimination of sex differences by young children. *Journal of Genetic Psychology*, 1955, *87*, 131–143.

KINSEY, A. C., POMEROY, W. B., and MARTIN, C. E. *Sexual behavior in the human male*. Philadelphia: Saunders, 1948.

KINSEY, A. C., POMEROY, W. B., MARTIN, C. E., and GEBHARD, P. H. *Sexual behavior in the human female*. Philadelphia: Saunders, 1953.

KLEEMAN, J. A. Genital self-discovery during a boy's second year: A follow-up. *Psychoanalytic Study of the Child*, 1969, *21*, 358–391.

KORNER, A. F. Neonatal startles, smiles, erections and reflex sucks as related to state, sex, and individuality. *Child Development*, 1969, *30*, 1039–1053.

KREITLER, H., and KREITLER, S. Children's concepts of sexuality and birth. *Child Development*, 1966, *37*, 363–378.

LEVIN, S. M., BALISTRIERI, J., and SCHUKIT, M. The development of sexual discrimination in children. *Journal of Child Psychology and Psychiatry*, 1972, *13*, 47–53.

LEWIS, M. Psychosexual development and sexual behavior in children. *Connecticut Medicine*, 1968, *32*, 437–443.

MARTINSON, F. M. Sexual knowledge, values, and behavior patterns of adolescents. In H. L. Gochros and L. G. Schultz (Eds.), *Human sexuality and social work*. New York: Association Press, 1972.

MARTINSON, F. M. *Infant and child sexuality: A sociological perspective*. St. Peter, Minnesota: The Book Mark, 1973. (Privately published, available from The Book Mark, GAC, St. Peter, Minnesota 56082).

MONEY, J. Too early puberty. *Sexology*, 1961, *28*, 154–157.

MONEY, J., and EHRHARDT, A. A. *Man and woman, boy and girl: The differentiation and dimorphism of gender identity from conception to maturity*. Baltimore: Johns Hopkins, 1972.

MONEY, J., and WALKER, P. S. Psychosexual development, maternalism, nonpromiscuity, and body image in 15 females with precocious puberty. *Archives of Sexual Behavior*, 1971, *1*(1), 45–60.

MONEY, J., and WOLFF, G. Late puberty, retarded growth and reversible hyposomatotropinism (psychosocial dwarfism). *Adolescence*, 1974, *9*, 121–134.

MONTAGU, M. F. A. The acquisition of sexual knowledge in children. *American Journal of Orthopsychiatry*, 1945, *15*, 290–300.

OFFER, D. Sexual behavior of a group of normal adolescents. *Medical Aspects of Human Sexuality*, 1971, *5*(9), 40–49.

OSOFSKY, H. J. Adolescent sexual behavior: Current status and anticipated trends for the future. *Clinical Obstetrics and Gynecology*, 1971, *14*, 393–408.

RAMSEY, G. V. The sex information of younger boys. *American Journal of Orthopsychiatry*, 1943, *13*, 347–352. (a)

RAMSEY, G. V. The sexual development of boys. *American Journal of Psychology*, 1943, *56*, 217–233. (b)

REEVY, W. R. Child sexuality. In A. Ellis and A. Abarbanel (Eds.), *Encyclopedia of sexual behavior*. New York: Hawthorn, 1961.

RENSHAW, D. C. Sexuality in children. *Medical Aspects of Human Sexuality*, 1971, *5*(10), 62–74.

RUTTER, M. Normal psychosexual development. *Journal of Child Psychology and Psychiatry*, 1971, *11*, 259–283.

SIGUSCH, V., and SCHMIDT, G. Teenage boys and girls in West Germany. *Journal of Sex Research*, 1973, *9*, 107–123.

SORENSEN, R. C. *Adolescent sexuality in contemporary America: Personal values and sexual behavior, ages thirteen to nineteen*. New York: World, 1973.

SZASZ, G. Adolescent sexual activity. *Canadian Nurse*, 1971, *67* (October), 39–43.

THOMPSON, S. K., and BENTLER, P. M. The priority of cues in sex discrimination by children and adults. *Developmental Psychology*, 1971, *5*, 181–185.

TOUSSIENG, P. W. Psychosexual development in childhood and adolescence. *Journal of School Health*, 1965, *35*, 158–165.

VENER, A. M. Adolescent sexual behavior in Middle America revisited: 1970–1973. *Journal of Marriage and the Family*, 1974, *36*, 728–735.

WOLLMAN, L. Brief statistics on female adolescents. *Journal of Sex Research*, 1966, *2*(1), 25–26.

WOLMAN, B. Sexual development in Israeli adolescents. *American Journal of Psychotherapy*, 1951, *5*, 531–559.

SEXUAL PROBLEMS IN CHILDHOOD AND ADOLESCENCE

CHAPMAN, A. H. *Management of emotional problems of children and adolescents* (2nd ed.). Philadelphia: Lippincott, 1974.

OLIVEN, J. F. *Clinical sexuality* (3rd ed.). Philadelphia: Lippincott, 1974.

RENSHAW, D. C. Sexuality and depression in infancy, childhood, and adolescence. *Medical Aspects of Human Sexuality*, 1975, *9*(June), 24; 29–45.

WAGGONER, R. W., and BOYD, D. A. Juvenile aberrant sexual behavior. *American Journal of Orthopsychiatry*, 1941, *11*, 275–291.

Excessive Masturbation

BITTER-LEBERT, I. [A case of excessive masturbation.] *Praxis der Kinderpsychologie und Kinderpsychiatrie*, 1956, *6*(2/3), 44–48.

GILBERT, J. A. An unusual case of masturbation. *American Journal of Urology and Sexology*, 1916, *12*, 82–87.

LEVINE, M. I., and BELL, A. I. Psychological aspects of pediatric practice. II. Masturbation. *Pediatrics*, 1956, *18*, 803–808.

RUDOLF, G. de M. An experiment in the treatment of masturbation in oligophrenia. *American Journal of Mental Deficiency*, 1954, *58*, 644–649.

STIRT, S. S. Overt mass masturbation in the classroom. *American Journal of Orthopsychiatry*, 1940, *10*, 801–804.

Homosexual Behavior

BAKWIN, H., and BAKWIN, R. M. Homosexual behavior in children. *Journal of Pediatrics*, 1953, *43*, 108–111.

BENDER, L., and PASTER, S. Homosexual trends in children. *American Journal of Orthopsychiatry*, 1941, *11*, 730–743.

COX, W. Panel on "homosexuality in the male adolescent." *International Mental Health Research Newsletter*, 1962, *4*(1/2), 7; 10.

DAVENPORT, C. W. Homosexuality—its origins, early recognition and prevention. *Clinical Pediatrics*, 1972, *11*, 7–10.

FRAIBERG, S. Homosexual conflicts. In S. Lorand and H. I. Schneer (Eds.), *Adolescents: Psychoanalytic approach to problems and therapy*. New York: Hoeber, 1961.

GADPAILLE, W. J. Homosexual experience in adolescence. *Medical Aspects of Human Sexuality*, 1968, *2*(10), 29–38.

GADPAILLE, W. J. Could that youngster become a homosexual? *Medical Economics*, November 24, 1969. (a)

GADPAILLE, W. J. Homosexual activity and homosexuality in adolescence. *Science and Psychoanalysis*, 1969, *15*, 60–70. (b)

GADPAILLE, W. J. Male "physique" magazines. *Medical Aspects of Human Sexuality*, April 1971, 45; 48; 51; 54–57; 60–61. (a)

GADPAILLE, W. J. A psychiatrist discusses myths about childhood homosexuality. *Today's Health*, 1971, *49*(1), 45–47; 65. (b)

GADPAILLE, W. J. Brief guide to office counseling: Adolescent concerns about homosexuality. *Medical Aspects of Human Sexuality*, 1973, *7*(11), 105–106.

GEBHARD, P. H. Homosexual socialization. *Excerpta Medica, International Congress Series*, 1966, *150*, 1028–1031.

GLICK, B. S. Homosexual panic: Clinical and theoretical considerations. *Journal of Nervous and Mental Disease*, 1959, *129*, 20–28.

GUNDLACH, R. H. Childhood parental relationships and the establishment of gender roles of homosexuals. *Journal of Consulting and Clinical Psychology*, 1969, *33*, 136–139.

HARRISON, S. I., and KLAPMAN, H. Relationships between social forces and homosexual behavior observed in a children's psychiatric hospital. *Journal of American Academy of Child Psychiatry*, 1966, *5*, 105–110.

HESTON, L. L., and SHIELDS, J. Homosexuality in twins: A family study and a registry study. *Archives of General Psychiatry*, 1968, *18*, 149–160.

KESTENBAUM, C. J. Brief guide to office counseling: Adolescent homosexual experiences. *Medical Aspects of Human Sexuality*, 1975, *9*(1), 99–100.

KINSEY, A. C. Homosexuality: Criteria for a hormonal explanation of the homosexual. *Journal of Clinical Endocrinology*, 1941, *1*, 424–428.

LITKEY, L. J., and FENICZY, P. An approach to the control of homosexual practices. *International Journal of Neuropsychiatry*, 1967, *3*(1), 20–23.

LURIE, L. A. The endocrine factor in homosexuality. *American Journal of Medical Sciences*, 1944, *208*, 176–186.

PARKER, W. *Homosexuality: A selective bibliography of over 3,000 items*. Metuchen, New Jersey: Scarecrow Press, 1971.

ROESLER, T., and DEISHER, R. W. Youthful male homosexuality: Homosexual experience and the process of developing homosexual identity in males aged 16 to 22 years. *Journal of the American Medical Association*, 1972, *219*, 1018–1023.

SHEARER, M. Homosexuality and the pediatrician, early recognition and preventive counseling. *Clinical Pediatrics*, 1966, *5*, 514–518.

SPRINCE, M. P. A contribution to the study of homosexuality in adolescence. *Journal of Child Psychology and Psychiatry*, 1964, *5*(2), 103–117.

SYMONDS, M. Homosexuality in adolescence. *Pennsylvania Psychiatric Quarterly*, 1969, *9*(2), 15–24.

WEINBERG, M. S., and BELL, A. P. *Homosexuality: An annotated bibliography*. New York: Harper & Row, 1972.

Gender Identity and Behavior Disturbance

BAKWIN, H. Transvestism in children. *Journal of Pediatrics*, 1960, *56*, 294–298.

BAKWIN, H. Deviant gender-role behavior in children: Relation to homosexuality. *Pediatrics*, 1968, *41*, 620–629.

BATES, J. E., and BENTLER, P. M. Play activities of normal and effeminate boys. *Developmental Psychology*, 1973, *9*, 20–27.

BATES, J. E., BENTLER, P. M., and THOMPSON, S. Measurement of deviant gender development in boys. *Child Development*, 1973, *44*, 591–598.

BATES, J. E., SKILBECK, W. M., SMITH, K. V. R., and BENTLER, P. M. Gender role abnormalities in boys: An analysis of clinical ratings. *Journal of Abnormal Child Psychology*, 1974, *2*, 1–16.

BERG, I., NIXON, H. H., and MACMAHON, R. Change of assigned sex at puberty. *Lancet*, 1963, *2*, 1216–1217.

BROWN, D. G. Development of sex-role inversion and homosexuality. *Journal of Pediatrics*, 1957, *50*, 613–619.

CHARATAN, F. B., and GALEF, H. A case of transvestism in a six-year-old boy. *Journal of the Hillside Hospital*, 1965, *4*, 160–177.

COHN, L. S., and ZUGER, B. Scrutiny of parental relationships in affecting the behavior of effeminate boys. *American Journal of Psychiatry*, 1970, *127*(1), 107–108.

DON, A. Transvestism and transsexualism: A report of 4 cases and problems associated with their management. *South African Medical Journal*, 1963, *37*, 479–485.

EPSTEIN, A. W. Relationship of fetishism and transvestism to brain and particularly to temporal lobe dysfunction. *Journal of Nervous and Mental Disease*, 1961, *133*, 247–253.

FRIEND, M. R., SCHIDDEL, L., KLEIN, B., and DUNAEFF, D. Observations on the development of transvestitism in boys. *American Journal of Orthopsychiatry*, 1954, *24*, 563–575.

GEORGE, G. C. W., and BEUMONT, P. J. V., Transsexualism in a fourteen-year-old male. *South African Medical Journal*, 1972, *46*, 1947–1948.

REKERS, G. A. *Atypical sex-role development: Assessment, intervention, and ethics*. Paper presented at the meeting of the Society for Research in Child Development, Emeryville, Cal., April 1976. (Available from the author, 190 North Oakand Ave., Pasadena, Cal. 91101).

REKERS, G. A. Atypical gender development and psychosocial adjustment. *Journal of Applied Behavior Analysis*, in press.

REKERS, G. A., AMARO-PLOTKIN, H., and LOW, B. P. Feminine sex-typed mannerisms in normal boys and girls as a function of sex and age. *Child Development*, 1977, *48*, in press.

REKERS, G. A., BENTLER, P. M., ROSEN, A. C., and LOVAAS, O. I. Child gender disturbances: A clinical rationale for intervention. *Psychotherapy: Theory, Research, and Practice*, in press.

REKERS, G. A., and LOVAAS, O. I. Behavioral treatment of deviant sex-role behaviors in a male child. *Journal of Applied Behavior Analysis*, 1974, *7*, 173–190.

REKERS, G. A., LOVAAS, O. I., and LOW, B. P. The behavioral treatment of a "transsexual" preadolescent boy. *Journal of Abnormal Child Psychology*, 1974, *2*, 99–116.

REKERS, G. A., and VARNI, J. W. Self-monitoring and self-reinforcement processes in a pretranssexual boy. *Behaviour Research and Therapy*, in press.

REKERS, G. A., WILLIS, T. J., YATES, C. E., ROSEN, A. C., and LOW, B. P. Assessment of childhood gender behavior change. *Journal of Child Psychology and Psychiatry*, 1977, *18*, 53–65.

REKERS, G. A., and YATES, C. E. Sex-typed play in feminoid boys vs. normal boys and girls. *Journal of Abnormal Child Psychology*, 1976, *4*, 1–8.

REKERS, G. A., YATES, C. E., WILLIS, T. J., ROSEN, A. C., and TAUBMAN, M. Childhood gender identity change: Operant control over sex-typed play and mannerisms. *Journal of Behavior Therapy and Experimental Psychiatry*, 1976, *7*, 51–57.

SKILBECK, W. M., BATES, J. E., and BENTLER, P. M. Human figure drawings of gender-problem and school-problem boys. *Journal of Abnormal Child Psychology*, 1975, *3*, 191–199.

STOLLER, R. J. Etiological factors in male transsexualism. *Transactions of the New York Academy of Sciences, Series II*, 1967, *29*, 431–433.

STOLLER, R. J. Male childhood transsexualism. *Journal of American Academy of Child Psychiatry*, 1968, *7*, 193–209. (a)

STOLLER, R. J. *Sex and Gender*. New York: Science House, 1968. (b)

TAYLOR, A. J. W., and MCLACHLAN, D. G. Transvestism and psychosexual identification. *New Zealand Medical Journal*, 1964, *63*, 369–372.

ZUGER, B. Gender role determination: A critical review of the evidence from hermaphroditism. *Psychosomatic Medicine*, 1970, *32*, 449–467. (a)

ZUGER, B. The role of familial factors in persistent effeminate behavior in boys. *American Journal of Psychiatry*, 1970, *126*, 1167–1170. (b)

ZUGER, B. Effeminate behavior in boys. III. Parental age and other factors. *Archives of General Psychiatry*, 1974, *30*, 173–177.

ZUGER, B., and TAYLOR, P. Effeminate behavior present in boys from early childhood. II. Comparison with similar symptoms in non-effeminate boys. *Pediatrics*, 1969, *44*, 375–380.

Sexual Asphyxias

COE, J. L. Sexual asphyxias. *Life-threatening Behavior*, 1974, *4*, 171–175.

EDMONDSON, J. S. A case of sexual asphyxia without fatal termination. *British Journal of Psychiatry*, 1972, *121*, 437–438.

RESNIK, H. L. P. Erotized repetitive hangings: A form of self-destructive behavior. *American Journal of Psychotherapy*, 1972, *26*, 4–21.

SHANKEL, L. W., and CARR, A. C. Transvestism and hanging episodes in a male adolescent. *Psychiatric Quarterly*, 1956, *30*, 478–493.

STEARNS, A. W. Cases of probable suicide in young persons without obvious motivation. *Journal of the Maine Medical Association*, 1953, *44*(1), 16–23.

Prostitution, Exhibitionism, and other Sex Offences

ATCHESON, J. D., and WILLIAMS, D. C. A study of juvenile sex offenders. *American Journal of Psychiatry*, 1954, *111*, 366–370.

CLARK, R. A. Sexual deviates in out-patient psychiatry. *Pennsylvania Psychiatric Quarterly*, 1964, *4*(1), 35–41.

CLEMENT, P. W. Parents, peers, and child patients make the best therapists. In G. Williams and S. Gordon (Eds.), *Clinical child psychology: Current practices and future perspectives*. New York: Behavioral Publications, 1974.

CRAFT, M. Boy prostitutes and their fate. *British Journal of Psychiatry*, 1966, *112*, 1111–1114.

DEISHER, R. W. The young male prostitute. *Pediatrics*, 1970, *45*, 153–154.

DEISHER, R. W., EISNER, V., and SULZBACHER, S. I. The young male prostitute. *Pediatrics*, 1969, *43*, 936–941.

GANDY, P., and DEISHER, R. Young male prostitutes: The physician's role in social rehabilitation. *Journal of the American Medical Association*, 1970, *212*, 1661–1666.

GINSBURG, K. N. The "meat-rack": A study of the male homosexual prostitute. *American Journal of Psychotherapy*, 1967, *21*, 170–185.

HACKETT, T. P. The psychotherapy of exhibitionists in a court clinic setting. *Seminars in Psychiatry*, 1971, *3*, 297–306.

HARTMANN, L. Some uses of dirty words by children. *Journal of the American Academy of Child Psychiatry*, 1973, *12*, 108–122.

MOHR, J. W., and TURNER, R. E. Sexual deviations. Part III. Exhibitionism. *Applied Therapeutics*, 1967, *9*, 263–265.

NADLER, R. P. Approach to psychodynamics of obscene telephone calls. *New York State Journal of Medicine*, 1968, *68*, 521–526.

PITTMAN, D. J. The male house of prostitution. *Trans-Action*, 1971, *8*(5/6), 21–27.

RAVEN, S. Boys will be boys: The male prostitute in London. In H. M. Ruitenbeek (Ed.), *Problem of Homosexuality in Modern Society*. New York: E. P. Dutton, 1963.

REISS, A. J. Social integration of queers and peers. In H. M. Ruitenbeek (Ed.), *Problem of Homosexuality in Modern Society*. New York: E. P. Dutton, 1963.

ROBERTS, R., MCBEE, G. W., and BETTIS, M. C. Youthful sex offenders: An epidemiologic comparison of types. *Journal of Sex Research*, 1969, *5*, 29–40.

RUSSELL, D. H. On the psychopathology of boy prostitutes. *International Journal of Offender Therapy*, 1971, *15*(1), 49–52.

SALFIELD, D. J. [Juvenile fetishism.] *Zeitschrift für Kinderpsychiatrie*, 1957, *24*(6), 183–188.

SHOOR, M., SPEED, M. H., and BARTELT, C. Syndrome of the adolescent child molester. *American Journal of Psychiatry*, 1966, *122*, 783–789.

VANDEN BERGH, R. L., and KELLY, J. F. Vampirism: A review with new observations. *Archives of General Psychiatry*, 1964, *11*, 543–547.

Child Victims of Sexual Crimes

BRUNOLD, H. Observations after sexual traumata suffered in childhood. *Excerpta Criminologica* (Netherlands), 1964, *4*(1), 5–8.

MANGUS, A. R. Sex crimes against children. In K. M. Bournen, *Sexual deviation research*. Sacramento: Assembly of the State of California, March, 1932.

SCHULTZ, L. G. Psychotherapeutic and legal approaches to the sexually victimized child. *International Journal of Child Psychotherapy*, 1972, *1*(4), 115–128.

SCHULTZ, L. G. The child sex victim: Social, psychological and legal perspectives. *Child Welfare*, 1973, *52*, 147–157.

WEISS, J., ROGERS, E., DARWIN, M. R., and DUTTON, C. E. A study of girl sex victims. *Psychiatric Quarterly*, 1955, *29*, 1–27.

Observation of Adult Sexual Behavior and Pornography

BENDER, L., and GRUGETT, A. E. Follow-up report on children who had atypical sexual experience. *American Journal of Orthopsychiatry*, 1952, *22*, 825–837.

KATZMAN, M. Early sexual trauma. *Sexual Behavior*, 1972, *2*(2), 13–17.

MANGUS, A. R. Sexual deviation and the family. *Marriage and Family Living*, 1953, *15*, 325–331.

Sexual Seduction of Children

BENDER, L., and BLAU, A. The reaction of children to sexual relations with adults. *American Journal of Orthopsychiatry*, 1937, *7*, 500–518.

LANGSLEY, D. G., SCHWARTZ, M. N., and FAIRBAIRN, R. H. Father-son incest. *Comprehensive Psychiatry*, 1968, *9*, 218–226.

LITIN, E. M., GIFFIN, M. E., and JOHNSON, A. M. Parental influence in unusual sexual behavior in children. *Psychoanalytic Quarterly*, 1956, *25*, 37–55.

Veneral Disease, Pregnancy out of Wedlock, Sexual Delinquency, Premature Ejaculation, Impotence, and Effects of Media and Pornography on Sexual Development

BROWN, F. Sexual problems of the adolescent girl. *Pediatric Clinics of North America*, 1972, *19*, 759–764.

GROVER, J. W. Problems of emerging sexuality and their management. *Rhode Island Medical Journal*, 1973, *56*, 274–279; 298.

HAMELSTEIN, H. Youth and *their* sexual problems. *Journal of Clinical Child Psychology*, 1974, *3*(3), 31–33.

MCCOY, K. Adolescent sexuality: A national concern. Report on the Wingspread Conference on adolescent sexuality and health care. *Journal of Clinical Child Psychology*, 1974, *3*(3), 18–22.

MILLER, W. B. Sexuality, contraception, and pregnancy in high-school population. *California Medicine*, 1973, *119*(2), 14–21.

MOSSE, H. L. The influence of mass media on the sex problems of teenagers. *Journal of Sex Research*, 1966, *2*(1), 27–35.

ROBERTS, R. E., ABRAMS, L., and FINCH, J. R. Delinquent sex behavior among adolescents. *Medical Aspects of Human Sexuality*, 1973, *7*(1), 162–175.

SALZMAN, L. Sexual problems in adolescence. *Contemporary Psychoanalysis*, 1974, *10*, 189–207.

ZELNIK, M., and KANTNER, J. J. Probability of premarital intercourse. *Social Science Research*, 1972, *1*, 335–341. (a)

ZELNIK, M., and KANTNER, J. J. Sexuality, contraception, and pregnancy among young unwed females in the United States. In C. Westoff and R. Parke (Eds.), *Demographic and social aspects of population growth*. Washington, D. C.: U. S. Government Printing Office, 1972. (b)

18

ANTISOCIAL BEHAVIOR: BEHAVIOR MODIFICATION[1]

Dennis M. Maloney, Dean L. Fixsen, & Karen B. Maloney

The purpose of this chapter is to provide an overview of the current dimensions of behavior modification with youths who exhibit antisocial behavior. These dimensions include selecting those clients for therapy who are most in need of treatment, selecting problem behaviors that are socially significant, and selecting treatment procedures that are effective yet intrude as little as necessary into the lives of youths. Also discussed are legal and ethical issues that relate to the treatment of antisocial youths and issues relevant to evaluating treatment programs. These issues were derived from a review of the behavior modification literature as it pertains to antisocial behavior. However, a detailed review of the literature is not provided in this chapter. We refer the interested reader to several recent reviews that cover the literature quite adequately (i.e., Braukmann & Fixsen, 1975; Braukmann, Fixsen, Phillips, & Wolf, 1975; Gentry, 1975; Berkowitz & Graziano, 1972; Kazdin & Bootzin, 1972). Instead, we have attempted to describe the general practical considerations that therapists and program developers must face when they work with antisocial youths.

SELECTING CLIENTS FOR THERAPY

Behavior that violates accepted norms of society is not rare. One needs only to be a casual observer of human behavior to see children hitting one another or adolescents disobeying their parents or adults abusing the people around them. In these cases, if one were to continue to observe the situations, one might see the children being separated by an adult, the disobedient adolescent being disciplined, and the abusive adult being socially ostracized by those around him. Society has no organized or systematic methods for correcting occasional norm-violating behaviors but, in general, the "natural solutions" that are applied seem to be sufficient to socialize most of us adequately.

In some cases the informal socialization methods are either not applied or are ineffective and the child or youth becomes a persistent "norm violator." If the problems become serious,

[1]The preparation of this manuscript was supported by The Boys Town Center for the Study of Youth Development but the views represented do not necessarily reflect those of The Boys Town Center. The authors wish to thank Joan Fixsen, Janelle Maston, and Bess Melvin for their assistance in preparing the manuscript.

the youth is labeled as "antisocial," and some of the formal mechanisms of society are brought to bear to correct the problem behavior. These formal mechanisms include special classrooms in the public schools, probation in a juvenile court, out-patient care in a mental health center, or commitment to a mental hospital, reformatory, or training school, to name only a few. The incidence of antisocial behavior is substantial. For example, Wolfgang, Figlio, and Sellin (1972) studied *all* the boys born in 1945 who lived in Philadelphia from age 10 to age 18, a total of 9,945 boys. They found that 35% (3,475) of the boys in this "birth cohort" had at least one officially recorded contact with the police and that these youths were responsible for 10,214 delinquent acts between the ages of 10 and 17. They also found that 54% of the 3,475 antisocial youths committed at least two offenses, 35% committed at least three offenses, 25% at least four offenses, and 18% (625 boys) five or more offenses. In fact, these researchers reported that the 625 "chronic offenders"—those with five or more offenses—accounted for about 52% of the *total* number of offenses committed by all 3,475 youths. In England, West and Farrington (1973) conducted a longitudinal study of all 8- to 9-year-old boys who attended six elementary schools in a working-class area of London, a total of 411 boys. They found that between the ages of 8 and 16, 20% (84) of the youths had been found guilty of non-traffic offenses and that these youths were responsible for 255 delinquent acts. Of the 84 delinquents, 53% committed two or more offenses. These two studies are important because they give us estimates of the extent of antisocial behavior that occurs in the general population of youths during adolescence. Wolfgang and collaborators (1972) found that one youth out of three had at least one contact with the police, while West and Farrington (1973) found that one youth out of five had at least one formal court adjudication. The difference in the recorded incidence of antisocial behavior between the two studies may be due to the fact that the court adjudication criterion used by the British researchers was more stringent than the police contact criterion used by the Americans. If these findings are true for the general population, the number of male youths alone who might be classified as "antisocial" would be staggering. For example, 1970 census data indicated there were about 16,600,000 boys between the ages of 10 and 18 in the United States. Using the 35% rate of antisocial behavior found by Wolfgang et al. (1972), this would mean that about 5,800,000 of these youths would have at least one contact with the police before they reach age 18.

Given this high incidence of antisocial behavior in the general population, our next question would be, What kinds of adolescent antisocial behavior are most predictive of adult antisocial behavior? Robins (1966) reported the results of a remarkable 30-year follow-up study of 524 children who had been referred to a child guidance clinic and 100 matched control children who had no history of childhood behavior problems. A total of 406 of the children had been referred to the clinic for antisocial behavior such as theft, incorrigibility, sexual offenses, runaway, truancy, aggression, and vandalism. The remaining 118 children had been referred for reasons other than antisocial behavior. Robins found that 71% of the 260 boys referred for antisocial behavior problems had one or more arrests during the 30-year follow-up period compared to 30% of the 90 boys referred for other problems and 22% of the 69 boys in the control group. She also found that 49% of the antisocial boys, 18% of the other referral boys, and 4% of the control boys had been arrested three or more times and that 43%, 13%, and 0%, respectively, had served time in a jail or an institution for their offenses. After surveying a wide variety of measures of the behavior of the subjects as both children and adults, Robins concluded that "the best single predictor of [adult antisocial behavior] was the degree of juvenile antisocial behavior. [Adult antisocial behavior] could be about equally well predicted by three measures of antisocial behavior: (1) the variety of antisocial behavior. . .; (2) the number of episodes; and (3) the seriousness of the behavior, as measured by whether or not the behavior was of the kind for which children appear in Juvenile Court" (p. 296). As juveniles, these children had "a history of juvenile theft, . . . incorrigibility, running away from home, truancy, associating with bad companions, sexual activities, and staying out late. Most of them were discipline problems in school and [had] been held back at least one grade by the time they appeared in the clinic . . . they were described as aggressive, reckless, impulsive, slovenly, enuretic, lacking guilt, and lying without cause" (p. 293). As adults, they "had a poor work history, had been financially dependent on social agencies or relatives, and had marital problems. Three-quarters of them had multiple arrests leading to prison terms. They drank excessively, were impulsive, sexually promiscuous, had been vagrant, were belligerent, delinquent in paying their debts, and socially isolated. . . . At time of follow-up, about age 44, 12% of the . . . group had given up their antisocial behavior, and an additional 27% had reduced it markedly. The remaining 61% were still seriously antisocial" (p. 296).

Robins' data provide important indicators of the types of adolescent problems that are likely to lead to adult antisocial behavior. It is precisely these kinds of adolescent problem behaviors that must be identified for therapy if we are to intervene in the lives of adolescents in a way that can produce long-term benefits to our clients and to society. Both the American and British studies cited earlier found that nearly half of the youths had only one contact with the police. Thus, a social intervention program designed to treat every youth who had contact with the police or juvenile court might unnecessarily treat a large number of antisocial youths who "naturally" stop violating the law after their first offense. If we were to follow Robins' advice, we would first establish social intervention programs for those youths whose antisocial behavior is varied, occurs often, and is serious. Instead of attempting to deal with 35% of all adolescents, we might be able to focus on only the 6% (625/9945) who are "chronic offenders" but who commit over half of all offenses (Wolfgang et al., 1972) and have the highest probability of becoming antisocial adults (Robins, 1966).

We are not suggesting that nothing be done for youths who have mild forms of antisocial behavior or who have only one or two contacts with law enforcement agencies. However, we are suggesting that clinicians begin examining longitudinal data on the life course of youths who display antisocial behavior to help them decide which children to accept for treatment. Given the practical and clinical considerations involved in treating large numbers of youths, the greatest benefits to society will occur when we can treat those problems that are most likely to persist into later adolescence and adulthood. While the data provided by Robins (1966), Wolfgang et al. (1972), West and Farrington (1973), and others are helpful, we can only hope that more longitudinal studies will be conducted to provide more definitive guidance in selecting those antisocial adolescents who are most in need of therapy.

SELECTING PROBLEM BEHAVIORS FOR THERAPY

The problem of selecting the most critical behaviors for therapy is in some ways even more difficult than selecting clients. As has been implied in all the studies cited, the number of police and court contacts is one measure that could be used to select antisocial clients for therapy. However, police and court contacts are low-rate behaviors and are, therefore, problematic aims for therapy that must be conducted on a frequent basis. Robins' data suggested other antisocial behaviors that can occur more often (e.g., incorrigibility), but even that list of behaviors did not include a number of potential behaviors that might also be important foci for treatment. Once again, we will have to look to future research to provide guidance in selecting the most appropriate goals for therapy.

One promising procedure for determining which behaviors are important for therapy has been developed by Haase and Tepper (1972) and used by Werner, Minkin, Minkin, Fixsen, Phillips, and Wolf (1975). This procedure involves having relevant individuals view real or simulated interactions involving adolescents and asking the individuals to rate the interactions on several dimensions. The simulated interactions can be performed "live," recorded on audio and videotape, or written as interaction scenes to be rated. Those behaviors that are seen as important dimensions of the interaction are then rated by the relevant individuals to determine their social importance. For example, the Werner study (1975) selected delinquent youths and police officers as "relevant individuals" and asked them to describe the important aspects of police-youth encounters. Their responses were then used to develop a questionnaire that was designed to identify the specific appropriate behaviors a youth should engage in when interacting with a police officer. In this way, some general categories of behavior (e.g., cooperation, politeness) and some specific behaviors (e.g., looking at the officer, listening attentively, not arguing) were identified as important components of a youth's interaction with the police. This approach reduces the likelihood that selection of therapy goals will be biased by individual therapist's theories concerning which behaviors should be treated.

At this point, one cannot be sure that the component behaviors selected are the functional behaviors in a police-youth interaction—that is, the behaviors identified by the relevant individuals may not be those behaviors that really influence the outcome of police-youth interactions. However, a social validation procedure (Braukmann & Fixsen, 1975; Fawcett & Miller, 1975) can be used to establish the functional importance of the behaviors. This procedure consists of having relevant individuals rate the quality of the interactions, then training the youths to engage in those behaviors that were originally identified as socially important in the interaction, and then having relevant individuals again rate the quality of the interaction. If the ratings by the relevant individuals show a pre-post improvement in the quality of interaction and if there is a correlated change in the behavior of the youths, then the behaviors are socially valid and are reasonable foci for therapy. In the Werner et al. study videotapes were made of each youth's interaction with a police officer before and after the youths were taught how to interact appropriately with police officers. A sample of police officers then viewed the videotapes and rated each segment on several dimensions (e.g., cooperation, suspiciousness, labeling as a troublemaker). The results showed that the police officers gave more positive ratings to the youths' behavior in the post-training tapes than in the pre-training tapes. The videotapes also were scored for the presence of the behaviors that were determined to be socially important and this measure was correlated with the social validity ratings. The correlation was +.85, indicating that higher ratings by the police were associated strongly with the presence of the socially important behaviors.

The procedures for identifying socially important behaviors and for socially validating them have been used for youth's conversation behaviors (Minkin, Braukmann, Minkin, Timbers, Timbers, Fixsen, Phillips, & Wolf, 1976) and for staff behaviors (Willner, Braukmann, Kirigin, Fixsen, Phillips, & Wolf, in press). The social validation procedures also have been used for conversation-related behaviors (Maloney, Harper, Braukmann, Fixsen, Phillips, & Wolf, 1976), classroom behavior (Meichenbaum, Bowers, and Ross, 1968), and school-related behavior (Bednar, Zelhart, Greathouse, & Weinberg, 1970).

SELECTING TREATMENT PROCEDURES

The selection of appropriate treatment procedures for therapeutic intervention is as difficult and complex as identifying appropriate client populations and socially valid therapeutic goals. In the past, therapists were relatively free to choose among a variety of treatment procedures that might constitute appropriate remedies for a youth's antisocial behavior. However, recent court decisions (e.g., *Wyatt* v. *Stickney*, 1972) have stated that children and youth have the right to "least restrictive treatment." The principle of least restrictive treatment establishes that the therapist must use mild forms of intervention restricting the client's freedom as little as possible. In addition, the therapist must assess the effectiveness of the least restrictive treatment procedure before attempting to utilize more intrusive or more aversive techniques. For example, the therapist should first employ minimally intrusive positive reinforcement procedures such as contingent praise and attention. However, if the evidence indicates that the less obtrusive procedure rarely facilitates changes in the youth's antisocial behavior, then the therapist is obligated to implement a more obtrusive and potentially more effective procedure.

The concerned therapist is presented with a paradox of values in attempting to select treatment procedures. He or she is obliged, on the one hand, to help the antisocial youth as quickly and effectively as possible and, on the other hand, according to ethical and legal sanctions, to interfere minimally in the life of the youth. It is again apparent that longitudinal studies are needed to determine the relative "success rates" of various procedures and therapies for treating antisocial adolescents. Such studies will assist therapists in selecting appropriate treatment procedures that are most effective and least restrictive.

The following section details the usefulness of various treatment procedures as well as some necessary cautions to be exercised by the therapist.

BEHAVIOR MODIFICATION PROCEDURES

A number of clinical and experimental procedures have been subsumed under the general heading of "behavior modification," but some of the techniques mentioned in the literature do not really fall into the category. Agras (1973) has listed a number of procedures and discussed the problem of incorrectly designating some therapeutic procedures as behavior therapy or behavior modification. For example, the inclusion of "implosion therapy" or "flooding" as a behavioral therapy was considered inappropriate. Implosive therapy claims to be based on the behavior modification principle of extinction (Stampfl & Levis, 1967), yet extinction is a phenomenon observed under conditions considerably different from the clinical setting where implosion therapy is practiced. The transition from the laboratory to the applied setting is actively encouraged in behavior modification, but a number of analytic components must remain—including the analysis of treatment effectiveness and the specification of factors responsible for the measured effects of therapy.

Review of the existing behavior modification literature reveals that there appears to be a "core group" of techniques most often used when working with antisocial adolescents. These procedures are contingent praise and attention; behavioral contracting; token economy; a wide variety of teaching methods and skill-training techniques to impart pro-social behaviors; and isolation and time-out from positive reinforcement. These procedures have been used singly and in varying combinations with each other. While these procedures are useful, some pose such a host of moral, ethical, and legal concerns that they are *not* recommended for general use. Later sections of this paper contain such recommendations, along with evaluations of the effectiveness of these techniques.

CONTINGENT PRAISE AND ATTENTION

The most common form of positive reinforcement is contingent praise and attention. The technique includes praise statements such as "That's good" or "All right!" and verbal or nonverbal attention such as friendly conversation or an affectionate "pat on the back" that are contingent upon the occurrence of desired pro-social behaviors. In clinical practice with antisocial adolescents, the behavior modifier in conjunction with the client (1) establishes a set of pro-social behaviors to be positively reinforced; (2) immediately gives and/or instructs significant others to give brief praise and attention to the youth when those behaviors occur; and (3) ignores and/or instructs significant others to ignore the youth's antisocial behaviors. Using what has since become a classical use of praise and attention, Hall, Lund, and Jackson (1968) instructed teachers systematically to vary their positive social attention toward disruptive students in the classroom. During pretherapy "baseline" conditions, measures were taken of the amount of study behavior exhibited by disruptive youths in selected classrooms. In the first therapy "reinforcement" condition, teachers were instructed to approach these students when they were engaging in study behavior (and *not* displaying any antisocial behaviors) and make some positive verbal comment to the youths, pat them on the shoulder or use some positive physical contact. In the second baseline condition of the "reversal" research design (Sidman, 1960), the teachers stopped the experimental praise and attention and returned to their former pattern of usually attending to the antisocial behaviors. In the next reinforcement condition, the teachers were once again instructed to praise and attend to pro-social behavior and ignore antisocial and non-study behavior. The results clearly showed that the students' disruptive antisocial and nonstudy behaviors *decreased* when ignored by the teachers. Concurrently, the youths' pro-social and study behaviors *increased* when immediately followed by teacher praise and attention. Occasional "post checks" during the rest of the school year showed that the youths' appropriate behavior was sustained at a high level.

Although no normative studies have appeared describing how much positive teacher attention should be used to increase youths' pro-social behaviors, the value of positive attention in the classroom appears to be clear. Thomas, Becker, and Armstrong (1968) instructed teachers to vary systematically their use of praise for pro-social student behavior and their use of typical verbal reprimands for antisocial behavior. They reported that if teachers withheld all approval and used only reprimands to control antisocial student behaviors, the class conduct was poor. Moreover, if the teachers increased their reprimands in attempting to control the class, conduct became even worse. Thus, a high ratio of contingent positive attention to reprimands appears useful in working with adolescent antisocial behaviors in school settings. Praise and attention contingent upon appropriate, pro-social behavior has been used also for antisocial adolescents in nonschool settings such as institutions for the retarded (e.g., Doubros, 1966) and with families in the home environment (e.g., Patterson, Cobb, & Ray, 1973).

It should be noted that attention that is contingent upon the occurrence of a youth's antisocial behavior can conceivably increase the incidence of antisocial behavior, albeit unintentionally. Even when the perceived valence of the attention is negative (e.g., reprimands, lectures) the attention may still function as positive reinforcement for the youth. Because of the importance of attention as a factor influencing adolescent behavior, special care should be taken in treatment environments where staff can inadvertently increase youths' antisocial behaviors (Buehler, Patterson, & Furniss, 1966). In this sense, even staff who are not specifically designated as therapists still modify the behavior of clients with whom they interact.

Behavioral Contract

"Behavioral contracting" is another behavior modification procedure used in working with antisocial youth (Stuart, 1971, 1976; Stuart & Lott, 1972; Tripodi, Jayaratne, & Canburn, 1976). Stuart (1971) listed five elements of good behavioral contracts that describe how an adult and an adolescent can make an agreement that will influence their interpersonal interactions. The five elements are: (1) *detailed privileges* that each party of the contract expects to earn after fulfilling his or her responsibilities; (2) *detailed responsibilities* that should be kept to a minimum (if the number of responsibilities is increased without an equal increase in the value of offered privileges, then little or no reinforcement will be provided for the new responsibilities and they are unlikely to be met); (3) *sanctions* for failing to meet responsibilities; (4) a *bonus clause* that assures positive reinforcement for compliance with the contract itself; and (5) a *provision for feedback* so that progress of the participants can be recorded (e.g., by use of a checklist where participants check off fulfillment of responsibilities).

Jayaratne, Stuart, and Tripodi (1974) reported the results of three behavioral contracting projects spanning the years from 1970 to 1973. Of 94 families referred to the project by school personnel because of severe antisocial displays of the students in those families, 79 families agreed to participate. Additional families were added in subsequent years as comparison groups. Each of ten therapists worked with 3 to 15 families in helping natural parents and their junior high school children negotiate contracts involving both school and home behaviors of the youths.

Research data on the effectiveness of the

behavioral contracts were difficult to analyze, since different interaction styles were employed by various therapists. A separate experiment revealed that "fixed" contracts, which more clearly specified contracting procedures, produced no differences in treatment *approach* by different therapists. However, "open contracts" not specifying contractual procedures did produce differences between therapists' interaction styles. The more typical fixed contract as used by Jayaratne et al. (1974) included five responsibility and privilege areas: school attendance, school performance, school behavior, (natural) home chores, and other home behaviors. For example, under the attendance *responsibility* area would be specified the number of classes per day a youth must attend in exchange for *privileges* such as allowance. The therapist's primary role was to monitor and guide the negotiations between the parent and the youth. Continuing consultation was provided by therapists after contracts were negotiated to solve conflicts or assist in renegotiating unworkable agreements. A number of follow-up measures were obtained after the conclusion of therapy. One result showed that after one year of follow-up, those youths not under contract with their families had approximately three times as many court contacts as did the contract therapy youths. However, other measures revealed mixed results and the authors themselves noted problems that are relevant to program evaluation. Behavior contracting—like other treatment procedures—must be evaluated further to assess its long-term effectiveness.

Behavior contracting also has been used in other settings, such as correctional institutions (Musante, 1975). This technique may well represent a significant advance toward solving some of the ethical and "who controls whom" issues of behavior modification. Ayllon and Skuban (1973) listed four parts of a therapeutic contract that appear to divide responsibility *and* reward *equally* between client and therapist: (1) an overview of the client problem (tantrums in this case) and the therapist's modification program; (2) explicit pro-social behavioral objectives for the youth; (3) specification of the time and place of therapeutic intervention; and (4) withholding by the client of one-third of the prepaid therapy fee until successful completion of the contractual therapy. These and similar innovations can only promote more equitable therapies and more ethical uses of behavior modification procedures.

TOKEN ECONOMY

The token economy developed by Ayllon and Azrin (1968) for hospitalized psychiatric patients has been adapted to a large number of environments dealing with a variety of clients. A token economy can be viewed as an elaborate behavioral contract used with a number of clients in contrast to the client–parent–therapist triad typical of many behavior contracts. In a typical token economy, a number of youth behaviors are identified for which the client can earn or lose tokens ("points" marked on a card, plastic markers, or whatever). The token "balance" (i.e., tokens earned minus tokens lost) is computed after a specified time period, and the balance may be used by the client to purchase a variety of tangible items or privileges. The token economy is clearly one of the most prevalent behavior modification procedures used in psychiatric hospitals (Foreyt, 1975). Foreyt reported the existence of bibliographies listing 271 articles and papers about token economies, and there are reports of its use in hospitals in England and Ireland (Turton & Gathercole, 1972).

Phillips (1968) investigated the usefulness of a token economy in a Teaching-Family group home (Phillips, Phillips, Fixsen, & Wolf, 1974) for predelinquent boys. Phillips (1968) examined the effectiveness of token ("point") fines upon such behaviors as verbal aggression (e.g., "I'll kill you") by the boys. While "corrective" statements by the group home houseparents such as "That's not the way to talk" or "Stop that kind of talk" reduced aggressive statements somewhat, the point losses were more effective. Point losses were effected by "fining" the boys after each aggressive statement. Boys' access to privileges, such as allowance and permission to stay up late, could be limited if they did not make up these point losses. It should be noted that the "back-up reinforcers" were *special* privileges, and the token system was designed so that no youth would be without privileges for an extended period of time. If either condition had not been present (i.e., if the back-ups were normal rights due clients such as food or shelter, or if it had been difficult for clients to regain their lost points), then the token economy would have become an obtrusive, aversive system. Token economies also have been used in school classrooms (e.g., O'Leary, Becker, Evans, & Saudargas, 1969) and to a lesser degree in natural families of problem children (e.g., Sloop, 1975).

Practitioners should use caution when implementing a token economy, for they can be difficult to operate and can be abused to the detriment of an adolescent. Basic necessities such as food or shelter should never be used as back-up rewards for token economies, yet problems arise in some settings (e.g., correctional institutions) in providing acceptable reinforcers. In addition, complex relationships between earned tokens, token savings, and client behavior over time may be similar to problems (e.g., inflation) experienced in monetary economies (Winkler, 1972, 1973). Furthermore, Kazdin and Bootzin (1972) discussed several obstacles impeding the successful use of a token economy, including inadequate staff training prior to token economy implementation, client resistance, client circumvention of the approved contractual methods of earning tokens, and nonresponsiveness of clients. These problems can be alleviated—for example, by staff training programs (Gardner, 1972)—but are diffcult to remedy in large institutions (Musante & Gallemore, 1973).

Teaching Pro-Social Behaviors

Most of the behavior modification procedures thus far described are typically used to increase or decrease the occurrence of behavior *already in the adolescent's repertoire*. In these cases, researchers have not questioned *whether* the youth is able to engage in a pro-social behavior (since he has displayed the behavior at some point in the past) but only *how often* or *where* the youth will engage in pro-social behaviors instead of antisocial behaviors. However, a number of behavior modifiers theorize that many youths display antisocial behaviors because they have never adequately learned the pro-social alternatives required by society. Thus, incentives such as praise and attention or a token economy alone cannot possibly operate to improve behaviors that simply do not exist.

Various skill-teaching methods are sometimes added to the token economies to instill alternative pro-social behaviors and hopefully to better prepare patients for normal living (Kazdin & Bootzin, 1972; Wolfensberger, 1970). For example Martin, England, Kaprowy, Kilgour, and Pilek (1968) reported that the use of tokens plus "prompting" and "fading" decreased tantrums and increased appropriate pro-social behaviors of four hospitalized youths between 8 and 13 years of age. "Prompting" refers to the technique of introducing a stimulus (e.g., a visible cue) into an environmental setting to increase the probability that a particular behavior will occur (Geller, Farris, & Post, 1973). Prompts have been used with behaviors other than antisocial behaviors and have been cited often in working with retardates (e.g., Kazdin, Silverman, & Sittler, 1975) although it has been implemented with other client groups as well (McClannahan & Risley, 1975). "Fading" is a technique whereby a stimulus is gradually and systematically removed from an environment to increase the probability that a learned behavior will continue to occur even without the stimulus. As the stimulus is "faded out," the therapist checks the desired behavior for persistence. Fading has been used to describe the reduction of an experimenter's physical guidance of retarded youths paired with positive reinforcement of youth responses so that the children no longer required the experimenter's direct prompting to use the newly acquired skill (Whitman, Zakaras, & Chardos, 1971). This technique has been used as a way of reducing therapist-youth token exchanges over time so that more natural reinforcers can gradually be substituted and treatment effects will be generalized beyond the group home setting (Phillips, Phillips, Fixsen, & Wolf, 1971).

Some research efforts have attempted to assess the effects of various procedures used to inculcate pro-social behaviors in group home settings (e.g.,

Braukmann, Maloney, Fixsen, Phillips, & Wolf, 1974; Maloney, et al., 1976; Minkin, et al., 1976). Many of the procedures are based on previous studies on teacher training methods (e.g., McKnight, 1971), among them prompting, fading, and "shaping," which refers to the positive reinforcement of small components or approximations of a behavior until the client learns the complete behavior. Shaping has been used also in several settings to teach a variety of complex social and physical motor skills other than prosocial behaviors (Azrin and Foxx, 1971; Horner, 1971; Mahoney, Van Wagenen, & Meyerson, 1971). In addition, "behavior rehearsals" (Gittelman, 1965; Kaufmann & Wagner, 1972) are often used to allow staff trainees or clients to practice clearly defined pro-social behaviors and then receive some form of feedback from the behavior modifier (via audio- or videotape playback, feedback graphs, etc.). Such precise feedback assists the trainee or client in learning the new skill.

The importance of adding skill-training to a token economy for antisocial adolescents was suggested in two experiments by Ford, Christopherson, Fixsen, Phillips, and Wolf (1973). These researchers found that the combination of skill-training sessions plus token incentives (points) was more effective than either procedure alone in teaching a number of household maintenance and pro-social behaviors to adolescents in a group home. Research in behavior modification has necessarily involved training the *staff* to use the specific skill-teaching procedures (Kirigin, Ayala, Braukmann, Brown, Fixsen, Phillips, & Wolf, 1975; Maloney, Fixsen, Maloney, and Phillips, in press; Maloney, Phillips, Fixsen, & Wolf, 1975). In addition to the typical skill-teaching procedures, Teaching-Family group home programs (Phillips, et al., 1974) have included in their training programs for "teaching-parents" how to present rationales to youths explaining why they should change their behavior. Evidence exists that youths prefer this use of rationales by adults (Elder, 1963; Pikas, 1961).

It is also becoming evident that some antisocial behaviors can apparently be decreased *without* recourse to a token economy. For example, one study (Kifer, Lewis, Green, & Phillips, 1974) was designed to teach conflict negotiation skills to three youth-parent pairs. Two of the youths were residents in group homes, and the third was an eligible candidate for group home placement. The study consisted of three phases: (1) observations in the *natural homes* to collect data about parent-youth interactions during actual conflicts; (2) *classroom* sessions, consisting of behavioral rehearsals with experimenter feedback, plus discussions and practice of the Situations–Options–Consequences–Simulation (SOCS) model for negotiation of conflicts (Roosa, 1973) and testing of parent and youth negotiation skills before and after training; and (3) observations in the *natural home* again to measure generalization of trained behaviors into the home. The results showed a clear improvement in negotiation skills on both sides and an increase in fulfilled parent-youth agreements in the home setting.

ISOLATION AND "TIME-OUT"

A common consequence used by natural parents for adolescent behavior problems is sending the youth to his or her room, "grounding" (i.e., the youth is forbidden to leave the house for a period of time), and similar restrictions on youth activities. When deliberately used as a therapeutic procedure for antisocial behavior, the therapist, school teacher, or trained parent (1) establishes a set of inappropriate behaviors that will be "punished" with restrictions; (2) immediately restricts the activities of the youth when the identified antisocial behaviors occur, and (3) attends to or ignores other appropriate or inappropriate behaviors as usual.

The use of time-out in correctional and other settings has been reported in the past (e.g., Burchard & Tyler, 1965; Tyler & Brown, 1967). In Tyler and Brown's (1967) study, institutionalized delinquents were placed in a room for 15 minutes immediately following any display of antisocial behaviors. In phase two of the experiment, time-out was dropped and staff substituted such phrases as "Now cut it out!" Following reinstitution of the time-out procedure, it was concluded that time-out was far more effective than verbal admonitions in reducing antisocial behaviors. However, some experiments on time-out have indicated that it does not always decrease antisocial behaviors of all youths and it actually can *increase* them under certain conditions (Burchard & Barrera, 1972; White, Nielson, & Johnson, 1972).

Since Leitenberg's (1965) review of the behavior modification technique known as time-out, a number of practitioners have used the same term to refer to a much more obtrusive technique that would be more appropriately called isolation. The difference between time-out and isolation is not merely one of semantics. Time-out is an abbreviation for "time-out from positive reinforcement" and refers to *temporary removal from positive reinforcement* following client display of some inappropriate behavior. Isolation is simply the removal of a client from an environment for a long period of time.

Except in rare instances of violent behavior, isolation can deprive clients of legal rights. The use of time-out is not recommended except when the usefulness of removing the client from positive reinforcement for a brief period of time can be clearly demonstrated. Neither time-out nor isolation should be attempted unless all less restrictive alternatives have been documented as ineffective. In practice, it is very difficult to exhaust *all* less restrictive alternatives, and it is even more difficult to document thoroughly the ineffectiveness of these techniques. Such documentation requires adequate research designs to control for the effects of nontreatment variables, computation of the reliability of the measures used to assess the client's responses to the milder procedures, and so forth. Unfortunately, isolation and time-out are such relatively "easy" procedures to implement (e.g., it is not very difficult to train staff to lock an adolescent in a room) that they are often used as substitutes for more acceptable behavior modification procedures.

ETHICAL AND LEGAL ISSUES

As behavior modification has developed as a science, various problems have arisen (May, 1975). Initial *ethical* objections were that behavior modification treated only "symptoms" rather than the true underlying causes of human disorders. These fears were generally addressed satisfactorily (Eysenck, 1959), only to be replaced by fears of the *moral* nature of behavior modification; i.e., "who will control the controllers?" These concerns, the subject of much discussion during the 1960s (e.g., Ullman & Krasner, 1965) are presently being attended to with various contractual agreements and the inclusion of consumer feedback systems. Recently, *legal* questions have emerged about behavior modification (Halleck, 1974; Stepelton, 1975; Wexler, 1973). While many of these legal issues apply equally to other treatment modalities, there is little doubt that the publicity of occasional abuses has put the spotlight on behavior modification. May (1975) lists four procedures that behavior modification programs can use to help prevent such abuses. First, adequate staff training with supervised practical experience should be given to anyone responsible for therapeutic intervention (American Psychiatric Association, 1973). Second, behavior modification techniques should be used only with consenting clients. Third, the use of highly aversive or unusual punishment procedures should be minimized or avoided entirely. Fourth, behavior modification procedures should be constantly monitored so that the "good" programs may prosper and "bad" ones can be justifiably terminated. May (1975) states that behavior modification programs should follow these steps since "... too many abuses could lead to an untimely and unnecessary end to a treatment approach that has demonstrated its worth in many settings, with many types of clients ..." (p. 159).

Ethical and Moral Issues

Roos (1974) argues that some of the ethical concerns with behavior modification are exaggerated, since the American legal system itself is an elaborate functioning of aversive consequences. Behavior modification procedures, Roos points out, are probably more ethical than normal societal regulations since behavior modifiers use aversive consequences on a more limited basis, as part of an overall research strategy with knowledge of its possible effects, and only after careful evaluation of alternatives. It should be stressed, however, that the aversive consequences discussed by Roos are only a small part of the behavior modification literature and that some relevant moral issues pertain to even the more acceptable positive techniques. These additional issues involve the role of human values in behavior modification and how the behavior modifier influences his or her client. All therapies can be viewed as attempts to persuade the client to behave differently and to exert some control over the client (Strupp, 1974). Thus, ethical and moral concerns with behavior modification in particular typically focus on the manner in which the client is controlled.

Although the direct but limited deprivation of an inmate's food and clothing has been suggested as a means to modify prisoners' behavior (Musante, 1975) it is not generally recommended. Instead, the more popular token economy is often used where clients receive tokens and exchange them for *special* privileges beyond their basic necessities. Despite the difficulties in implementing a token economy (Sherman and Baer, 1969), it is a useful behavior modification technique and—when supplemented with additional components such as skill-training for youths and consumer feedback—it can be a humane and effective therapy for anti-social adolescents.

LEGAL ISSUES

Right to Treatment. In a landmark decision (*Donaldson* v. *O'Connor*, 1974), it was affirmed that hospital patients have a "right to treatment" and must be released if no treatment is provided by an institution. This decision did not pose immediate problems for behavior modification, since the demonstrated effectiveness of behavioral programs in some institutions had suggested that behavior modification programs could help institutionalized patients. However, it did raise the question of how an organization and a potential or actual client are to choose among available therapies. There is no question that this issue is actively discussed in the legal field (Bazelon, 1969; Katz, 1969) and will continue to be important in coming years.

Right to Refuse Treatment. Another court decision (*Wyatt* v. *Stickney*, 1972) held that patients have the right to *refuse* treatment. Wexler (1973) stated that this decision threatens the use of token economies in institutions since it guarantees the patient access to reinforcers that formerly were available only through token rewards for prosocial behavior. Wexler recommended that the decision in *Wyatt* v. *Stickney* be reevaluated if it adversely affects patient progress in token economy environments. While this problem can be partially solved by the development of reinforcers other than basic necessities, the decision has led to further questioning of what are "rights" and what are "privileges." As long as effective treatment does not become impossible, this increased scrutiny of rights versus privileges can be considered a healthy concern.

Conflict of Two "Rights." Begelman (1975) discussed the legal conflicts that may arise between the ethical obligation and legal mandate to provide treatment on the one hand, and the patient's right to refuse treatment on the other. Theoretically, involuntarily committed patients (with whom the legal decisions were originally concerned) who refuse treatment could later sue the program for lack of treatment! Peck's (1975) solution to the paradox is two-fold: (a) a limitation on involuntary commitments to "dangerous persons" or to those adjudicated incompetent—thereby reducing the number of hospitalized patients and perhaps reducing the number of people who would want to exercise the right to refuse treatment; and (b) granting the right to refuse treatment to *all* committed persons. While the proposed solution has merit, there remains the possibility that involuntarily committed "dangerous" persons may well refuse treatment and thus the problem of conflicting laws would persist. Begelman (1975) has suggested that behavioral scientists distinguish between the phenomena of "custodial care" and "treatment" for future legal decisions. Such an approach would focus on the behavioral impact of treatment environments upon individual clients and would thus insure that future mental health laws are written in the best interests of the client.

PROGRAM EVALUATION

Distinctions have been made between "formative" and "summative" evaluation in social science research (Weiss, 1972). Formative evaluation is roughly equivalent to "procedure" evaluation (Braukmann et al., 1975) where the short-term effectiveness of specific treatment techniques is assessed and the day-to-day operation of a program is monitored. Summative evaluation, or "program" evaluation, attempts to determine the overall impact a program has on its clients. Program evaluation—especially long-term follow-up of released clients—is urgently needed for behavior modification programs in all settings, but is a difficult research activity to perform (Wortmanm, 1975). It is suggested that a minimum of three types of program evaluation data be collected to assess any treatment program: effectiveness, cost, and consumer satisfaction.

EFFECTIVENESS

Although behavior modification has been recognized as the only treatment methodology that routinely produces quantitative and analyzable client records (May, 1975), more evaluation should be performed. The most crucial need is for follow-up evaluations to assess the long-term effects of different kinds of treatment approaches. Braukmann et al. (1975) recommended several measures for use in follow-up studies with antisocial youths. Among the recommendations are (1) that post-release institutionalization rates be obtained for the youths, with provision for measuring the relative "seriousness" of offenses that result in their being sent to an institution (Sellin & Wolfgang, 1964); (2) that school grades and attendance records of released adolescents be assessed; and (3) that employment and vocational functioning be evaluated (Shah, 1968). Importantly, all released youths, not just selected subjects, should be included in follow-up studies (Lerman, 1975).

The few follow-up studies of behavioral programs reported in the literature (Davidson & Seidman, 1975) generally cover only a 2-year follow-up period. Examples of these reports indicate that specially trained parents of 27 aggressive boys maintained low rates of antisocial behaviors for a one-year follow-up period (Patterson, 1974); delinquents of behavior-contracting families showed lower recidivism rates than two comparison groups over a 6 to 18 month follow-up (Alexander & Parsons, 1975); and sixteen youths who had resided in Teaching-Family group homes had fewer police and court contacts, lower recidivism, higher grades, and were attending school more regularly over a two-year follow-up period than were a comparison group of boys who had been on probation or who had been institutionalized (Phillips, Phillips, Fixsen, & Wolf, 1973). All of these studies contain certain methodological deficiencies pointed out by their authors, but they do demonstrate that such evaluations are possible and can help assess the usefulness of treatment programs.

Generalization. It is clear that researchers need to investigate more thoroughly the generalization of treatment effects. Sloop (1975), for example, presented generalization as one of the three main future directions for behavior modification work with parents and families. While Sloop noted the existence of some data indicating the generalization of behavior modification treatment, there is also evidence that it does not generalize (e.g., Patterson, Cobb, & Ray, 1973; Wahler, 1969).

There can be no question that generalization of behavior modification treatment effects is an important issue. However, one of the reasons why research results on generalization appear to be so contradictory may rest in the terminology itself. Generalization commonly refers to the maintenance of appropriate client behavior in nontreatment conditions, that is, where the behavior modifier is no longer in a position directly to reinforce the appropriate behavior. The assumption is that if the therapist has modified the crucial client behaviors, the "natural" reinforcers in the nontreatment environment will maintain the new behaviors.

The degree of generalization that occurs is obviously dependent upon the degree of similarity between the treatment and nontreatment setting. Generalization may occur differentially between environmental components within the same setting, between different settings, and between different consecutive settings. One example of generalization between environmental components within the same setting is that between different classes in the same school (Schwarz & Hawkins, 1970). Generalization between different settings can take place between two highly dissimilar settings on a frequent, regular basis during treatment; e.g., between school and the natural home of a youth while the youth is receiving treatment at school. Generalization between different consecutive settings refers to highly dissimilar treatment and nontreatment settings where a single transition takes place, such as between an institutional treatment setting and a normal community living setting. Because of the two-fold adjustment involved in generalization between different consecutive settings (Feldman, Wodarski, Flax, & Goodman, 1972), this is perhaps the most difficult adjustment to achieve. However, the importance of follow-up studies in evaluating programs has necessitated perhaps an overemphasis on methods for achieving generalization between different consecutive settings.

A number of methods have been suggested for achieving generalization. Most of the generalization methods described by Braukmann et al. (1975), DeVoge and Downey (1975), and Musante (1975) assume that the pro-social behaviors taught to clients will be supported by natural consequences in nontreatment settings. The methods for increasing generalization can be summarized as follows: (1) construct the treatment environment to be as similar to the post-treatment environment as possible (through direct placement of the treatment setting within the community, as has been done with group homes); (2) gradually "fade out" treatment support systems such as token economies and replace them with increasing amounts of "normal" reinforcers while the client is still in treatment in order to facilitate the changeover to the new setting; and (3) do not depend solely on the two previous methods but include working closely with significant others in the client's post-release environment—training such persons if necessary to deliberately foster continuation of youths' pro-social behavior in nontreatment settings. These three methods require considerable program planning and staff training commitments, but all three have been implemented for antisocial adolescents (Phillips et al., 1974).

COST

The financial burden of mental health programs has been criticized (Stuart, 1970; Park, 1967), and there can be little doubt that funding agencies and state legislatures look closely at program costs when deciding which programs to fund. It is extremely difficult to weigh effectiveness against cost when judging the social value of an overall program (Adams, 1974), but cost-effectiveness research is emerging as a new field within the social sciences.

Certainly the issues in evaluating program costs are complex: Should one include capital expenditures? What are included in operating costs (staff time, overtime, use of already available services, etc.)? And how can one relate costs—adjusted for inflation—to various client benefits during different follow-up years? Despite their inherent complexities, and despite the typical lack of economic expertise of treatment personnel, these factors must be assessed. The cost of programs is considered by political bodies, whether or not social scientists wish it were otherwise (Maloney, 1974).

CONSUMER SATISFACTION

A shared concern of therapists and clients is how to assure a client of receiving proper care. Legal remedies have already been touched upon, but other methods exist to ensure citizens that behavior modifiers are using appropriate therapy. The general intent of these methods is to enable various "consumers" of social service programs to provide frequent feedback to treatment program managers about how "satisfied" they are with the program. For discussion purposes, consumers are divided into the *clients* receiving treatment (antisocial adolescents) and the *significant others* who play some role in the lives of these youth (parents, teachers, agency representatives, etc.).

Satisfaction of the Client. Clients should be able to express their satisfaction with any proposed treatment mode before, during, and after treatment. Such feedback should theoretically tend to modify treatment techniques over time. Client satisfaction with proposed therapeutic procedures *before* treatment is currently apparent to a limited extent in contracts of various kinds. In the business world, explicit contractual agreements have been used for centuries to support mutual satisfaction of the parties, but only recently has the concept of contracting been used in social sciences. Client satisfaction *during* treatment is also important. Phillips, Phillips, Wolf and Fixsen (1973) conducted a series of nine experiments with antisocial adolescents in a Teaching-Family group home and evaluated different youth-manager systems according to their effectiveness in achieving the goals and according to "preference" measures by the youths. A system that was effective *and* preferred by the boys was adopted. Thus the youths' "satisfaction" became another dimension in evaluating the procedures. Other research has demonstrated that it is possible to develop "self-government" systems that allow youths to express their degree of satisfaction with a program during residency and even facilitate cooperative and rational decision making by antisocial adolescents in a group home (Fixsen, Phillips, & Wolf, 1973). Youths also can fill out questionnaires during their treatment to express their degree of satisfaction with all aspects of the program (Phillips et al., 1974). Measures of client satisfaction with a program expressed *after* treatment are rare but could be a valuable measure for program evaluation. It is possible that post-release satisfaction would be more objective than in-program satisfaction measures since released clients would be free from any potentially biasing constraints. Such satisfaction measures could be an integral part of longitudinal follow-up evaluations, although it should be noted that follow-up evaluations are not yet part of most treatment programs.

Satisfaction of Significant Others. Persons who play important roles in the adolescent's life should have the opportunity to express their satisfaction with a program. Ratings by such persons also could serve as a form of program evaluation (Fischer, 1973). Phillips et al. (1974) outlined procedures whereby members of the juvenile court (probation officers, court counselors, and judges), agency representatives (social workers, mental health officials), school personnel (teachers, counselors, principals), members of a community Board of Directors (neighbors, club members, lawyers, etc.), and the parents of the youths could express the extent of their satisfaction with the care given to antisocial adolescents in Teaching-Family group homes during the youths' residency. This information is then added to the satisfaction ratings given by the adolescents themselves and used to improve the treatment program and to certify the staff who operate Teaching-Family homes (Braukmann et al., 1975b). While the validity of satisfaction ratings from such a diverse group of consumers is currently being studied, it already has been shown that there is a high degree of agreement between parent ratings of their child's improvement over time and the ratings recorded by the professional therapist (O'Leary, Turkewitz, & Taffel, 1975).

CONCLUSIONS

There are many dimensions to conducting therapy with antisocial youths. The therapist must decide whom to treat and what behaviors to establish as goals for therapy. It was noted that the therapist's decisions should be based on the results of longitudinal studies that provide normative data on the long-term outcomes of client groups who exhibit various problem behaviors. However, only a few such studies have been conducted and these are limited in scope. The therapist also must decide which treatment procedures to use to accomplish the goals of therapy. Again, the therapist's decisions should be based on empirical evaluations of a variety of treatment procedures as they are used with client groups. Considerable data have been collected to evaluate the immediate effects of treatment procedures on youths' antisocial behavior but only a few studies have looked at the long-term effects of treatment procedures. A therapist's choice of treatment procedure is further limited by legal and ethical issues that have only recently been articulated. A youth's "right to least restrictive treatment," "right to treatment," and "right to refuse treatment" must be given careful attention whenever treatment procedures are chosen and implemented.

Evaluation has been a hallmark of behavior modification treatment for antisocial youths. Such evaluation has focused on the immediate effects of treatment procedures on specific behaviors. While these procedure evaluations are necessary, they are not sufficient to demonstrate the overall value of behavior modification treatment programs. It has been suggested that evaluations be conducted to determine the long-term effects of programs on the lives of the youths after they leave a program, the costs of the program, and the satisfaction of the youths and other consumers with a program.

REFERENCES

ADAMS, S. Measurement of effectiveness and efficiency in corrections. In N. D. Glaser (Ed.), *Handbook of criminology*. Chicago, Ill.: Rand McNally, 1974.

AGRAS, W. S. Toward the certification of behavior therapists? *Journal of Applied Behavior Analysis*, 1973, *6*, 167–173.

ALEXANDER, J. F., and PARSONS, B. V. Short-term behavioral intervention with delinquent families: Impact on family process and recidivism. In A. M. Graziano (Ed.), *Behavior therapy with children II*. Chicago, Ill.: Aldine Publishing Co., 1975.

AMERICAN PSYCHIATRIC ASSOCIATION, *Behavior therapy in psychiatry*. Task Force Report, 5, 1973.

AYLLON, T., and AZRIN, N. H. *The token economy: Motivational system for therapy and rehabilitation*. New York: Appleton-Century-Crofts, 1968.

AYLLON, T., and SKUBAN, W. Accountability in psychotherapy: A test case. *Journal of Behavior Therapy and Experimental Psychiatry*, 1973, *4*, 19–30.

AZRIN, N. H., and FOXX, R. M. A rapid method of toilet training the institutionalized retarded. *Journal of Applied Behavior Analysis*, 1971, *4*, 89–99.

BAZELON, D. L. Implementing the right to treatment. *University of Chicago Law Review*, 1969, *36*, 742–754.

BEDNAR, R. L., ZELHART, P. F., GREATHOUSE, L., and WEINBERG, S. Operant conditioning principles in the treatment of learning and behavior problems with delinquent boys. *Journal of Counseling Psychology*, 1970, *17*, 492–497.

BEGELMAN, D. A. Ethical and legal issues of behavior modification. In M. Hersen, R. M. Eisler, and P. M. Miller (Eds.), *Progress in behavior modification* (Vol. I). New York: Academic Press, 1975.

BERKOWITZ, B. P., and GRAZIANO, A. M. Training parents as behavior therapists: A review. *Behaviour Research and Therapy*, 1972, *10*, 297–317.

BRAUKMANN, C. J., and FIXSEN, D. L. Behavior modification with delinquents. In M. Hersen, R. M. Eisler, and P. M. Miller (Eds.), *Progress in behavior modification* (Vol. I). New York: Academic Press, 1975. (a)

BRAUKMANN, C. J., FIXSEN, D. L., KIRIGIN, K. A., PHILLIPS, E. A., PHILLIPS, E. L., and WOLF, M. M. Achievement Place: The training and certification of teaching-parents. In W. S. Wood (Ed.), *Issues in evaluating behavior modification.* Champaign, Ill.: Research Press, 1975. (b)

Braukmann, C. J., Fixsen, D. L., Phillips, E. L., and Wolf, M. M. Behavioral approaches to treatment in the crime and delinquency field. *Criminology*, 1975, *13*, 299–331. (c)

Braukmann, C. J., Maloney, D. M., Fixsen, D. L., Phillips, E. L., and Wolf, M. M. An analysis of selection interview training package for pre-delinquent boys at Achievement Place. *Criminal Justice and Behavior*, 1974, *1*, 30–42.

Buehler, R. E., Patterson, G. R., and Furniss, J. M. The reinforcement of behavior in institutional settings. *Behaviour Research and Therapy*, 1966, *4*, 157–167.

Burchard, J. D., and Barrera, F. An analysis of time-out and response cost in a programmed environment. *Journal of Applied Behavior Analysis*, 1972, *5*, 271–282.

Burchard, J., and Tyler, V., Jr. The modification of delinquent behavior through operant conditioning. *Behaviour Research and Therapy*, 1965, *2*, 245–250.

Davidson II, W. S., and Seidman, E. Studies of behavior modification and juvenile delinquency: A review, methodological critique, and social perspective. In A. M. Graziano (Ed.), *Behavior therapy with children II.* Chicago, Ill.: Aldine Publishing Co., 1975.

DeVoge, J. T., and Downey, W. E. A token economy program in a community mental health day treatment center. In W. Doyle Gentry (Ed.), *Applied behavior modification.* St. Louis, Mo.: C. V. Mosby, 1975.

Donaldson v. *O'Connor*, 493 F.2d (5th Cir.), 1974.

Doubros, S. Behavior therapy with high level institutionalized, retarded adolescents. *Exceptional Children*, 1966, *33*, 229–233.

Elder, G. H. Parental power legitimation and its effects on the adolescent. *Sociometry*, 1963, *26*, 50–65.

Eysenck, H. J. Learning theory in behavior therapy. *Journal of Mental Science*, 1959, *105*, 61–75.

Fawcett, S. B., and Miller, L. K. The experimental analysis and social validation of the training of public speaking behaviors. *Journal of Applied Behavior Analysis*, 1975, *8*, 125–135.

Feldman, R. A., Wodarski, J. S., Flax, N., and Goodman, M. Treating delinquents in traditional agencies. *Social Work*, 1972, *17*, 71–78.

Fischer, J. Is case work effective? A review. *Social Work*, 1973 (Jan.), 5–20.

Fixsen, D. L., Phillips, E. L., and Wolf, M. M. Achievement Place: Experiments in self-government with pre-delinquents. *Journal of Applied Behavior Analysis*, 1973, *6*, 31–47.

Ford, D., Christopherson, E., Fixsen, D. L., Phillips, E. L., and Wolf, M. M. Parent-child interaction in a token economy. Unpublished manuscript, University of Kansas, Lawrence, Kansas, 1973.

Foreyt, J. P. Behavior modification in mental institutions. In W. Doyle Gentry (Ed.), *Applied behavior modification.* St. Louis, Mo.: C. V. Mosby, 1975.

Gardner, J. M. Teaching behavior modification to non-professionals. *Journal of Applied Behavior Analysis*, 1972, *5*, 517–521.

Geller, E. S., Farris, J. C., and Post, D. S. Prompting a consumer behavior for pollution control. *Journal of Applied Behavior Analysis*, 1973, *6*, 367–376.

Gentry, W. D. (Ed.), *Applied behavior modification.* St. Louis, Mo.: C. V. Mosby, 1975.

Gittelman, M. Behavior rehearsal as a technique in child treatment. *Journal of Child Psychology and Psychiatry*, 1965, *6*, 251–255.

Haase, R. F., and Tepper, D. T. Nonverbal components of empathic communication. *Journal of Counseling Psychology*, 1972, *19*, 417–424.

Hall, R. V., Lund, D., and Jackson, D. Effects of teacher attention on study behavior. *Journal of Applied Behavior Analysis*, 1968, *1*, 1–12.

Halleck, S. L. Legal and ethical aspects of behavioral control. *American Journal of Psychiatry*, 1974, *131*, 381–385.

HORNER, R. D. Establishing use of crutches by a mentally retarded spina bifida child. *Journal of Applied Behavior Analysis*, 1971, *4*, 183–189.

JAYARATNE, S., STUART, R. B., and TRIPODI, T. Methodological issues and problems in evaluating treatment outcomes in the Family and School Consultation Project, 1970–1973. In P. O. Davidson, F. W. Clark, and L. A. Hamerlynck (Eds.), *Evaluation of behavioral programs*. Champaign, Ill.: Research Press, 1974.

KATZ, J. The right to treatment—an enchanting legal fiction? *University of Chicago Law Review*, 1969, *36*, 755–783.

KAUFMANN, L. M., and WAGNER, B. R. Barb: A systematic treatment technology for temper control disorders. *Behavior Therapy*, 1972, *3*, 84–90.

KAZDIN, A. E., and BOOTZIN, R. R. The token economy: An evaluative review. *Journal of Applied Behavior Analysis*, 1972, *5*, 343–372.

KAZDIN, A. E., SILVERMAN, N. A., and SITTLER, J. L. The use of prompts to enhance vicarious effects of non-verbal approval. *Journal of Applied Behavior Analysis*, 1975, *8*, 279–286.

KIFER, R. F., LEWIS, M. A., GREEN, D. R., and PHILLIPS, E. L. Training pre-delinquent youths and their parents to negotiate conflict situations. *Journal of Applied Behavior Analysis*, 1974, *7*, 357–364.

KIRIGIN, K. A., AYALA, H. E., BRAUKMANN, C. J., BROWN, W. G., FIXSEN, D. L., PHILLIPS, E. L., and WOLF, M. M. Training teaching-parents: An evaluation and analysis of workshop training procedures. In E. Ramp and G. Semb (Eds.), *Behavior analysis: Areas of research and application*. Englewood Cliffs, N. J.: Prentice-Hall, 1975.

LEITENBERG, H. Is time out from positive reinforcement an aversive event? *Psychological Bulletin*, 1965, *64*, 428–441.

LERMAN, P. *Community treatment and social control*. Chicago: University of Chicago Press, 1975.

MAHONEY, K., VAN WAGENEN, R. K., and MEYERSON, L. Toilet training of normal and retarded children. *Journal of Applied Behavior Analysis*, 1971, *4*, 173–181.

MALONEY, D. M. *Evaluation of community-based treatment facilities*. Chapel Hill, N. C.: Developmental Disabilities Technical Assistance Systems, 1974.

MALONEY, D. M., HARPER, T. M., BRAUKMANN, C. J., FIXSEN, D. L., PHILLIPS, E. L., and WOLF, M. M. Teaching conversation-related skills to pre delinquent girls. *Journal of Applied Behavior Analysis*, 1976, *9*, 371.

MALONEY, D. M., PHILLIPS, E. L., FIXSEN, D. L., and WOLF, M. M. Training teachniques for staff in group homes for juvenile offenders: An analysis. *Criminal Justice and Behavior*, 1975, *2*, 195–216.

MALONEY, K. B., FIXSEN, D. L., MALONEY, D. M., and PHILLIPS E. L. Behavior technology in child-care: The Teaching-Parent and the Teaching-Family Model. In J. Beker (Ed.), *The child-care worker in the United States: A comparative analysis of evolving role models*. New York: Human Sciences Press, in press.

MARTIN, G. L., ENGLAND, G., KAPROWY, E., KILGOUR, K., and PILEK, V. Operant conditioning of kindergarten-class behavior in autistic children. *Behaviour Research and Therapy*, 1968, *6*, 281–294.

MAY, JR., J. G. Moral, ethical, and legal considerations in behavior modification. In W. Doyle Gentry (Ed.), *Applied behavior modification*. St. Louis, Mo.: C. V. Mosby, 1975.

MCCLANNAHAN, L. E., and RISLEY, T. R. Design of living environments for nursing-home residents: Increasing participation in recreation activities. *Journal of Applied Behavior Analysis*, 1975, *8*, 261–268.

MCKNIGHT, P. C. Microteaching in teacher training: A review of research. *Research in Education*. Manchester University Press, No. 6, November 1971.

MEICHENBAUM, D. H., BOWERS, K. S., and ROSS, R. R. Modification of classroom behavior of institutionalized female adolescent offenders.

Behaviour Research and Therapy, 1968, *6*, 343–353.

MINKIN, N., BRAUKMANN, C. J., MINKIN, B. L., TIMBERS, G. D., TIMBERS, B. J., FIXSEN, D. L., PHILLIPS, E. L., and WOLF, M. M. The social validation and training of conversation skills. *Journal of Applied Behavior Analysis*, 1976, *9*, 127–139.

MUSANTE, G. J. Behavior modification in prisons and correctional facilities. In W. Doyle Gentry (Ed.), *Applied behavior modification*. St. Louis, Mo.: C. V. Mosby, 1975.

MUSANTE, G. J., and GALLEMORE, JR., J. L. Utilization of a staff development group in prison consultation. *Community Mental Health Journal*, 1973, *9*, 222–230.

O'LEARY, K. D., BECKER, W. C., EVANS, M. B., and SAUDARGAS, R. A. A token reinforcement program in a public school: A replication and systematic analysis. *Journal of Applied Behavior Analysis*, 1969, *2*, 3–13.

O'LEARY, K. D., TURKEWITZ, H., and TAFFEL, S. J. Parent and therapist evaluation of behavior therapy in a child psychological clinic. In A. M. Graziano (Ed.), *Behavior therapy with children II*. Chicago, Ill.: Aldine Publishing Co., 1975.

PARK, C. C. *The Siege*. New York: Harcourt Brace and World, 1967.

PATTERSON, G. R. Retraining of aggressive boys by their parents: review of recent literature and follow-up evaluation. In F. Lowy (Ed.), Symposium on the Seriously Disturbed Pre-School Child. *Canadian Psychiatric Association Journal*, 1974, *19*, 142–161.

PATTERSON, G. R., COBB, J. A., and RAY, R. S. A social engineering technology for retraining the families of aggressive boys. In H. E. Adams and I. E. Unikel (Eds.), *Issues and trends in behavior therapy*. Springfield, Ill.: Charles C. Thomas, Publisher, 1973.

PECK, G. L. Current legislative issues concerning the right to refuse versus the right to choose hospitalization and treatment. *Psychiatry*, 1975, *38*, 303–317.

PHILLIPS, E. L. Achievement Place: Token reinforcement procedures in a home-style rehabilitation setting for "pre-delinquent" boys. *Journal of Applied Behavior Analysis*, 1968, *1*, 213–223.

PHILLIPS, E. L., PHILLIPS, E. A., FIXSEN, D. L., and WOLF, M. M. Achievement Place: Modification of the behaviors of pre-delinquent boys within a token economy. *Journal of Applied Behavior Analysis*, 1971, *4*, 45–59.

PHILLIPS, E. L., PHILLIPS, E. A., FIXSEN, D. L., and WOLF, M. M. Behavior shaping works for delinquents. *Psychology Today*, 1973 (June), 74–79.

PHILLIPS, E. L., PHILLIPS, E. A., FIXSEN, D. L., and WOLF, M. M. *The Teaching-Family handbook* (rev. ed.). Lawrence, Kan.: University of Kansas Printing Service, 1974.

PHILLIPS, E. L., PHILLIPS, E. A., WOLF, M. M., and FIXSEN, D. L. Achievement Place: Development of the elected manager system. *Journal of Applied Behavior Analysis*, 1973, *6*, 541–561.

PIKAS, A. Children's attitudes toward rational versus inhibiting parental authority. *Journal of Abnormal and Social Psychology*, 1961, *62*, 315–321.

ROBINS, L. N. *Deviant children grown up*. Baltimore, Md.: Williams & Wilkins, 1966.

ROOS, P. Human rights and behavior modification. *Mental Retardation*, 1974, *12*, 48–66.

ROOSA, J. B. *SOCS: Situations, options, consequences, and simulation. A technique for teaching social interaction*. Paper presented to the American Psychological Association, Montreal, Canada, 1973.

SCHWARZ, M. L., and HAWKINS, R. P. Application of delayed reinforcement procedures to the behavior of an elementary school child. *Journal of Applied Behavior Analysis*, 1970, *3*, 85–96.

SELLIN, T., and WOLFGANG, M. E. *The measurement of delinquency*. New York: John Wiley, 1964.

SHAH, S. A. Preparation for release and community follow-up. In H. L. Cohen, I. Goldiamond, J. A. Filipczak, and R. Pooley (Eds.), *Training professionals in procedures for the establishment of educational environments.* Silver Springs, Md.: Institute for Behavioral Research, Educational Facility Press, 1968.

SHERMAN, J. A., and BAER, D. M. Appraisal of operant therapy techniques with children and adults. In C. M. Franks (Ed.), *Behavior therapy: Appraisal and status.* New York: McGraw-Hill, 1969.

SIDMAN, M. *Tactics of scientific research.* New York: Basic Books, 1960.

SLOOP, E. W. Parents as behavior modifiers. In W. Doyle Gentry (Ed.), *Applied behavior modification.* St. Louis, Mo.: C. V. Mosby, 1975.

STAMPFL, T. G., and LEVIS, D. J. Essentials of implosive therapy: A learning-theory-based psychodynamic behavioral therapy. *Journal of Abnormal Psychology*, 1967, *72*, 496–503.

STEPELTON, J. V. Legal issues confronting behavior modification. *Behavioral Engineering*, 1975, *2*, 35–43.

STRUPP, H. H. Some observations on the fallacy of value-free psychotherapy in the empty organism: Comments on a case study. *Journal of Abnormal Psychology*, 1974, *83*, 199–201.

STUART, R. B. *Trick or treatment.* Champaign, Ill.: Research Press, 1970.

STUART, R. B. Behavioral contracting within the families of delinquents. *Journal of Behavior Therapy and Experimental Psychiatry*, 1971, *2*, 1–11.

STUART, R. B. Experimental validation of contract based techniques for the control of delinquent behavior and communication. *Journal of Behavioral Science*, 1976, *8*, 132–144.

STUART, R. B., and LOTT, L. A. Behavioral contracting with delinquents: A cautionary note. *Journal of Behavior Therapy and Experimental Psychiatry*, 1972, *3*, 161–169.

THOMAS, D. R., BECKER, W. C., and ARMSTRONG, M. Production and elimination of disruptive classroom behavior by systematically varying teacher's behavior. *Journal of Applied Behavior Analysis*, 1968, *1*, 35–45.

TRIPODI, T., JAYARATNE, S., and CANBURN, D. An experiment in social engineering in serving the families of delinquents. *Journal of Abnormal Child Psychology*, 1976, *4*, 243–261.

TURTON, B. K., and GATHERCOLE, C. E. Token economies in the U.K. and Eire. *Bulletin of the British Psychological Society*, 1972, *25*, 83–87.

TYLER, V. O., and BROWN, G. D. The use of swift, brief isolation as a group control device for institutionalized delinquents. *Behaviour Research and Therapy*, 1967, *5*, 1–9.

ULLMAN, L. P., and KRASNER, L. A. *Case studies in behavior modification.* New York: Holt, Rinehart & Winston, 1965.

WAHLER, R. G. Setting generality: Some specific and general effects of child behavior therapy. *Journal of Applied Behavior Analysis*, 1969, *2*, 239–246.

WEISS, C. H. (Ed.). *Evaluating action programs: Readings in social actions and education.* Boston, Mass.: Allyn-Bacon, 1972.

WERNER, J. S., MINKIN, N., MINKIN, B. L., FIXSEN, D. L., PHILLIPS, E. L., and WOLF, M. M. Intervention package: An analysis to prepare juvenile delinquents for encounters with police officers. *Criminal Justice and Behavior*, 1975, *2*, 55–84.

WEST, D. J., and FARRINGTON, D. P. *Who becomes delinquent?* London, England: Heinemann Educational Books, Ltd., 1973.

WEXLER, T. B. Token and taboo: Behavior modification, token economies, and the law. *California Law Review*, 1973, *61*, 81–109.

WHITE, G. D., NIELSON, G., and JOHNSON, S. M. Time-out duration and the suppression of deviant behavior in children. *Journal of Applied Behavior Analysis*, 1972, *5*, 111–120.

WHITMAN, T. L., ZAKARAS, M., and CHARDOS, S. Effects of reinforcement and guidance procedures on instruction-following behavior of severely retarded children. *Journal of Applied Behavior Analysis*, 1971, *4*, 283–290.

WILLNER, A. G., BRAUKMANN, C. J., KIRIGIN, K. A., FIXSEN, D. L., PHILLIPS, E. L., and

Wolf, M. M. The training and validation of youth-preferred social behaviors of child-care personnel. *Journal of Applied Behavior Analysis*, in press.

Winkler, R. A theory of equilibrium in token economies. *Journal of Abnormal Psychology*, 1972, *79*, 169–173.

Winkler, R. An experimental analysis of economic balance, savings and wages in a token economy. *Behavior Therapy*, 1973, *4*, 22–40.

Wolfensberger, W. The principle of normalization and its implications to psychiatric services. *American Journal of Psychiatry*, 1970, *127*, 291–297.

Wolfgang, M. E., Figlio, R. M., and Sellin, T. *Delinquency in a birth cohort*. Chicago, Ill.: The University of Chicago Press, 1972.

Wortmann, P. M. Evaluation research: A psychological perspective. *American Psychologist*, 1975 (May), 562–575.

Wyatt v. *Stickney*, 344 F. Supp. 373 (M.D. ALA., 1972).

19

THE ANTISOCIAL AGGRESSIVE SCHOOL AGE CHILD: DAY HOSPITALS

Louis C. Zang

Until recently the child whose antisocial, aggressive behavior was of such magnitude that he was permanently excluded from the community's schools was dealt with ultimately in an institutional setting—be it a highly structured boarding school, a residential treatment center, a state psychiatric hospital, or a training school. A large percentage of these children can now be successfully treated in the community in the day hospitals and day treatment programs which are currently proliferating in the United States and elsewhere.

The concept of partial hospitalization in the treatment of mental illness and emotional disorders was first described in the report of a program begun in Moscow in 1933 and extended to include children in this country as early as 1943. Partial hospitalization is utilized in the treatment of emotionally disturbed children in many day hospital programs here and abroad, but there has been a paucity of reports on these ventures available to those who would launch a new program.

A children's psychiatric day hospital may be differentiated from other day treatment programs by the broader range of diagnostic and therapeutic resources available for the emotionally disabled child. While the day hospital affiliated with a medical school may offer the broadest range of resources convenient under one umbrella, most programs developed in such a hospital can be applied by other day treatment centers.

The rationale for day hospitalization of children with severe emotional disabilities may be described under four main headings: First, it maintains the existing home intact and avoids removing the child from a home which might never accept his return after experiencing life without him. Second, it permits treatment of the home itself. Third, it avoids giving the child the message that he is so evil he cannot be maintained or tolerated at home. And, fourth, it creates a better community awareness of the problems of emotionally disturbed children and prompts the community to develop services needed by child and family.

The necessary conditions for the successful treatment of an emotionally disturbed child in a day hospital setting are: First, a home that provides some semblance of safety for the child. Second, a home where there is some chance of change for the better taking place, however minimal. And, third, a child who is young enough to be supervised in the home when not in the day hospital.

THE CHILDREN'S DAY HOSPITAL AS A MODEL TREATMENT APPROACH

The title *day hospital* necessitates a medical model, and a children's day hospital should be under the overall supervision of a medical director who is a qualified child psychiatrist. The medical director is responsible for the quality of care of the patients in the hospital program. The director is assisted by a multi-disciplinary team including a pediatric neurologist, a pediatrician, a psychologist, a social worker, teachers, and the primary child-caring agents, who in this instance will be referred to as counselors. The medical director is responsible for all aspects of treatment including medical and psychotherapeutic care, behavior modification, and education, and, therefore, the selection of the most qualified staff available is of vital importance. Since the teachers and counselors are with the children throughout the day every day, it is imperative that the best qualified people fill these positions.

The educational component of a day hospital program may be provided in either of two ways. The day hospital can operate its own school in which case the medical director can assume full responsibility for the selection of qualified teachers, which has an obvious advantage. The alternative is to have a cooperative program with the public school system in which district the day hospital is situated. This may pose problems in the selection of personnel, but it provides one very positive feature in that the school has a vested interest in the continuing successful performance of the child who leaves the day hospital program. Since its inception in 1970, the Children's Day Hospital of the Westchester Division of New York Hospital Cornell Medical Center has been a cooperative project with the White Plains Board of Education. The program to be described is based on this cooperative project.

The Children's Day Hospital treats children with severe emotional disabilities. It has a maximum census of 32 patients, 5 to 13 years in age. About one-third of the patients are girls. Roughly half the patients are black. Most are of average or above-average intelligence but, on occasion, a mildly retarded child is accepted. Eighty percent of the children are referred because of extreme antisocial behavior. Impulse ridden, physically assaultive, destructive, verbally assaultive, and defiant are terms frequently used by referring agencies. Twenty percent have autistic features, although children without language are not deemed appropriate. There is severe family pathology in a large percentage of cases.

The organizational structure gives the director the responsibility for all aspects of the day hospital, which consists of a lower program for children ages 5 to approximately 10 and a middle program for children through age 13. Immediately responsible to the director are the teacher-coordinator, who supervises all school activities in both divisions, an assistant to the director, or chief counselor, for each of the two divisions, and the director of art therapies who is in charge of an extensive and varied arts program in each division. Each division is staffed by teachers, who are responsible to the teacher-coordinator, counselors, who are responsible to the chief counselor, and an extremely talented core of volunteers who work under the supervision of the counselors, teachers, and art therapist.

SELECTION OF STAFF

In the beginning, the counselors were selected by the director acting alone. Since then a selection process has evolved which provides additional safeguards and facilitates entry into the program for the new counselor. An equal opportunity advertisement is placed in the health care section of a large metropolitan newspaper. The educational requirements stated are a bachelor's degree. After the written applications are screened, the more promising candidates are given one or more personal interviews with members of the senior staff. From these, the top ten or so contenders are invited to spend a day on the job with children and staff. Following this, the director meets with the counselors, who have been asked to rate the candidates one to ten. There is almost complete unanimity about the top contenders. The director looks for sincere dedication to a lifetime career working with children, emotional stability, maturity, intelligence, and an abundance of energy.

The counselors look for the ability to communicate with the children and a willingness to reach out to them. Once a selection has been made, the candidates are interviewed by the director of special education programs for the school. If he concurs, an official offering is made, and the prospective counselor is asked to commit him or herself to the program for at least two years. In addition to the safeguards such a selection process offers, it obviates the need for the new counselor to prove himself to the seasoned members of the staff.

The counselor is the person who is ever present with the children from the time of their arrival in the morning until the bus takes them away in the afternoon. The counselor's responsibilities are to monitor the flow of children from activity to activity, to intervene in crisis situations, to set limits, to conduct the diversity of activities, to work with families, to participate in the selection of children for the program, to supervise volunteers, to assist in the in-service training activities, to act as individual psychotherapists for three or four children, to prepare the children for reentry into the regular schools, and to continue to follow the children after discharge—a multifaceted program of activities.

Counselors were first utilized as primary psychotherapists because they were the only staff members who could be expected to stay with the patients from entry to discharge. Although there was a concern whether one person could simultaneously cope with the dual role of therapist and disciplinarian, the counselors from the beginning have had the character, sensitivity, intelligence, and motivation to be good therapists and they have been able skillfully to balance the two roles. The children also have been quite able to separate the two roles in which the counselor acts.

THEORETICAL FRAMEWORK FOR THERAPY

The director supervises all of the psychotherapy done by the counselors. Before describing the methods used in supervision, it seems important to discuss the theoretical frame of reference which underlies all aspects of the children's day hospital. While we are concerned with the practical application of therapies, a theoretical frame of reference is useful in enabling the therapists to understand the concepts that give rise to the practical applications and recommendations they employ in endeavoring to help the children, whether the method be psychotherapy, behavior modification, activity therapy, milieu therapy, crisis intervention, family therapy, or community action. Eclecticism, a seemingly comfortable way of making use of parts of several theories, has not made for really clear understanding. Lester Havens (1973) of Harvard has made an appeal for a pluralistic approach and this has much logic for treating profoundly disturbed children. However, it is unrealistic to expect many therapists to be equally proficient in all the major therapies. Therefore, while a pluralistic approach is ideal, it is imperative that there be a consistent underlying point of view which can be called upon to explain what is taking place in the process of therapy.

"Psychoanalytic theories of personality development and structure of the mind are the most inclusive." Jane Kessler states in her textbook on childhood psychopathology (1966) that it is impossible for her "to discuss the full range of deviations in child behavior without making use of explanatory principles provided by psychoanalytic theory." She does not believe that there is a fundamental incompatibility between learning theory and psychoanalytic theory. "The principles of learning would have to do with ego-functioning." The basic drives postulated in psychoanalytic theory can also serve as the motivation for learning. Both psychoanalytic theory and learning theory embrace the developmental point of view; but neither accepts the theory that development and maturation alone can account for all of the intricacies of individual development.

To the critics who sight determinism as their major objection to psychoanalytic theory, David Rappaport supplies the best answer in balancing drive with drive restraint. Gill and Klein (1967) in introducing Rappaport's collective papers point out that "he was profoundly concerned with the question of how to reconcile strict determinism, the coercive claims of man's inescapable drives and immutable reality on the one hand, while on the other, his personal belief that man does play a role in shaping his own destiny. He found the solution of the paradox in a principle that wise men have always known. Freedom lies in control and in the awareness of necessity." Hartman (1976) has similarly said "in the ego's relative autonomy lies a measure of freedom and a base from which to enlarge the scope of freedom. The normal ego must be able to control, but it also must be able to must." Although psychoanalytic theory provides a frame of reference on which it is convenient to mount the hypotheses for our therapeutic techniques, it must be stressed that the therapy carried out in the day hospital is neither psychoanalysis nor psychoanalytic psychotherapy. In Reider's (1959) terms, this therapy is "often directed towards meeting derivative needs and strengthening pathogenic defenses and it, therefore, cannot be called psychoanalysis."

As soon as a child is accepted into the program, that child is assigned for individual psychotherapy. Within the first 2 weeks, a formal treatment plan is prepared. The official form for the original treatment plan provides a description of the current condition of the child under four headings: "Emotional," "Behavioral," "Cognitive," and "Neurological-physical." There are spaces for brief dynamic formulation, for statement of the long-range goals, the short-range goals, and for treatment methods and procedures. In stating the problem, formulating the dynamics that are operating, setting goals and initating a treatment plan, the assumptions upon which psychoanalytic theory is based are kept in mind.

SUPERVISION OF PSYCHOTHERAPY

Five Points of View as Helpful Constructs

Rappaport and Gill (1959) outline five points of view. In recognizing the drives, both aggressive and libidinal, the *economic point of view* is accepted. The derivatives of the aggressive and sexual drives are repeatedly observable by anyone present with the children for any time in the day hospital. It has been of no practical importance whether there is one drive with aggressive and libidinal components or multiple drives.

The *genetic point of view* is helpful in the developmental assessment of the child. Whether Anna Freud's (1965) Developmental Lines or other approaches to developmental profiling are used, the genetic concepts that there is an epigenetic ground plan for maturation and development and that earlier forms of psychological phenomena remain potentially active even after being superseded by later forms, are particularly helpful in explaining the ebb and flow of development.

The genetic point of view has been referred to as the accumulation of all past dynamics and the *dynamic point of view* is helpful in explaining psychological forces at work at any particular time.

The *adaptive point of view* states that psychological processes of adaptation to the environment exist at every point of life, that man adapts to the environment and that adaptation relationships are mutual. In essence, this gives a reason to expect that much of the work with the child can yield results.

Finally, and probably most important to the understanding of the treatment plan and procedures, there is the *structural point of view*. The structural point of view states that there are hypothetical structures of the mind, slow to undergo change, within which, between which, and by means of which mental processes take place. Moreover, structures are held to be hierarchically ordered, and this is important. The ego is the structure with which we are usually and most immediately concerned. We certainly are not unaware of the superego. It must be remembered that the idea of structure, and particularly the idea of an ego, is an abstraction but one which nonetheless has been found useful in understanding personality and character. It is in fact the concept which has made possible the development of the whole area of ego psychology which has been found to be so invaluable. Ego psychology is actually the arena in which most of the debates about what goes on in the day hospital take place.

The Ego and Its Functions

The ego is defined by its function. David Beres published a paper in 1956 that clarified this concept by spotlighting the main ego apparatuses and their functions. Fundamental to all ego activity is the synthetic function. It is felt that damage to the synthetic function is the result of a flawed early mother-child relationship. Certainly synthesis is impaired by stress and one of our primary therapeutic efforts is to improve synthesis.

The autonomous functions of the ego, perception, memory, and motor activity, depend on the ability to synthesize. Rappaport (1959) also includes with the autonomous functions a threshold capacity. Therapy also aims at improving perceptual skills, motor skills, and memory.

Co-existing with the autonomous functions are those functions which emerge out of conflict. These are reality testing, impulse control, object relations, thinking, and the defense mechanisms. In supervision, the child's level of functioning in each area is explored.

Dr. George Vaillant (1974) of Harvard has attempted to establish a hierarchy of defense mechanisms going from the psychotic to the immature defenses to the neurotic defenses and on to the mature coping mechanisms. The day hospital children mostly use immature methods in reacting to stressful situations. These, in Dr. Vaillant's scheme, are schizoid fantasy, projection, somatization, passive aggression, and acting out. The latter two are the most frequently observed.

In determining whether a child's behavior is psychotic, many of the day hospital staff become very defensive of the child and try to avoid this diagnosis. The checklist of psychotic symptoms published by the Working Party of the British Psychiatric Association (1961) has been found useful. When a child's behavior is described in terms of the nine behaviors on the checklist, the therapist finds it more acceptable to diagnose psychosis, in which case use of medication might be one option. It should be emphasized that medication is rarely used in the day hospital and then only as one part of the overall treatment plan when there are very specific medical reasons and never merely to suppress unacceptable behavior.

In attempting to understand, and to help the therapist understand, what technically is happening in therapy and what curative processes are taking place, the supervisor has found most useful Edward Biebring's five technical and curative principles (1954). The first and second principles—suggestion and abreaction—need no great elaboration. The third principle, manipulation, will be discussed shortly. The fourth principle, clarification, is of great importance. This is the assistance the therapist gives the patient in understanding what he is doing, how this behavior appears to others, and the consequences of what he is doing for himself. The fifth principle, interpretation, is less frequently used in working with the children but is occasionally called for particularly in the later phases of therapy.

Returning to the third principle, manipulation, let it be stressed how much of the therapy involves technical and curative manipulation. This does not refer to such crude forms of manipulation as advice, guidance, or other similar ways of running a patient's life. In Biebring's words, manipulation can be defined as the employment of various emotional systems existing in the patient for the purpose of achieving therapeutic change. Either in the technical sense of promoting the treatment or in the curative process, the corrective emotional experience which the therapist attempts to provide for the patient is a technical manipulation in that it attempts to produce a favorable attitude toward treatment and to remove obstructive attitudes. The children in the day hospital have never before had the experience of being really listened to by an adult. The therapist who makes a sincere effort to understand what the child is saying is providing the child with a corrective emotional experience and is thereby utilizing the manipulative technique. Much of the treatment in the day hospital may be explained in terms of technical manipulation. These principles of Biebring are applicable to all schools of psychotherapy not just to those based on psychoanalytic theory.

To sum up, the supervision of psychotherapy by the counselors is structured on the five points of view of psychoanalytic theory, the ego apparatuses described by Beres, the defense hierarchy of George Vaillant, the British Working Party's checklist of psychotic symptoms in children, and Biebring's five technical and curative principles.

THE THERAPIST—PATIENT RELATIONSHIP

In the first supervisory session, it is pointed out to the novice therapist that few of the patients have ever had the opportunity to relate to a trustworthy adult who is not preoccupied with problems of her or his own survival. Therefore, the first goal of our therapy is the building of a mutually trusting relationship with the child. As a first step toward attaining trust, the therapist is urged to consider that the therapeutic session with the child takes absolute precedence over any other duties in the program and is not to be delayed, postponed, or cancelled except for the direst emergency. It is pointed out to the counselor that it is not unusual for it to take months for a child to be convinced that he has really found someone he can trust.

This simple introduction puts the counselor at ease, to the extent that he or she can now approach the first session with only a reasonable amount of anxiety. Each therapy session is dealt with in detail in supervision. Although each counselor was selected for his stability and sincere interest in children, it has been extremely rewarding to observe the growth of the therapeutic skills of the counselors. This has far exceeded original expectations. The question of whether a counselor could carry out simultaneously the dual roles of therapist and disciplinarian was answered by a child who in one breath expressed anger to a counselor because of a disciplinary action and in the next breath asked expectantly when his next individual therapy session would take place.

Admission Procedures

The majority of the referrals to the day hospital come from schools. All resorces in the schools have already been exhausted in attempting to help these children when the referral is made. However, some children have been referred by other mental health agencies and others have entered the program after a trial of therapy in the hospital's outpatient clinic. The first call from the referring person gives the intake social worker an opportunity to begin preparing the child and family for the best possible introduction to the day hospital. Any misconceptions that the referring person has about the day hospital should be corrected. It should be urged that the parent be made to understand clearly that the first call and subsequent visit is solely for the purpose of the sharing of information and does not in any way commit the family to send their child to the day hospital, nor does it commit the day hospital to accept the child.

When the parent then calls to make application for the child's admission to the day hospital, the intake worker should ask what the family has been told about the day hospital and any false impressions should be set straight. One weeping mother asked how long was her son going to be kept locked up before she could see him again. At this time it should be emphasized that should the child be found appropriate for the program and accepted, the parents still have full freedom to admit the child or not, according to their own wishes and best judgment. The nature of the evaluation process should be explained and the parents should be given an appointment to come in without the child and talk.

The history is taken and the examination of the child is done by a counselor under the supervision of the director or the chief social worker. When possible, the same counselor who may later become the child's therapist does the evaluation. During the first visit the counselor makes sure that the parents understand the nature and scope of the program. A skilled counselor can use this first visit to explore the parents' feelings about the child, about the school or other community authorities by whom they may have felt intimidated, and about the need for such intensive psychiatric care and any attendant stigma.

In addition to a complete psychiatric evaluation, each candidate receives a neurological examination and appropriate psychological testing to serve as a baseline. If the psychiatric examination establishes a clear case for admission to the day hospital, these other tests may be postponed until after admission. Reports are obtained from the school, family doctor, and others who may have relevant information. Finally, a conference attended by the director , the counselor who did the evaluation, and social worker, representatives of the referring school, other interested agencies, and the parents is held. The parents are again given the opportunity to discuss their own feelings and how to prepare the child for the new experience.

Much valuable information may be obtained from the school, which is often the referring agency. Rather than send a request for school reports, which usually yields xeroxed report cards, it is helpful to send a questionnaire that has been compiled in an effort to obtain from the teacher observations about all of the child's areas of function, including ego, superego, and affect. The questionnaire is sent to the principal of the school with the request that he ask the teacher, and in effect give the teacher permission, to fill out the questionnaire, providing the teacher with the assistance, if necessary, of the school psychologist and social worker. By requesting information in this way, the quality of the responses is greatly improved. After the questionnaire is returned, a phone call to the teacher is often helpful.

The Children's Therapeutic Needs

The therapeutic potentials of the milieu are limited only by the imagination and energy of the staff. Bill Hartman (1976) has written "the task of milieu therapy is to identify critical elements in the mutual adaptation process between patient and environment and to manipulate them so as to facilitate personality growth. Three major areas are identified. First the children need to curtail their acting out behavior. The environment must move quickly to establish control when the individual child cannot contain himself. The child must know, for example, that we will not let him hit or be hit by another child; that we will establish control when he loses the ability to do so."

"Second, the children need acceptance on an emotional level, especially from adult figures. The day hospital staff works hard to reach past the child's pathological behavior and offer emotionally close relationships. It is clear that the children and staff like each other and moments of joy occur almost as frequently as do struggles. The children's sense of basic trust is enhanced as they interact within an environment structured to provide both consistent controls and acceptance. As anxiety is lowered they become more able to engage in increasingly more organized patterns of activity."

"This leads us to our third major concern, the child's need to work. Our children need to spend sufficient periods of time engaged in doing or making things so that they can begin to experience the rewards of focusing their energy and attention. Working gives one a sense of being able to have an effect on things. For our children, this means an increased feeling of power and mastery vis-a-vis the environment, and a greater appreciation of their own worth as they experience themselves being successful. This, then, lays the foundation for a heightened sense of autonomy, industry, and initiative."

The physical facilities of a children's day hospital are important but will vary to reflect the community's resources. The important atmosphere of the milieu is set by the sincerity of concern which each member of the staff has for every child. The milieu must provide appropriate facilities for assisting the child to control his or her behavior. Children with such a wide span of ages can feel secure together because strict limits are imposed on physical aggression. All forms of sexual acting out including sexually stimulating conversations are discouraged. A seven-year-old boy from a home where sexual acting out was rampant was greatly relieved to find that our staff, while not permitting public acting out or sexually stimulating discussions, was quite ready to talk to him privately about activities that were appropriately private affairs. He seemed more comfortable when he understood that these limits would be enforced. In addition to aggression and sexual acting out, destruction of property and verbal abuse are strictly prohibited.

After a child has been in the program for a period of observation, specific pathological behaviors are listed and a behavior control prescription is suggested. The staff discusses each of the pathological behaviors and agrees on both a unified approach in dealing with the behavior and the specific goals to be sought. The prescription includes an attempt to isolate the dynamic factors resulting in the behavior; the staff also attempts to estimate the percentage of time each child is engaged in each of the specifically identified behaviors.

Dealing with Unacceptable Behavior

A hierarchy of techniques for dealing with unacceptable behavior is established. At the extreme end of this hierarchy is contacting the child's parent and possibly sending the child home. During the first year of the program, the teacher would frequently want to employ the regular school's technique of suspending the child for up to five days for insupportable behavior. Though it was pointed out that hospital patients are not sent home when their symptoms worsen, the pressure to utilize this legalistic approach persisted. To counter this the hospital staff proposed that if a child's behavior became so aggressive that it seemed unlikely that he would be able to regain self control, he could be sent home, but only until a parent could return with him to have a conference with the teacher, the counselor, and the director. Hopefully this would take place on the same day. The child would then be returned to the therapeutic program. In this way the parent is not relieved of all responsibility for the child's behavior; and since the child and the parent are both present at the conference there is no confusion about what happened. Since this technique was adopted, no child has been sent home more than three times and most have not been sent home at all. Lesser crises are dealt with on the spot by whatever staff person is available, usually by separating the child from the group and staying with him until the loss of control has passed and the child can return to the group without embarrassment.

A Varied Program of Activities

In addition to the corrective emotional experiences the milieu offers the children outside of the psychotherapy session and the relief provided them by an atmosphere in which they are safe from their own behavior and the behavior of others, the milieu should provide the children with a varied program of activities in which they can experience a sense of accomplishment. A heavy emphasis on sports to promote the development of motor control leads to a rapid improvement of self-image, which in turn enhances peer object relations in a low stress setting where success is most likely. Important activities in art, crafts, music, and animal care are enriching to a program. Frequent parties may be given by the children who are involved in the planning, execution, and hosting. It must be pointed out that parties, when inappropriate, can have a devastatingly destructive effect; however, parties for departing children and staff members can ease the problems of separation for both children and staff. More and more recognition is given to the importance of separations when a staff member or patient leaves. It is just as important for the staff to deal actively with their feelings arising from separations as it is for them to encourage the children to recognize and resolve separation problems. Field trips to parks, beaches, museums, nature centers, and the interesting areas of the city are a frequent part of the school year and the summer. Activities involving cooking have proven invaluable in their therapeutic potentials.

Volunteers when properly employed can render much service to a program. However, when the staff is so continuously occupied with regular responsibilities, care must be taken to avoid unnecessary confusion. One elementary rule should be that no volunteer is accepted for the program unless a clear function has been identified that the volunteer can carry out. In the program a counselor can be appointed as coordinator of volunteer activity. Anyone who has an idea of how a volunteer might be utilized in enriching the program may take this idea to the coordinator of volunteer activities who in turn takes the responsibility for exploring the feasibility of the proposal when it is discussed at the staff meeting. If it is agreed that an additional volunteer would be an asset to the program, then the coordinator of volunteer activities recruits someone through the hospital's director of volunteer services. The New York Hospital program has made use of volunteers ranging from high school students to the head of the section of child psychology at a major university. A resourceful coordinator has been able to establish contracts with several universities both near and far for full-time volunteers doing off-campus independent studies, on the one hand, and field placements of from 12 to 16 hours a week in conjunction with courses in psychology, on the other. By offering the volunteers an exceptional experience, we can expect the contracting universities to send their best students, and the hospital should have the privilege of screening all volunteers for character and appropriate motivation.

THE EDUCATIONAL COMPONENT OF THE PROGRAM

Since few of the children can be expected to attain high levels of achievement academically, a work motivation program is desirable. This should be individualized for each child and can begin at the first-grade level.

There are advantages in following the community school calendar during the school year. A one-week recess following the termination of the school year is followed by a summer program based on a day camp model. No academic work is involved in the summer program. There is a three-week recess before the beginning of the next school year in September. Staff members are expected to take their vacations when the children are on holiday.

There are many advantages in having the day hospital a cooperative project with the local public school. However, it is vital that the director of the day hospital participate in the selection of the teachers and have absolute authority to veto any teacher proposed for the program whom he deems unsuited. The senior teacher must be immediately responsible to the director and furthermore must be clearly aware that she or he is so responsible. The only responsibility which the hospital program should have to the local board of education is that the children who are patients of the day hospital be in regular attendance.

A good treatment plan helps to put the educational component of therapy into proper perspective. Nevertheless it is an extremely important ongoing responsibility of the director to provide a large amount of support for the teacher so that she will find it easier to shift her role toward a more therapeutic approach. It is often difficult for the teacher to understand that the patient is in the hospital program primarily because of an emotional disorder of real consequence and that the learning disability that is almost invariably present is a symptom of the emotional conflict and not vice versa. When the teacher's educational prescription for each child takes this into account, the patient is spared the stress of being expected to perform tasks in school of which he or she is not capable. This seems like a simple and self-evident concept, but it takes continuous and sympathetic support for the teacher to help her refrain from placing impossible expectations on her accomplishments with the child. When she can accept that the child's emotional disorder takes precedence over his learning disability and that the latter is a symptom of the former, the child will reward everyone by showing progress.

To plan clearly for the child's academic program, a detailed teaching prescription is developed in regular conference between the teacher, the hospital's educational coordinator, and the psychologist. These prescriptions are subject to ongoing amendment and are reviewed by the psychiatrist and the entire staff when the child is presented at the weekly clinical meeting. The prescription encompasses an outline of the child's assets, a list of the objectives, a discussion and enumeration of the teaching materials, all reinforced by references. As clear as possible a differentiation is made between learning disabilities due to perceptual or specific cognitive disorders and those that arise from nonspecific interference or blocking of the learning processes because of anxiety or preoccupation with overwhelming and more immediate problems.

In the first days after admission some patients may be asked to do no school work. A child who cannot tolerate working alongside another child may be given 20 to 30 minutes of individual attention daily by the teacher in a room away from other children. A child may begin with only one session a week. The teacher may then find that he or she can attend two sessions a day alone, but still cannot tolerate the presence of another child. Or again the teacher may find that the pupil can progress to work paired with another child but still can only tolerate one session a day. A child may be able to work paired with one special child while not being able to tolerate another. At some later date the child may progress to work in a small group. Frequent meetings of teachers and counselors under the guidance of the psychologist and the director enable the decisions for each child's teaching prescription to be highly individualized and fluid, amenable to observations from all members of the staff.

Role Flexibility

It is also helpful to have the counselors assume some teaching functions, enabling the teachers to reciprocate by stepping out of the strictly academic role into a more therapeutic one. Some children come into the program lacking the most basic equipment for family living. In this area the counselors have developed valuable teaching skills. Time must often be spent teaching a child to understand what a family is, what a mother is, what a father is, what breakfast is, and so forth. So many children come to the hospital without breakfast that it was found necessary to begin the day by serving cereal with fruit and milk the first thing upon arrival. This may lead to the child's developing the ability to bargain with a parent for breakfast at home on Saturday and Sunday. Cooking class is popular and provides many openings to deal with elementary life situations. One day after the cooking class had prepared pizza and applesauce the group of two girls and two boys sat down with the counselor to eat the food. One 8-year-old girl only saw her mother in passing, because the mother always left for work as the child returned from the hospital. When she sat down to eat with the counselor and children she exclaimed, "Gee! This must be what a family is like!" One child would regularly come to the hospital smelling so foul that the other children and staff alike found it difficult to endure. The hygiene teacher found a clever solution to this by starting a class in clothes washing. Each child in the class was asked to bring into school extra underwear and socks. The class learns proper care of clothing in relation to other matters of hygiene. Naturally some tact was required in proposing this to the parents.

Liaison Work with the Families

In the beginning of the program a social worker was assigned to work with the day hospital families. Although the social worker was both dedicated and skilled, her attempt to involve the families was more often than not totally unsuccessful. At present the counselor-therapist is on the front line in working with the families and with remarkable results. The counselor rapidly becomes one of the most significant persons in the child's life and his first name soon becomes a household word with the family. Frequent home visits enable the counselor to get to know the parents and other members of the patient's family. The visit may involve a meal with the family or an activity with the children in the family or neighborhood. A relationship of mutual trust and concern is eventually established. In many cases the counselor is called upon for advice and help in a variety of family problems and crises. At all times the counselor is supervised by, and has the back-up and guidance of, the chief social worker. Recently, on a weekday evening a mother called her son's counselor in a state of agitation. She announced that she had called the police to report her son for having purchased four packages of fireworks, that she could no longer handle him, and wanted him institutionalized, and that she was afraid he was going to run away, all in one breath. The counselor went immediately to their home, where he found the mother literally sitting on the 11-year-old boy. The counselor talked to the mother until she regained her composure. He then took the enraged boy for a walk. Several children in the neighborhood were exploding fire crackers. They talked about the boy's feeling of the unfairness of his mother's actions. Before the counselor departed from the family everyone had calmed down. The next day the boy came to the hospital on the bus as usual.

Occasionally parents may refuse to become involved until they notice some evidence of the child's improvement, which then alters their feeling about the day hospital. Our technique in working with the families of the younger patients is to attempt to win their cooperation with a minimum of overt coercion. Since the older child has a shorter time left to be treated in the day hospital, an agreement on the part of the parent to be involved in the program is a condition of admission.

The social worker is available at all times for on-the-spot consultation with the counselors about their work with the families. She has a supervisory session with each counselor once a week, and she conducts a group meeting with all the counselors in which they are encouraged to express their feelings about their work with the families. In addition, since most of the counselors are male and one-third of the patients are girls, she has assumed the role of advocate for the girls, and she attempts to make the counselors more aware of the reality of being a girl. In this she solicits the help of the one female counselor, the teachers, and many of the volunteers.

THE RETURN OF THE CHILD TO THE COMMUNITY

Proper preparation for the return of a child to the community is one of the most important tasks of the day hospital. Timing is important. Experience has shown that in approximately a two-month period there develops an agreement amongst the staff that a child has made the significant movement that will allow him or her to succeed in a regular school. The child shares this awareness of readiness and if steps are not begun for the actual return, the child's trust in the staff is diminished and he or she may regress. It is important to have a good working relationship with the director of special programs in the local school. With his assistance the first task is to select the proper school. In any community two factors are important. One is the personality and character of the principal of the school. The second is the relationship of the elementary school to the junior high school if the child is going into a fifth or sixth grade. If an elementary school shares a campus with a junior high school this is of value. It is helpful if the junior high school has a special class for emotionally disturbed students which can act as a supporting back-up in case the child has serious difficulties making the transition from elementary to junior high school in a regular class. Just the child's awareness of such a class has motivational value.

When the school is selected, the child's counselor, the teacher, and the day hospital director sit down with the principal to select the teacher and the class where the child will have the best chance to succeed. Occasionally the best teacher may have a class that already has a disproportionate number of behavior problems, and a less stressful class with the second best teacher is the wisest choice. It should be pointed out that the teacher who is best for one child is not necessarily the best teacher for the next child. One child may need a large, loving lap when another may function better with someone who is more structured and firm.

The teacher is prepared for the child and is assured of the day hospital's intention to continue to work with the child and to provide her with any support which might be necessary. A date is set, the child visits the school with the counselor and meets the new teacher and class. Later the counselor accompanies the parent to the school to meet the teacher, principal, and social worker. At first the child goes only in the morning, returning to the day hospital in the afternoon. Usually, after two or three weeks, both teacher and child are ready for a full day. After this the counselor sees the patient once a week and continues contact with the family, school teacher, school psychologist, and social worker. The day hospital staff assists the family in planning the child's summer. After school resumes in the fall, if the child seems to make a satisfactory adjustment to the next grade and there seem to be no other indications for psychotherapy, the process for termination of therapy may be begun by the counselor. After a belated discovery that one of the early apparent outstanding successes in the day hospital had gotten into serious trouble, a much more rigorous follow-up program was developed. Now the therapist of every patient who has returned to the community is in weekly contact with the patient, his family, and the school for at least a year after the child has been discharged from therapy. With this intensive interest in the patient's progress after leaving the program, it has been possible to intervene early when it was sensed that a problem was brewing, thus making it possible to follow through with the day hospital's early, hard-won success.

STAFF LEARNING PROGRAMS AND PROGRAM EVALUATION

In-service training enriches the experience of the staff. In addition to the psychotherapy supervision provided to each staff member who acts as therapist to a day hospital patient, each counselor receives supervision for one therapy case carried in the out-patient clinic. This enables the counselor to have a more rounded view of the psychopathology of children. Several counselors have acted as assistant therapists to senior staff members in conducting children's out-patient therapy groups, and counselors assist senior staff members in parent groups. At present there is a 2-year training program encompassing growth and development, case study, mental examination of children, ego psychology, psychopathology, psychological evaluation of the child, family dynamics, and community mental health.

Counselors act as mental health consultants to community agencies serving children. Each counselor is encouraged to participate in research projects. They have also been encouraged to participate in such outside training activities as a total emersion course in psychomotricity and a seminar in outdoor teaching techniques in order to attain special competence in a particular area that can later be shared with the other counselors. The counselor who is a specialist in outdoor teaching techniques has found that children who cannot comprehend the more abstract presentation in the classroom are often able to grasp a principle that is demonstrated in a more concrete way using the infinite variety of teaching material found out of doors.

A formal program evaluation project has been put into effect. Those children who enter the program primarily because of aggressive acting out behavior are the experimental group, and all children admitted to the day hospital for other disorders are the control group. Those children who are able to return to the community in a less structured program are considered successes. Those who leave the day hospital for a more structured program or for other causes are considered not to have benefitted from the program. Two hypotheses are being tested. The first is that day hospital treatment is beneficial to emotionally disabled children; the second is that the experimental group and the control group are benefitted equally by day hospitalization. Many other interesting research projects are possible in a day hospital setting.

CONCLUSIONS

There are many models for treatment. The one described here is clearly a day hospital. There are many advantages in not camouflaging this fact. Against the argument that calling this treatment, hospitalization, stigmatizes the patient, it can be contended that every child who is admitted is quite aware of being affected with some serious disability. Furthermore those parents who have a great proclivity to deny are helped to accept the seriousness of their child's disorder. The community is better able to accept the fiscal investment when the program of treatment is recognized as hospitalization. Each member of the staff has a clearer idea of his or her responsibility when every undertaking can be interpreted within the concept of hospital treatment. Early in the program one child was accepted with the agreement that his private neurologist would supervise anticonvulsant medication. Communication between the neurologist and hospital was less than satisfactory. The patient's overall progress was hindered until the conflict in the management of therapies was resolved. After anticonvulsant medication given for two years because of an EEG abnormality was discontinued and the hospital assumed total management, the overall condition of the patient began to improve for the first time.

When the staff clearly understands that the

program is hospital treatment, they are able to help the patient and the parent deal with feelings about this. The children have encountered little neighborhood ridicule, and what little they have encountered they have been able to handle with the help they have received from the counselors.

The director who learns how to make full use of his staff's many talents and skills, and who uses their eyes and their ears and their cognitive and intuitive skills, not only serves the patients better but also helps each staff member grow toward his or her potential and he finds that his own experiences are more exciting.

The day hospital concept is already leading to new applications. The local school personnel are requesting that counselors trained in the day hospital be made available to work in regular school classes for emotionally disturbed children alongside the special education teacher to give individual and group therapy to the children and to their families and to act in the capacity of consultants. The counselors are becoming expert in community mental health education. They are becoming recognized and accepted in the neighborhood and youth centers. Recently several counselors were invited to a school in a nearby district to participate in a junior high school mental health day. The children were disarmed to find the shrinks in blue jeans, sneakers, and with long hair, and they kept the counselor overtime in small rap sessions where they eagerly asked serious, intelligent questions about mental illness and mental health. The day hospital has enabled the parent hospital to feel comfortable admitting children as young as eight years old to in-patient units. In a day hospital program, success in working with severely disturbed children depends on choosing front line personnel who combine an overriding dedication to children with stability, maturity, youth, and vigor, and in providing them with supervision, guidance, and support from a skilled clinical professional team. Most of the personnel who have left the Children's Day Hospital have gone up the ladder in the helping professions.

REFERENCES

BERES, D. Ego deviation and the concept of schizophrenia. *In the psychoanalytic study of the Child* New York: International Universities Press, 1956.

BIEBRING, E. Psychoanalysis and the dynamic psychotherapies. *Journal of the American Psychoanalytic Association*, 1954, *2*, 745–770.

FREUD, A. *Normality and pathology in childhood.* New York: International Universities Press, 1965.

GILL, M. A., and KLEIN, G. S. *The structuring of drive and reality. Collected papers of David Rappaport.* New York: Basic Books, 1967.

HARTMAN, B. Unpublished paper delivered at the Symposium on Innovations in Developing Human Power to Help Emotionally Disabled Children, New York Hospital, Westchester Division, White Plains, New York, 1976.

HARTMAN, H. *Ego psychology and the problem of adaptation* (1939). New York: International Universities Press, 1958.

HAVENS, L. *Approaches to the mind.* Boston: Little, Brown, & Co. 1973.

KESSLER, J. W. *Psychopathology of childhood.* Englewood Cliffs, N.J.: Prenctice Hall, 1966.

RAPPAPORT, D., and GILL, M. M. The points of view and assumptions of metapsychology. *International Journal of Psychoanalysis*, 1959, 153–162.

REIDER, N. A type of psychotherapy based on psychoanalytic principles. *Bulletin of the Menninger Clinic*, 1959, 153–162.

VAILLANT, G. Theoretical hierarchy of adaptive ego mechanisms. *Archives of General Psychiatry*, 1974, *24*, 107–118.

A Working Party of the British Psychiatric Association. Schizophrenic syndrome in childhood. *British Medical Journal*, Sept. 30, 1961, pp. 889–891.

20

SOCIAL WITHDRAWAL AND NEGATIVE EMOTIONAL STATES: BEHAVIOR THERAPY[1]

Donna M. Gelfand

This review will focus on behaviorally based techniques used in the treatment of children's avoidance (phobic) behavior, social withdrawal, and negative emotional states such as reported or observed anxiety and fear. Behavioral methods have also been used to treat sleep disturbances and compulsive, ritualized behavioral routines, but the published accounts of such interventions have typically taken the form of anecdotal case studies. Consequently, treatment for these latter problems cannot yet be adequately evaluated or reviewed. For the most part, the studies considered here are experimentally controlled evaluations of behavioral treatment techniques in either a group comparison or a within-subject replication design.

Many of the problem behaviors exhibited by children are predictable and preventable. Educational and therapeutic techniques currently available could be used to forestall the occurrence of problems that befall a great many children and their families. Some prevention programs in current use will be described, and suggestions for new directions will be presented for use with children who are at high risk of developing specific behavioral problems.

[1]I am greatly indebted to Donald P. Hartmann and to Terry Wade for their prompt, critical reading of this manuscript and for their helpful comments.

TREATMENT OF COMMON CHILDHOOD FEARS

Perhaps as many as 90% of all children develop specific fears at some point in their early years (Macfarlane, Allen, & Honzik, 1954). Preschool children are commonly reported to fear animals, particularly dogs and snakes, storms and darkness, and doctors, as well as strange persons and unfamiliar social situations (Agras, Sylvester, & Oliveau, 1969; Hagman, 1932; Jersild & Holmes, 1935; Jersild, Markey, & Jersild, 1933; Macfarlane, et al., 1954; Miller, Barrett, Hampe, & Noble, 1972). Some of these fears decline sharply with the child's increasing age. In their longitudinal study, Macfarlane and her colleagues found that fear of dogs was the predominant fear of 3-year-olds, but that this specific fear had largely disappeared among the same children five years later. A recent epidemiological survey conducted by Agras, Chapin, and Oliveau (1972) revealed that children who had been psychiatrically diagnosed as phobic improved markedly over a 5-year period without any professional treatment interventions. This 100% improvement rate for children was markedly superior to the improvement rate of only 43% shown by the phobic adults sampled. Although the particular, very small sample surveyed may have yielded a misleadingly high rate of improvement for children, it appears that no treatment is necessary in many instances.

Whether or not intervention is necessary can be determined by considering both the predicted duration and the potential seriousness of the problem. Some fears are more tenacious than others. Miller and his associates (1972) have determined that fear of physical injury and psychic stress carry through much of the individual's life span, but that fear of natural events such as storms and darkness tends to mitigate during maturation. Jersild and Holmes (1936) noted that fears of animals are less likely to be outgrown than are some other fears such as those of strange objects, people, and situations. The longer lasting fears would certainly justify professional treatment. Moreover, although the prognosis for children who develop specific fears appears to be relatively good, a short-term, inexpensive treatment method would be desirable to provide immediate relief for fearful children and their parents, and thus avoid several years of needless distress. Early intervention would also benefit those few individuals who will not experience a reduction or disappearance of fears as they grow older. The behavioral treatment methods available are relatively brief and inexpensive to administer and would thus warrant use in many cases, even with predictably short-lived, but intense fears.

FEARS OF ANIMALS

A variety of treatment methods has been reported to be useful in counteracting children's fears of animals. Such methods as counter-conditioning, exposure to fearless models, graded exposure to the feared stimulus, and guided participation were used as early as the 1920s (e.g., Holmes, 1936; Jones, 1924a, 1924b; Jersild & Holmes, 1936). Improved descendants of these fear-reduction techniques are in present-day clinical use. Table 20-1 summarizes the various behavioral treatments used in combating children's fear of animals and provides information on the relative speed and effectiveness of each method.

Counter-conditioning. The counter-conditioning procedure consists of pairing a positive emotional response such as pleasure with a graded sequence of presentations of the feared stimulus. The presentation sequence is carefully arranged so that the positive emotional state is maintained while the client's proximity to the fear stimulus is gradually and progressively increased. Eventually the formerly avoided stimulus loses its aversive properties for the child and the original conditioning that produced the phobic reaction is reversed. Bandura (1969) has presented a description of the theory and empirical information underlying this technique.

Jones (1924a, 1924b) provided a now classic account of the counter-conditioning of a child's fear of small animals. In Jones' procedure, a rabbit was slowly moved toward a table at which the child was eating. It was presumed that pairing the sight of the feared rabbit with the pleasant emotional state produced by eating would result in a reconditioning or counter-conditioning process which would eliminate the phobic reaction. Counter-conditioning techniques usually are combined with the shaping of approach responses using the therapist's expressions of approbation as a reinforcer, or with the presentation of peer models successfully approaching situations which the child avoids and fears. Counter-conditioning appears to be a component of the modeling and reinforced practice techniques to be discussed in following sections.

Systematic desensitization and emotive imagery. More recently, Wolpe (1958, 1961) has used counter-conditioning procedures in a systematic desensitization technique which has been widely used in the treatment of phobic reactions in adults. As originally formulated, systematic desensitization required that a response antagonistic to anxiety be evoked in the presence of anxiety-arousing stimuli. This procedure presumably resulted in the suppression of the anxiety reaction

Table 20-1 SUCCESS AND DURABILITY OF BEHAVIORAL TREATMENTS FOR CHILDREN'S FEAR AND AVOIDANCE OF ANIMALS

INVESTIGATORS	TREATMENT METHOD	TREATMENT LENGTH	OUTCOME	FOLLOW-UP
Bandura, Blanchard & Ritter (1969)	a. Systematic desensitization	a. Average of $4\frac{1}{2}$ hrs	a. 25% of children performed terminal item on snake approach test	a. None
	b. Self-administered film modeling	b. About 2 hrs	b. 33% performed terminal items	b. None
	c. In vivo modeling with guided participation	c. About 2 hrs	c. 92% performed terminal items	c. None
Bandura, Grusec & Menlove (1967)	In vivo peer modeling	Maximum of 80 mins	Significant increase in dog approach scores	Improvement maintained at 1-month follow-up
Bandura & Menlove (1968)	Filmed peer modeling	Eight 3-min films	Significant increase in dog approach scores	Maintained or increased at 1-month follow-up
Blanchard (1970 a, b)	In vivo modeling with guided participation	Maximum of 8 sessions, about 2 hrs	Participant modeling most increased approaches to snake; modeling produced greatest generalization	None, but post-tests were 1–7 days after final treatment session
Hill, Liebert & Mott (1968)	Filmed peer modeling	11-min film	Significant increase in dog approach scores	None
Holmes (1936)	Reinforced practice, in vivo peer modeling	5–11 brief treatment sessions	13 of 14 children entered dark room; 1 of 2 children overcame fear of height	None
Jones (1924 b)	Counterconditioning and in vivo peer modeling	45 experimental sessions	Complete control of animal phobia in 1 child treated	None
Kornhaber & Schroeder (1975)	Filmed peer and adult modeling	Two 6–7 min films	Significant increase in snake approach scores, greater for peer models	None

Lazarus & Abramovitz (1962)	Emotive imagery	Average of 3.3 treatment sessions	Complete control of phobic reactions in 7 of 9 children	Maintained at 1 year follow-up
Murphy & Bootzin (1973)	Contact desensitization	Maximum of four 8-min sessions	93% of children performed terminal item on snake approach test	Maintained at 10-day follow-up
Ritter (1968)	Contact desensitization	Two 35-min sessions	Significant increase in snake approach scores for 12 of 15 children	None
Weissbrod & Bryan (1973)	Filmed peer modeling	10 mins of film viewing	Significant increase in snake approach scores	None

and the weakening of the association between these stimuli and the anxiety reaction (Wolpe, 1958). The most frequently used antagonistic response is relaxation, which is paired with the client's imagining progressively more threatening confrontations with the aversive stimulus. It is presumed that once the negative emotional reaction to the stimulus is controlled, then the individual will cease attempting to escape from and avoid the object of his previous fears.

The systematic desensitization technique requires that the client admit to and report accurately his or her fears, that the client follow relatively complex instructions regarding the construction of a hierarchy of anxiety-provoking mental images, that he achieve a state of muscular relaxation upon command (or in response to a drug), and that he summon clear mental images of anxiety-arousing stimuli. Because young children are not usually able to perform these demanding actions, age-appropriate versions of systematic desensitization techniques have been developed for younger clients. Lazarus and Abramovitz (1962) devised an emotive imagery procedure in which pleasant mental images are paired with imaginary approximations to the feared stimulus. They reported that children as young as seven years could be trained to imagine particularly pleasant scenes of themselves at the wheel of powerful racing cars or consorting with their favorite film or story heroes. These pleasant images are then associated with progressively more threatening mental images of the feared situation. As in systematic desensitization, the child is instructed to raise a finger to indicate feeling anxiety, whereupon the child is to cease imagining that scene and instead to visualize a less arousing item from the fear hierarchy. Lazarus and Abramovitz reported that this emotive imagery technique was successful in controlling various fears, including dog phobia, in children who had proved unable to complete relaxation training preparatory to systematic desensitization therapy. In seven of nine children treated, complete control of phobic responding was accomplished in an average of only 3.3 treatment sessions. One unsuccessfully treated child was unable to concentrate on the emotive imagery and could thus not profit from the technique. Tasto (1969) also reported systematic desensitization to be ineffective in the treatment of a 4-year-old boy's fear of loud sounds because the boy apparently failed to comprehend the imagery instructions. Because this problem may be shared by many children, emotive imagery, like systematic desensitization, probably has limited utility in child therapy.

Rimm and Masters (1974) have also advised against sole reliance on desensitization techniques unless the therapist is certain that the client has all of the appropriate behavioral skills required to cope with the feared stimulus, but is inhibited by anxiety. Otherwise, a procedure aimed at the acquisition of skills, perhaps through modeling or reinforced practice, may be more appropriate than desensitization as a treatment measure. Socially inexperienced young children are far less likely than adults to have acquired the requisite skills, so neither systematic desensitization nor emotive imagery is usually the treatment of choice with children.

Modeling. To date, the most successful methods of reducing children's fears of animals have employed modeling demonstrations. Typically, the child is shown either live or filmed children engaging in increasingly active encounters with the animal that the child fears, and without adverse consequences to the peer models. The procedure desensitizes the child to the sight and sound of the animal and reduces his motivation to avoid contact with the animal (Bandura, 1969, 1971). The model's positive affective expressions provide an additional source of vicarious extinction of fear arousal for the observer (Bandura, 1969, chap. 3) and inform him that interacting with the animal can be rewarding. The model's behavior also instructs the observing child in techniques appropriate for handling the animal. For example, the observer learns how to approach, pet, and romp with a dog, or how to lift and hold a snake. Knowledge of these handling skills would increase the probability of the animal's positive response to the observer's first attempts at approaching the animal, and would increase the likelihood of a positive experience. Observation of a competent and fearless model may be particularly important in the instruction of young children who most probably lack handling skills, and who might otherwise elicit barking, hissing, and pursuit by the very animal they fear as a result of their panicky attempts at escape. The likely result of such an encounter would be an exacerbation of the child's fear.

Everyday observations of the behavior of others who do not share the child's fear probably do not suffice to allay the child's apprehensions, because the child may still avoid witnessing fear-provoking, active encounters with the animal. Also, the child may reject the possibility of emulating models who are so obviously successful and thus quite dissimilar to himself (see Bandura, 1969, chap. 3, for a discussion of this issue).

The popularity of modeling techniques in the treatment of fear and avoidance behavior stemmed from Bandura's (Bandura, 1969; Bandura & Walters, 1963) influential social learning theory and from numerous experimental demonstrations of the power and potential clinical utility of modeling presentations. Excellent reviews of clinical applications have been presented by Bandura (1971), by Rosenthal (1976), and by Marlatt and Perry, (1975). Bandura, Grusec, and Menlove (1967) demonstrated that a dramatic and stable reduction in preschool children's fear of dogs could be produced through observing another child display progressively more prolonged and more intimate interactions with a dog. Initially, the dog was confined in a playpen, and the child model merely talked to and occasionally petted Chloe, a friendly cocker spaniel, while a small group of fearful children observed. In a carefully controlled experiment, the children participated in eight 10-minute treatment sessions, during which the 4-year-old boy who served as the model petted, fed, and walked the dog. During the final two sessions, the boy climbed into the playpen with Chloe, then petted, hugged, and fed her. During a behavioral post-test, the children who had received the vicarious extinction (modeling) treatment interacted fearlessly not only with the now familiar experimental dog, but with an unfamiliar dog as well. One month later, they continued to approach and interact with the formerly feared animals. To ensure that the treatment did not prove too effective for the children's safety, they were warned to confine their friendly approaches to familiar dogs, or to animals whose owners had vouched for them. This study also revealed that the addition of a counter-conditioning procedure in the form of a party did not significantly aid in fear reduction beyond that achieved by the modeling procedure alone. Modeling was equally effective with or without an additional counter-conditioning procedure.

Symbolic modeling. The in vivo modeling technique has limitations, however. Both Jones (1924a) and Bandura (1967) have noted that the modeling demonstrations must be carefully controlled to prevent the peer models from imitating the fearful behavior of the target child, and to ensure that the demonstrations are carefully graduated so the observer does not become frightened at the sight of too vigorous an interaction between model and animal. Of course, it would prove therapeutically disastrous should the animal confirm the fearful observer's apprehensions by snarling at or biting one of the models.

Modern technology has provided motion picture and videotape recording devices that can greatly aid the therapist. Carefully selected models, docile animals, and graded sequences of interactions can be filmed, and each scene can be viewed any number of times by an individual child or by separate groups of children (e.g., Bandura & Menlove, 1968; Hill, Liebert, & Mott, 1968). This innovation has great clinical promise, as Mischel (1968, p. 262) has pointed out.

In a carefully controlled study, Bandura, Blanchard, and Ritter (1969) evaluated the relative effectiveness of three different treatments for snake phobia in persons between 13 and 59 years of age. Individuals matched on the basis of behavioral tests of reaction toward snakes were randomly assigned to the following treatment conditions: (a) standard systematic desensitization, (b) graduated live modeling combined with guided participation, in which the therapist first demonstrated and then assisted the subject in handling a snake, (c) self-administered symbolic modeling in which each person viewed a film showing adults and children in progressively more fearless interactions with snakes, and (d) a no-treatment control condition. Some of the symbolic modeling subjects were also trained to relax while they viewed the film, while others received no relaxation training. Whenever they became uncomfortable, they reversed the film and viewed a scene that was not anxiety arousing. Individuals were thus able to proceed at their own pace through the hierarchy of modeling displays. As can be seen from Table 20-1, approach behavior was most facilitated by live, or in vivo, modeling with guided participation; 92% of this group was able to complete the terminal approach task of sitting motionless for 30 seconds while the snake crawled on the person's lap. In contrast, only comparatively few of the persons who had received the symbolic modeling or the systematic desensitization were able to perform this task, and none of the control group could do so. Also, as compared to systematic desensitization, the modeling procedures produced greater reductions in self-rated fear arousal and in negative attitudes about snakes. Modeling procedures also produced more generalized behavior change as reflected in approaches to an unfamiliar snake encountered for the first time.

Clinicians choosing a treatment technique will wish to know just how effective the various alternatives might be. In an examination of the relative contributions of modeling, provision of factual information, and physical contact in the control of snake phobic behavior, Blanchard (1970b) has found that modeling was the most powerful influence over actual approach behavior. Modeling was also the most potent factor in promoting generalized approach toward an unfamiliar snake, and accounted for approximately 80% of the variance in the attitude change concerning reptiles. Direct contact in the form of guided participation also contributed significantly to approach behavior and self-reported fear reduction, but not to attitude change. In confirmation of popular belief, factual information concerning the innocuous nature of nonpoisonous snakes was ineffective in reducing fear, and may actually have increased observers' fear levels. Blanchard's study indicates that modeling demonstrations may well be the most effective single method currently available for treating phobic behavior. If a modeling procedure does not sufficiently reduce or eliminate a fear reaction, guided participation or reinforced practice of the feared activity can be undertaken.

Reinforced practice. Leitenberg and his colleagues (Leitenberg, 1976; Leitenberg & Callahan, 1973) have contended that the prior elimination of anxiety through direct or vicarious desensitization is not an essential prerequisite to the reduction of avoidance behavior. Rather, Leitenberg suggests treating the avoidance responding directly through a technique he terms reinforced practice. The technique includes a number of components such as graduated, repeated practice in approaching the aversive stimulus, praise from the therapist and from family members for successful approach attempts, charting of the client's behavior to provide highly salient evidence of improvement, and therapeutic instructions designed to arouse expectations of success. As yet, no component analysis of this technique has been reported, so it is impossible to identify the effective elements and to rule out possible placebo effects produced by the therapist's optimistic statements to the clients. Nevertheless, the promising results of preliminary studies (reviewed by Leitenberg, 1976) warrant consideration of the use of reinforced practice in the treatment of children's avoidance behavior. A very similar technique, stimulus fading, will be discussed in the following review of behavioral treatments of separation anxiety and school phobic behavior.

School Phobia

Fearful avoidance of school attendance, often termed school phobia, is a fairly common problem among school age children. Kennedy (1965) estimates the incidence of school phobia at 17 per 1000 children each school year, and school phobia remains a prevalent problem among adolescents (Coolidge, Willer, Tessman, & Waldfogel, 1960; Johnson, 1957). The prognosis for improvement is extremely good with nearly any type of treatment if the child receives professional attention before failure to attend school becomes a chronic pattern (Coolidge, Hahn, & Peck 1957). Forced school attendance followed by supportive psychotherapy resulted in regular school attendance in 89% of a sample of children younger than 11 years (Rodriguez, Rodriguez, & Eisenberg, 1959). Kennedy (1965) also reported 100% success in the early treatment of 50 school phobic children. Kennedy's program featured forced school attendance, parental praise for the child's school attendance so long as it lasted at least 30 minutes on the first day, a party held by the family to celebrate the child's return to school, and systematic extinction of the child's somatic complaints and expressions of fear or anxiety. Potential medical problems were not ignored, however. The children's complaints of abdominal pains or headaches were dealt with by scheduling medical examinations before or after school hours, and did not serve as a means for the children to avoid going to school. This combination of ignoring the child's complaints and enforcing and rewarding his school attendance appears effective, especially when there is a strong operant component to the child's avoidance which is maintained by reinforcing consequences—e.g., those provided by parents who support or inadvertently encourage the child's staying home from school.

Operant components. Several other groups of investigators have also treated school phobia by concentrating on the operant aspects of the problem. Hersen (1968, 1970), Ayllon, Smith, and Rogers (1970), and Brown, Copeland, and Hall (1974) have all reported success in treatments based on contingency management programs. Of course, the decision to employ these methods stems from a careful observation and assessment that confirms that the child is receiving positive reinforcement for avoiding school. Typically, the child's parents are instructed to cease attending to and encouraging the child's complaints and failure to attend school (Tahmasian & McReynolds, 1971). This action is intended to place the child's inappropriate behavior on an extinction schedule by removing consequences suspected to serve as reinforcers. Teachers and school administrators also receive similar instructions, and all of the child's adult caretakers are trained to respond positively to the child's presumed school participation. In addition to social reinforcement, treats and trinkets may be used as back-up reinforcers (Ayllon, et al., 1970; Kennedy, 1965). Forced school attendance prevents the child's avoidance maneuvers, but if used alone, is perhaps unnecessarily stressful in comparison to the employment of positive consequences.

Respondent components. Other treatment tactics have focused on the respondent or emotional reactions that may motivate avoidance of school. In treating a 7-year-old boy, Patterson (1965) assumed that separation from his mother functioned as an eliciting stimulus for an anxiety reaction that led to escape and avoidance of school. Patterson carried out a counter-conditioning program in which the eliciting stimulus was paired with a response incompatible with anxiety. In a series of structured doll play situations, the boy was given candy for bold assertions that the boy doll was not afraid when left in a strange situation without his mother. In a combination of respondent and operant conditioning procedures, the parents also praised the child for independent play and for saying that he wished to return to school. The boy was attending classes regularly at the end of the 6 weeks of treatment and at a 3-month follow-up assessment.

Counter-conditioning and desensitization treatments are more time consuming than enforced return to school. Patterson's procedure required 23 sessions, or a total of 10 hours of staff time. Garvey and Hegrenes (1966) used an in vivo desensitization procedure to reintroduce a 10-year-old boy gradually to his school over a period of 20 consecutive days. This procedure required 20 to 40 minutes of adult attention per day. At first, the therapist escorted the boy to school, then the father did, and finally, the school principal helped carry out the treatment program.

In an effort to reduce the time required by in vivo desensitization and to minimize the duration of the child's stress in a forcible return to school, Smith and Sharpe (1970) attempted implosive therapy (Stampfl & Levis, 1967) with a 13-year-old boy. Their approach was based on the presumption that the high-intensity, relatively brief presentation of the anxiety provoking stimulus would result in the rapid extinction of the anxiety response. In six brief sessions, the boy was asked to imagine scenes that illustrated his worst apprehensions regarding the school situation and his fellow students' reactions to him. For example, he was told to imagine that the other students were encircling him, pressing closer and closer, calling him stupid, and pummeling him. The actual school situation the boy would encounter pales in comparison to this dreadful scene, and therefore appears less terrifying. After the first such treatment session, the boy was able to attend the following day's math class, and he returned to school full time after the fourth session.

Many clinicians, however, would be reluctant to stress young children in this fashion if effective, alternative treatment methods are available. There is the risk, too, of the child's finding the treatment situation so aversive that he will refuse to cooperate or to return for a second session. As Ullmann and Krasner (1975, p. 278) have cautioned, the successful use of implosive techniques requires considerable clinical skill and sensitivity so the highly aversive treatment experience is associated with the avoided object and not with the therapist.

A central issue in the choice of treatments for school avoidance concerns the identification of the factors responsible for the child's behavior. Lazarus, Davison, and Polefka (1965) pointed out that avoidance behavior could be motivated either by intense fear of the school situation or by various positive reinforcing consequences such as attention received from adults and from peers. These separate maintaining conditions can co-exist for an individual child, in which case more than one type of treatment procedure might be required. Lazarus and his colleagues used emotive imagery and in vivo desensitization procedures to reduce a 9-year-old boy's fear of school, and a token reinforcement program to promote school attendance. The boy's parents were provided with detailed instructions for supporting his approaching the school and for ignoring his inappropriate behavior. The treatment efforts took place over a period of 4½ months, and were successful in reestablishing the child's regular school attendance.

Unresolved issues. It is likely that over the long run attention to both operant and respondent features of the avoidance responding will optimize treatment results. Attending only to the operant features by extinguishing avoidance attempts and reinforcing school attendance may not sufficiently reduce emotional arousal. Alternatively, reducing fear and anxiety may not suffice to reinstate school attendance. And frightening the child or forcibly returning him to the school may inadvertently provide the child with a model of callousness and disregard for the feelings of others that may be reflected in his own future interpersonal behavior (Bandura, & Walters, 1963, p. 194; Gelfand, Hartmann, Lamb, Smith, Mahan, & Paul, 1974).

The fact remains, however, that in the absence of controlled treatment comparisons we cannot very well choose among the various clinical alternatives. Some possible treatments for school phobia such as modeling techniques have not yet been investigated. Also, as Hersen (1972) has pointed out, we have no information regarding the expected duration and outcome of untreated school phobia. As a result, it is impossible to ascertain whether any professional treatment is necessary in most cases. Perhaps within the next few years this topic will receive the research attention that its incidence and seriousness merit.

Other Common Childhood Fears

The early behaviorists anticipated modern treatment techniques for another common fear of early childhood, the fear of darkness. John B. Watson (1928) recommended using counter-conditioning procedures. His advice to parents of apprehensive youngsters was as follows:

> Start unconditioning at once. Put the child to bed at its usual time. Leave a faint light in the hall and leave the door open. Then every night after putting the child to bed close the door a little more and dim the light still more. Three or four nights usually suffice. (p. 67)

Parents and practitioners could still profit from such advice.

Reinforced practice. Leitenberg and Callahan (1973) used reinforced practice to treat nursery school and kindergarten children's fear of the dark. Children were treated individually in the laboratory and were instructed to remain in a darkened room for increasing periods of time. A poster depicting a thermometer indicated the amount of time the child had spent in the darkened room. Each increase in the time spent in the dark earned the child a small prize. On a behavioral post-test, four of seven children given reinforced practice remained voluntarily in the unlighted room for the maximum designated time of five minutes. In contrast, non-treated control children decreased the time they spent in the dark during the post-test, confirming the treatment's effectiveness.

Role playing and self-descriptions. Kanfer, Karoly, and Newman (1975) treated fear of the dark by training children to utter competence statements such as, "I am a brave girl. I can take care of myself in the dark." The 5- and 6-year-olds trained to describe themselves as competent surpassed two comparison groups in the toleration of darkness during a post-test. Both the competence group and a stimulus comparison group trained to say. "The dark is a fun place to be," performed significantly better than did a control group on a generalization task which required each child to darken a room as much as he could tolerate.

The source of this treatment's effectiveness is not yet known. Kanfer and his colleagues have suggested that the child's new self-description as a brave person could serve as a guiding standard or intention that the child fulfills by tolerating exposure to darkness. An additional consideration is the powerful experimental demand made of the children in the self-statement and the stimulus statement groups. The therapist clearly expected that these children would stay in the dark as long as possible.

The use of therapist-determined self-descriptions resembles Kelly's (1955) fixed-role therapy and Wolpe and Lazarus's (1966) exaggerated role training in which clients are instructed to enact prescribed roles as competent persons while facing fear-arousing situations. It appears that children, as well as adults, benefit from such instructions if they have a prior acquaintance with the specific behaviors required to deal competently with a feared stimulus.

A reinforced role-playing procedure was used by Hosford (1969) to reduce a sixth-grade girl's anxiety over giving oral reports and participating in classroom discussions. The girl first role-played giving oral reports under low-stress conditions with only the counselor present. In weekly counseling sessions over a period of 6 weeks, the length and realism of the girl's presentations were increased, and the counselor praised her speaking attempts. With the aid and encouragement of her teacher and classmates, she was gradually able to increase her participation in classroom presentations.

Because Hosford and Sorenson (1969) found that about 25% of a large sample of fourth- through sixth-grade pupils reported experiencing anxiety over participating in class discussions, these investigators produced an 8-minute modeling film for routine classroom use. The film features a coping model (Meichenbaum, 1971), a child who experiences speech anxiety which he overcomes through behavioral counseling involving role-playing class presentations. Hosford and Sorenson report that the film is well received by students and teachers, but offer no evidence that it actually reduces stage fright in academic situations.

Water phobia. Children's fear of water has been successfully treated through counter-conditioning (Bentler, 1962) in just the manner that Watson (1928) suggested. An interesting modeling and participation treatment has been developed by Lewis (1974) who compared various behavior therapy techniques for reducing boys' fear and avoidance of swimming instruction. She found that a procedure that combined symbolic modeling and graduated, reinforced practice (participation) was the most effective intervention. The 8-minute modeling film showed three initially hesitant peers overcoming their apprehensions and praising their own bravery as they swam joyously in a pool. In the reinforced practice procedure, an adult spent 10 minutes in the pool with each boy encouraging him to attempt swimming readiness tasks and praising his successes. The improvement displayed by the children who received both the film modeling and the reinforced practice significantly exceeded that of groups given either the modeling or the practice alone. Thus, in three comparative evaluations (Bandura, Blanchard, & Ritter, 1969; Blanchard, 1970b; Lewis, 1974), a combination of modeling and subsequent successful participation proved more effective than the other methods tested, and so may be considered the treatment of choice.

Test anxiety. It has been estimated that approximately 20% of school children dread tests and examinations to an extent that may seriously impair their academic performance (Eysenck & Rachman, 1965). There is some evidence that simple meditation training can reduce children's test anxiety (Linden, 1973). Linden viewed meditation as a technique for training attention and resistance to distraction as well as for combating anxiety. Third-grade children who were taught a breathing exercise to induce meditation scored significantly lower on a test anxiety scale than did either children who received instruction in study skills or a no-treatment control group. The children tested, however, were not reported to have suffered from test anxiety, so it is not yet certain how well meditation would work with a clinical population.

Adolescents with severe examination anxiety have responded well to direct and vicarious desensitization procedures. Mann and Rosenthal (1969) found that whether they were treated individually or in groups, and whether they underwent or merely observed a systematic desensitization procedure, treated clients improved relative to untreated control subjects. In fact, the vicarious treatment groups tended to surpass the direct groups in magnitude of improvement, thus once again demonstrating the efficacy of modeling procedures. In a replication study, Mann (1972) found that presenting videotaped peer models progressing through the fear hierarchy items was as effective as was portrayal of the entire desensitization procedure.

Behavior Under Stimulus Control of Parents' Presence

Some children's appropriate social behavior, e.g., speaking, occurs only in their parents' presence. Like the experimental bird that pecks only at a lighted key, these children speak, or maintain eye contact, or play rather than cry, only when they are accompanied by their parents. This pattern of behavior is sometimes labeled separation anxiety when a dominant feature is emotional outbursts. When the major component is failure to speak under certain appropriate circumstances such as in the classroom, the problem is termed selective, elective, or situation-specific mutism.

Stimulus fading. The stimulus fading technique described by Terrace (1966) has obvious application to the situation in which the child's social responding occurs in the presence of the parents, but not in the presence of teachers or others. Neisworth, Madle, and Goeke (1975) successfully used a stimulus fading procedure to treat a 4-year-old girl's refusal to allow her mother to leave her presence. Whenever her mother left her to go to work or delivered her at her preschool, the girl would cry and tantrum until her mother returned. At first the therapist separated the mother and child for a few seconds only, then gradually and progressively increased the time the child spent at the preschool without her mother. The treatment was accomplished in a total of 7 hours (18 sessions) during which the child exhibited only 10 minutes of anxious behavior. At a 6-month follow-up, the problem had not recurred.

Stimulus fading procedures have also been employed with positive results in the treatment of situation-specific mutism. Both Montenegro (1968) and Conrad and associates (Conrad, Delk, & Williams, 1974) have reported case studies in which the child was reinforced with food and ate while the mother slowly moved further away from, and the therapist and others moved nearer to the child. The Conrad group's (1974) procedure required 12 treatment sessions. An 11-year-old girl who never spoke in class was first asked to state solutions to math problems presented on flash cards and received candy for responding. The treatment began in her home with her mother present. In successive phases, she continued to respond aloud and to receive candy in her home with her mother absent, then in the clinic with the therapist and a classmate, then with a teacher also present, next in the classroom with the teacher and five classmates, and finally in her regular classroom with the entire class. The use of candy was also progressively decreased and finally eliminated. This stimulus fading technique has typically required 12 to 18 treatment sessions.

Reid and his associates (Reid, Hawkins, Keutzer, McNeal, Phelps, Reid, & Mees, 1967) employed a marathon procedure in which a 6-year-old girl's situation-specific mutism was eliminated in just one day. The girl was brought to the clinic one morning without breakfast and was first required to ask her mother for bites of her breakfast, then to ask for food from a single therapist who was gradually moved closer to the eating child. Gradually, additional unfamiliar adults and children were introduced until, in the afternoon, the somewhat satiated little girl had a party with seven adults and two children.

Another group of investigators (Wulbert, Nyman, Snow, & Owen, 1973) analyzed the separate effects of stimulus fading and reinforcement contingency management in the treatment of selective mutism. This study also illustrates the utility of within-subject and single-subject experimental analysis in investigating treatment methods for relatively rare behavioral problems. These single-subject replication procedures allow therapists to identify effective treatment procedures without accumulating the large number of equivalent cases necessary for group comparisons. Wulbert and associates found that the stimulus fading procedure of gradually removing the mother and introducing other adults into the situation was a necessary component of the treatment process. A 1-minute isolation time-out period contingent upon the child's failure to answer aloud proved ineffective when used alone, but was found to facilitate the treatment when combined with stimulus fading procedures.

These latter results suggest that for practical as well as ethical reasons, clinicians should not rely solely on aversive methods (Gelfand & Hartmann, 1975, chap. 6). When a competently conducted positive method such as stimulus fading proves inadequate, however, the therapist might wish to consider adding a brief time-out period contingent on the child's inappropriate responding. If stimulus fading is accomplished in sufficiently gradual steps, there should be little need for any type of coercion.

Contingency management. A considerably more stressful procedure has been described by Halpern, Hammond, and Cohen (1972). Children who spoke at home but not at school were at first required to gesture in response to teachers' questions, then to whisper or speak the word "go" in order to be excused with the rest of the class. Although this escape conditioning procedure was successful in inducing the children to speak in class, one child waited with the teacher in the classroom until 6:00 p. m. before saying the required word on the first day. This procedure seems unduly aversive for all concerned, so most practitioners prefer to rely on positive reinforcement procedures.

Therapists have successfully administered shaping programs using various reward consequences for approximations to classroom recitation. Reinforcing stimuli that have been employed include token reinforcers with toys as back-up reinforcers (Bauermeister & Jemail, 1975), special school activities (Rasbury, 1974), praise and positive attention (Brison, 1966), toys and art materials (Reynolds & Risley, 1968), treats and pocket money (Nolan & Pence, 1970), and points toward a party for the child's entire class (Straughan, Potter, & Hamilton, 1965). In most instances in which tangible reinforcers were used, the child also received positive attention and praise.

Various treatment techniques may be employed to deal with several co-existing behavioral problems. Although children are somewhat more likely than adults to display a single, discrete behavioral problem (Gelfand & Hartmann, 1968), some children suffer from multiple problem behaviors. Patterson and Brodsky (1966) used four different conditioning and instructional programs to treat a 5-year-old boy's various behavioral deviancies. The procedures included an extinction procedure to control the boy's temper tantrums, an extinction and counter-conditioning procedure to reduce his anxiety upon separation from his mother, a positive reinforcement program to train him to initiate social approaches to children, and instruction of his parents in contingency management to reduce his negativistic and immature behaviors. The treatment methods used for controlling multiple problems are essentially the same as those aimed at isolated, specific deviant behaviors. Although the intervention program is necessarily more complex, and perhaps lengthier, no unique principles or practices are involved in the treatment of multi-problem children.

SHYNESS AND SOCIAL WITHDRAWAL

Shyness is a frequently observed childhood problem which, unless overcome, can continue to affect the individual during adulthood. Among a large sample of California high school and college students, over 40% labeled themselves as presently shy, and 25% reported having been shy for most of their lives (Zimbardo, Pilkonis, & Norwood, 1974). Only 1% of those surveyed reported themselves as never having experienced shyness. As in the case of childhood fears, a fairly large proportion of those affected seem to overcome their problems with shyness with increasing age. Zimbardo and associates reported that 41% of their sample stated that they were shy as children, but are not presently troubled by shyness. The young people reported a number of problems associated with their shyness such as depressed mood and inability to make friends, express opinions, or enjoy social occasions.

Apparently, informal efforts to aid socially retiring children meet with relatively little success. Bonny (1971) reported limited effectiveness for a variety of "socialization experiences," such as involving socially isolated children in collaborative efforts with other children, offering advice to their parents, or enrolling the children in nondirective, individual play therapy. Since socially awkward children are likely to have equally socially inept parents (Sherman & Farina, 1974), it is not surprising that offering advice to the parents proved ineffective. And most treatment efforts that do not directly address the problem and remedy the child's social skill deficit are doomed to failure.

Modeling

Psychologists have long been aware of the beneficial effects of modeling on children's social assertiveness (Anderson, 1937; Page, 1936). In an early study, Jack (1934) taught nursery school children to become generally less inhibited by providing them with demonstrations of methods for coping with tasks of increasing difficulty and by praising them for good performance.

More recently, O'Connor (1969, 1972) has developed a symbolic modeling treatment for the modification of nursery school children's social withdrawal. In a well-conducted study, O'Connor (1969) selected nursery school children nominated by their teachers as being socially withdrawn and then verified the child's low peer interaction rates by means of classroom observations. Non-isolate classmates were also observed for comparison purposes. The socially withdrawn children were then randomly assigned to see either a peer-modeling film or a control film featuring performing dolphins. The 23-minute peer-modeling film portrayed 11 scenes of young children in progressively more active interactions while a woman narrator described the action and the positive outcomes for the initially shy peer models. The modeling film proved highly effective; in fact this group's behavior was indistinguishable from that of socially normal classmates in observations conducted in the classroom immediately following the film. In contrast, the withdrawn children who viewed the control film did not become more socially assertive. The results of O'Connor's study are particularly impressive because the raters were unaware of each child's treatment condition and whether the child was considered a social isolate.

In a subsequent study, O'Connor (1972) found that the beneficial effects of modeling remained evident at a 3-week follow-up observation at which the treated children's interaction rates were at normal levels. In contrast, a successive approximation procedure in which women graduate students praised children for social approaches to peers produced less durable improvements. At the 3-week follow-up assessment, the children treated by shaping procedures had returned to their own low initial base rates of interaction. This comparison between modeling and shaping may unduly favor the modeling treatment, however, since the reinforcement schedules used were not those that would produce durable responding during extinction in the absence of praise (see Ferster & Skinner, 1957, for information on reinforcement schedule effects).

Sources of treatment failure. A word of caution. Some attempts to treat social withdrawal by symbolic modeling have not succeeded (e.g., Kelly, 1975; Walker, Hops, Greenwood, & Todd, 1975). Clement, Roberts, and Lantz (1970) employed a series of 20 5-minute videotapes showing popular fourth-grade boys in progressively more assertive interactions. Small groups of shy, withdrawn boys received play therapy either with or without exposure to the modeling tapes and with or without receiving token reinforcers from the therapist for their social approach behavior. None of the treatments used was particularly effective, and the modeling tapes failed to add significantly to the therapeutic impact of the play therapy alone. The authors suggested that their failure to include an accompanying narrative sound track or to use coping models who visibly increased in social skills may have reduced the symbolic modeling's effectiveness. Additionally, it may not be advisable to treat withdrawn children in groups because they may not attend to the films (Kelly, 1975) or may imitate each other's social awkwardness rather than the symbolic model's skills (Walker, et al., 1975). Consequently, Clement and his associates (Clement, Roberts, & Lantz, 1976) now treat shy children in groups with normally assertive peers rather than together with other social isolates.

Modeling films designed for nursery school children may fail to effect positive changes in older children. Walker and his fellow investigators (Walker, et al., 1975) found that O'Connor's film did not increase the interaction rates of groups of 7- to 10-year-old social isolates. This treatment failure could have occurred because the social skills demonstrated were appropriate for younger children, but not for schoolage viewers. Alternatively, the observing children could have considered the preschool models as of such low status and so dissimilar to themselves as to be unworthy of emulation. Investigators are beginning to determine the stimulus characteristics affecting the power of modeling treatments for various behavioral problems. It may be that effective components of modeling displays will vary with the nature of the problem to be treated. The type of narration accompanying the modeling film may also be an important determinant of treatment outcome. In a recent study, Jakibchuk and Smeriglio (1975) found that with a young child as the narrator, videotapes showing a coping peer model will be effective in enhancing social interactions only if the narrative takes a self-speech, first person form. When the child narrator described herself or himself as the initially shy central figure in the tapes, observers became significantly more socially assertive, and remained so at a 3-week follow-up evaluation. When the child narrator used the third person form to describe the behavior of the videotaped model, observers displayed no subsequent behavioral improvement. The previously discussed work of Clement and Walker and their associates indicates that an essential feature of the modeling procedure may be the establishment of similarity between the model and the observer. Laboratory research (see Bandura, 1969, chap. 3 for a review of this research) has also indicated that this similarity factor may enhance modeling effects because observers may reject highly competent models as unrealistic objects for emulation. The contrast between the suave child-about-town and the shy, inhibited observer may only serve to confirm the observer's convictions that his case is hopeless.

REINFORCEMENT PROCEDURES

The beneficial effects of modeling demonstrations may be lost rapidly unless the observer engages in reinforced practice (Bandura, Jeffery, & Wright, 1974). Keller and Carlson (1974) reported that post-treatment increases in withdrawn preschool children's interaction rates had vanished within 3 weeks following a symbolic modeling treatment. Consequently, many therapists have combined modeling with shaping procedures designed to promote and maintain appropriate social responding. Such studies have not yielded definitive results, however. Evers and Schwarz (1973) found that the addition of a shaping procedure using teachers' praise for peer interactions did not significantly add to the improvements achieved through O'Connor's modeling film alone. Of course, the teachers may not have been very skillful or systematic at administering the praise consequation program.

In a series of experiments, Walker and Hops (1973) contrasted the effects of various contingency management schemes as supplements to showing O'Connor's peer-modeling film to withdrawn first and second graders. Each shy child's social interactions reliably increased when either the child or the child's classmates received token reinforcers for increased rates of interaction involving the target child. The treatment was more effective when both the target child and the other children were informed of the reinforcement contingency in effect. Thus, for children who had viewed the modeling film, social activity rates could be systematically varied by introducing or withdrawing reinforcement contingencies. When reinforcement was contingent on interactions, such behaviors were frequent, but the rates dropped abruptly during extinction periods. Unfortunately, no follow-up data were provided, but the prompt return to interaction base rates during reversal periods is discomforting (see Hartmann & Atkinson's [1973] discussion of this frequently encountered clinical dilemma). Perhaps the treatment's durability could be increased by a more gradual thinning and fading of reinforcement schedules, or a greater reliance on social than on material reinforcement as suggested by O'Leary, Poulos, and Devine (1972). Various methods for enhancing the generalization and the durability of behavioral treatments have been reviewed by Gelfand and Hartmann (1975, chap. 9).

Sometimes the manipulation of incentives suffices to increase the social participation of social isolates, and no modeling demonstrations are required. Allen and her colleagues (Allen, et al., 1964) reliably increased the peer interactions of a retiring 4-year-old girl by having her nursery school teachers attend to her only when she approached and interacted with the other children. In a similar vein, Buell's group (Buell, Stoddard, Harris, & Baer, 1968) demonstrated that increasing the rate of play equipment usage by an inactive nursery school child also increased such desirable social encounters as talking to and playing with other youngsters. Once again in this study, teacher attention was found to act as a powerful reinforcing stimulus for preschool children. Older children may require tangible as well as social reinforcers (Clement, 1968; Clement & Milne, 1967), and nearly all children can profit from explicit statements of the contingency between approach behavior and reinforcement (Clement, Roberts, & Lantz, 1976). When yougsters are so inhibited that they cannot bring themselves even to speak in the classroom, it is necessary to shape appropriate responding in a less public setting. Then stimulus fading procedures can be used to introduce cues from the natural environment in a graduated fashion (Jackson & Wallace, 1974).

Physical prompting. When shaping programs are used to increase social participation, it may prove necessary to provide physical prompts for the child's first reinforceable responses. In training the preschool girl to use outdoor play equipment, Buell and her associates (Beull et al., 1968) first prompted the child by lifting her onto a piece of play equipment and holding her there briefly. Once she was in this position, she received social reinforcement in the form of attention and approval from the teachers. Retarded children who are unresponsive to verbal instructions are particularly likely to require physical prompting, for example, in developing hand waving as a social greeting behavior (Stokes, Baer, & Jackson, 1974), or in learning to participate in a ball-rolling game with another child (Whitman, Mercurio, & Caponigri, 1970). Once the child has been physically or verbally assisted in making the first few responses and has received reinforcement, the prompts can be progressively removed so long as the reinforcement continues.

INDIRECT METHODS

An imaginative use of candy incentives was reported by Kirby and Toler (1970). These investigators increased a 5-year-old boy's rate of interaction with classmates by the simple tactic of having him pass out candy. His interactions with other children increased markedly during the periods he provided them with candy. Such a manipulation could have long-term beneficial consequences. If the children become accustomed to speaking to and playing with the target child and find interactions with him mutually reinforcing, he could become a permanent member of the peer-interaction system. Baer and Wolf (1967) have termed this entry into natural communities of reinforcement a behavioral trap. The child's therapeutically-instated desirable behavior naturally draws reinforcement, and this itself further stimulates and maintains the behavior without continuing professional intervention.

CHARACTERISTICS OF SUCCESSFUL INTERVENTIONS

In summary, some symbolic modeling and shaping procedures have proved effective in increasing social participation rates among shy and withdrawn children. Effective modeling demonstrations have presented peer models as initially highly similar to the unskilled observers, but as increasingly assertive and successful. There is some evidence that even brief symbolic modeling treatments can have long lasting effects, but are particularly likely to effect long-term improvement when combined with shaping and contingency management programs.

To be effective, both the models and the contingencies must be age-appropriate for the children treated. Treatment failures can be extremely instructive. McCullough (1972) reports such a case in which an attempt was made to increase high-school students' discussion participation rates through a modeling and reward procedure. Exemplary students were chosen to serve as peer models. The teacher praised each model for participating and put a mark opposite the student's name on the blackboard as a record of participation. In response to this manipulation, the adolescent observers further reduced their participation in discussions, and stated that they found the teachers' comments and public recording of participation to be childish and silly. The intended teacher reinforcement actually served as a punishing stimulus. Such a procedure might work well with young children but insult older ones. More subtle modeling and reinforcement procedures and a greater reliance on self-monitoring and self-regulation would be appropriate for use with older children, teenagers, and adults.

NEGATIVE REACTIONS TO MEDICAL AND DENTAL TREATMENT

Many medical diagnostic and treatment procedures are painful, and few children relish a trip to the dentist or doctor. Children's fears are based not only on their own painful experiences, but also on their observations of the fearful reactions of others. They are very likely to overhear their parents and siblings expressing apprehension about and avoidance of medical treatment, and these models help determine the observing child's own reactions. Studies of correlates of children's behavior during dental treatment support this view. Children who are uncooperative or fearful during dental visits tend to have mothers with similar apprehensions (Johnson & Baldwin, 1969), and to have families who have unfavorable attitudes toward dentistry and unfortunate dental experiences (Shoben & Borland, 1954). Moreover, children receive negative expectations from others, including symbolic models presented in cartoons and on television (Kleinknecht, Klepac, & Alexander, 1973). Additionally, if a child has been led to believe that she or he has dental problems, the child will be less cooperative during the first dental visit (Wright & Alpern, 1971). All of these interpersonal influences help to determine the child's emotional and cooperative behavior during dental treatment.

Many pedodontists unwittingly contribute to the child's fear because of their beliefs concerning the sources of the child's resistance to treatment, and because of the methods sometimes used to ensure the child's cooperation. A recent survey of opinions held by diplomates in pedodontics (Association of Pedodontic Diplomates, 1972) reveals that pediatric dentists view children's attempts to escape painful treatment techniques as motivated by willfullness rather than by fear. Accordingly, many dentists reported using physical restraints and coercion such as blocking the child's mouth and sometimes also his nostrils with a hand or a towel (see Craig, 1971) in order to force the child to cease resisting. These tactics are likely to terrify young children. It is not surprising, therefore, to find that at least 5% to 6% of the population is too fearful to make necessary dental visits (Freidson & Feldman, 1958; Gale & Ayer, 1969), and that possibly as many as 16% of school-age children exhibit serious fear and avoidance reactions to dental treatment (Stricker & Howitt, 1965).

Behavioral Treatments

This doleful outlook should improve, however, with the increasing use of behavior therapy techniques based on principles of modeling and reinforcement. Only within the past several years have practitioners recognized the potential merit of the application of learning principles in the treatment of medical management problems (Katz & Zlutnick, 1975). Both in vivo systematic desensitization (Machen & Johnson, 1974) and emotive imagery (Ayer, 1973) have been demonstrated to be useful in overcoming children's fears of and resistance to dental treatment. Systematic desensitization combined with reinforcement for stoic behavior has been reported to decrease resistance to hemodialysis (Katz, 1974) and panicky refusal of oral medication for asthma attacks (Miklich, 1973).

Both live modeling (White & Davis, 1974) and symbolic modeling in the form of brief films portraying coping peer models have been repeatedly demonstrated to be useful in reducing fear-related dental and medical management problems (Adelson & Goldfried, 1970; Adelson, Liebert, Poulos, & Herskovitz, 1972; Johnson & Machen, 1973; Liebert, 1973; Machen & Johnson, 1974; Melamed, Hawes, Heiby, & Glick, 1975; Melamed, Weinstein, Hawes, & Katin-Borland, 1975). In an excellent experimental study, Melamed and Siegel (1973) found a symbolic modeling treatment to be effective in reducing children's pre-surgery anxiety and postoperative adjustment problems during recovery from various common elective surgical procedures.[2]

PREVENTION OF FEAR AND AVOIDANCE REACTIONS

We are rapidly acquiring the theoretical and empirical knowledge needed to devise large-scale prevention programs. It may prove possible to protect children from developing needless fears and anxieties concerning animals, unfamiliar persons and situations, medical and dental treatments, and from other common childhood anxieties. Experimental studies with both animal and human learners have indicated that non-reinforced preexposure to a stimulus can result in a decrement in conditioning of avoidance responses to that stimulus (see Poser, 1970, and Poser & King, 1975, for a review of this literature). Thus, familiarizing a child with a particular stimulus object such as a snake should make it more difficult for the child to acquire a conditioned fear and avoidance reaction to snakes. In fact, King (1975) has found just such an effect in young children who were initially unacquainted with snakes. Those children who observed child models in fearless interactions with snakes exhibited lower levels of physiological arousal indicative of fear and greater approach behavior on a behavioral test than did either untreated children or children who observed initially fearful coping models. The latter children may well have imitated the timidness originally displayed by the coping models. In contrast, the fearless models provided observers both with exposure to potentially frightening stimuli and with demonstrations of appropriate behavior.

Other investigators have reported that preexposure to the dental office and its associated equip-

[2]The film used by Melamed and Siegel, entitled, *Ethan Has an Operation*, may be obtained from the Health Services Communication Center, Case Western Reserve University, Cleveland, Ohio 44106.

ment prevented children from becoming fearful during their first dental visits (Surwit, 1972), and that symbolic modeling treatments are particularly effective in this regard. Melamed and her associates (Melamed, Hawes, Heiby, & Glick, 1975; Melamed, Weinstein, Hawes, & Katin-Borland, 1975) have found that youngsters who received the usual dental handling increased their disruptive behavior, such as complaining, kicking, and crying, as much as 256% from their initial examination visit to the more stressful restorative treatment visits. In contrast, children who witnessed a film of a brave peer model either maintained or actually decreased their rates of disruptive behavior during treatment by a margin as great as 23%. These results suggest that videotape casettes featuring exemplary child patients could usefully replace the dog-eared comic books and outdated magazines typically to be found in the waiting rooms of pediatricians and pedodontists. The experiments just described are true prevention studies in that a population at high risk of acquiring fear and avoidance reactions is shown to display fewer such reactions as a result of a treatment administered prior to their first experience with a particular stressor.

These initial demonstrations are promising ,but considerably more research is required, as Poser (1975) has suggested. We cannot yet determine the risk factor for many childhood behavioral problems, nor can we identify the mechanisms responsible for stress inoculation effects. Poser and his associates (Poser & King, 1975) are undertaking an ambitious project to identify high-school students susceptible to behavior disorders, but who are still functioning adequately. In successive phases of the project, the investigators hope to determine the particular types of maladaptive reactions likely to be developed by high-risk adolescents, and to devise and test preventive interventions such as those involving preexposure or symbolic modeling techniques.

Other investigators may choose to focus on the development of behavioral prevention measures that could be applied to youngsters now known to be highly vulnerable to acquiring negative reactions to medical treatment, to separation from parents, or to other common experiences. The research studies reviewed in this paper suggest that we may already be well on the way to the prevention of behavioral problems which have plagued generations of children.

REFERENCES

ADELSON, R., and GOLDFRIED, M. R. Modeling and the fearful child patient. *Journal of Dentisty for Children*, 1970, *37*, 476–489.

ADELSON, R., LIEBERT, R. M., POULOS, R. W., and HERSKOVITZ, A. A modeling film to reduce children's fear of dental treatment. *Journal of Dental Research*, 1972, *51*, 1708 (Abstract).

AGRAS, W. S., CHAPIN, H. H., and OLIVEAU, D. C. The natural history of phobia. *Archives of General Psychiatry*, 1972, *26*, 315–317.

AGRAS, W. S., SYLVESTER, D., and OLIVEAU, D. The epidemiology of common fears and phobias. *Comprehensive Psychiatry*, 1969, *10*, 151–156.

ALLEN, K., HART, B., BUELL, S., HARRIS, R., and WOLF, M. Effects of social reinforcement on isolate behavior of a nursery school child. *Child Development*, 1964, *35*, 511–518.

ANDERSON, H. H. Domination and integration in the social behavior of young children in an experimental play situation. *Genetic Psychology Monographs*, 1937, *19*, 341–408.

Association of Pedodontic Diplomates. Technique for behavior management: A survey. *Journal of Dentistry for Children*, 1972, *39*, 368–372.

AYER, W. A. Use of visual imagery in needle phobic children. *Journal of Dentistry for Children*, 1973, *40*, 125–127.

AYLLON, T., SMITH, D., and ROGERS, M. Behavioral management of school phobia. *Journal of Behavior Therapy and Experimental Psychiatry*, 1970, *1*, 125–138.

BAER, D. M., and WOLF, M. M. *The entry into natural communities of reinforcement.* Paper presented at the meeting of the American Psychological Association, Washington, D. C., September 1967.

BANDURA, A. The role of modeling processes in personality development. In W. W. Hartup and M. L. Smothergill (Eds.), *The young child* (Vol. 1). Washington, D. C.: National Association for the Education of Young Children, 1967.

BANDURA, A. *Principles of behavior modification.* New York: Holt, Rinehart & Winston, 1969.

BANDURA, A. Psychotherapy based upon modeling principles. In A. E. Bergin and S. L. Garfield (Eds.), *Handbook of psychotherapy and behavior change.* New York: John Wiley, 1971.

BANDURA, A., BLANCHARD, E. B., and RITTER, B. Relative efficacy of desensitization and modeling approaches for inducing behavioral, affective, and attitudinal changes. *Journal of Personality and Social Psychology*, 1969, *13*, 173–199.

BANDURA, A., GRUSEC, E., and MENLOVE, F. L. Vicarious extinction of avoidance behavior. *Journal of Personality and Social Psychology*, 1967, *5*, 16–23.

BANDURA, A., JEFFERY, R. W., and WRIGHT, C. L. Efficacy of participant modeling as a function of response induction aids. *Journal of Abnormal Psychology*, 1974, *83*, 56–64.

BANDURA, A., and MENLOVE, F. L. Factors determining vicarious extinction of avoidance behavior through symbolic modeling. *Journal of Personality and Social Psychology*, 1968, *8*, 99–198.

BANDURA, A., and WALTERS, R. H. *Social learning and personality development.* New York: Holt, Rinehart & Winston, 1963.

BAUERMEISTER, J. J., and JEMAIL, J. A. Modification of "elective mutism" in the classroom setting: A case study. *Behavior Therapy*, 1975, *6*, 246–250.

BENTLER, PETER M. An infant's phobia treated with reciprocal inhibition therapy. *Journal of Child Psychology and Psychiatry*, 1962, *3*, 185–189.

BLANCHARD, E. B. The generalization of vicarious extinction effects. *Behaviour Research and Therapy*, 1970, *8*, 323–330. (a)

BLANCHARD, E. B. The relative contributions of modeling, informational influences, and physical contact in the extinction of phobic behavior. *Journal of Abnormal Psychology*, 1970, *76*, 55–61. (b)

BONNY, M. E. Assessment of effort to aid socially isolated elementary school pupils. *Journal of Educational Research*, 1971, *64*, 359–364.

BRISON, D. W. Case studies in school psychology: A non-talking child in kindergarten: An application of behavior therapy. *Journal of School Psychology*, 1966, *4*, 65–69.

BROWN, R. E., COPELAND R. E., and HALL, R. V. School phobia: Effects of behavior modification treatment applied by an elementary school principal. *Child Study Journal*, 1974, *4*, 125–133.

BUELL, J., STODDARD, P., HARRIS, F. R., and BAER, D. M. Collateral social development accompanying reinforcement of outdoor play in a preschool child. *Journal of Applied Behavior Analysis*, 1968, *1*, 167–173.

CLEMENT, P. W. Operant conditioning in group psychotherapy with children. *Journal of School Health*, 1968, *38*, 271–278.

CLEMENT, P. W., and MILNE, D. C. Group play therapy and tangible reinforcers used to modify the behavior of 8-year-old boys. *Behaviour Research and Therapy*, 1967, *5*, 301–312.

CLEMENT, P. W., ROBERTS, P. V., and LANTZ, C. E. Social models and token reinforcement in the treatment of shy withdrawn boys. *Proceedings of the 78th Annual Convention of the American Psychological Association*, 1970, *5*, 515–516.

CLEMENT, P. W., ROBERTS, P. V., and LANTZ, C. E. Mothers and peers as child behavior therapists. *International Journal of Group Psychotherapy*, 1976, *26*, 335–359.

CONRAD, R. D., DELK, J. L., and WILLIAMS, C. Use of stimulus fading procedures in the treatment of situation specific mutism: A case study. *Journal of Behavior Therapy and Experimental Psychiatry*, 1974, *5*, 99–100.

COOLIDGE, J. C., HAHN, P. B., and PECK, A. L. School phobia: Neurotic crisis or way of life. *American Journal of Orthopsychiatry*, 1957, *27*, 296–306.

COOLIDGE, J. C., WILLER, M. L., TESSMAN, E., and WALDFOGEL, S. School phobia in adolescence: A manifestation of severe character disturbance. *American Journal of Orthopsychiatry*, 1960, *30*, 599–607.

CRAIG, W. Hand over mouth technique. *Journal of Dentistry for Children*, 1971, *38*, 387–389.

EVERS, W. L., and SCHWARZ, J. C. Modifying social withdrawal in preschoolers: The effects of filmed modeling and teacher praise. *Journal of Abnormal Child Psychology*, 1973, *1*, 248–256.

EYSENCK, H. J. Learning theory and behaviour therapy. *Journal of Mental Science*, 1959, *105*, 61–75.

EYSENCK, H. J., and RACHMAN, S. *The causes and cures of neurosis*. San Diego, Cal.: Knapp, 1965.

FERSTER, C. B., and SKINNER, B. F. *Schedules of reinforcement*. New York: Appleton-Century-Crofts, 1957.

FREIDSON, E., and FELDMAN, J. J. The public looks at dental care. *Journal of the American Dental Association*, 1958, *57*, 325–331.

GALE, E. N., and AYER, W. A. Treatment of dental phobias. *Journal of the American Dental Association*, 1969, *78*, 1304–1307.

GARVEY, W. P., and HEGRENES, J. R. Desensitization techniques in the treatment of school phobia. *American Journal of Orthopsychiatry*, 1966, *36*, 147–152.

GELFAND, D. M., and HARTMANN, D. P. Behavior therapy with children: A review and evaluation of research methodology. *Psychological Bulletin*, 1968, *67*, 204–215.

GELFAND, D. M., and HARTMANN, D. P. *Child behavior analysis and therapy*. New York: Pergamon Press, 1975.

GELFAND, D. M., HARTMANN, D. P., LAMB, A. K., SMITH, C. L., MAHAN, M. A., and PAUL, S. C. The effects of adult models and described alternatives on children's choice of behavior management techniques. *Child Development*, 1974, *45*, 585–593.

HAGMAN, E. A study of fears of children of preschool age. *Journal of Experimental Education*, 1932, *1*, 110–130.

HALPERN, W. I., HAMMOND, J., and COHEN, R. A therapeutic approach to speech phobia: Elective mutism reexamined. In S. Chess and A. Thomas (Eds.), *Annual progress in child psychiatry and child development*, 1972. New York: Brunner/Mazel, 1972.

HARTMANN, D. P., and ATKINSON, D. Having your cake and eating it too! A note on some apparent contradictions between therapeutic achievements and design requirements in $N = 1$ studies. *Behavior Therapy*, 1973, *4*, 589–591.

HERSEN, M. Treatment of a compulsive and phobic disorder through a total behavior therapy program: A case study. *Psychotherapy*, 1968, *5*, 220–225.

HERSEN, M. Behavior modification approach to a school-phobia case. *Journal of Clinical Psychology*, 1970, *20*, 395–402.

HERSEN, M. The behavioral treatment of school phobia: Current techniques. Is S. Chess and A. Thomas (Eds.), *Annual progress in child psychiatry and child development*, 1972. New York: Brunner/Mazel, 1972.

HILL, J. H., LIEBERT, R. M., and MOTT, D. E. W. Vicarious extinction of avoidance behavior through films: An initial test. *Psychological Reports*, 1968, *22*, 192.

HOLMES, F. B. An experimental investigation of a method of overcoming children's fears. *Child Development*, 1936, *7*, 6–30.

HOSFORD, R. E. Overcoming fear of speaking in a group. In J. D. Krumboltz and C. E. Thoresen (Eds.), *Behavioral counseling*. New York: Holt, Rinehart, & Winston, 1969.

HOSFORD, R. E., and SORENSON, D. L. Participating in classroom discussions. In J. D. Krumboltz and C. E. Thoresen (Eds.),

Behavioral counseling. New York: Holt, Rinehart & Winston, 1969.

JACK, L. M. An experimental study of ascendant behavior in preschool children. *University of Iowa Studies in Child Welfare*, 1934, *9*, 3–65.

JACKSON, D. A., and WALLACE R. F. The modification and generalization of voice loudness in a fifteen-year-old retarded girl. *Journal of Applied Behavior Analysis*, 1974, *7*, 461–471.

JAKIBCHUK, Z., and SMERIGLIO, V. L. *The influence of symbolic modeling on the social behavior of preschool children with low levels of social responsiveness*. Paper presented at the meeting of the Society for Research in Child Development, Denver, March, 1975.

JERSILD, A. T., and HOLMES, F. B. Children's fears. *Child Development Monographs*. New York: Bureau of Publications. Teachers College, Columbia University, 1935.

JERSILD, A. T., and HOLMES, F. B. Methods of overcoming children's fears. *Journal of Psychology*, 1936, *1*, 75–104.

JERSILD, A. T., MARKEY, F. V., and JERSILD, C. L. Children's fears, dreams, wishes, daydreams, likes, dislikes, pleasant and unpleasant memories. *Child Development Monographs*. New York: Bureau of Publications. Teachers College, Columbia University, 1933.

JOHNSON, A. M. School phobia. *American Journal of Orthopsychiatry*, 1957, *27*, 307–309.

JOHNSON, R., and BALDWIN, D. C., JR. Maternal anxiety and child behavior. *Journal of Dentistry for Children*, 1969, *36*, 87–92.

JOHNSON, R., and MACHEN, J. B. Behavior modification techniques and maternal anxiety. *Journal of Dentistry for Children*, 1973, *40*, 272–276.

JONES, MARY C. The elimination of children's fears. *Journal of Experimental Psychology*, 1924, *7*, 382–390. (a)

JONES, MARY C. A laboratory study of fear: The case of Peter. *Pedagogical Seminar*, 1924, *31*, 308–315. (b)

KANFER, F. H., KAROLY, P., and NEWMAN, A. Reduction of children's fear of the dark by competence-related and situational threat-related verbal cues. *Journal of Consulting and Clinical Psychology*, 1975, *43*, 251–258.

KATZ, R. C. Single session recovery from a hemodialysis phobia: A case study *Journal of Behavior Therapy and Experimental Psychiatry*, 1974, *5*, 205–206.

KATZ, R. C., and ZLUTNICK, S. *Behavior therapy and health care: Principles and applications*. New York: Pergamon, 1975.

KELLER, M. F., and CARLSON, P. M. The use of symbolic modeling to promote social skills in preschool children with low levels of social responsiveness. *Child Development*, 1974, *45*, 912–919.

KELLY, G. A. *The psychology of personal constructs*. New York: Norton, 1955.

KELLY, M. P. *Modification of preschool social isolate behavior through the use of videotape modeling techniques*. Unpublished Master's thesis, University of Utah, 1975.

KENNEDY, W. A. School phobia: Rapid treatment of fifty cases. *Journal of Abnormal Psychology*, 1965, *70*, 285–289.

KING, M. *The prevention of maladaptive avoidance responses through observational learning: An analogue study*. Unpublished doctoral dissertation, McGill University, 1975.

KIRBY, F. D., and TOLER, H. C., JR. Modification of preschool isolate behavior: A case study. *Journal of Applied Behavior Analysis*, 1970, *3*, 309–314.

KLEINKNECHT, R. A., KLEPAC, R. K., and ALEXANder, L. D. Origins and characteristics of fear of dentistry. *Journal of the American Dental Association*, 1973, *86*, 842–848.

KORNHABER, R. C., and SCOROEDER, H. E. Importance of model similarity on extinction of avoidance behavior in children. *Journal of Consulting and Clinical Psychology*, 1975, *43*, 601–607.

LAZARUS, A. A. New methods in psychotherapy: A case study. *South African Medical Journal*, 1958, *33*, 660.

LAZARUS, A. A. The elimination of children's phobias by deconditioning. *Medical Proceed-*

ings, South Africa, 1959, *5*, 261–265 (also in Eysenck, 1960).

LAZARUS, A., and ABRAMOVITZ, A. The use of "emotive imagery" in the treatment of children's phobias. *Journal of Mental Science*, 1962, *108*, 191–195.

LAZARUS, A. A., DAVISON, D. C., and POLEFKA, B. A. Classical and operant factors in the treatment of school phobia. *Journal of Abnormal Psychology*, 1965, *70*, 225–229.

LEITENBERG, H. Behavioral approaches to treatment of neuroses. In H. Leitenberg (Ed.), *Handbook of behavior modification and behavior therapy*. Englewood Cliffs, N. J.: Prentice Hall, 1976.

LEITENBERG, H., and CALLAHAN, E. J. Reinforced practice and reduction of different kinds of fears in adults and children. *Behaviour Research and Therapy*, 1973, *11*, 19–30.

LEWIS, S. A comparison of behavior therapy techniques in the reduction of fearful avoidance behavior. *Behavior Therapy*, 1974, *5*, 648–655.

LIEBERT, R. Observational learning: Some applied implications. In P. Elich (Ed.), *Social learning*. Bellingham: Western Washington State College Press, 1973.

LINDEN, W. Practicing of meditation by school children and their levels of field dependence-independence, test anxiety, and reading achievement. *Journal of Consulting and Clinical Psychology*, 1973, *41*, 139–143.

MACFARLANE, J. W., ALLEN, L., and HONZIK, M. P. *A developmental study of the behavior problems of normal children between 21 months and 14 years*. Berkeley: University of California Press, 1954.

MACHEN, J. B., and JOHNSON, R. Desensitization, model learning, and the dental behavior of children. *Journal of Dental Research*, 1974, *53*, 83–87.

MANN, J. Vicarious desensitization of test anxiety through observation of videotaped treatment. *Journal of Counseling Psychology*, 1972, *19*, 1–7.

MANN, J., and ROSENTHAL, T. L. Vicarious and direct counterconditioning of test anxiety through individual and group desensitization. *Behaviour Research and Therapy*, 1969, *7*, 359–367.

MARLATT, G. A., and PERRY, M. A. Modeling methods. In F. H. Kanfer and A. P. Goldstein (Eds.), *Helping people change*. New York: Pergamon, 1975.

MCCULLOUGH, J. P. An investigation of the effects of model group size upon response facilitation in the high school classroom. *Behavior Therapy*, 1972, *3*, 561–566.

MEICHENBAUM, D. Examination of model characteristics in reducing avoidance behavior. *Journal of Personality and Social Psychology*, 1971, *17*, 298–307.

MELAMED, B. G., HAWES, R. R., HEIBY, E., and GLICK, J. The use of filmed modeling to reduce uncooperative behavior of children during dental treatment. *Journal of Dental Research*, 1975, *54*.

MELAMED, B. G., and SIEGEL, L. J. Reduction of anxiety in children facing hospitalization and surgery by use of filmed modeling. *Journal of Consulting and Clinical Psychology*, 1975, *43*, 511–521.

MELAMED, B. G., WEINSTEIN, J., HAWES, R., and KATIN-BORLAND, M. Reduction of fear-related dental management problems with use of filmed modeling. *Journal of the American Dental Association*, 1975, *90*, 822–826.

MIKLICH, D. R. Operant conditioning procedures with systematic desensitization in a hyperkinetic asthmatic boy. *Journal of Behavior Therapy and Experimental Psychiatry*, 1973, *4*, 177–182.

MILLER, L. C., BARRETT, C. L., HAMPE, E., and NOBLE, H. Factor structure of children's fears. *Journal of Consulting and Clinical Psychology*, 1972, *39*, 264–268.

MISCHEL, W. *Personality and assessment*. New York: John Wiley, 1968.

MONTENEGRO, H. Severe separation anxiety in two preschool children successfully treated by reciprocal inhibition. *Journal of Child Psychology and Psychiatry*, 1968, *9*, 93–103.

MURPHY, C. M., and BOOTZIN, R. R. Active and

passive participation in the contact desensitization of snake fear in children. *Behavior Therapy*, 1973, *2*, 203–211.

NEISWORTH, J. T., MADLE, R. A., and GOEKE, K. E. "Errorless" elimination of separation anxiety: A case study. *Behavior Therapy and Experimental Psychiatry*, 1975, *6*, 79–82.

NOLAN, J. D., and PENCE, C. Operant conditioning principles in the treatment of a selectively mute child. *Journal of Consulting and Clinical Psychology*, 1970, *35*, 265–268.

O'CONNOR, R. D. Modification of social withdrawal through symbolic modeling. *Journal of Applied Behavior Analysis*, 1969, *2*, 15–22.

O'CONNOR, R. D. Relative efficacy of modeling, shaping, and the combined procedures for modification of social withdrawal. *Journal of Abnormal Psychology*, 1972, *79*, 327–334.

O'LEARY, K. D., POULOS, R. W., and DEVINE, V. T. Tangible reinforcers: Bonuses or bribes? *Journal of Consulting and Clinical Psychology*, 1972, *38*, 1–8.

PAGE, M. L. The modification of ascendant behavior in preschool children. *University of Iowa Studies in Child Welfare*, 1936, *9*, 3–65.

PATTERSON, G. R. A learning theory approach to the treatment of the school phobic child. In Leonard P. Ullmann and Leonard Krasner (Ed.), *Case studies in behavior modification*. New York: Holt, Rinehart & Winston, 1965.

PATTERSON, G. R., and BRODSKY, G. A behavior modification program for a child with multiple problem behaviors. *Journal of Child Psychology and Psychiatry*, 1966, *7*, 277–295.

POSER, E. G. Toward a theory of "behavioral prophylaxis". *Journal of Behavior Therapy and Experimental Psychiatry*, 1970, *1*, 39–43.

POSER, E. G. *Strategies for behavioral prevention*. Paper presented at the 7th Banff International Conference on Behavior Modification, Banff, Alberta, March 23–27, 1975.

POSER, E. G., and King, M. C. *Primary prevention of fear: An experimental approach*. Unpublished manuscript, McGill University, Montreal, 1975.

RASBURY, W. C. Behavioral treatment of selective mutism: A case report. *Journal of Behavior Therapy and Experimental Psychiatry*, 1974, *5*, 103–104.

REID, J. B., HAWKINS, L., KEUTZER, C., MCNEAL, S. A., PHELPS, R. E., REID, K. M., and MEES, H. L. A marathon behavior modification of a selectively mute child. *Journal of Child Psychology and Psychiatry*, 1967, *8*, 27–30.

REYNOLDS, N. J., and RISLEY, T. R. The role of social and material reinforcers in increasing talking of a disadvantaged preschool child. *Journal of Applied Behavior Analysis*, 1968, *1*, 253–262.

RIMM, D. C., and MASTERS, J. C. *Behavior therapy: Techniques and empirical findings*. New York: Academic Press, 1974.

RITTER, B. The group desensitization of children's snake phobias using vicarious and contact desensitization procedures. *Behaviour Research and Therapy*, 1968, *6*, 1–6.

RODRIGUEZ, A., RODRIGUEZ, M., and EISENBERG, L. The outcome of school phobia: A follow-up study based on 41 cases. *American Journal of Psychiatry*, 1959, *116*, 540–544.

ROSENTHAL, T. L. Modeling therapies. In M. Hersen, R. M. Eisler, and P. M. Miller (Eds.) *Progress in behavior modification* (Vol. 2). New York: Academic Press, 1976.

SHERMAN, H., and FARINA, A. Social inadequacy of parents and children. *Journal of Abnormal Psychology*, 1974, *83*, 327–330.

SHOBEN, E. J., JR., and BORLAND, L. An empirical study of the etiology of dental fears. *Journal of Clinical Psychology*, 1954, *10*, 171–174.

SMITH, R. E., and SHARPE, T. H. Treatment of a school phobia with implosive therapy. *Journal of Consulting and Clinical Psychology*, 1970, *35*, 239–243.

STAMPFL, T. G., and LEVIS, D. J. Essentials of implosive therapy: A learning theory-based psychodynamic behavioral therapy. *Journal of Abnormal Psychology*, 1967, *72*, 496–503.

STOKES, T. F., BAER, D. M., and JACKSON, R. L. Programming the generalization of a greeting response in four retarded children. *Journal of Applied Behavior Analysis*, 1974, *7*, 599–610.

STRAUGHAN, J. H., POTTER, W. K., and HAMILTON, S. H. The behavioral treatment of an elective mute. *Journal of Child Psychology and Psychiatry*, 1965, *6*, 125–139.

STRICKER, G., and HOWITT, J. W. Physiological recording during simulated dental appointments. *New York State Dental Journal*, 1965, *31*, 204–213.

SURWIT, R. *The anticipatory modification of the conditioning of a fear response in humans.* Unpublished doctoral dissertation, McGill University, 1972.

TAHMASIAN, J., and MCREYNOLDS, W. Use of parents as behavioral engineers in the treatment of a school-phobic girl. *Journal of Counseling Psychology*, 1971, *18*, 225–228.

TASTO, D. L. Systematic desensitization, muscle relaxation and visual imagery in the counterconditioning of a four-year-old phobic child. *Behaviour Research and Therapy*, 1969, *7*, 409–411.

TERRACE, H. S. Stimulus control. In W. Honig (Ed.), *Operant behavior: Areas of research and application.* New York: Appleton-Century-Crofts, 1966.

ULLMANN, L. P., and KRASNER, L. *A psychological approach to abnormal behavior* (2nd ed.). Englewood Cliffs, N. J.: Prentice-Hall, 1975.

WALKER, H. M., and HOPS, H. Group and individual reinforcement contingencies in the modification of social withdrawal. In L. A. Hamerlynck, L. Handy, and E. Mash (Eds.), *Behavior change: Methodology, concepts and practice.* Champaign, Ill.: Research Press, 1973.

WALKER, H. M., HOPS, H., GREENWOOD, C. R., and TODD, N. M. *Social interaction: Effects of symbolic modeling and individual and group reinforcement contingencies on the behavior of withdrawn children.* (Report No. 15). Eugene, Oregon: Center at Oregon for Research in the Behavioral Education of the Handicapped, Center on Human Development, August, 1975.

WATSON, J. B. *Psychological care of infant and child.* New York: Norton, 1928.

WEISSBROD, C. S., and BRYAN, J. H. Filmed treatment as an effective fear-reduction technique. *Journal of Abnormal Child Psychology*, 1973, *1*, 196–201.

WHITE, W. C., JR., and DAVIS, M. T. Vicarious extinction of phobic behavior in early childhood. *Journal of Abnormal Child Psychology*, 1974, *2*, 25–32.

WHITMAN, T. L., MERCURIO, J. R., and CAPONIGRI, V. Development of social responses in two severely retarded children. *Journal of Applied Behavior Analysis*, 1970, *3*, 133–138.

WOLPE, J. *Psycho-therapy by reciprocal inhibition.* Stanford: Stanford University Press, 1958.

WOLPE, J. The systematic desensitization treatment of neuroses. *Journal of Nervous and Mental Disease*, 1961, *132*, 189–203.

WOLPE, J., and LAZARUS, A. A. *Behavior therapy techniques: A guide to the treatment of neuroses.* Oxford: Pergamon, 1966.

WRIGHT, G. Z., and ALPERN, G. D. Variables influencing children's cooperative behavior at the first dental visit. *Journal of Dentistry for Children*, 1971, *38*, 124–128.

WULBERT, M., NYMAN, B. A., SNOW, D., and OWEN, Y. The efficacy of stimulus fading and contingency management in the treatment of elective mutism: A case study. *Journal of Applied Behavior Analysis*, 1973, *6*, 435–441.

ZIMBARDO, P., PILKONIS, P., and NORWOOD, R. *The silent prison of shyness.* Unpublished manuscript, Stanford University, 1974.

21

CHILDHOOD PSYCHOSIS: PSYCHOTHERAPY

Clarice J. Kestenbaum

Ideally the term *medical treatment* implies knowledge of a specific illness of known etiology, and of a pathogenic agent for which a specific remedy is administered with a predictable outcome. Unfortunately, for the group of disorders we subsume under the heading of *childhood schizophrenia* we are far from being able to supply simple conclusive answers. The nomenclature of psychotic disorders in children is undergoing change with each new edition of the American Psychiatric Association's *Diagnostic and Statistical Manual*. There is continued disagreement concerning differential diagnosis, etiology of the various syndrome complexes, and treatment methods.

Disagreement regarding a psychodynamic versus an organic etiology goes back to the first decade of the 20th century. In 1906 DeSanctis described young children who regressed to a "feeble-minded" condition and exhibited negativism and stereotyped movements. His syndrome was an early form of Kraepelin's dementia praecox which he named "dementia praecoccissima."

Thomas Heller who, between 1908 and 1930, collected 28 cases of a disease he called "dementia infantilis" took issue with DeSanctis, especially with the latter's assumption that dementia praecoccissima was an early form of dementia praecox in childhood. Heller believed that DeSanctis was actually dealing with post-encephalitic states and progressive forms of mental deficiency. His own "dementia infantilis" described children previously normal in development who became, at age three or four, anxious and destructive and who, in addition, lost previously acquired speech and developed tics and grimaces, regressing to the level of idiocy. Kanner (1935) wrote in his classic textbook, *Child Psychiatry:*

> It was customary to list Heller's disease among the varieties of infantile schizophrenia. However, it is more plausible that this condition represents a cerebral degenerative process akin to Tay Sachs disease.

He went on to quote Schilder as having stated categorically:

> I assume as a matter of course that dementia infantilis has nothing to do with schizophrenia but is an organic progress. (p. 280)

A number of workers in the 1930s described cases of children with severe developmental disturbances (c.f. Despert, 1938; Kasanin and Kaufman, 1929; Richmond, 1932; Potter, 1932) but it was not until the 1940s that *childhood schizophrenia* began to attract attention as a serious and not uncommon disorder. A number of overlapping but related clinical syndromes began to be included in this general category.

MAJOR CLINICAL SYNDROMES

NUCLEAR SCHIZOPHRENIA

Lauretta Bender (1942) writing of her vast experience on the children's ward of the psychiatric division of Bellevue Hospital wrote that in her definition, *childhood schizophrenia* is a clinical entity occurring before puberty which "reveals pathology in behavior of every level and in every area of integration of patterning within the functioning of the central nervous system, be it vegetative, motor, perceptual, intellectual, emotional or social." (p. 139) She holds that the disorder is based on dysmaturation of the central nervous system, and that there is a strong constitutional factor. The onset is frequently within the first two years of life, but more commonly in the first year. Development is uneven. Neurological "soft signs" are common with motor awkwardness; a motility disorder with whirling, flapping hands is prominent. There are problems of identity, body image, and bodily functions. There are perceptual problems, emotional instability (irritability, excitement, tantrums), phobias, extreme anxiety, and a severe language disorder characterized by echolalia, pronomial confusion, etc. Bender holds that the final clinical picture is determined by the age of onset and the mechanism of defense utilized by the child. She labels any given child as exhibiting (a) the pseudo-defective, (b) the pseudo-neurotic, or (c) the pseudo-psychopathic variety of the disorder.

EARLY INFANTILE AUTISM

In 1943 Leo Kanner presented his detailed and carefully documented case histories of eleven children, whose symptoms of extreme aloneness and desire for preservation of sameness (with distress at any change) occurred within the first two years of life. He did not find a history of mental illness in the families, but described the parents as "intelligent, obsessive, and aloof." From an early age, the children showed profound withdrawal from people and seemed more interested in objects than people. All showed a severe disturbance in language acquisition, and those who had speech did not use language for communication (showing echolalia, neologisms, or reversal of pronouns as in Bender's cases). Kanner felt the children were intelligent despite the low level of intellectual function. Rote memory was often excellent. Absent or inadequate responses to sound often simulated deafness. Kanner found no neurological impairment and originally felt the disorder was nonorganic in origin. However, he concludes his paper with the observation:

> We must assume that these children have come into the world with innate inability to form the usual, biologically provided affective contact with people.

SYMBIOTIC PSYCHOSIS

In 1952 Margaret Mahler described an entity she considered as distinct from autistic psychosis. Using developmental psychoanalytic theory as a model, she theorized:

> . . . the early mother-infant symbiotic relationship is marked, but does not progress to the stage of object-libidinal cathexis of the mother. The mental representation of the mother remains, or is regressively fused with the self.

The onset of symbiotic psychosis, Mahler maintained, was during the separation-individuation phase from age 2½ to about the fourth year of life. Boundaries of self and non-self are blurred. There is a strong clinging attachment to adults, particularly to the mother. The child's body contour melts, as it were, into that of the other person. The child exhibits primary-process thinking, magical omnipotence, and uses private language. There are often hallucinations aimed at restoring symbiosis. There are severe panic reactions with rage and violent destructiveness, and abnormally low frustration tolerance. Some children exhibit deviations in motility patterns, e.g., whirling. Although her argument is largely for environmentally induced psychopathology, she has written:

> These children are constitutionally vulnerable and predisposed toward the development of a psychosis. It is the very existence of the constitutional ego defect in the child that helps create the vicious cycle of the pathogenic mother-child relationship by stimulating the mother to react to the child in ways that are deleterious to his attempts to separate and individuate. (1955, p. 201)

Unusual Sensitivity

Bergman and Escalona (1949) reported on five severely disturbed children who demonstrated unusual sensitivity to sensory stimulation such as light, sound and color, a marked unevenness in intellectual development, and excessive vulnerability to stress. Many could not tolerate change, were negativistic, had temper tantrums and outbursts of rage. The authors felt that the "protective stimulus barrier" was possibly constitutionally weak.

Borderline Psychotic Child

Rudolf Ekstein (1954) described a case of a child with atypical development in whom there were marked, sudden fluctuations in ego states without observable cause. Such children fit neither neurotic nor psychotic categories. Conflict is handled by flight and regression to a safer distance while maintaining contact with the therapist, with whom the relationship is autistic or symbiotic, tenuous, and easily disrupted.

Atypical Development

Beata Rank's description (1949) of severe emotional disorders of childhood emphasized the mother's role in the child's arriving at a state of marked emotional deprivation.

It is obvious that confusion is bound to exist with such a plethora of overlapping syndromes. The work of the last 15 years has been directed toward establishing more objective criteria for diagnostic evaluation.

In 1961 a British Working Party in an effort to achieve stricter diagnostic criteria formulated nine points which they felt distinguished the schizophrenic syndrome of childhood (Creak, 1961).

The nine criteria in essence are:

1. gross and sustained impairment of relationships with people;
2. apparent unawareness of his own personal identity to a degree inappropriate to his age;
3. pathological preoccupation with particular objects or certain characteristics of them without regard to their accepted functions;
4. sustained resistance to change in the environment and a striving to maintain or restore sameness;
5. abnormal perceptual experience (in the absence of discernible organic abnormality);
6. acute, excessive and seemingly illogical anxiety as a frequent phenomenon;
7. speech either lost or never acquired, or showing failure to develop beyond a level appropriate to an earlier age;
8. distortion in motility patterns;
9. a background of serious retardation in which islets of normal, near normal, or exceptional intellectual function or skill may appear.

Goldfarb's (1970) review of the major studies of childhood schizophrenia noted that all the symptoms that had been used in them for arriving at the diagnosis were coincidentally included in these nine points. Barbara Fish (1971) concluded that gross impairment in human relationships and noncommunicative speech were the two symptoms both necessary and sufficient to make the diagnosis of childhood schizophrenia.

Currently many workers are using the age of onset of symptoms as a primary criterion in classification, thus "lumping" together many of the well-established clinical syndromes of the past thirty years.

GROUP A: Onset between birth and three years
GROUP B: Onset between three and five years
GROUP C: Onset after five years

The child with late onset schizophrenia may have a formal thinking disorder, hallucinations, and delusions similar to adult schizophrenia. Rutter (1967) and Kolvin (1971) contend that early onset psychosis is a separate disease entity distinct from the adult form and other forms of childhood schizophrenia. Barbara Fish (1975), on the other hand, feels that childhood schizophrenia represents that particular subgroup of schizophrenia exhibiting the most severe biological disorder. She believes, with Bender and Kanner (who made the point in 1954) that:

> The differences in the way these cardinal symptoms are expressed by adults and children depend upon the degree of immaturity. The form of the children's psychotic speech is limited by their mental age and can be analyzed quantitatively. . . . When the psychotic process begins in the first years as in early infantile autism, the absence of any normal experience inevitably leads to major mental retardation. The severe cognitive disorder reflected in the beginnings of his speech indicate that the two to three year old, severely schizophrenic child does not respond to the meaningful patterns and relationships in the world around him in the same way the normal child does. (p. 50)

ETIOLOGICAL CONSIDERATIONS

PSYCHOGENIC VIEW

Few issues have been so widely contested, with opinions so sharply polarized, as the nature/nurture controversy regarding childhood schizophrenia. Many earlier workers took issue with Lauretta Bender's findings and looked toward the environment—particularly to the role of the mother as being causative in producing disordered children. Eisenberg and Kanner (1956) noted the "emotional refrigeration" in the parents of the autistic children they studied. Boatman and Szurek (1960) held that the parents demonstrated marked pathology, that "the disorder of the psychotic child represents its identification with and futile rebellion against the disorder of the parent."

Bettelheim (1956) is probably the strongest proponent of a psychogenic theory of childhood autism. He stated "the child senses the mother's destructive wishes toward him" and tries to "blot out what is too destructive an experience" for him. The autism, he believes, is a defense against a sense of total helplessness.

The family as a primary pathological agent has been implicated primarily by Bateson, Jackson Haley, and Weakland (1956), Lidz (1965), and Singer and Wynne (1963). Many of their studies were impressionistic and uncontrolled but rich in clinical vignettes of pathological family interaction.

BIOLOGICALLY ATYPICAL ORGANISM

Genetic Studies. A large body of evidence is accumulating which suggests that schizophrenia is a genetically determined illness affecting the central nervous system.

Since Kallman's initial exploration of genetic factors in the transmission of schizophrenia (1946) a vast amount of evidence points to a combined gene-environment interaction which is responsible for disordered behavior. While the estimated risk for the development of schizophrenia among the general population is 1 to 2%, the child of one schizophrenic parent has a 10 to 16% likelihood of developing schizophrenia (Kallman, 1946; Hesten, 1970).

Heston's studies (1966) of adopted children who had been separated from their schizophrenic mothers at birth have demonstrated that the rate of schizophrenia for these adopted children is high even when there has been no contact whatsoever with the biological parents. Children with two affected parents have a 35 to 44% chance of becoming schizophrenic (Erlenmeyer-Kimling, 1968).

The probability of a monozygotic co-twin's becoming schizophrenic is higher still. Concordance rates have been reported from 35 to 88% (Kallman, 1946; Stabenau, 1967), with most modern studies converging around the 35 to 40% range.

Although most studies involve post-adolescent schizophrenic breakdown, studies of the parents of schizophrenic *children* (with mid- or late-onset) have shown that the rate for schizophrenia in their parents is as high as for parents of adult schizophrenics (Kallman & Roth, 1956; Bender, 1972; Goldfarb, 1968). The genetic studies for early-onset schizophrenia (under age 2), however, are still questionable. The exact mechanism or the mode of operation of the genic error is unknown and intermediary neurophysiological mechanisms remain unclarified. Recent prospective studies of children at-risk for schizophrenia are, however, helping to cast light on this hitherto dark area (c.f. Mednick, 1965; Anthony, 1972; Kimling, 1973).

Primary Central Nervous System Abnormality. A number of anomalies have been found in schizophrenic children. Miller (1975, p. 367) has summarized those factors which point to a primary central nervous system abnormality:

1. Perinatal at-risk factors;
(Perinatal complications associated with childhood schizophrenia and infantile autism have been found by many researchers.)
2. Presence of neurological "soft" or "hard" signs;
3. Presence of abnormal EEG findings;
4. Higher incidence of below-average IQ;
5. Presence of perceptual and motor disorder similar to those found in patients with clear evidence of CNS impairment.
6. Association of infantile autism with various diseases, including rubella, toxoplasmosis, syphilis, retrolental fibroplasia, and hypsarrhythmia;
7. Presence of abnormal developmental patterns;
8. Biochemical abnormalities—increase in platelet serotonin has been reported in childhood autism.

An extensive bibliography has been prepared by Miller (1975), who points out that arguments for causality based on these studies are still inconclusive.

One important question in regard to children with schizophrenic symptoms and associated anomalies is yet unanswered: Is a perinatal insult (such as anoxia) by itself enough to produce childhood schizophrenia or is a genetic predisposition a necessary though not sufficient component? Stated otherwise, is the genotype indistinguishable from a phenocopy produced by exogenous factors?

Some Speculations Regarding Intervening Mechanisms. A number of important theories on the perceptual and cognitive dysfunction in childhood schizophrenia have been elaborated in recent years.

Anthony (1958 a,b) wrote that autistic children have a derangement of sensory input. Following a Piagetian model, he feels that such children do not achieve object-constancy, have no sense of temporal or spatial organization, and cannot organize the world in a meaningful manner. Moreover, without language, they are unable to conceptualize. Hermelin and O'Connor (1970) in their careful clinical and experimental studies of autistic children came to similar conclusions—that the basic cognitive deficit of autistic children lay in their inability to encode stimuli in a significant way. They confirmed Goldfarb's earlier observations (1956) that schizophrenic children used proximal rather than distal receptors. Goldfarb found abnormal patterns of receptor response and disturbances in active integration of sensory impressions (1961). There were extremes of either hyper- or hyposensitivity in all sensory modalities (eg., pain, auditory). Wing (1966) noted the importance of perceptual and motor deficiencies, viewing them as a primary impairment. For instance, he considers the need for sameness a result of the autistic child's inability to organize disordered perceptual stimuli.

Rimland (1964) feels that childhood psychosis results from a lack of integration of sensory input. He notes that the psychotic child stores memories which reemerge unmodified without accompanying associative linkages, resulting in a lack of ability to generalize. Rimland speculates that annoxia to the reticular activating system is a possible causal agent.

Hutt, Hutt, Lee, and Ounsted (1964) hypothesize that a chronically high arousal level in the reticular activating system causes the symptoms of autism (sterotopy, preservation of sameness), apparently as a means of avoiding a new situation which might provoke even greater activation of an already overactive RAS.

Ornitz and Ritvo (1968) have renamed infantile autism "the syndrome of perceptual inconsistency." According to these authors "disturbances of perception are shown to be fundamental to the other aspects of the disease and to be manifested by early developmental failure to distinguish between self and environment, to imitate, and to modulate sensory input." Furthermore, they hold that the illness is characterized by alternating states of excitation and inhibition. They point to the motility patterns of autistic children—whirling, darting, handflapping—alternating with posturing and motor inhibition and believe that central vestibular mechanisms may be involved in the deficiency in sensory-motor integration.

Rutter's theory (1971) holds that the language disorder of autism is primary and is similar to receptive aphasia. He feels that disturbances in affect and relatedness are secondary to the basic impairment in language skills. The inability to understand the meaning of spoken words he feels is more in keeping with a cognitive defect than with motivational failure.

Shapiro, Chariandini, and Fish (1974) note that schizophrenic children do not transform phrases into new sentences nor use them in new contexts. In their molecular analysis of the language of psychotic children, they find the speech patterns rigid and stereotyped. The child uses words in an idiosyncratic fashion and cannot seem to symbolize.

It is important to keep in mind that the speech of the schizophrenic child is at no time like that of his normal (same-aged or even younger) counterpart. These children are not simply retarded, Shapiro feels, for their communication disorder is unique. Neither does Shapiro believe that it resembles the disorder of aphasic children. Rather it seems to represent a central cognitive disorder involving disturbances of association and conceptualization.

Interactional View

As more systematic research during the last 15 years, has led to greater knowledge of biological mechanisms, even the most avid "environmentalists" acknowledge the presence of "inborn constitutional factors."

Margaret Mahler, discussing the constitutional-versus-experiential controversy wrote:

> . . . looking at autistic and symbiotic psychotic children, . . . the psychotic child's primary defect in being able to utilize (to perceive) the catalyzing mothering agent for homeostasis, is inborn, constitutional, and very probably hereditary, or else acquired very early in the first days or weeks of extrauterine life. (1968, p. 48)

By now it is almost universally accepted that biological impairment and life experiences *interact* to produce the clinical syndrome we call childhood schizophrenia.

Goldfarb (1961) describes two groups of schizophrenic children—an "organic" group with evidence of neurological dysfunction, and a "nonorganic" group who demonstrated a higher level of intellectual capacity. The parents of the non-organic group were shown to be far more psychologically disturbed than the "organic" children's parents. Goldfarb feels these sicker parents were not able to offer their children a stable and predictable environment. His term "parental perplexity" refers to this type of parental functioning which in his opinion can cause the psychotic child to react with fear and perceptual avoidance (Behrens & Goldfarb, 1958).

THERAPEUTIC INTERVENTIONS

The foregoing discussion of the various syndromes and multiple etiological theories of childhood schizophrenia should render more vivid the complexity of evaluating a psychotic child and formulating an adequate treatment plan.

There are many similarities among the heterogeneous group of schizophrenic children, yet each child is different in his own individual way. Therapeutic approaches have often been empirical: whatever works, works! The type of treatment has typically been shaped to the theoretical orientation of the therapist; it has not always been based on methodical study of all the neurological and psychological deficits in a particular child.

It is of the utmost importance to obtain as much data as possible: genetic and developmental history, psychiatric examination, neurological and psychological tests, before selecting a therapeutic plan.

For a psychoanalytically oriented therapist, verbal communication (interpretation, clarification, etc.) is the sine qua non of treatment, but where childhood schizophrenia is concerned the precondition—namely, that the child be able to understand what the therapist is saying—cannot so readily be taken for granted.

Des Lauriers and Carlson (1969) write: "With the autistic child how can one insure that some interaction and communication will take place, without knowing what (are) the specific obstacles to the communication . . . ?" (p. 71)

Therapy can occur in a number of settings: in a total therapeutic milieu, such as a hospital or residential treatment center; in a part-time therapeutic milieu (the therapeutic nursery or special school); or in a psychotherapist's office. The therapeutic model may be psychotherapy, individual and family therapy, behavior therapy, educational therapy or combinations of the above, with or without adjunctive pharmocotherapy. In some cases many of these modalities must be employed simultaneously; whereas in others, several modalities may need to be used "in series," chosen so as to meet the phase-specific requirements of the child. Behavior therapy tailored to counteract a socially alienating symptom or character trait may be required, for example, until the undesirable traits are under the child's control. The child may then be ready to benefit from individual psychotherapy of a sort that might have been fruitless had it been attempted first. Whatever the treatment model, in each instance the therapist must look at his "case" as an entity unto itself with his mind open to careful clinical observation. He must attempt to understand the meaning of the child's particular deviant behavior before he can hope to reach him and offer help.

CASE HISTORIES

I have selected four cases to describe in some detail in order to demonstrate the treatment approaches I have found most useful in working with schizophrenic children.

Each therapist brings to the treatment situation his own unique personality, experience, theoretical orientation, and countertransference problems. It is not easy to treat psychotic children without awakening the conflicts and painful memories of our own childhood.

It is very useful for an inexperienced child therapist to approach his first case armed with the histories of famous patients from the past, such as "Victor," the wild boy of Aveyron (Itard, 1801), Renée (Sechèhaye, 1947), or the "Space-Child" (Ekstein, 1954), but no amount of reading can equal one hour in a room with an autistic child.

1. Childhood Schizophrenia—Early Onset

Harry: A Six-year-old Boy With Features of Early Infantile Autism. The first time I saw Harry he was in the midst of a group of children on the children's ward of a psychiatric institution where I was a first-year Child Fellow. All of the children in this diffuse and disconnected "group" were there because of serious emotional disturbances. Yet six-year-old Harry was immediately noticeable for his peculiar machine-like quality, as if a robot's mechanism had taken over his mind and body. I had a sudden déjà-vu and realized I was reminded of Joey, the "mechanical boy" of Bettelheim (1959), junior version. Harry was a handsome, chubby, freckled-faced child with short blond hair and an impish smile. He was marching wooden fashion in a circle, holding a page of the local newspaper: the automobile exchange page, in fact, and he was reading in a loud, high-pitched monotone. "In-ex-pen-sive ware-house stor-age trai-lers for rent Mor-ris Leasing Co. Orange, Conn. Call Coll. 203-792–8661."

The floor nurse brought me over for introductions. "Harry, this is your new doctor, Dr. Kestenbaum." "Hello, Harry," I said. "Large-est sel-ech-shun of road trai-lers N. Y. area. 516–725–6001," he continued to read. "Harry, my name is Dr. Kestenbaum." He ignored me. I repeated my name five times and told him I would come back later.

Daily-rates-65-dollars-from-noon-to-Mon.-11-A.-M.," he said.

Harry was first brought to the attention of the local mental hygiene authorities in his home town when he was five. He had lasted $2\frac{1}{2}$ days in kindergarten. The teacher noted that he was hyperactive, had almost no communicative speech in spite of his ability to read aloud (apparently without comprehension). In addition he was extremely socially retarded. The clinic felt a longer in-patient evaluation in a "big city hospital" was required.

Harry's parents had three other children, boys of 11 and 4 and a girl of 8, and many nieces and nephews. "Harry always stood out from the rest like a sore thumb. We don't know where he came from."

Mr. Smith was a 50-year-old carpenter with a good business he developed himself. He was a hard working, outdoor type who enjoyed fishing, hunting, working with his hands. Mrs. Smith, aged 43, was a music teacher who worked part time, enjoyed taking care of her children, and was active in town affairs. She seemed warm and outgoing. They knew Harry was "different" but the pediatrician had said "he would outgrow his strange ways." They were patiently waiting for that day to come. The other children looked as if they were cut out from the mold labelled "normal as apple pie."

The only family pathology we elicited was that Mr. Smith's mother had been institutionalized twenty years before for "involutional melancholia" and had committed suicide (a careful genetic history was not taken, however).

Mrs. Smith recalled that her pregnancy and delivery had been uneventful. Harry was a full-term, 7-lb baby and was declared healthy and sound. "Still," she related, "I noticed from the first that he was different from the other two. He did not seem affectionate or cuddly. He was irritable and cried a lot.

"Even as an infant he did not show much of a startle response. We had to change his formula at least three times. He didn't smile as the other children had at three or four months of age, and in fact he always seemed to be 'into himself.' It was as if he didn't want or need us. He could not be comforted in the usual way, such as being patted on the shoulder or rocked." Apparently the only object to which Harry became attached was his pacifier. Harry sat alone at six months, stood up at nine months, and walked at ten months. "From that time on, he was constantly on the go, running, insatiably curious, into everything," Mrs. Smith recalled. He was toilet trained by age $1\frac{1}{2}$ with little difficulty.

"He seemed to be more interested in things than people," Mrs. Smith continued. "He was never destructive but he would examine calendars, clocks, toy cars; when he discovered television he would watch it for hours. We think he learned to read from watching TV, because certainly I never taught him. He wouldn't sit still with me long enough, but he would sit quietly in front of the TV or when he was being driven in the family car. He seemed to love the feeling of motion."

Harry's speech was delayed. He didn't speak at all until age $3\frac{1}{2}$ or 4; when he did, it was to repeat words he heard on TV. He rarely responded to his name, or called people by their names either. Yet he would recite nursery jingles and TV commercials endlessly to himself. At 3 he became extremely attached to books. He began to collect all the newspapers and magazines in the house and stack them in his room. "He became very set in his ways and had to follow a very rigid routine, counting dishes, books, light bulbs. If everything in the house was not in its place he became upset —in fact, he would have a screaming tantrum." The need for sameness carried over to articles of clothing and food. He had certain foods (cereal, milk, fruit, sandwiches) and would not try anything else. Harry's parents let him have his way, so that in effect he was running the household. "He never related to either one of us," Mrs. Smith noted. He probably didn't even recognize other adults, although at six months he would scream at any stranger and seemed unapproachable. He noted his father's going to and from work without a comment except when the routine was broken. Once Mr. Smith returned home half an hour early and Harry said, "go away and come back at the right time." When Harry's younger brother Ben was born, Harry loved riding to the hospital in the car but completely ignored the new baby, paying no attention to him whatsoever. He became more negativistic at this time "but maybe that was just an exaggeration of the terrible two's." He would get very frustrated when he didn't get his way and that lasted more than an hour.

Ben was a very happy, affectionate baby who giggled and cooed and reached up his arms to be held. "Harry tried to do what Ben did," Mrs. Smith said sadly, "but when he did it, it seemed like an imitation of a happy feeling—not real."

"Punishment does not work at all," Mr. Smith noted. "A good swat doesn't faze him the way it does the others. You can't take away love or toys to teach him a lesson either. He just didn't seem to care about anyone or anything—even Spotty, the family dog."

He was first brought to the institute for a 3-day evaluation. The neurologist felt that Harry demonstrated some soft signs (clumsiness, poor heel-toe walking, dysmetric finger-nose test, poor rapid succession movements) compatible with non-motor brain damage; his EEG was negative. During the first psychological testing situation, however, Harry was virtually untestable by the usual criteria.

"What is your name," the psychologist asked him.

"What is your name," he echoed.

The psychologist noted his flow of irrelevant, meaningless conversation. Standing before the office calendar, he babbled, "In 60 seconds go to the next and now we count the date, the first day of the year, Tuesday. January first will be world wonder, a trick. The password belongs to quack." In spite of this, the psychologist felt he was potentially of *superior intelligence*.

The overall staff impression was "childhood schizophrenia, organic substrate, with autism," and Harry was admitted for treatment. Except for summer vacations, he remained for 2 years.

The treatment plan was built into the living-in situation. Harry would attend school in the hospital (a one-to-one situation for him); he also was to attend all ward activities, including group experiences in physical education, occupational therapy, and individual psychotherapy (the latter consisting of three office visits a week and daily ward visits of briefer duration). The family met every other week with a social worker, and monthly for conjoint family sessions with the therapist and Harry. Frequent staff conferences helped coordinate the day-to-day therapeutic goals, the first of which was to attempt to help foster an attachment to his doctor, to the ward nurse (who was his principal caretaker), and to his teacher.

It is all too easy to formulate a plan and expect others to follow through, but where does one begin with a child who, as it seemed, came from Mars—aloof, alone, and appearing to need no other human being? How easy for the staff in charge of Harry to become like the mother, "turned off" by his rejection. For one noted in him no eye contact, no body molding, and none of the attachment systems one associates with the normal child. Even retarded children cuddle, and symbiotic children cling, giving their therapists a feeling of being needed, or at least important.

The first tasks were to break through the wall of aloneness and make Harry comfortable enough to acknowledge his need of the other. One had to foster in him a sense of body integrity through which a sense of self would one day evolve; there was also the need to teach him to recognize his own feelings and to use language for communicating these needs to others.

Among the therapeutic staff there could be no strict division of roles. In the beginning, all those working with him had to concentrate on helping Harry "understand." Therefore, the psychiatrist served as "educational therapist," nurse, teacher, primary object until he had enough comprehension of language to understand verbal interpretation.

During the early sessions I strove to establish myself as a real person. The second day, for example, I took Harry by the hand as he followed me into the elevator to my office. He counted all the floors out loud, repeated the numbers on the offices. "What is my name, Harry?" After five such questions he answered, "You're Mrs. Robinson (his teacher). "No, I'm Dr. Kestenbaum." He brought his newspaper with him but I said "in the office we play games like these" (I pointed to a group of some children's picture books, paper and crayons, mini-dolls and a dollhouse). I firmly shut the newspaper, gently folded it and put it on the table. He screamed. I said, "No, here we will play with toys," as firmly as possible and without raising my voice. Although he had little experience with limit-setting, he stopped screaming instantly and went toward the cars.

But what if he had not stopped screaming, what if he had kicked and spat and had remained otherwise uncontrolled.

That would be, in essence, a different case, and I would have "miscalculated" and had to "make adjustments" in the treatment plan—a common occurrence.

As it was, Harry moved the cars back and forth on the radiator, the window sill, over the telephone, the floor, as if defining for himself the space in the small room. I told him, "This is my office, Harry; you and I will play here. Now show me the red car." After five attempts he showed me a blue car. I realized he had no color awareness. "This is a red car like *your* red sweater." I touched his sweater. "Like the red crayon." (I knew he did not know pronouns, but one has to start somewhere). For the next two weeks we played the "naming" games as he did in class—for example, pointing out pictures of boys in books and repeating the word, "boy" then pointing to him and other children in the ward. He read the word "car" in the news and I asked him, "What is a car, Harry?" With a sudden shock of recognition he ran to get his favorite office toy.

He had made a connection between the word and the object and seemed excited by the discovery.

During the first month Harry began to show interest in the blackboard and the "dollhouse," and he seemed to enjoy his sessions. He would not say hello to me if he saw me on the ward, but I would always intrude on his world with "Hello, Harry." At last he would respond by repeating my name.

He became fascinated with the telephone and I explained its use. He could be on the ward and talk from the nurses' station to me from my office.

The disembodied voice seemed very mysterious to him, especially when I would appear by his side five minutes later "in the flesh." The telephone game was as fascinating as the "news" and had for reasons of practicality to be "controlled" to once a day. Harry had a tantrum in my presence when I would not allow a second "telephone game" one afternoon. I put my arm around him and noted that he did not pull back. "You feel mad and sad when you can't do something you want," I told him. Later he pointed out another child having a tantrum. "Jimmy feels mad and sad." It was several months before he could distinguish "mad" from "sad," and soon thereafter he was able to integrate the idea of "glad."

One of the advantages of residential in-patient treatment is that both patient and therapist are required to be "on location" at times not usually designated for treatment. As a resident I had weekly on-call night duty and took advantage of my free time. I began visiting Harry during his bath and bedtime rituals. He was so unaware of his body he hardly recognized his mirror image and several sessions were spent in front of the bathroom mirror naming the various parts of his body and their reflections. He was soon able to answer the question, "Where is Harry's nose?" He would point to his face and the mirror. "Where is Dr. Kestenbaum's nose?" It took another 6 months for him to respond to "Where is *your* nose and *my* nose?"

Harry seemed to enjoy jumping up and down on his bed. He began catching my glances—the beginning of eye contact—when I would throw him down in mock wrestling and look him "straight in the eye." I would cover my face with a pillow, attempting to imitate peek-a-boo—the infant's first social game. He began to play peek-a-boo with the night nurses and attendants which led to his hiding under the bed and under the covers. An embryonic pleasure-sense began to develop. Soon I began tucking him in and giving him a hug and good night kiss. He began to have a vague concept of play and of games. I would say, "Harry, let us play a kissing game. I kiss your cheek like this. That is a kiss. And you put your arms around my neck like this. That is a hug." He asked for the kissing game nightly for two weeks. A rather moving transaction occurred during the next family session. Harry, his mother, father, three siblings, the social worker, and I met in my office. Harry as usual made no attempt to greet his family as they entered but continued to draw pictures on the blackboard. He did not respond to "Hello, Harry" until his five-year-old brother, Ben, went up to him and pulled his sleeve. "Hello, Harry. Say, hello." On the fifth try Harry answered, "Hello, Ben, see the red car. See the telephone," pointing to his favorite objects. Mrs. Smith sat somewhat wooden and detached with a fixed "pleasant" smile on her face, as she usually did in Harry's presence. Suddenly Harry in an effort to display his repertoire of accomplishments, or so it seemed to me, walked to his mother and climbed into her lap. "Kissing game," he said and placed his lips mechanically on her cheek. Mrs. Smith suddenly seemed transformed—her face blushed—tears sprung to her eyes, her arms enfolded him as if he were a lost baby newly found. She rocked him back and forth. "This is a hug," he said continuing to play the game. "Is that what they teach them now in school?" Mr. Smith asked in a choked voice.

From that moment a true affectionate bond began to develop between Harry and his mother. He wanted to sit on her lap, cling to her, follow her around. He became jealous of attention she showed to Ben or the other children. On the ward he began to notice other child patients and would call them by their names. At the same time he became resentful of any attention the teachers or I gave to them.

Harry continued to make great strides in his cognitive development. He was, after one year's treatment, reading age-appropriate books with comprehension. He had a far greater attention span and was able to verbalize his feelings. He was more playful in his social interaction and looked forward to being home with his family on weekends.

The summer of his first treatment year he spent at home with his family. That fall he returned with what seemed a new personality. He was as negativistic as a two-year-old. Tantrums, for example, became daily occurrences. He wouldn't play with any child on the ward and was even upset that other children shared his birthday cake at his own birthday party. More rigid controls were established so that he could learn that what he did could effect a change in the environment. On one occasion that winter he came to my office saying, "I had to leave the classroom today and go to the ward. No gym." I asked him why he couldn't go with the other children to his favorite activity. "Because." Because why? "Because I threw a fork." So why can't you go to the gym? "The fork hit Billy so I had to go to the ward. It is against the rules to throw a fork." Nor could Harry hit, kick, spit, throw a book, or break any rule with which he was familiar. He was upset, however, when he was restricted for pushing Mary "because pushing is not against the rules." Pushing had to be dutifully added to his list of forbidden activities. Harry's extreme concreteness and total lack of empathy continued to be a major problem.

Two years after Harry first entered the institute he was discharged with plans to attend a special boarding school for emotionally disturbed children. He was retested and obtained an IQ score of 120.

On the last day Harry shook hands with the assembled staff. "I am going to miss all my friends." He turned to me and said, "I am going to miss you like my mother—Mrs.—Mises—Kestenbaum—you!"

2. George: A Seven-Year-Old Boy With Features of Symbiotic Psychosis

George was referred for in-patient treatment at a psychiatric hospital after a one-year trial in a therapeutic nursery for severely disturbed children.

He was the second of three children born into a normal family, the Johnsons, in whom there was no known history of mental illness. The parents were middle-class professionals, the 9-year-old sister extremely bright and friendly, the 4-year-old brother quick and outgoing. Mrs. Johnson had kept very careful "baby books" on all her children.

She reported that in spite of an uneventful planned pregnancy and full-term normal birth, she noticed that George was different from the other children "from the first day." He rarely cried and seemed content to remain in his crib or playpen. Mrs. Johnson noted that he either felt very soft to pick up—floppy at times—or very stiff, arching his back and seeming to dislike being held. George liked to rock and smiled when he rocked himself. At two, he spoke only 15 words. He did cuddle with his mother, to whom he became deeply attached and demanding. "He'd scream a lot, pulling my hand to reach for things he wanted. Away from me, he was fearful of anything or anyone new, or of being left alone in his room."

Tantrums became a daily occurrence. He was punished at first by being left alone "but it only made him scream louder." George was very resentful of his two-month-old brother Tim and became more demanding of his mother's attention. The Johnsons attributed this to normal sibling rivalry in a sensitive child. The pediatrician assured the family that George was a slow starter and "would outgrow it."

By age four it was clear that George was not about to "outgrow" his difficulties. He was increasingly withdrawn or, when not clinging to mother, enraged and out of control each time his desires were frustrated. His vocal production was limited to echolalic imitations and strange noises as if imitating automobile horns, trains, or vacuum cleaners. He could not play with other children, relating only to his mother and older sister. Declared "retarded," he was sent for a work-up at a local clinic. The child psychiatrist noted that he could be absorbed in music for hours, watching the turntable while he listened to records; also that his speech—unintelligible jargon—was delivered in a monotone and that he had no understanding of pronouns. He was preoccupied with turning light switches on and off, or with locking doors and pushing elevator buttons.

George was enrolled in a therapeutic day nursery where he made some progress in speaking and comprehension. He always had great difficulty separating from his mother and seemed depressed and fearful much of the time.

At age six he pushed his hand through a window during a tantrum that followed his having been refused a second piece of cake. He did not cry nor did he show any reaction either to the blood streaming down his arm or to the stitches he received in the emergency room. It was at this time his school recommended in-patient treatment.

There was a question about George's diagnosis. The neurologist found incoordination, poor balance, spinning, flailing arm movements and "soft signs" like those associated with minimal cerebral dysfunction. The psychologist, although George was untestable by usual criteria, noted perceptual deficits and overall retardation but felt he was only "pseudo-retarded" and capable of intellectual growth. A working diagnosis was finally established—childhood schizophrenia, organic type, with symbiotic psychotic syndrome.

George was placed in individual psychotherapy, educational therapy (school), and the usual therapeutic milieu. The family was to meet with the therapist every week. George became attached to his female therapist, but she became pregnant and left the service the following summer. He was able to grasp that she was leaving and became very upset: "I don't want babies. I don't like babies." He began to mutilate himself, scratching his face with his fingernails, and regressed to the point of urinating and defecating on the floor. He would stay alone in his room, rocking, repeating to himself "Daddy's angry."

I first saw George in that state when he was reassigned for individual psychotherapy. I knelt down beside him and introduced myself. He kicked me. "Go away. I hate you. I don't want you." "Even so, I am going to sit outside the room so you won't be alone anymore." It took several weeks of such daily visits outside his room before George would even look at me. "You are very mad that Dr. Beth went away and that I am your new doctor instead. I will come to see you many, many days."

George seemed to love music, so I started bringing him to the music room. At first I used drums and shakers to facilitate his coming to feel comfortable with me. Rocking in time to the music, he finally sat on my lap. Next I played tunes on the piano and sang the words to him, "I like Georgie. Does Georgie *like* me?" in a singsong rhythm.

George responded by singing back words to the tune of "Jingle Bells" and "Row Your Boat." The negativism and withdrawal disappeared. After 3 months, George had made a complete attachment, would smile with pleasure during the music games in office sessions, and was beginning to relate to his teachers and nurses. I began having sessions outside the office. He would take my hand and lead me to the hospital coffee shop for a shared snack, saying to any adult in the snack bar, "I am George Johnson. I am a boy. You are a man (lady)."

During this period George developed some affection for two dolls, whom he named Bleeny and Bloony, and who had to accompany him everywhere. His teacher reported that his ability to concentrate on a book or listen in class was 15 to 20 minutes and that his diction was becoming increasingly better. George still had a marked perceptual problem. I was not aware of its extent until one day, when he was sitting on my lap looking at a picture of an inviting mountain lake, he said, "Take me to the lake. I want to go in the lake," and literally dived from my lap into the postcard. He was shocked and disappointed to land on the office floor and not in the mountain lake. He cried and hit me despite my explanations and withdrew into his silent world for several hours.

George often would speak jargon—comprehensible perhaps only to him. I would say, "Speak English, George. I don't understand that other speech," and he would repeat more clearly and simply what he was trying to say. Much work was done explaining and "interpreting" so that after one year he was completely understandable.

I was concerned about George's reaction to my 3-week summer vacation. I told him I would be back and would send him three postcards. He refused to greet me on the last session before the vacation. "I don't like you." During my absence, I learned from the ward staff, he carried the postcards I sent to all his activities and put them under his pillow while he slept. He ran to greet me with a hug and kiss. "I like you. I'm your Georgie. You went away and you came back."

George was still very concrete but he began making simple jokes and playing tricks ("It's sunny," he would say on a rainy day, laughing). He developed a concept of sharing and taking turns. He still had no concept of what others experienced. Once, for example, he pulled my hair to see if it would come off like Silky, the puppet's hair. I yelled 'ouch' and told him he hurt me. He laughed and wanted to pull my hair and hear the funny 'ouch' sound again. "It hurts when you do that." He seemed surprised and pulled his own hair, repeating "ouch, it hurts" in imitation. From that time he would say 'it hurts, ouch' when he accidentally fell and scraped a knee or cut himself.

He began to identify feelings. George's home visits became increasingly more rewarding. He would ask to go home and wept on returning. One day he said "I don't want you, Dr. Kestenbaum. I want my mother. Can I go home?" I explained that it was all right to love more than one person. George could love mother and Daddy and Timmy and Mary (his siblings) *and* me. George merely put his hands over his ears to shut out the words and began making his old "noises" so he would not hear me. "You *can* love mother *and* me," I yelled and hugged him.

While George was learning to interact with others and master basic cognitive skills to the best of his limited ability, his parents were engaged in weekly sessions with me. At first I attempted to help them understand their own feelings about their damaged child. Underneath the cool exterior, Mr. Johnson was angry and resentful that his son should be defective in any way. George's mother felt shame and guilt for producing a sick child. The parents had never shared their deep disappointment with one another. After several months George began to participate in family sessions. The family learned to handle deviant behavior following the example set by the staff. They rarely isolated him for punishment but discouraged his occasional outbursts by saying, "I don't like you to scream. I will wait here until you can tell me in words what you want." They held him forcibly the few times he attempted to strike his head on the floor. After a number of months George was able to go home for weekend visits without undue difficulties.

After 2 years of in-patient treatment, the staff felt George had benefited all he could from hospitalization. He had learned to read at first grade level. He could communicate in simple sentences. George was still considered "pseudo-retarded" but was clearly trainable. He was no longer bizarre, fearful, and unhappy, but presented a picture of a playful, friendly contentment much of the time. No longer psychotic, he was sent to an institution for retarded children. He was retested and the overall IQ was 48. George had made friends among staff and patients. Everyone who had been involved in his case missed him and was sorry to see him go.

3. CHILDHOOD SCHIZOPHRENIA—LATE ONSET

LUBA: A NINE-YEAR-OLD "NUCLEAR SCHIZOPHRENIC" GIRL. Luba, a nine-year-old girl, was transferred to a state psychiatric institute following a seven-month hospitalization in a city hospital. The chief complaint at the time of admission was a severe personality change from a girl who was outgoing and spontaneous to a withdrawn, morose youngster occupied with death fantasies.

According to her parents and late-teenage brothers, Luba Cohen was a normal child without apparent problems until the family arrived in the United States when she was six. The parents were Hungarian-Jewish emigrees who had left their home "in order to forget the tragedy." Their seven-year-old daughter Marta had died shortly before of a ruptured appendix following a mistaken diagnosis of gastroenteritis.

Mrs. Cohen became deeply depressed and would not speak of Marta. In fact the week following her death she removed all photographs of the child from the walls and scrapbooks. Mr. Cohen arrived in the United States first in order to find work as a housepainter and find suitable living quarters.

Luba was enrolled in a parochial school and had difficulty adjusting to the English language and to the new peer group. She began to fight physically with her brothers and to throw objects at schoolmates, spitting at them and kicking them. She developed fear of the dark, fears of "dirt" in her food, and she expressed fear of dying because of poisoned food. Such was the "unreliability" of the informants, that all questions concerning her were answered "normal." Little was actually known about her developmental landmarks. She had reportedly been sociable, excellent in school, and sensitive to the needs of others. For instance, she had been aware of her mother's wish to "forget Marta" and had once told her neighbors not to mention Marta's name in front of the mother.

Luba was finally hospitalized at the school's insistence, the parents having been unaware of the severity of the symptoms she was demonstrating at school.

Physical and neurological work-up, including EEG, were essentially negative. Luba was a tall, well built, pretty girl. Her constant spitting, lip-biting, and expressions of disgust, however, made her appear ugly and deformed. She would lie on the floor clutching herself, kicking at an approaching nurse or physician. Her arms and legs were bruised from self-inflicted injuries (slapping or biting herself). She was grossly delusional, one manifestation of which was that she thought she was burning in hell. Another manifestation: she had lost twenty pounds in 4 months because she refused to swallow much of her food, fearing that her own saliva would poison her. During the first 6 months of her hospitalization Luba was cared for by a male psychiatrist. She was somewhat more manageable on Thorazine 300 mg/day and the therapist was able to unravel the threads of the delusional material so that her behavior at least became understandable. He learned that much of the oral activity was accompanied by genital masturbation for which she felt inordinately guilty. She believed, for example, that by touching her clitoris (a small harmful, dirty "animal" in her view) and subsequently touching her mouth—thereby contaminating the dishes—that she had been directly responsible for Marta's infection and death. She touched her clitoris in the first place in order to "make her penis grow." Girls were "weak" and "died," she felt, while boys, preferred by her parents, were strong and would live. She was preoccupied with getting fat, since getting big would mean her subsequent death. She openly expressed oral impregnation fantasies.

While the therapist attempted to interpret some of this behavior to her, it soon became apparent that she was reluctant to speak of Marta and in general felt guilty about thoughts concerning her sister. "If I talk about Marta, mother will get sick and die." She sometimes dreamed of Marta and thought she would be punished in hell for making her mother sad.

Her behavior was increasingly difficult to manage. She would strike out at children and female staff members whom she said were trying to hurt her. She was transferred to my care after 8 months of in-patient therapy.

After several weeks she became comfortable with me. I told her I would help her control all those symptoms which were harmful to herself or to others—pinching, hitting, etc. I forbade such antisocial acts as spitting. Use of a behavioral model (rewarding her with walks to the coffee shop, the park, or ice cream parlor) eventually helped control the symptoms.

In a short time the bruises disappeared and she stopped mutilating herself altogether. She began to discuss other aspects of her delusion. Her preoccupation with fat was actually based on the supposition that since fat "burns in fire," if she were sent to hell, she "would burn longer" if she were fat. She spoke at length about her jealousy of Marta, whom mother loved more, and described her mother's beating her chest and pinching herself when Marta died. She would accept psychodynamic interpretations at least intellectually and with some apparent understanding.

At this time Luba became involved in group therapy with three other psychotic children. The pressure from the other children acted as a deterrent to her "disgusting" behavior. This was far more effective a way of social control than the threats and punishments of the adult staff members. She became more socially acceptable, gained weight, and was no longer a "ward management problem." The treatment plan at that time was directed toward bringing Luba more in contact with reality, toward answering her delusional questions only briefly and perfunctorily, without getting involved in her constant "intellectual" struggles about which foods would make her fat and what fats burned the fastest.

The social worker assigned to the family noted the parents' blanket denial regarding the seriousness of Luba's condition, along with their own depression. Family treatment was extremely difficult. Luba returned from her infrequent home vists as delusional as before. Her parents made no efforts to control her behavior at home and, as usual, mother wept whenever Luba tried to speak of Marta.

In family sessions Luba attempted to speak of her jealousy toward her sister. Her father could not accept "hatred" in her, however, and remonstrated "the Bible says it is a sin to hate." Nonetheless, the social worker and I encouraged Luba's expression both of past bottled up feelings and of her impressions about the meaning of past events. The sessions eventually proved beneficial, and Luba began to show real improvement. She began to draw pictures of her feeling states, whereas before she was content merely to act them out. Most of her psychotic outbursts seemed to be controlled by this maneuver.

A staff conference one year after admission actually ended on a hopeful note. The social worker felt some headway had been achieved in breaking down the extreme denial and emotional isolation within the family (although 6 years had passed) and especially with respect to Marta's death. Luba's attempt to get care and attention was always extremely apparent, as was her conviction that her mother could only care for someone who was sick or dead. Luba's art work—which consisted of a series of paintings dating from the time of admission—had begun to show greater form and structure. Her body image still showed distortions. She thought of herself as a sick, deformed, ugly girl. Meanwhile her ideal self was that of a beloved boy possessing a penis (which would render her strong and safe from the fate of her sister). It was felt that Luba was more aware of her feelings and was beginning to distinguish between fantasy and reality. Shortly after this staff conference, however, an event occurred that precipitated a downhill course from which Luba was never to recover.

During a family session Luba lost control and struck her mother in the face. Her mother burst into tears and left the room. Luba was inconsolable. She became convinced she had killed her mother, whom she viewed as "God's wife." She had to be placed in a camisole to keep her from biting her own arms and tearing her hair. She was placed on the acute ward. Thorazine was increased up to 1600 mg/day (with little effect). She became more delusional than ever. Her thoughts were of "evil deeds," she was a "monster" who would "burn in hell forever." Seeing staff members, myself, or her mother had no calming effect. She would grimace in the mirror making infantile sounds—ma–mee–moo–milk–mommy. She played at being a "bee-a-baby-bee" and tried to touch the nurse's breasts. She was at this time developing breasts and pubic hair of her own, which she tried to hide. Growing up she misconstrued as a sign she would "die." She appeared intermittently hebephrenic, with silly smiles, giggles and dancing. Her gross thinking disorder had by now also included flight-of-ideas. After 6 weeks with no improvement she was given 20 ECT with minimal response. Other phenothiazines were also administered, both alone and in combination but to no avail.

The staff felt hopeless: Luba was by now convinced that the spirit of her dead sister had invaded her body. Apparently, that was why she was hurting herself—to punish her sister who had caused her so much pain. In a last effort to reach the child, a rabbi was called in to perform a ritual exorcism.

When the rabbi, in the presence of the family and few staff members, commanded the spirit of the sister to leave Liba's body, the child fell to the floor. She awoke from that state less troubled, convinced that the spirit of Marta had passed from her. The family was greatly relieved and actually thankful that everything possible had been done to help their daughter. Luba no longer mutilated herself and sat quietly, staring blankly for long periods, apparently hallucinating quietly. She remained several months longer in that state with little change in her symptomatology. Finally 20 months after her admission, Luba was discharged to a state hospital. Her prognosis could only be considered most guarded.

4. CHILDHOOD SCHIZOPHRENIA—LATE ONSET

DAN: A NINE-YEAR-OLD BOY WITH PSEUDONEUROTIC SYMPTOMS. Dan was first seen by a psychiatrist at the age of nine in the mid-fifties. He had been referred by his pediatrician after he had become conspicuously preoccupied with death, with feelings that he was "stupid," and that he didn't deserve to live. His parents had noted that he was becoming increasingly fearful of being alone, of the dark, and of animals, particularly spiders. He had been terrified at a younger age of children's fairy tales, such as *Hansel and Gretel* and *Snow White*. These fears had not diminished with time; in fact, he was unable to sit through the *Wizard of Oz* without becoming "hysterical" at the sight of the wicked witch—an unusual occurrence, in his parents' opinion, for a child as old and intelligent as Dan.

The oldest son of a highly intelligent but "shrewish" woman and a passive man of average abilities and meager accomplishments, Dan achieved an IQ score at the time of that psychiatric evaluation of over 150. He was noted to be small and clumsy, with a lumbering, awkward gait. He exhibited a number of "soft signs" similar to those found in non-motor brain damage. He behaved more like a miniature adult than a child. He was clearly quite brilliant intellectually but he alienated all his peers by continually correcting and criticizing them. He had no close friends and was always the last one to be chosen for any team. The parents reported that he had a number of obsessive rituals and, if something prevented him from performing them, he would become extremely anxious. He would bow his head, holding his hands in front of him, looking up and down, and praying silently. He felt God would strike him or his mother dead if he did not follow God's wishes, and several times he felt God had "spoken" audibly to command him. He was particularly fearful of contracting cholera, which he had read about in school.

The therapist at the time felt that Dan was most likely a childhood schizophrenic, borderline type, whose superior intellectual endowment enabled him to function as well as he did. Psychotherapy was begun on a twice weekly basis.

The therapist, using techniques of play therapy and story telling, learned that Dan was greatly confused about his gender identity and about sex and reproduction in general. He had interrupted his parents during intercourse when he was four and had received a long and thorough explanation of the reproductive functions of which he understood nothing. He believed "the man urinates inside the lady, only the pee has invisible bugs in it that makes babies grow." Dan was preoccupied with thoughts of bodily injury. He had seen his mother use menstrual pads in the bathroom on one occasion and believed his father had hurt her and caused her to bleed. Dan's mother, so the therapist learned, frequently used him as a sounding board about the unfairness of men toward women, about her lot in life, and her husband's neglect of her needs. Dan felt close to his mother but was frightened of her angry scolding and the verbal attacks on his father.

After 2 years of therapy Dan's symptoms had abated considerably; he was able to adopt a more social attitude toward peers, although he was still considered "odd" or "a brilliant weirdo" by schoolmates. The parents felt the symptomatic relief was sufficient and, against the therapist's advice, treatment was discontinued.

Dan first came to my attention at the age of 28 when he was sent to me for an emergency consultation. He had been at a party where a number of friends were smoking marijuana. Dan, who did not smoke, felt himself suddenly "going mad"—as if the marijuana fumes were making his body "disintegrate" and his thoughts fly out of his head. He complained that he had no sensation whatsoever in his genitals. He had had other episodes of acute anxiety, particularly while traveling, but nothing akin to this one.

Dan impressed others as strange looking: the sort of person the elevator operator in the medical office building would immediately size up as the one who "needs to see a shrink." Though of average height, he walked stooped over, usually scanning a newspaper so that he appeared considerably shorter than he was. His gait was jerky; his movements uncoordinated. His hair was long and unkempt, his mustache untrimmed. He was dressed in "counter-culture" jeans. He looked, as a colleague of his commented, "like a fawn who had lost his way." When Dan spoke he never looked directly at his listener, but would avert his eyes, usually selecting a spot several feet away. Equally striking was his obvious intelligence: he was a gifted and skillful language instructor, who, despite his mannerisms, could hold his class spellbound—albeit from a distance. He was a respected and creative academician.

He had had, however, some difficulty functioning because his compulsive behavior was of such severity as to interfere with many everyday activities. He had, for example, to read every word on a page no matter what the material, whether it were want ads, box tops, etc. He had innumerable fears—many persisting from childhood, which had still not abated (fear of the dark, fear of crowds, fear of being alone [and he lived alone], fear of flying) and some of which were distinctly idiosyncratic. Thus he was deathly afraid of contracting cholera, and as a result assiduously avoided any trips to tropical climates. He had obsessional thoughts about tarantulas which might sting him to death, for which reason he refused to travel to the Southwest. The psychologist who tested him shortly after his panic reaction felt he had a marked homosexual conflict and sexual confusion about his gender. Actually he had never had overt homosexual experiences of any kind (nor heterosexual either). In fact, he denied ever having masturbated during his entire life. The idea was repellent to him and, moreover, frightening inasmuch as he believed he could do irreparable harm to his penis.

Despite superior functioning at work, his self-esteem was inordinately low. His successes did not in any way affect this situation. On the other hand, he elaborated grandiose fantasies and manifested a strong need to control (as if to compensate for feelings of worthlessness). One had the impression his high intelligence protected him from a more gross break with reality, although under emotionally charged circumstances (such as the marijuana incident) he experienced a brief psychotic episode (schizophrenic in type).

Dan's academic performance had been outstanding throughout his college and postgraduate years, despite his lack of social relationships. There, as in grade school, he was tolerated as a brilliant "oddball." Since his therapy in childhood he had not felt the need to seek psychiatric help, but he eventually came to feel he should try to "get at the roots of the problem." He began intensive psychotherapy with me and remained in treatment for over 5 years.

DISCUSSION

All schizophrenic children show great diversity. Harry and George were as different from each other as they were from the mainstream of normal children. Both boys were felt to be "different" from birth. In Harry's case, he did not "cuddle" or mould to the mother; he seemed alone and in need of no one. He had not succeeded in mastering the first task of infancy—attachment to a human object. Bowlby (1958) speaks of built-in attachment systems with which the infant is fully equipped at birth and upon which subsequent learned behavior is organized. The normal baby at birth can suck, grasp, cling, follow with his eyes, cry, and within a few weeks, smile.

Kestenbaum (1973) writes:

> We now recognize that the baby craves more than food or relief from pain. He needs the warmth of his mother's body. The touching, caressing, fondling, the sound of her voice and the gazing at her face. She needs him, too . . . each comes to know the other's rhythms in a wordless communication which flows from one to the other. The mother becomes acutely sensitive, tuned into the baby's needs. The attachment . . . is the cornerstone of successful adaptation. The mother-child bond is the prototype for all future relationships. (Introduction, xxiii)

The causes of nonattachment may arise out of factors inherent in the mother, depression or psychosis, for example. But in Harry's case the problem in all likelihood lay deep within Harry. The mother's quiet detachment in his presence, it was felt by all who became familiar with the case, was a defense against her feelings of rejection and disappointment.

The first task of the therapist is at all events to foster attachment, to form a bond with the child, through which we hope he will ultimately develop a sense of trust in another human being.

The therapist must be emotionally equipped and prepared to provide the autistic child with those early tactile, proprioceptive and kinesthetic experiences he has missed. The presence of this nurturing figure should be comforting and accepting and should help alleviate the episodes of panic such children experience in unfamiliar situations. These attempts to pass through the autistic barrier must be gradual and nonintrusive. Paraverbal techniques (Heimlich 1965, 1972), such as the use of rhythms, music, and body movements to foster communication until such time as language is understood, may prove particularly useful. From pleasure in rhythmic movement a sense of body integrity eventually develops. Autistic children have a poorly defined body image as well as a lack of self-concept. There is no concept of "the other" before consciousness of a sense of "self." The unawareness of body boundaries and inner sensations was particularly marked both in Harry and in George. Defining the limits of the body was a primary task for Harry. George, like the Wild Boy of Aveyron, had to be taught even the perception of pain.

At the same time that the therapist is attempting to alter the affective state of the child and to help him establish object relationships, the cognitive level must also be carefully considered. Serious attention must be given to the particular ego deficits where they exist. Since cognition appears to follow perception, it must be borne in mind that perception of the mothering figure's *face* is, for the normal child, the beginning of associative thought. This point has been emphasized by the author elsewhere:

> At this point (three to six months) the social bond is fragile: mother's face is but a fleeting image. As with the rattle now dangled in front of him, now quickly removed, images tend to be 'out of sight, out of mind.' It appears (associated with comfort and relief of distress) and disappears without warning; but from the second six months of life to the end of the second year, the baby learns that objects have permanence. Even though mother disappears, for example, she will, indeed, return. Some babies, at around seven months, may scan the mother's face . . . intensely when a stranger appears. Others may scream with fright at the appearance of a new face, even in the presence of the mother. This 'stranger anxiety,' a prelude to 'separation anxiety' of a few months hence, is a sign that the baby is learning to discriminate Mother (who is all important) from Not Mother. It's only when the mother's image has been firmly internalized that we can speak of 'object constancy.' (Kestenbaum, ibid., xxvi)

Christ (1975) has focused attention on an understanding of the cognitive level of the psychotic child in the Piagetian sense. He feels many autistic children are fixated at the "sensory-motor" stage of development (4 to 8 months, before the beginning of object constancy) and can best be understood by taking into account the cognitive structure of this pathological behavior.

George, despite being a step higher in the object-relations scale (symbiotic rather than autistic), was retarded in all functions. Harry, on the other hand, was considered to have the potential for superior intelligence and demonstrated special skills, reminding staff of the "idiots savants" (Scheerer, Rothman, and Goldstein, 1945, Horowitz, Kestenbaum, Person and Jarvik 1965), who despite subnormal intelligence were endowed with superior capacity for eidetic imagery and could, perform amazing feats of calendar calculations without being able to generalize from the vast store of information they possessed.

Neither boy was capable of learning in the usual sense (i.e., of acquiring new information and mastering new skills). Bruner (1973) notes that competence requires (1) intention (directed action), (2) feedback, and (3) mediation of patterns of action. Capacity, he believes, is present from birth and is reinforced by the child's observation of his own acts.

During the first year of life the child becomes competent in the areas of feeding, perceiving, manipulating, locomoting, interacting with other members of the species and with controlling his inner state; where such innate capacity is lacking, the therapist has to be aware of the specific absent link in the chain. The teacher, the language therapist, and the psychotherapist must work as a team to select the proper educational approach to facilitate the child's acquisition of missing skills.

The game of peek-a-boo which Harry began to enjoy early in treatment is a way of fostering both attachment and cognitive development. Kleeman (1967) notes that peek-a-boo "is a form of interaction, play, a social game pleasurable to infant and adult. It represents a mutually responsive communication with a love object, whose attention the infant thus gains or whom the child may wish to please by playing the game. . . . There is pleasure of imitation and of accomplishment as well as the pleasure inherent in functioning or in rhythmic backward and foreward motions. . . . Peek-a-boo represents a form of exploration . . . the mastery of making an object go and come."

Although Harry had acquired the cognitive skills that would have enabled him to play the game during his first year—memory, anticipation, visual and auditory perception, control of motility—his inability to form human bonds prevented his developing the motiviation to play peek-a-boo.

The therapist must also help the deviant child develop a sense of time and space. Otherwise, the child will remain confused and unable to learn temporal sequences. Transitions for both George and Harry, for example, were difficult. A 3-week separation for George seemed to him a lifetime. Harry was also continually preoccupied with time. He would fly into a rage if his schedule were disturbed. Seeing his father return home a half hour early seemingly challenged his sense of omnipotence, his control of time, and created considerable confusion in his mind.

The therapist, moreover, must at all times present a clear picture of reality. He must interpret the child's inner sensations and life events as well as help him to communicate these experiences in a meaningful way.

A word must be said about behavioral modification treatment of autistic children. A number of workers (Treffert, 1973; Lovaas, Freitag, Gold and Kassokla, 1965) have reported success in increasing social responsiveness and reducing the self-destructive and self-mutilating behavior seen in some psychotic children using a system of rewards (e.g., candy) and, to a lesser degree, and only when absolutely necessary—punishments (e.g., removal of food or toys).

Lovass et al. (1965) has demonstrated that the degree of communicative speech can be increased and echolalic jargon reduced. He has reported that severe and self-mutilating self-destructive behavior can be greatly reduced by aversive conditioning with electric shocks. Positive reinforcement techniques described by Hintgten and Churchill (1970) have established an "imitative set" in the child.

Critics of behavior modification techniques suggest that one cannot make these new behaviors generalize outside the experimental situation. Furthermore, as Des Lauriers writes:

> Whatever therapeutic implications our neurophysiological model may have . . . in regard to his learning capabilities . . . any attempt at correcting these deviations . . . has to include . . . the human component. . . . Des Lauriers & Carlson, 1969, p. 83)

In other words, the primary therapeutic agent is the human being. Harry was certainly responsive to operant-conditioning techniques but the reinforcements were primarily the *attention* and *social rewards* of the staff and the love of his parents. After he had learned the "kissing game" his own mother responded to his "signals" with such spontaneous pleasure that Harry's initial act was reinforced a hundredfold. Working with parents, incidentally, is not only an opportunity for ventilation of feelings; it is also an opportunity to teach the parents how to understand the deviant communication of their child and respond to it as the therapists have learned to do. A normal parent, as was Harry's mother, needs only to follow his or her own intuitive feeling with a little help from the staff. George's parents were actively engaged in conjoint family therapy of the kind described by Berlin and Szurek (1973). As George's deviant behavior became more understandable to the staff, clarification and interpretations of his psychotic communication were made to the parents. For example, when George regressed to the point of scratching himself, urinating, and defecating on the floor after his therapist left, he would stay alone in his room, repeating the words "Daddy's angry."

George was punishing himself so it seems, in the way his father used to punish him—by isolation—for his rage toward Dr. Beth, which he both displaced and projected onto his father. The parents came to understand his profound fear of abandonment and never again used isolation as a means of punishment.

The first year of Harry's hospitalization was spent in helping Harry attach himself to a human object—first to myself which led subsequently to a clinging dependency on his mother. George had formed an early attachment but had not passed through a separation-individuation phase which normally occurs, according to Mahler (1965), between 5 and 36 months. George had no clear representation of his mother when she was "out of sight." Because he had not yet obtained object constancy, he reacted to separation with panic, aggressive outbursts, and regression. Concerning treatment of such children, Mahler speaks of a "corrective symbiotic experience":

> It is important to let the (symbiotic) child test reality very gradually and at his own pace. As he cautiously begins this testing of himself as a separate entity, he needs constantly to feel the support of an understanding adult, preferably the mother or the therapist as mother substitute. (1968, p. 168)

This auxiliary ego might be necessary for months or even years until complete autonomy is achieved.

It is obvious from the case examples that schizophrenic children show great diversity and lack of appropriate adaptive mechanisms required for coping successfully with the normal stresses of life. Goldfarb's (1969) method of achieving correction "lies in the process of human interaction." The therapeutic approach he calls "corrective socialization." This represents an attempt to

> . . . fill in the gaps in the development of his ego —that is, his capacity for self-regulation and self-direction. . . . We are encouraged by the repeated observation that each of his disordered functions is highly responsive to social stimulation. (p. 3)

Goldfarb states furthermore that a realistic correction of each child's impairment must take into account differences in capacity, motivation, level of communication, and the characteristic substantive features of his bewilderment.

The therapeutic setting is an integral part of the therapy, with clearly defined boundaries, structure, and regularity. It must supply more than custodial care, it must offer a remedial attitude 24 hours a day. Limit-setting is important. A child must be prevented from hurting others. An attempt to understand the child's communication is of course equally important.

If a child makes an assault against another person, for example, the act needs to be understood as well as controlled. One must then make an interpretation to the child about the action, tailored to his level of comprehension.

The case of Luba is illustrative of a schizophrenic child who had already obtained a high degree of intellectual competence before her psychosis prevented further development. Her breakdown resembled the adult pattern of schizophernic decompensation with primary process thinking, delusions, and hallucinations. She could not distinguish her aggressive fantasies from reality. She exhibited regression in every area of functioning. Seft-mutilation in schizophrenic children can be seen as a habit associated with defective perception, an idiosyncratic interpretation of pain, or an attempt to define body boundaries (Green, 1967). In Luba's case it may have been an attempt to expiate guilt for murderous wishes toward her mother and sister, whom she believed she had killed. She displayed extreme anxiety relating to object-loss and body fragmentation. The illusory penis represented her wish to repair and replace her own "damaged" genital, and also her wish to survive—since in her view, girls were weak and died. Strongly identified as she was with her dead sister, she also attempted reunion via incorporation of the total person (cf. Green, 1970).

Beres (1956) sees the core problem in schizophrenia as a failure in all aspects of ego functions. Luba's mechnaisms of defense were extremely primitive, consisting of marked denial, projection, and turning against the self. There was a total failure of repression either of sexual or of aggressive drives. The numerous treatment approaches failed to check the psychotic process. Phenothiazines in high doses did not stop the rapid downhill course. Even ECT, which is rarely used in children except in severely regressed adolescents, was employed here without success.

The case of Dan illustrates a point Bender has made for over 40 years, namely that "childhood" schizophrenia ends up uniformly as "adult" schizophrenia, expressed in a wide variety of clinical pictures (1970). Dan presented relatively mild symptomatology. He might even have been diagnosed (incorrectly) by some as severely neurotic. His poor reality testing, however, the persistence of magical thinking which permeated many areas of his life, and his severe identity confusion were all signs of serious ego weakness; one was dealing here with the persistence of psychotic structure, in Kernberg's sense of the term (1976).

The "pseudoneurotic" defenses (obsessive-compulsive behavior and multiple phobias) did not protect him from overwhelming anxiety. A psychoanalyst, if he relied entirely upon a psychological model, would contend that this patient was fixated at a preoedipal level of psychosexual development in which primitive oral and anal components predominated (Freud, 1905). Ekstein (Ekstein & Friedman, 1967) would have drawn attention to his rapidly fluctuating ego states as a manifestation of "borderline" pathology (using "borderline" here in a *clinical* sense).

The combination of primitive defenses, nonspecific signs of ego weakness (especially, low anxiety tolerance), and the syndrome of identity diffusion would have established the psychostructural diagnosis as borderline (Kernberg, 1976). But faulty reality testing was present also, establishing the structural diagnosis as psychotic. Dan's superior intellectual defenses permitted him to keep in better control of his aggressive and sexual drives, but stressful situations readily precipitated regression, with psychotic symptoms distinctly schizophrenic in quality. He was particularly concerned with bodily functions and conflicts relating to gender identity. The 2-year period of therapy during childhood helped strengthen his defenses to a degree but did not protect him from decompensation later on. Fear of losing control particularly of incestuous sexual impulses had led him to deny his own sexual urges. Thus, the clinical picture (in adult life) of an ascetic loner (characterologically speaking, Dan presented the picture of a *schizoid personality*).

In the provocative and seductive atmosphere of the "pot party" he could not control these impulses and experienced a "micropsychotic" episode, schizophrenic in nature.

As this case amply illustrates, proper diagnostic appraisal of a fairly well functioning patient in whom the vulnerability to schizophrenic decompensation is ever present requires a comprehensive approach that takes into consideration the hereditary, the psychostructural, and the characterological frames of reference. Such a diagnostic model has recently been elaborated by Stone (1976), in his description of a tri-axial method of psychodiagnosis. For precise definition of the psychostructural dimension the recent paper of Kernberg (1976) should be consulted.

The therapist working with the late-onset schizophrenic or borderline child has to be aware of fluctuating ego states, the propensity for rapid regression and decompensation. Typically, their intrapsychic conflicts are more intense than those of neurotic children. Magical thinking (e.g., thoughts *can* kill, wishes *are* deeds) must come to be replaced by good reality testing, one of the primary therapeutic goals.

There have been numerous carefully documented case reports describing in detail successful treatment with psychotic children (Klein, 1932; Despert, 1975; Geleerd, 1946; Ekstein, 1966, Wolman, 1970 to name a few). There is no "perfect method" or absolute solution. With a schizophrenic child the emphasis must be on strengthening the ego, supplying structure as well as interpreting conflict. One attempts to teach the child better adaptive mechanisms.

The therapist must often use himself as a real object, not merely as a transference object. Again and again the therapist will find himself acting as an "auxiliary ego," enlightening the patient about areas in which his awareness is deficient. Often, as we saw in the case of George, the child will need to be taught to recognize and to label something as elementary as his own emotional states.

COUNTERTRANSFERENCE ASPECTS

Intensive treatment of any kind with schizophrenic children of whatever type cannot help but evoke strong countertransference reactions in the therapist. These reactions will not so often be of a type specific to the individual patient (as reminders of past figures in the life of the therapist), as characteristically occurs in the analysis of neurotic patients. Rather the countertransference reactions will tend to be of a nonspecific sort, in response to the bizarre or menacing or fascinating aspects of the disturbed child—such as might evoke strong responses in any ordinary person. Some schizophrenic children, for example, will not have differentiated themselves from other forms of life, animal or vegetable, or even from certain inanimate objects, machines, and the like. If the therapist is a reasonably well-adjusted neurotic, he will have long since put behind him his own tendencies to identify himself, literally, with dogs, or trees, or robots, or for that matter, with cannibals or monsters. To this extent it will strain his empathic capacity to work with the psychotic child to whom the questions "Am I a boy or an automaton?"—"Am I a nice person or an ogre?" are still quite lively and unsettled. A moving exposition of these issues, particularly in regard to adult schizophrenics but also applicable to schizophrenic children, is to be found in Searles' *The Non-Human Environment* (1960, pp. 200–203; 234–235).

By the same token, working with a child who may spit at the therapist or fail to exercise bladder or bowel control in the office or playroom may evoke feelings not all therapists are equipped to deal with, let alone deal with empathically, effectively, and tactfully. Similarly, while one should never encourage acts of aggression, many schizophrenic children will at one time or another manifest gross dyscontrol, which may take the form of throwing objects, breaking windows, hitting the therapists or others in the therapeutic milieu, all of which requires deft handling to ensure that the destructive behavior is curbed without retaliation and, where possible, interpreted without rancor. Fascination with the eccentric or the grotesque may lead certain therapists, especially early in their training, to an exaggerated and counterproductive kind of tolerance for bizarre speech or behavior, such that the child is subtly encouraged to retain rather than to modify these symptoms. Therapeutic stalemates may develop in this way. The therapist must guard against feelings of fascination with the older schizophrenic child's fantasy world, which would impede progress in developing better reality testing. The child correctly perceives the therapist's wish for the delusional world to remain. Linder (1952) writes movingly of this phenomenon in his case "the jet-propelled couch," in which the patient had given up his fantasy world long before the therapist was ready to do so.

Lebovici, Diatkine, Favreau, and Luget-Paret (1959) have alluded to one countertransference manifestation that appears in the tendency for some childless women to gravitate toward work with chronically disturbed children. The field has in general been dominated by women, of whom Mahler and Sechèhaye are examples. It may be that the intuitiveness and maternal qualitites of some of these gifted women are necessary, along with the usual perseverance and analytic skills, if therapy with certain schizophrenic children is to continue and flourish. The situation is analogous to what Stone (1971) has written about the special countertransference manifestations noted in certain unusually successful therapists of adult schizophrenics. The most celebrated example of long-term intensive analysis of a childhood schizophrenic is that of the gifted Madame Sechèhaye (1956) whose work with a highly intelligent but (at first) grossly psychotic child spanned some thirteen years, until her patient, Renée, was able (at 19) to function well at a university. Sechèhaye's case illustrates qualities that are necessary in those who would dedicate themselves to the rehabilitation of schizophrenic children: the capacity to generate hope (and this can only arise from a genuine and spontaneous attitude of hopefulness present in some—but not all—therapists of such children) and, of course, infinite patience.

PROGNOSIS AND OUTCOME

Mainly because of three factors—(1) the lack of controlled studies of childhood schizophrenia, (2) the dissimilarity of diagnostic criteria used by different researchers, and (3) the rarity[1] of the illness—follow-up studies are for the most part unreliable and impressionistic.

Eisenberg and Kanner (1956) were the first to do a follow-up of 63 of their cases of early infantile autism. Only three had made a "good" adjustment (5%), while 46 were designated "poor" (still very severely disturbed), and of these 34 were institutionalized. Bennett and Klein (1966) followed up 14 cases of Potter's (1933) series of children hospitalized at New York State Psychiatric Institute. Eleven were institutionalized either in a state hospital or an institute for the severely retarded.

Creak (1963) described 100 children who had been diagnosed as autistic—17% had improved to an age-appropriate adult level.

Bender's follow-up studies (1970) of fifty autistic children noted that 5 to 10% functioned independently in adult life. Rutter's figures (1970) of "best outcome" were the same as Creak's 17%.

When the schizophrenic groups are further broken down into subgroups it is clear that determination of outcome is directly related to the presence or absence of speech by age five (Bettelheim, 1967; Eisenberg, 1956; Rutter, 1970). Rutter (1967) believes that IQ has prognostic significance: children having an IQ below 60, for example, have a poor outcome. Pollack (1966) in his review of 13 studies of childhood schizophrenia found that most of the children studied had evidence of cerebral dysfunction and low IQ scores. Almost half had IQ's lower than 70.

Etemad and Szurek (1973) describe a follow-up study of 84 autistic children who had been at the Langley Porter Neuropsychiatiric Institute between 1946 and 1961. They defined four classes of outcome based on (1) timing and amount of hospitalization and (2) level of functioning. Class I patients had not been hospitalized since termination of treatment and had functioned as independent adults. Class II patients had been hospitalized less than half the time since discharge and were enrolled in special classes, sheltered workshops, or similar structured programs. Class III patients had been hospitalized less than half the time since discharge but were hospitalized at follow-up and could not function independently Class IV patients had been hospitalized more than half the time since discharge.

Class I	28.6%
Class II	23.8%
Class III	15.5%
Class IV	32.1%

[1]Prevalence of the early-onset form of childhood schizophrenia is 4/9000 (Rutter, 1967).

Further subdivision comparing speech development and later outcome revealed the following:

	64 Children with Speech by Age 5	*20 Mute Children*
Class I	35.9%	5%
Class II	26.6%	15%
Class III	9.4%	35%
Class IV	28.1%	45%

In other words, two-thirds of the total number of children with communicative speech by age five were in Classes I and II, while only one-fifth of the mute children were in Classes I and II.

Follow-up studies of various treatment modalities are sparse and largely retrospective.

Goldfarb (1974) is one of the few investigators who is engaged in prospective research comprised of longitudinal studies of schizophrenic children from the Ittleson Center. He has selected 40 cases, using 65 carefully matched normal children as controls. Forty measured characteristics were divided into two categories: (1) "characteristics which . . . represent capacity levels in which normal children may be expected to improve solely on the basis of maturation. . . ," (e.g., perception, conceptualization, psychomotor performance); (2) "characteristics which reflect the primary influence of social and educational experience" (e.g., social competence).

> Overall, the most impressive findings of the present investigation are the many definite evidences of growth and change (in both of the above noted types of variables) which were demonstrated by the schizophrenic children during the three-year period of observation. They showed significant improvements in most functions which normally mature in childhood. They grew in level of perceptual response, conceptual behavior, orientation, ability to communicate, psychomotor ability, motor strength, and a variety of neurological functions embodying locomotor balance, inhibition of motor overflow, integration of multiple stimuli and coordination. They also improved in educational achievement and social competence. (p. 129)

Goldfarb makes the point that, despite significant change, after 3 years the children as a group remained below normal levels in most of the variables tested. Those abnormalities which changed the least were activity level and muscle tone, which "may be hypothetically related to the level of integrity of the schizophrenic child's nervous system."

FOLLOW-UP OF THE AUTHOR'S CASES

The four children presented here had distinctly different outcomes. Harry, twelve years after leaving the institute, went to a residential center where he completed high school with excellent grades. He did very well in subjects involving memory, especially computation, but made no friends among his peer groups. He returned home and has been able to remain outside an institution. He attends a junior college where he is studying accounting skills. His parents reported that he still becomes upset if he does not get his own way and is generally rigid and perfectionistic. The father mentioned that Harry "has no empathy—he never can see the other person's point of view." He is a large, clumsy young man who still speaks in a wooden monotone, very much like a robot: "Hel-lo-Doc-tor-Kes-ten-baum-I-am-very-glad-to-see-you!"

When I asked him about friends, he answered "friends . . . that is an area . . . of con-sid-er-able . . . dif-fi-cul-ty. I have a number of acquaintances. The news-paper-man-where-I-buy-my Daily Paper and the sand-wich-lady-at-the-del-i-ca-tes-sen."

If a psychiatrist evaluated him today without knowing his early history, he would undoubtedly be diagnosed as a nuclear or "core" schizophrenic. Socially, Harry is a complete isolate, preoccupied with an inner world of his own. Nevertheless, when Harry left my office following our reunion after twelve years, he suddenly threw his arms around me and kissed me. "I re-mem-ber the kiss-ing game. That is what I re-mem-ber the best of all."

When George left the hospital he was sent to an institution for retarded children. He was considered to be a happy, affectionate child. He made no progress in the six years of his institutionalization because of the custodial nature of his care (hundreds of children, few teachers). At the age of 14 his parents removed him and had him placed in a special enrichment program for trainable retardates, where after 2 years he learned to read and write at a third-grade level (his parents moved to a small town in the western United States). George was able to live at home and attend a daily community center for retarded adults. He walks to and from the center by himself; he has made many friends among the townspeople and seems happy. His IQ has remained stable (around 50). His parents told me George's greatest problem is his lack of judgment. He needs supervision at home and cannot be left alone for long. "For example," his mother said, "I had told George to study his lessons for half an hour while I went to the basement. When I returned, flames were emanating from the kitchen stove. George was still reading his book. I cried, 'George, there's a fire!' He answered, 'Yes, I know, but I still have five more minutes to study before the half hour is up.' "

George wrote me a long letter in a childish hand. He still kept the postcard I had sent him twelve years before. He wrote, "I remember all my friends at the hospital. I miss you. Love, your George."

Luba never recovered from her extremely regressed condition. She died in the "back ward" of a state hospital, at the age of eighteen, of "generalized debilitation and pneumonia."

Her course resembled the cases of *dementia* described by Kraepelin (1905) at the turn of the century. Even her superior intelligence could not protect her from her malignant illness despite the best psychiatric treatment of the day.

Dan was in psychoanalytically oriented therapy for a period of 4 years. He made a clinging ambivalent transference to me and eventually was able to work through part of the separation-individuation phase, this time achieving a greater sense of autonomy. During the course of therapy he began socializing and dating, at first with difficulty, but eventually he became engaged to a creative woman in his own field. He had lost his stilted mannerisms; the phobias and compulsive habits disappeared as did his bizarre behavior. He terminated treatment when he was offered a professorship at a leading university in a different city. In subsequent letters he reported an excellent adjustment to his new life.

CONCLUSION

It is obvious from the foregoing discussion that our understanding of childhood schizophrenia is still very limited. Treatment approaches still rely heavily upon the impressions, the intuition, and the clinical still of individual therapists. Clearly more longitudinal studies are needed to determine the best methods of helping each schizophrenic child approach his optimal level of functioning. How can we insure the smoothest transition for those children who might later be able to enter the mainstream of normal life?

As matters stand, it is hard to predict whether a patient such as Harry, for example, had he been able to continue individual psychotherapy in a residential school, would have developed effective social skills rather than merely isolated islands of superior intellectual functioning. Certainly George was capable of further cognitive development following discharge from the hospital. Instead he became isolated from family and community, and progress ceased. It was only after six wasted years of custodial care that the decision was made to bring him back home. There he demonstrated how the "retarded" can continue to develop emotionally and intellectually in a therapeutic milieu in their own community. The after-care of schizophenic children (when they leave the intensive treatment situation) is still a sorely neglected area and needs further study.

There are currently in existence a number of innovative programs for psychotic preschool children directed at helping the disturbed child return to a "normal" setting as soon as possible.

Williams (1974), for example, describes the unique treatment approach of the Julia Ann Singer Nursery in Los Angeles. Following careful diagnostic evaluation, a child deemed suitable for the program is admitted to a therapeutic day nursery. The mother becomes an integral part of the program and receives training from a special staff comprised, among others, of a language therapist and a teacher-therapist under the supervising psychiatrist's direction. She learns to work with her own child much as the school personnel do, while the child is under their care. After 3 to 6 months of intensive work (a considerable shorter time than most therapeutic nursery experiences) the child is sent to a normal nursery of kindergarten class. The new teacher will have had special training from the Julia Ann Singer staff and will also have become faimiliar with the child in the former nursery. In this fashion, the transition into the normal classroom is facilitated. In connection with this program it has been our experience that normal children often become the most effective co-therapists. The following brief vignette is illustrative.

Jamey was an intelligent autistic child who was able to make such a transition from the therapeutic nursery school of St. Luke's into a normal classroom. This child was in the habit of whirling objects and watching them spin hour after hour. The first day in the strange kindergarten he observed two boys playing with toy cars. He picked up a car and joined them. "The blue car goes fast," one of the boys exclaimed. "I have a fan at home; it turns round and round," Jamey rejoined. The second day a similar scene was enacted: Jamey spoke only of his fan. On the third day Jamey again mentioned his fan, and by now one of the boys turned to his companion and said, "Why does this kid keep talking about his fan? What's so good about a dumb old fan? C'mon play cars!" Jamey soon gave up all talk of spinning tops and whirling fans and became a regular member of the group, and in this manner he grew, little by little, indistinguishable from his normal peers.

We need to know how to establish more effective preschool programs for psychotic children. Even more important, however, would be the discovery of techniques to prevent the schizophrenic vulnerability, at least in some cases, from becoming activated in the form of chronic and disabling symptoms.

Barbara Fish (1975) has been studying from their infancy the highly vulnerable children of schizophrenic mothers, and she feels that the developmental lags noted in almost half of these children serve as a predictor of later difficulty. In other words, she believes the "transient pan-developmental retardation . . . appears to serve as an early 'marker' for the inherited neuro-integrative defect in schizophrenia" (1976, p. 62).

Fish contends that preventive efforts could be directed toward the children with early developmental deviations as well as toward those who have suffered a later decompensation.

If we could determine which children are most susceptible to the schizophrenic process (the most "at-risk," that is), we would then be in a position to introduce appropriate therapeutic measures, beginning in the earliest months of life, before maladaptive patterns are firmly established and before the child departs irrecoverably from the normal developmental track. In those children with the heaviest genetic loading or the most profound perinatal neurological disturbances, to be sure, our therapeutic efforts may continue to yield only meager results. But in the majority of cases early detection and vigorous treatment conducted in a systematic and comprehensive manner may well confer substantial and enduring improvement.

REFERENCES

ANTHONY, E. J. An experimental approach to the psychopathology of childhood: Autism. *British Journal of Medical Psychology*, 1958, *31*, 211–225. (a)

ANTHONY, E. J. An etiological approach to the diagnosis of psychosis in childhood. *Revue de Psychiatric Infantile*, 1958, *25*, 89–95. (b)

ANTHONY, E. J. A clinical and experimental study of high risk children and their schizophrenic parents. In A. R. Kaplan (Ed.), *Genetic Factors in Schizophrenia*. Springfield, Ill.: Charles Thomas Publisher, 1972.

BATESON, G., JACKSON, D. D., HALEY, J., and WEAKLAND, J. Toward a theory of schizophrenia. *Behavioral Science*, 1956, *1*, 151–264.

BEHRENS, M., and GOLDFARB, W. A study of patterns of interaction of families of schizophrenic children in residential treatment. *American Journal of Orthopsychiatry*, 1958, *28*, 300–312.

BENDER, L. Childhood schizophrenia. *The Nervous Child*, 1942, vol. 1, no. 2, pp. 138–140.

BENDER, L. The life course of schizophrenic children. *Biological Psychiatry*, 1970, *2*, 165.

BENDER, L., and FARETRA, G. The relationship between childhood schizophrenia and adult schizophrenia. In A. R. Kaplan (Ed.), *Genetic Factors in Schizophrenia*. Springfield, Ill.: Charles Thomas Publisher, 1972.

BENNETT, S., and KLEIN, H. Childhood schizophrenia thrity years later. *American Journal of Psychiatry*, 1966, *122*, 1121.

BERES, D. Ego deviations and the concept of schizophrenia. *The Psychoanalytic Study of the Child*. New York: International Universities Press, 1956, *11*, 164–235.

BERGMAN, P., and ESCALONA, S. K. Unusual sensitivities in very young children. *The Psychoanalytic Study of the Child*. New York: International Universities Press, 1949, *3–4*, 333–352.

BERLIN, I. Simultaneous psychotherapy with a psychotic child and both parents. In S. A. Szurek and I. N. Berlin (Eds.), *Clinical Studies in Childhood Psychosis*. New York: Brunner/Mazel, 1973.

BETTELHEIM, B. Schizophrenia as the reaction to extreme situations. *American Journal of Orthopsychiatry*, 1956, *26*, 507–518.

BETTELHEIM, B. Joey: A "mechanical" boy. *Frontiers of Psychological Research*, 1959, p. 223.

BETTELHEIM, B. *The Empty Fortress: Infantile Autism and the Birth of the Self*. New York: Free Press, 1967.

BOATMAN, M. J., and Szurek, S. A. A clinical study of childhood schizophrenia. In D. D. Jackson (Ed.), *The Etiology of Schizophrenia*. New York: Basic Books, 1960.

BOWLBY, J. The nature of the child's tie to his mother. *International Journal of Psychoanalysis*, 1958, 39.

BRUNER, J. S. Organization of early skilled action. *Child Development*, 1973, *44*, 1–11.

CHRIST, A. E. Cognitive assessment of the psychotic child: A Piagetian framework. Presented at the Annual Meeting of the American Academy of Child Psychiatry, St. Louis, Missouri, November 1975.

CREAK, M. Schizophrenic syndrome in childhood: Report of a working party. *British Medical Journal*, 1961, *2*, 889–890.

CREAK, M. Childhood psychosis: A review of 100 cases. *British Journal of Psychiatry*, 1963, *109*, 84–89.

DESANCTIS, S. Sopra alcune varietà della demenza precoce. *Revista Sperimentale di Freniatria*, 1906, *32*, 141–145.

DESANCTIS, S. [On some varieties of dementia praecox.] In "Three Historic Papers" (trans. by Maria-Livia Osborn) in John E. Howells (Ed.), *Modern perspectives in international child psychiatry*. New York: Brunner/Mazel, 1971.

DESLAURIERS, A. M., and CARLSON, C. F. *Your child is asleep: Early infantile autism*. Homewood, Ill.: Dorsey Press, 1969.

DESPERT, J. L. Schizophrenia in childhood. *Psychiatric Quarterly*, 1938, *12*, 366–371.

DESPERT, J. L. *Schizophrenia in children*. New York: Brunner/Mazel, 1975.

EISENBERG, L. The autistic child in adolescence. *American Journal of Psychiatry*, 1956, *112*, 607.

EISENBERG, L., and KANNER, L. Early infantile autism: 1943–1955. *American Journal of Orthopsychiatry*, 1956, *26*, 556–566.

EKSTEIN, R. The space child's time machine: On reconstruction in the psychotherapeutic treatment of a schizophrenic child. *American Journal of Orthopsychiatry*, 1954, *24*, 492–506.

EKSTEIN, R. *Children of time and space, of action and impulse: Clinical studies on the psychoanalytic treatment of severely disturbed children*. New York: Appleton-Century-Crofts, 1966.

EKSTEIN, R., and FRIEDMAN, S. Object constancy and psychotic reconstruction. *The Psycho-*

analytic Study of the Child. New York: International Universities Press, 1967, *22*, 357–374.

EKSTEIN, R., and WRIGHT, D. C. The space child. *Bulletin of the Menninger Clinic*, 1952, *16*, 211–224.

ERLENMEYER-KIMLING, L. Studies on the offspring of two schizophrenic parents. In D. Rosenthal and S. Kety (Eds.), *The transmission of schizophrenia*. New York: Pergamon, 1968.

ERLENMEYER-KIMLING, L. A prospective study of children at risk for schizophrenia: Methodological considerations and some preliminary findings. In R. Wirt, G. Winokur, & M. Roff (Eds.), *Life History Research in Psychopathology*. Minneapolis: University of Minnesota Press, 1976, *4*.

ETEMAD, J., and SZUREK, S. A modified follow-up study of a group of psychotic children. In S. Szurek and I. Berlin (Eds.), *Clinical Studies in Childhood Psychosis*. New York: Brunner/Mazel, 1973.

FISH, B. The "one child, one drug" myth of stimulants in hyperkinesis: Importance of diagnostic categories in evaluating treatment. *Archives of General Psychiatry*, 1971, *25*, 193–203.

FISH, B. Biologic antecedents of psychosis in children. In D. X. Freedman (Ed.), *The biology of the major psychoses* (Association for Research into Mental Disorders Publication No. 54). New York: Raven Press, 1975.

FISH, B. An approach to prevention in infants at risk for schizophrenia: Developmental deviations from birth to ten years. *Journal of the American Academy of Child Psychiatry*, 1976, *15*, 62–82.

FREUD, S. Three essays on sexuality. In *Standard Edition of Complete Works* (Vol. VII). London: Hogarth Press, 1964. (Originally published, 1905.)

GELEERD, E. A contribution to the problem of psychoses in children. *The Psychoanalytic Study of the Child*. New York: International Universities Press, 1946, *2*, 271–292.

GOLDFARB, W. Receptor preferences in schizophrenic children. *Archives of Neurological Psychiatry*, 1956, *76*, 643–653.

GOLDFARB, W. *Childhood schizophrenia*. Cambridge, Mass.: Harvard University Press, 1961.

GOLDFARB, W. Childhood Psychosis. In Carmichael (Ed.), *Manual of Child Psychology*, Third Edition, New York: J. Wiley & Sons, Inc., 1970, *2*, 765–830.

GOLDFARB, W. *Growth and Change of Schizophrenic Children: A Longitudinal Study*, New York: John Wiley & Sons, Inc., 1974.

GREEN, A. Self-mutilation in schizophrenic children. *Archives of General Psychiatry*, 1967, *17*, 234–244.

GREEN, A. The effects of object loss on the body image of schizophrenic girls. *Journal of the American Academy Child Psychiatry*, 1970, *9*, 3, 532–547.

HEIMLICH, E. P. The specialized use of music as a mode of communication in the treatment of disturbed children. *Journal of the American Academy of Child Psychiatry*, 1965, *4*, 86–122.

HEIMLICH, E. P. Paraverbal techniques in the therapy of childhood communication disorders. *International Journal of Child Psychotherapy*, 1972, *1*(1), 65–82.

HELLER, T. Ueber Dementia infantilis. *Ztschr. für die Erforschung und Behandlung des Jugendl. Schwachsinns*. 1908, *2*, 17–28.

HELLER, T. About dementia infantilis (translated by W. Hulse) *Journal of Nervous and Mental Disease*, 1954, *119*, 610–616.

HERMELIN, B. and O'CONNOR, N. *Psychological Experiments with Autistic Children*. Oxford: Pergamon Press, 1970, p. 60.

HESTEN, L. L. Psychiatric disorders in foster home reared children of schizophrenic mothers. *British Journal of Psychiatry*, 1966, *112*, 819.

HESTEN, L. L. The genetics of schizophrenia and schizoid disease. *Science*, 1970, *167*, 249.

HINTGTEN, J. and CHURCHILL, D. In D. Churchill, D. Alpern and M. Demyer (Eds.), *Infantile Autism, Proceedings of the Indiana University Colloquium*, Springfield, Illinois: Charles C Thomas, 1971.

HOROWITZ, W. A., KESTENBAUM, C. J., PERSON, E., and JARVIK, L. Identical twins—"idiot savants"—calander calculators. *American Journal of Psychiatry*, 1965, *121*, 11, 1075–1079.

HUTT, S. J., HUTT, C., LEE, D. and OUNSTED, C. Arousal and childhood autism. *Nature*, 1967, *204*, 908–909.

ITARD, J. M. G. *The Wild Boy of Aveyron* (translated by G. Humphrey 1932). New York: Appleton Century Press, 1801.

KALLMAN, F. J. The genetic theory of schizophrenia. *American Journal of Psychiatry*, 1946, *103*, 309.

KALLMAN, F. and ROTH, B. Genetic aspects of pre-adolescent schizophrenia. *American Journal of Psychiatry*. 1956, *112*, 599–606.

KANNER, L. *Child Psychiatry*. 3rd Edution, Springfield, Illinois: Charles C Thomas, 1935, p. 280.

KANNER, L. Autistic disturbances of affective contact, *Nervous Child*, 1943, *2*, 217–250.

KANNER, L. General concept of schizophrenia at different ages. (In *Neurology and Psychiatry in Childhood*) *Research Publications of the Association of Nervous and Mental Disease*. 1954, *34*, 451–453.

KASANIN, J. and KAUFMAN, M. R. A study of the functional psychosis in childhood. *American Journal of Psychiatry*, 1929, *86*, 307–384.

KERNBERG, O. F. "The structural diagnosis of borderline personality organization." Presented at the International Conference on Borderline Disorders, Topeka, Kansas, March 19, 1976.

KESTENBAUM, C. J. Introductory chapter in P. Brusiloff, and M. J. Witenberg (Eds.), *The Emerging Child*. New York, Jason Aronson, Inc., 1973.

KLEEMAN, J. A. The peek-a-boo game: Part I—Its origins, meanings and related phenomena in the first year. *The Psychoanalytic Study of the Child*, New York: International Universities Press, 1967, 239–273.

KLEIN, M. *The Psychoanalysis of Children*. New York: Grove Press, Inc., 1960. (Originally published by Hogarth Press and The Institute of Psychoanalysis, No. 22, London, 1932.)

KOLVIN, I., OUNSTED, C., HUMPHREY, M., MCNAY, A., RICHARDSON, L., GARSIDE, R., KIDD, J. and ROTH, M. Studies in the childhood psychosis: I–VI. *British Journal Psychiatry*, 1971, *1118*, 385–415.

KRAEPELIN, E. *Einführung in die Psychiatrische Klinik*. 2nd Edit. Leipzig: J. A. Barth–Verlag, 1905, 21–30.

LEVOBICI, S., DIATKINE, R., FAVREAU, J. A. and LUGET-PARET, P. The psychoanalysis of children. In S. Naeht, (Ed.) *Psychoanalysis of Today*. New York: Grune & Stratton, Co., 1959.

LIDZ, T., FLECK, S., and CORNELISON, A. R. *Schizophrenia and the Family*, New York: International Universities Press, 1965.

LINDNER, R. *The Fifty-Minute Hour*. New York: Bantam Books, 1952.

LOVAAS, O., FREITAG, E., GOLD, V. J. and KASSORLA, I. C. Experimental studies in childhood schizophrenia: Analysis of self-destructive behavior. *Journal of Experimental Psychology*, 1965, *2*, 67–84.

MAHLER, M. On child psychosis and schizophrenia: Autistic and symbiotic infantile psychosis. *Psychoanalytic Study of the Child*. *7*, 286–305. New York: International University Press, 1952.

MAHLER, M. On the significance of the normal separation-individuation phase with reference to research in symbiotic child psychosis. In McSchur (Ed.), *Drives, Affects, Behavior 2*, 161–169, New York: International Universities Press, 1965.

MAHLER, M. S. and FURER, M. *On Human Symbrosis and the Vicissitudes of the Individuation*. New York: International Universities Press, 1968.

MAHLER, M. and GOSLINER, B. J. On symbiotic child psychosis: Genetic, dynamic and restitutive aspects. *Psychoanalytic Study of the Child, 10*, 195–211, New York: International Universities Press, 1955.

MEDNICK, S. A. and SCHULSINGER, F. A longitudinal study of children with a high risk for schizophrenia: A preliminary report. In S. E. Vandenburg (Ed.), *Methods and Goals in Human Behavior Genetics* New York: Academic Press, 1965.

MILLER, R. Childhood schizophrenia: A review of selected literature. *International Journal of Mental Health*, Vol. 3, No. 1, 3–46; *Annual Progress in Child Psychiatry and Child Development* (1975), S. Chess and A. Thomas (Eds.). New York: Brunner/Mazel, Inc., 1974.

ORNITZ, E. and RITVO, E. Perceptual inconstancy in early infantile autism. *Archives of General Psychiatry*, 1968, *18*, 76.

POLLACK, M. Mental Subnormality and "childhood schizophrenia." In J. Zubin and G. Jervis (Eds.), *Psychopathology of Mental Development*. New York: Grune and Stratton, Inc.

POTTER, H. W. Schizophrenia in children. *American Journal Psychiatry*, 1933, *89*, 1253–1270.

RANK, B. Adaptation of the psychoanalytic technique for the treatment of young children with atypical development, *American Journal of Orthopsychiatry*, 1949 *19*, 130–139.

RICHMOND, W. The dementia praecox child. *American Journal of Psychiatry*, 1932, *88*, 1153–1159.

RIMLAND, B. *Infantile Autism*, New York: Appleton-Century-Crofts, 1964.

RUTTER, M. Psychotic disorders in early childhood. In A. Cooper and A. Walk (Eds.), *Recent Developments in Schizophrenia, British Journal of Psychiatry* (special publication) 1967, No. 1, 113–133.

RUTTER, M. Autistic children, infancy to adulthood. *Seminars in Psychiatry*, 1970, *2*, 435.

RUTTER, M., BARTAK, L. and NEWMAN, S. Autism —A central disorder of cognition and language? In (Ed. M. Rutter) *Infantile Autism* 148–171, London: Churchill and Livingstone, 1971.

SCHEERER, W., ROTHMAN, E. and GOLDSTEIN, K. A case of idiot savant. *Psychological Monographs*, 1945, *58*, No. 4.

SEARLES, H. F. *The Non-Human Environment in Normal Development and In Schizophrenia.* New York: International Universities Press, 1960.

SECHÈHAYE, M. A. *Symbolic Realization: A New Method of Psychotherapy Applied To A Case of Schizophrenia.* New York: International Universities Press, 1947.

SECHÈHAYE, M. *A New Psychotherapy in Schizophrenia*. New York: Grune & Stratton, 1956.

SHAPIRO, T., CHARIANDINI, I., and FISH, B. 30 Severely Disturbed Children: Evaluation of Their Language Development for Classification and Prognosis. *Archives of General Psychiatry*. 1974, *30*, 819–825.

STABENAU, J. R. and POLLIN, W. Early characteristics of monozygotic twins discordant for schizophrenia. *Archives of General Psychiatry*. 1967, *17*, 723–734.

STONE, M. H. Therapists' personalities and unexpected success with schizophrenic patients. *American Journal of Psychotherapy*, 1971, *25*, 543–552.

STONE, M. H. Psychodiagnosis and psychoanalytic psychotherapy. Presented at the Northwestern Branch, American Psychiatric Association, Spring Meeting, Vancouver, Canada on March 27th, 1976.

SZUREK, C. A. and BERLIN, I. N. Elements of psychotherapeutics with the schizophrenic child and his parents; (1961) *Psychiatry: Journal for the Study of Interpersonal Processes*, 1956.

TREFFERT, D. A., MCANDREW, J. and DREIFURST, P. Inpatient treatment program and outcome for 57 autistic and schizophrenia. *Journal of Autism and Childhood Schizophrenia*, 1973, *3*(2), 138.

WILLIAMS, F. In Div. of Child Psychiatry, Cedars-

Sinai Medical Center, L.A., In R. Glasscote and M. E. Fishman (Eds.), *Mental Health Programs for Pre-School Children: A Field Study*, P141, Joint Information Service of the American Psychological Association and the National Association for Mental Health, Washington, D.C., 1974.

Wing, J. K. *Diagnosis and Epidemiology, An Etiology in Childhood Autism: Clinical Educational and Social Aspects*, London: Pergamon Press, 1966.

Wolman, B. B. *Children without childhood: A study of childhood schizophrenia.* New York Grune and Stratton, 1970.

Wynne, L. O. and Singer, M. T. Thought disorder in the family relations of schizophrenics, *Archives of General Psychiatry*, 1963, *9*, 191–198.

22

CHILDHOOD PSYCHOSIS: BEHAVIORAL TREATMENT

O. Ivar Lovaas, Douglas B. Young and Crighton D. Newsom

Kanner (1943) is generally recognized as being the first to describe a distinct type of childhood psychosis, namely infantile autism. He felt that the crucial problems presented by these children were an inability to relate to people and to ordinary social situations that apparently dated from early infancy, as well as an obsessive desire for the maintenance of sameness. Since Kanner's criteria may appear somewhat general and difficult to replicate in diagnostic work, we have attempted to specify the syndrome in more behaviorally oriented terms. It should first be mentioned that there is considerable confusion about highly discriminated classifications within the general category of childhood psychosis. The labels childhood schizophrenia, symbiotic psychosis, autism, atypical development, and ego deviant are used, often indiscriminantly, throughout the literature. However, it can been argued that physiological, psychological, and behavioral variables have not as yet been adequately specified to warrant the use of many of the supposedly distinct categories mentioned above. What follows then is the behavioral picture of a psychotic condition of early childhood, and, in particular, infantile autism.

Severe Affective Isolation. Attempts to love, cuddle, and show affection to these children typically result in a profound lack of response on the child's part. The child may actively resist the parents' attempt to love him. He seems not to know or care whether he is alone or in the company of others. As small babies such children often do not cup or mold when they are held, nor do they respond with anticipation to being picked up. They manifest few of the feelings normal children do. Thus, they do not seem to be sad or depressed, hopeless, bewildered or confused, and they seem generally unaffected by the moods and feelings of those around them.

Compulsivity. The child shows a compulsive insistence that his environment remain unchanged. For example, he may become quite upset or frightened if a piece of furniture is moved or if he is required to take a new or different route when walking to a familiar place. This compulsivity may also include an extreme inflexibility in eating habits, an insistence that only certain words be used in a given situation, or the lining up of blocks, toys, or other objects in neat rows or patterns with the demand that they remain unchanged.

Apparent Sensory Deficit. One may move directly in front of the child, smile and talk to him, yet he may act as if no one were there. An observer may not feel that the child is avoiding or ignoring him, but rather that the child simply does not seem to see or hear. The parents often report that they have, in fact, incorrectly suspected the child to be blind or deaf. As one gets to know these children better, one becomes aware of the extreme variability in their attentional behavior. For example, although the child may give no visible reaction to a loud noise, such as a clapping of hands directly behind his ears (i.e., the child does not startle), he may orient to the crinkle of a cellophane wrapper or react fearfully to a distant and barely audible siren. Similarly, though he may not notice the comings or goings of people around him, or other major changes in his visual field (turning off the lights may have no visible effect on his behavior), he may spot a small piece of candy on a table some 20 feet away. This apparent sensory deficit is often not limited to the visual or auditory modalities alone. Many autistic children often do not seem to feel pain. For example, the child may burn himself on the stove without crying or even seeming to be aware that he has injured himself.

Self-Stimulation. Probably the most striking and frequently engaged in behavior in these children centers on the very repetitive and highly stereotyped, idiosyncratic acts, such as rocking their bodies when in a sitting position, twirling around, flapping their hands at the wrists, humming a set of three or four notes over and over again, spinning objects, twirling twigs or pieces of string, etc. The child may spend entire days, weeks, or months gazing at his cupped hands, staring at lights, or spinning ashtrays in a most repetitive and incessant manner.

Tantrums and Self-Mutilatory Behavior. Most autistic children evidence some form of self-destructive behavior, which in some cases becomes so severe that the child bites himself until he bleeds, or beats his head against walls or sharp pieces of furniture so forcefully that large lumps rise and his skin turns black and blue. He may beat his face with his fists. Some children bear scars from their self-mutilation so that one can observe skin discolorations that remain from bite wounds on their arms. One is likely to trigger self-mutilatory behavior by imposing some restriction on movement (e.g., demanding that the child sit in a chair), or some other minimal standard for appropriate behavior. Sometimes the child's aggression will be directed outward against his parents or teachers in the most primitive form of biting, scratching, kicking, and other tantrumlike behavior. Some of these children stay awake and scream all night, tearing curtains off the window, smearing feces, spilling flour all over the kitchen, etc. The parents are often at a complete loss as to how to cope with these outbursts.

Mutism and Echolalia. A good many of these children are mute; their speech production is limited to uttering simple sounds. The speech of those who do talk may be echos of others' speech. For example, if one addresses a child with the question, "What is your name?" the child may answer "What is your name?" (preserving, perhaps, the exact intonation of the person who spoke to him). At other times the echolalia is not immediate but delayed; the child may repeat parental statements, television commercials, or other announcements he has heard that morning or on the preceding day, or even years ago. Receptive language abilities are similarly retarded.

Behavioral Deficiencies. Although the presence of these behavioral problems is rather striking, it is equally striking to take note of many behaviors that the autistic child does *not* have. He often has few if any self-help skills, necessitating his being fed, dressed, and toileted by others. He may not play with toys but put them in his mouth, or tap them repetitively with his fingers. Affect is generally shallow or inappropriate. He exhibits little, if any, appropriate peer play. He shows little understanding of common dangers. For example, one has to be careful not to let the child walk in the street unassisted, because he may walk directly in front of an oncoming car.

Other Considerations. Many diagnosticians now consider it mandatory that the child's motor development fall within the normal range in order to classify him as autistic rather than retarded. Thus, he must have turned over, sat up, walked, etc., at a normal age. In addition, many diagnosticians look for signs of average or perhaps above-average intellectual performance in certain limited areas. For example, some autistic children appear to be particularly clever at manipulating their parents by throwing tantrums; others are very skillful in assembling and disassembling mechanical objects such as clocks, watches, or intricate toys. Some are extremely clever at arranging objects for self-stimulatory purposes. Others give evidence of unusual memory, in that they detect minor changes in the furniture arrangement of their living room (even though they were not there when the changes were made) and become extremely upset. Others may be able to recite songs, series of numbers, or other kinds of material, which suggests an extensive rote memory. This last diagnostic task, of inferring intact intellectual functioning in limited areas, is admittedly a most difficult one, which no doubt contributes significantly to the problem of discriminating autistic children from other types of children with severe behavioral retardation. Finally, for the child to receive a primary diagnosis within this category, there is a general consensus that the behavioral picture presented above should occur in the absence of any presently detectable brain tissue impairment.

Although Kanner refrained from postulating a specific etiology, he did report that the parents of the children in his sample appeared detached, unaffectionate, cold, emotionally insulated, and intellectualizing. Some psychoanalytically oriented clinicians, such as Bettelheim (1967), were quick to seize upon a possible causal relationship between child deviance and parental rejection. From this point of view, autism is seen as a defense against a parental environment that is singularly cold and potentially destructive. This presumed parental psychopathology, combined with the child's conviction that he is threatened with total destruction by insensitive and irrational powers, causes the child to withdraw into his "inner autistic world." Angry parental rejection of the child is seen as the cause behind the child's failure to form normal relationships toward people; as a result, he never moves on developmentally to relate ("cathect") to the external world. His peculiar behaviors are viewed as manifestations ("symptoms") of this combined effect of fear of his parents' anger toward him and the correlated failure of ego development. For example, the autistic child's excessive preoccupation with rotating and spinning both himself and other objects is seen as symptomatic of the inescapable, vicious circle he is caught in—a cycle of longing and fear, of wanting and needing so much from other people and, at the same time, of being mortally afraid to let that longing be known, either to the other people or to himself. Insistence on sameness is thought to be an expression of a feeling of helplessness about influencing the external environment and is thus an attempt to reaffirm a limited hold on an otherwise fluctuating and frightening world. Self-destructive behaviors are often considered to reflect the child's attempts to injure his mother because she had hurt him. When he hurts himself, he is retaliating on his own terms.

The treatment prescribed by such an etiological assumption would consist of attempts to create an unconditionally accepting, loving, understanding, and warm adult-child relationship with the hope that the child would accept the adult in this therapeutic relationship. In order to insinuate himself into the behavior patterns of the child, and thus presumably increase the probability that the child will accept him, the therapist often actively participates in and mirrors the child's "primitive magical language," gestures, stereotypies, and fantasies. Once the child has accepted the adult, he would then be expected to move out toward the world, relate himself to that world, and concurrently lose the various "symptoms" of autism. Finally, as a result of this new emotional relationship with the adults around him, the child would be expected to acquire appropriate, normal behaviors as a matter of course, without anyone explicitly teaching them to him. As we shall see, this traditional psychodynamic view of infantile autism runs completely contrary to the approach reported in this chapter, but is presented here because it helps illustrate the behavioral approach by contrast.

Perhaps due to the imprecision with which the psychodynamic theory of autism has been stated, such attempts to understand the disorder and other childhood psychoses have not been adequately evaluated, and they may never be. But for the practicing clinician, it is important to be aware that on the empirical level, the outcome studies on traditional forms of psychotherapy with these children have failed to yield significant results. Brown (1960), Creak (1962), Kanner and Eisenberg (1955), and Rutter (1966) have all reported data demonstrating that autistic children treated according to psychoanalytic principles did not do significantly better than children receiving no treatment at all. Merely providing an unconditionally loving, understanding milieu does not seem to help these children. Furthermore, research has failed to identify parents of autistic children as emotionally cold and detached, or as belonging to any other emotionally deficient type (Creak & Ini, 1960; Pitfield & Oppenheim, 1964; Rimland, 1964; Schopler & Reichler, 1972; Wolff & Morris, 1971).

What we have, then, during the 1940s and 1950s, was the appearance of Dr. Kanner's suggestion that a distinct group of psychotic children be singled out and labeled "autistic," followed by a great deal of vigorous support for the creation of a new diagnostic category to recognize this condition, for which people like Bettelheim postulated a distinct psychogenic etiology and prescribed a supposedly distinct treatment. By the early 1960s, as data failed to support these earlier etiological and treatment formulations, an attitude of reservation and pessimism characterized those who considered treating autistic children; therapists felt they were giving a lot but not getting much back. It was in this atmosphere, of a pessimistic prognosis and confusion about etiology, that the first behavioral approach to the treatment of autistic children was begun.

BEHAVIOR THEORY AND AUTISM

Ferster (1961) made the first attempt to understand autistic children within a behavioral framework. He argued that autism could be viewed as a failure of the child to learn, and in particular, that the behavioral deficiency could be viewed as a consequence of social stimuli failing to acquire reinforcing properties for these children. Ferster's theoretical argument was very succinct and was followed by a series of experiments (Ferster & DeMyer, 1961, 1962) in which autistic children were exposed to very simple but highly structured environments where they learned very simple behaviors, including pulling levers and matching to sample for reinforcers (e.g., as food) that were functional in maintaining these behaviors over time. These studies were the first to show that the behavior of autistic children could be lawfully and predictably related to certain explicit environmental events and that these children could, in fact, be taught to learn or otherwise comply with certain aspects of reality.

Let us briefly summarize a behavioral analysis of autism in terms of learning theory. Within a learning theory framework, one can view a child's development as consisting of the acquisition of (1) behavioral repertoires and (2) stimulus functions. The behavioral repertoires of autistic children are strikingly deficient. That is, they have little, if any, adaptive behavior which would help them function in society. Therefore, a therapeutic program for autistic children may focus on how to strengthen certain behaviors, such as appropriate play, social interaction, and speech. One way to strengthen such behaviors is by *reinforcing* their occurrence; when they are initially absent, such behaviors may be *prompted* and gradually *shaped* by rewarding successive approximations to their final form. We shall give numerous examples of procedures designed to increase the behavioral repertoires of autistic children. Conversely, some behavior patterns are too strong in autistic children. This is particularly true of tantrums, self-destructive behavior, and self-stimulation, and we attempt to decrease their frequency and strength. One may attempt to decrease these patterns either by withholding those reinforcers which may be maintaining them (*extinction*), by removing the child to a place where no reinforcement can be obtained (*time-out*), or by systematically applying aversive stimuli contingent upon their occurrence (*punishment*). In short, it is quite possible to develop treatment programs where one works directly with the child's behaviors, increasing some and decreasing others by the use of whatever reinforcers (such as food) and punishers (such as physical pain) are functional for that particular child. In the procedures which we will discuss in this chapter, the major emphasis lies in the development of appropriate behaviors with the use of positive reinforcers in conjunction with shaping, prompting, and prompt-fading techniques.

As new appropriate behaviors are learned, the child's environment begins to acquire "meaning," or what we technically refer to as "stimulus functions," for him. Internal and external events to which the child attends when he responds acquire the capacity to evoke those responses in the future. These internal and external events are called *discriminative stimuli* (S^Ds) when they "set the occasion" for certain behaviors to be reinforced. We say that *stimulus control* exists to the extent that a given behavior reliably occurs when a given stimulus is present and does not occur when it is absent. Another aspect of the acquisition of stimulus functions has to do with symbolic rewards and punishers, which are known technically as secondary, acquired, or *conditioned* reinforcers and punishers. During normal development, certain aspects of the child's environment which were neutral when he was born come to acquire reinforcing or punitive functions for him. One can think of many good examples to illustrate this point, and it is particularly obvious that within the area of social functioning a great deal of such learning takes place. For example, the presence or absence of an approving smile, although probably neutral to the newborn infant, gradually assumes reinforcing functions as the child interacts with people around him. The primary reason for being concerned with these conditioned reinforcers lies in their contribution to the acquisition of complex social and intellectual behaviors. Children appear to acquire normal behaviors to the extent that there exists a variety of conditioned reinforcers to support such behavioral development. Since autistic children generally do not respond to praise, smiles, hugs, interpersonal closeness, being correct, and other events which seem to establish and maintain so much behavior in normal children, it is reasonable to expect their behavioral development to be correspondingly deficient. Thus, much of an autistic child's failure to acquire appropriate behavior can be viewed as the result of a failure of his environment to acquire motivational meaning for him; that is, his environment occasions few age-appropriate behavior patterns because it has acquired few appropriate stimulus functions (meanings), and these in turn result from a lack of development of "normal" conditioned reinforcers. This was the essence of Ferster's (1961) theoretical analysis of autism. One may conceive of conditioned and unconditioned reinforcers as being "causes" of behavior. Without any knowledge of an organic causative factor, to address one's therapeutic work to the development and rearrangement of reinforcing stimuli would seem to strike at the base of the autistic child's problem. Yet there has been surprisingly little work done in this area. We will consider this point again in more detail when we discuss motivation.

Soon after Ferster's theoretical paper appeared, several important studies were published describing therapy with autistic children using a behavioral approach. Methodologically powerful research designs characterized these studies, and much of the thrust of behavior therapy continues to derive from its adherence to such sound research designs. Typically, these studies have used single-subject, or within-subject, replication designs, so that one may be reasonably certain that the intervention that was given did in fact help the child.

But since the early studies were limited to a single child or just a few children, or limited themselves to interventions with just a few behaviors, it was difficult to assess the overall clinical effectiveness of behavior therapy from these studies. Within a short time, however, the early findings were independently replicated and extended by investigators in other laboratories and clinics. Let us very briefly review several of the early studies which employed behavioral techniques in the treatment of psychotic children.

In one of the best-known of the earlier studies, Wolf, Risley, and Mees (1964) used shaping, extinction, and time-out to treat a $3\frac{1}{2}$-year-old autistic boy who would not eat or sleep properly, lacked normal social and verbal repertoires, was very tantrumous and self-destructive, and refused to wear glasses necessary to preserve his macular vision. The child's behavior improved markedly during treatment, and a subsequent follow-up study (Wolf, Risley, Johnston, Harris, & Allen, 1967) showed that he continued to improve after discharge from the program, to the point where he was able to take advantage of a public school education program. In another early study, Hewett (1965) described a procedure for building speech in autistic children who were speech deficient or mute. He used a shaping procedure to increase the child's attending behavior, then systematically rewarded the child for vocalizations that eventually matched those modeled by the therapist. Under this procedure the child acquired the beginnings of meaningful language.

Around the time that this work was being conducted, there appeared two conceptually important studies, one demonstrating errorless discrimination learning (Terrace, 1963), the other generalized imitation (Bear & Sherman, 1964). These studies led to the development of techniques which enormously increased the therapeutic power of behavioral procedures with psychotic and retarded children. Consider imitative behavior as an example. As Bandura (1969) has argued, it may be literally impossible to shape highly complex behaviors one step at a time. Complex behaviors often seem to be acquired through imitation, but until the Bear and Sherman (1964) study appeared, we had no technology for establishing imitation. These investigators showed that if one reinforced a child for imitating some of a model's behaviors, the child would also begin to imitate the model's other behaviors, even though he had not been explicitly reinforced for imitating these. They thus demonstrated generalized imitation. Bear and Sherman viewed imitation as a discrimination: the child discriminates the similarity between his and the model's behavior as the occasion for reinforcement. Although the Bear and Sherman study dealt with normal children who already imitated, it provided a conceptual and methodological basis for building imitative behavior in nonimitating children. Thus, Metz (1965) demonstrated how one could use reinforcement to build nonverbal imitative behaviors in autistic children. Similarly, Lovaas, Freitas, Nelson, & Whalen (1967) established nonverbal imitative repertoires in autistic children and demonstrated how this greatly facilitated the acquisition of complex social, intellectual, and self-help skills. Lovaas, Berberich, Perloff, and Schaeffer (1966) showed that it was possible, through the use of a discrimination-learning paradigm, to build imitative verbal behavior in previously mute autistic children. These early behavioral studies showed that it was quite possble to take learning principles which had been discovered and developed in basic research laboratories and apply them to socially and clinically relevant behaviors in humans, such as self-help skills and language. From these studies has come a foundation for more comprehensive treatment programs for psychotic children (Kozloff, 1974; Lovaas, 1977). In the short span of about 15 years, from Ferster's (1961) theoretical argument to the present day, it is obvious that we have moved very quickly in helping a difficult clinical population.

UNDERSTANDING AND MANAGING SELF-MUTILATION

At one time or another in their lives, a significant proportion of psychotic and retarded children exhibit some form of self-injurious behavior. Usually this consists of head-banging, arm-banging, beating themselves on their heads and faces with fists or knees, and biting themselves on the hands, wrists, arms, and shoulders. Sometimes the self-destruction can be severe enough to pose a major problem for the child's safety. Such children often remove large quantities of flesh from their bodies, tear out their fingernails, open wounds in their heads, break their noses or fingers, and so on. Restraint, either by the use of camisoles ("strait-jackets") or by tying the child's feet and arms to his bed, is often required in severe cases. Sometimes the self-mutilation is sporadic; in other children it is long lasting, requiring such prolonged use of restraints that structural changes can be observed, such as demineralization, shortening of tendons, or arrested motor development, secondary to limb disuse. Obviously, such a child poses major psychological problems for those who take care of him, in the form of anxiety, demoralization, and hopelessness. We know of no form of treatment that invariably alleviates self-multilation.

Typically, intervention has consisted of some combination of tranquilizing drugs, supportive verbal therapy, and occasionally electroconvulsive therapy. There are no data demonstrating that any of these forms of treatment is particularly effective.

Some early observations from behavioral work indicated that the withdrawal of attention may reduce self-destructive behavior. For example, Wolf, Risley, and Mees (1964) reported the effectiveness of placing a 3½-year-old autistic boy in isolation whenever he threw tantrums or injured himself. Similarly, Hamilton, Stephens, and Allen (1967) used social isolation to eliminate head and back banging in a severely retarded institutionalized girl. Their technique was to physically confine the patient in a chair located away from ward activities, and hence social reinforcement, for a 30-minute period contingent upon each occurrence of self-injurious behavior. Such responding was eliminated very rapidly and did not recur over a 9-month follow-up period.

It could be argued that the experience of being contingently placed in isolation reduces self-destruction because it involves an interruption of ongoing behavior and a possibly aversive social interaction, and not necessarily because it involves the removal of social attention. However, the hypothesis that self-destruction is maintained by its social consequences would be directly supported by evidence that the contingent removal of all social consequences results in the elimination of self-destructive behavior. Such data is presented in the record of the self-destructive behavior of an 8-year-old boy, where the self-destruction is plotted as cumulative curves in Figure 22-1. Shown are the first eight extinction sessions. Each session consisted of a 90-minute period in which the child was left alone and unrestrained. At first his rate was very high; he hit himself more than 2,700 times during the first extinction period. Observe, however, that half an hour into the first session his rate began leveling off slightly, our first clue that the technique might work. Over these first eight sessions, the rate of his self-destructive behavior gradually decreased until it reached zero in the eighth session. Such evidence from our clinic sup-

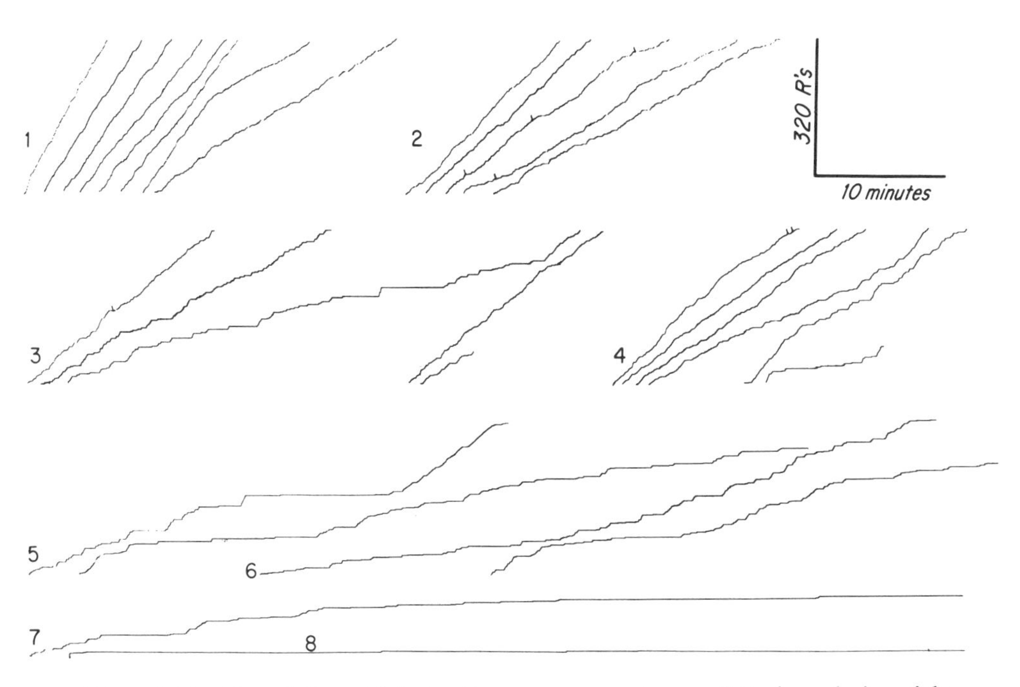

Figure 22-1 Cumulative self-destructive responses of an autistic boy during eight successive extinction sessions.

porting this effect of extinction on self-multilation was presented in papers by Lovaas, Freitag, Gold, and Kassorla (1965) and Lovaas and Simmons (1969).

If self-destruction in these children is learned social behavior, then it should show an opposite effect (i.e., increase in strength) if social reinforcement in the form of attention, concern, etc. is presented contingent on its occurrence. In an early study (Lovaas et al., 1965) we quite accidentally observed that on days when we attended to a child's self-destructive responding by verbalizing our concern about the child, the self-destruction increased, only to decrease on the days when we did not similarly attend to these behaviors. A singularly poignant demonstration of how detrimental such attention can be is provided in Figure 22-2 which gives data on an 11-year-old self-destructive boy (Lovaas & Simmons, 1969). The data are again presented as cumulative curves. The first and second 10-minute sessions formed a base rate of self-injurious responses and are referred to by the numbers 1 and 2. During these periods, the child was left free to hit himself and no one did anything about it. Gregg's self-destructive responding was at a very low level because he had just completed a prolonged series of extinction sessions. During the third 10-minute session (number 3), the approach was changed so that on the average of every fifth time Gregg hit himself, we would immediately attend to him for 30 to 60 seconds by comforting, hugging, and generally expressing concern for him. This type of intervention is shown by the diagonal hatchmarks. When we administered such "treatment," his rate of self-mutilation increased. In the fourth session, we again withdrew our comments and attention and his self-destructive responding extinguished. We then reintroduced the comments and attention contingent upon self-destruction in session 5. Once again note how detrimental this "therapeutic" approach was: self-injurious responses increased and were maintained at an alarmingly steady rate. But the effect was reversible, as can be seen in sessions 6 and 7, where we refrained from reinforcing his self-destruction; his rate again decreased to manageable levels. Unintentional shaping of self-mutilation by well-intentioned but naive parents and therapists can probably occur in natural settings and produce similar harmful effects.

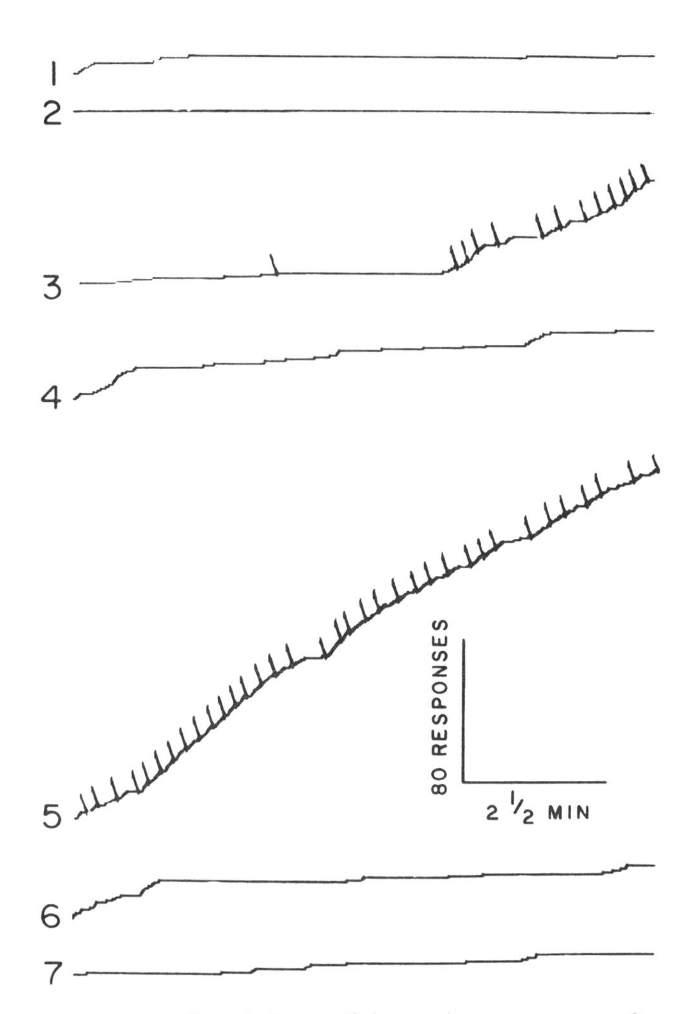

Figure 22-2 Cumulative self-destructive responses of Gregg during seven successive sessions. Diagonal hatchmarks in sessions 3 and 5 indicate occurrences of adults' attention contingent on self-destruction. Extinction was in force during the other sessions.

The most compelling evidence to support the social operant nature of self-mutilation can be found in the high degree of situational or stimulus control which the environment exerts over such patterns of responding. Because self-destruction appears most often to be maintained by social reinforcement, we can expect it to come under the control of those stimuli in the environment which signal the availability of social reinforcement. Since it is the social environment that shapes and maintains such behavior patterns and since people are not available to reinforce the behavior in all situations, some situations will be discriminative for self-destruction while others will not. The Lovaas and Simmons (1969) paper amply illustrates this "situationality" in self-destruction. Similar examples of such narrow stimulus control over self-mutilation are provided by children whose self-injury seems to serve as an escape response. That is, to get out of situations where demands are placed on them, self-injurious, psychotic children often appear to "use" self-destruction, much like normal children "use" whining, fussing, and throwing tantrums. For example, Carr, Newsom, and Binkoff (1976) reported on an autistic boy whose rate of self-hitting was very high when simple requests were made of him, but whose rate of self-mutilation dropped immediately to negligible levels when requests were withdrawn. The possibility that self-mutilation may serve as an escape response for some children suggests that extinction may not be an effective procedure for reducing such behavior. In fact, it may worsen it, thus underscoring the importance of assessing the stimulus conditions which maintain self-mutilation in order to discover effective treatments in all cases.

It is now necessary to turn to studies dealing with the punishment of self-injurious behavior. In terms of rapid and probable success, this technique currently constitutes the most significant form of intervention for severe forms of self-destruction in psychotic children. Essentially, we have observed that when a physically aversive stimulus is given contingent upon a self-destructive response, then that response decreases sharply or ceases to be emitted altogether. Lovaas, Schaeffer, and Simmons (1965) first reported such an effect in which a very brief but painful electric shock was applied to the leg contingent on self-destructive and other psychotic behaviors in two 5-year-old autistic boys. Almost immediately, their psychotic behavior decreased to zero. This finding has been replicated both by us and by investigators in a number of other clinics and laboratories (Corte, Wolfe, & Locke, 1971; Lovaas & Simmons, 1969; Merbaum, 1973; Risley, 1968; Tate, 1972; Tate & Baroff, 1966).

Clearly, the use of a physical punishment, like electric shock, with children who have psychological handicaps introduces a wide range of ethical and moral questions which have to be answered. Unfortunately, many of these questions lie beyond the scope and space limits of this chapter, which must primarily concern itself with the evaluation of empirical data. Suffice it to say that there are times when a child is so severely self-destructive that extinction operations cannot be undertaken for the simple reason that the child may kill himself during an extinction run. There may also be times when extinction and other procedures, such as strengthening incompatible behavior, do not work. In situations where one does use pain therapeutically, it has to be a last resort, and justified on the basis that a relatively small pain in the present can be used to prevent a relatively large and enduring pain in the future. The large pain we are referring to could include a lifetime spent in full bodily restraints as well as self-destructive acts leading to permanent tissue damage. Many forms of therapeutic intervention in medicine and dentistry are based on precisely this kind of rationale.

We cannot overemphasize the idea that one should use physical punishment, like shock, only as a last resort. Extinction, time-out, and teaching alternative and incompatible responses must all be tried before it is decided to employ punishment procedures. In addition, placing the child in a new environment or attempting some form of drug regime in combination with the above-mentioned procedures may offer effective alternatives. However, if all these methods fail to eliminate or substantially reduce the self-mutilation, we recommend that the medical and psychological professionals responsible for the case meet with the child's parents to discuss the use of punishment as well as to specify the exact conditions under which it is to be administered. Informed consent from the parents is essential. If it is decided to use shock, each adult should self-administer it several times in order to know just what the child is going to be subjected to. For a more comprehensive presentation of the guidelines to be followed under these circumstances, the reader is referred to the work of May et al. (1974).

Let us present the data on an 8-year-old boy, John, who received such aversive stimulation, because the case illustrates some of the problems one may encounter in doing this work. John had a history of self-destruction going back to the time he was age two, was institutionalized as psychotic and retarded, and had been kept in physical restraints most of his life to prevent excessive self-injury. He had received extensive and unsuccessful prior treatments. In the first treatment situation, "John on lap," John's restraints were removed and the attending nurse sat him on her lap. In the second situation, "John in room," he was left free to move about in his bedroom in the company of two adults. These observations took place on the same ward and were made on a daily basis, each lasting 5 minutes. We recorded the frequency of his self-destructive behavior as well as the amount of time that he attempted to avoid the nurse (defined as struggling to get off her lap) and the amount of time he whined and cried.

The upper half of Figure 22-3 shows the data on John during the lap sessions. On the abscissa are the days, the therapist-experimenter (one of four adults) present during each session, and condition (S denotes a shock punishment session). The frequency of self-destruction and the percent of time that John was avoiding and whining during the session are given on the ordinate. (Due to mechanical failures in the recording apparatus, some data are missing for some sessions.)

The first 15 days were used to obtain John's base rates for these various behaviors. Observe that these rates stayed about the same over this period, neither improving nor getting worse. Punishment, in the form of a one-second electric shock on the leg, was delivered contingent upon self-destructive responding by a hand-held inductorium. The shock was introduced in session 16 with an immediate decrease in self-destruction.

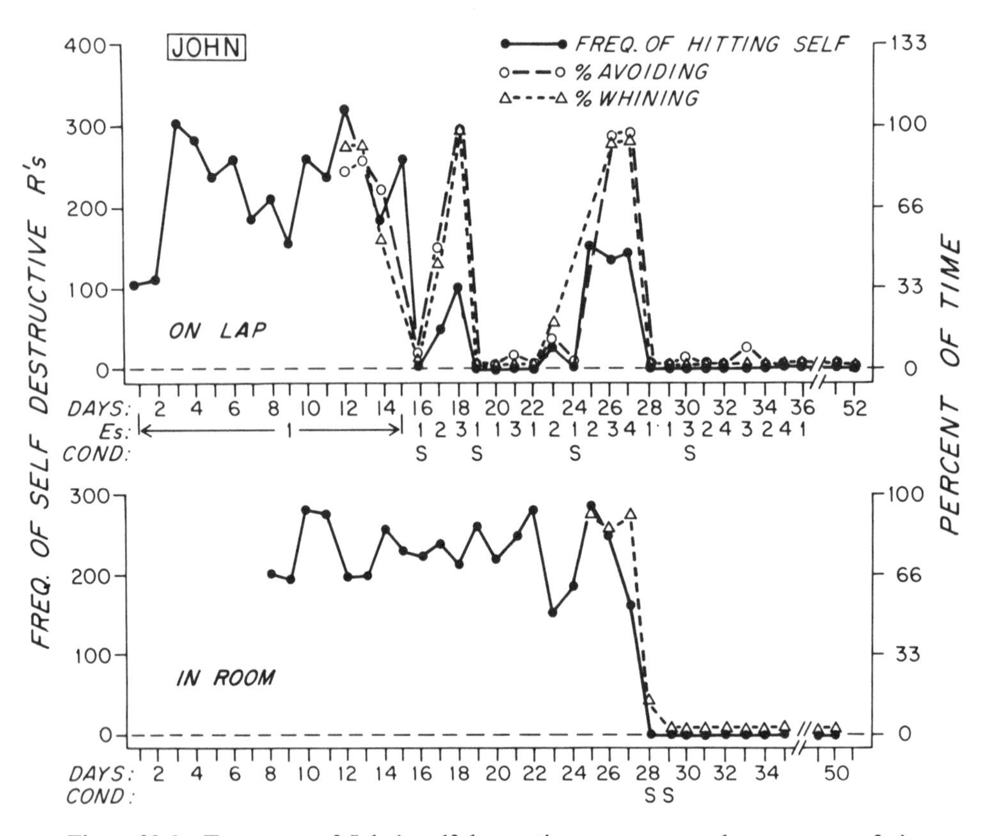

Figure 22-3 Frequency of John's self-destructive responses and percentage of time spent avoiding adults and whining during sessions with and without shock punishment. (Top: 5-minute sessions when John was on nurse's lap. Bottom: 5-minute sessions in a separate room.) The abscissa gives the daily sessions, the attending experimenter, and shock sessions (S).

One observation of interest concerns the generalization of the suppression effect across different adults. Up to session 29, John was punished for self-destruction only by adult 1. Note that the suppression effected by adult 1 generalized only partly to the other adults. John's rate of self-mutilation with the non-punishing adults was climbing alarmingly by sessions 25, 26, and 27. That is, he began to form a discrimination between the adult who punished his self-destruction and those who did not. Adult 3 also punished John for self-destruction in session 30, with the effect of producing generalization across the other adults.

A second important observation pertains to the generalization of shock effects to behavior patterns that were not punished. As the frequency of self-destruction decreased, John avoided the attending adult less and whined less. It would thus appear that avoiding, whining, and self-destruction fell within the same or a similar response class. John's data suggest that the side effects of contingent punishment were desirable. These findings were further confirmed by informal clinical observations (John was observed by some 20 staff members); the nurses' notes reported less psychological distance and less fussing.

There are a number of critical questions left to be explored:

1. In order to effectively suppress self-destruction, what level and distribution of aversive stimulation are optimal? Occasionally, a child is brought to our attention who has received a series of shocks without concomitant suppression of his self-destruction. It is our clinical guess that unless the child shows marked suppression within at least one situation or with one person after 5 to 10 shocks, he will not suppress to shock, and it is pointless to continue. Similarly, self-injurious behavior may be controlled by very different variables in children diagnosed as neurotic rather than psychotic, so that the procedures we have outlined for psychotic children may not apply to other populations.

2. Given a choice, which operation, punishment or extinction, produces the most durable results with the least undesirable side effects? When the child's life is in immediate danger, one clearly cannot employ extinction. But when one does have a choice, extinction may be more effective, since it allows the child to discriminate that the conditions which maintained his self-destruction have been removed. However, the complete answer to this question is simply not known.

3. Is it possible to reduce the high degree of situationality (discriminability) of the punishment and extinction effects? It appears that such situationality varies across children. The older children, especially those with long, varied, and complex reinforcement histories for self-destruction seem to demonstrate the most discriminated effects. We also know that with such children the contingent aversive stimulus has to be administered by more than one person and in more than one environment in order to be maximally effective. It would obviously be very detrimental if the child were simultaneously positively reinforced for self-destruction by other persons or in other situations. Other than using punishment in several different settings and delivered by several different persons, exactly how we might maximize generalization (in order to minimize punishments) is not known.

4. Even though contingent punishment reduces self-mutilation, is it really worth subjecting the child to this pain if he develops other, perhaps more serious, problems as a result of being punished? Surprisingly, all the available evidence indicates that the side effects of proper administration of punishment are desirable. Typically, there is an immediate increase in appropriate, socially directed behavior, such as physical contact and eye contact, as well as a simultaneous decrease in a large number of inappropriate responses, such as whining, fussing, self-isolation, and self-stimulation (Bachman, 1972; Hamilton, Stephens, & Allen, 1967; Kushner, 1970; Lovaas et al., 1965; Lovaas & Simmons, 1969; Risley, 1968; White & Taylor, 1967).

However, there are data clearly suggesting that situations where aversive stimuli are used should be separated from those where one wishes to facilitate language acquisition. We noted a decrease in a child's babbling and an increase in echolalia when the child was observed in a situation where aversive stimuli were used (Bucher & Lovaas, 1968, p. 129, figure 12). Although we are not sure why this occurred, we are obtaining increasing evidence of similar effects with other children.

5. In the face of follow-up data that do not exceed more than one year, when suppression of self-destruction can be observed, can one be optimistic about more long-term behavioral change? If social reinforcement controlled self-destruction in the first place, then that cluster of variables, being unaltered in strength through punishment operations, should retain the power to build other equally undesirable behaviors as

well as to reinstate self-destruction. That is, if the child had to respond self-destructively to gain some attention from his attending adults, then it seems reasonable that these adults, unless specifically taught to respond to the child's more appropriate behavior, may perhaps repeat past mistakes and begin shaping some similarly alarming behavior such as feces smearing, aggression toward other children, and the like. Therefore, we strongly recommend that no one undertake to punish self-destructive responding unless he is prepared to invest a considerable amount of time and effort in explicitly building and maintaining adaptive behaviors which will have a chance of displacing self-mutilation as a means of obtaining social reinforcers. The degree to which reinforcement for behaviors incompatible with self-destruction enhances the durability of the punishment-suppression effects is not known, although the basic research literature suggests it to greatly extend the effects (Azrin & Holz, 1966).

6. Why does the very brief pain over a small area, as is associated with shock delivery, terminate the self-destructive responding which in itself entails a much more prolonged and widespread pain? One reason may be that the child has not adapted to the pain of the shock, as he may have to the pain of his self-mutilation. Self-destructive responses usually build up gradually and to full intensity over a period of months or years. It is known that an organism will continue responding despite a high-intensity punishing stimulus whose full intensity is approached gradually, but will stop responding if a less intense punisher is presented at full strength right from the start (Masserman, 1946; Miller, 1960). Another possible reason is that stimuli which would ordinarily serve as punishers can become discriminative for reinforcement if they are differentially associated with reinforcement (e.g., Azrin & Holz, 1966, pp. 419–424, 428). That is, if the child receives sympathy and attention more reliably when he is self-injurious than when he is not, the presence of pain will become associated with reinforcement, whereas the absence of pain will become associated with non-reinforcement. The pain from self-injury for such a child, then, may acquire positive reinforcing properties.

ANALYSIS AND CONTROL OF SELF-STIMULATORY BEHAVIOR

One of the most peculiar and readily noticeable characteristics of the psychotic child is his large repertoire of stereotyped, repetitive behavior, such as spinning, rocking, hand-flapping, head-rolling, gazing, teeth-grinding, grimacing, saliva-swishing, toe-walking, etc. These behaviors maintain for months and years at very high intensities, and often seem quite unique and set for a particular child. We have referred to such behavior as *self-stimulatory*, because the child appears to "use" the behavior to stimulate himself. Furthermore, these idiosyncratic mannerisms appear to have no observable effect upon the child's social environment, instead providing the child with sensory input from the movements of his own body. Although slightly fewer than half of all psychotic children engage in self-mutilation, and even fewer require specific psychological or medical treatment for such behavior, all the psychotic children we have seen exhibit some pattern of self-stimulatory behaviors.

We paid little attention to self-stimulation in our earlier studies because it often decreased, without any direct intervention, when appropriate behavior was shaped up. Conversely, when the appropriate behaviors extinguished, the self-stimulation would invariably return. Apparently one can also observe a similar reciprocal relationship between appropriate (social, intellectual) behaviors and self-stimulation in normal children. In preliminary work we have placed normal 5- to 6-year-old children in situations not conducive to social or intellectual activity, such as a barren room, and they engaged in various patterns of self-stimulation which were virtually indistinguishable from those exhibited by the psychotic children. One can also observe similar self-stimulation in infants before they acquire true social behavior.

Such an inverse relationship between these two classes of behavior (self-stimulatory motor behavior and appropriate social, affective, and intellectual behavior) led us to suppose that the sensory feedback (proprioceptive, kinesthetic, visual, and auditory) from the self-stimulatory behavior was reinforcing to the child. Since most psychotic and severely retarded children have impoverished social and intellectual repertoires, it hardly seems surprising that they develop strong and elaborate response patterns for sensory consequences. We considered the hypothesis that the central nervous system requires a certain level of sensory input to function adequately (cf. Leuba, 1955; Zubek, 1969), and that behavior (including self-stimulatory behavior) generates the sensory input necessary to maintain some optimal level of activity in the CNS. Under this latter hypothesis, self-stimulation would seem to be rendered biologically useful and meaningful; one may view the sensory stimulation produced as a primary reinforcer, analogous to food and water. Similarly, we came to view psychodynamic attempts to "interpret" self-stimulation, on the premise that it has symbolic, communicative functions, as definitely nontherapeutic.

It soon became apparent that the child's self-stimulation would often actively interfere with the acquisition of new, appropriate behaviors. An example from one of our early studies (Lovaas et al., 1965) will help demonstrate this point. By walking across a room and into the arms of an adult within 5 seconds of a signal, the children could either obtain food or avoid shock. This is an extremely simple task, and the children were hungry and the shock startling. Thus, it was quite incredible to observe that when the child was halfway across the room, and literally inches and seconds away from safety, that he would visually fixate on a shiny door handle, cock his head, and start flapping his arms. The child would in some instances thus miss the opportunity to eat, despite his hunger, or, in other instances, he would receive shock. In fact, we observed no substantial improvement on these tasks until we had *first* directly punished self-stimulation.

Such observations led us to study the blocking effect of self-stimulation on responsiveness to external stimuli. Auditory responsivity of mute autistics, autistics with echolalic speech, and normals was studied under two conditions: when the children were engaged in self-stimulation and when they were free from such behavior (Lovaas, Litrownik, & Mann, 1971). At the sound of a tone, the children were taught to approach a dispenser for candy. Response latency was defined and measured as the time interval between the onset of the tone and the child's approach to the dispenser. We found that (1) in the mute autistics, increased response latencies were associated with the presence of self-stimulation; (2) as the mute autistics received increased training in responding to the auditory stimulus, response latencies decreased; (3) the amount of self-stimulation varied inversely with the magnitude of reinforcement for other behavior; (4) we were able to exert some control over response latencies by experimentally manipulating the amount of self-stimulation.

Particularly strong support for the notion that self-stimulation interferes with the acquisition of new behaviors is provided by Koegel and Covert (1972). Three autistic children characterized by high levels of self-stimulatory behaviors were unable to learn a very simple discrimination *until* the experimenters suppressed the self-stimulation. The children were required to respond by pressing a bar in the presence of a light and a tone, and *not* to respond in the absence of these stimuli. Correct responses were reinforced with food. They made no progress on this task until their self-stimulation was suppressed by the experimenter's yelling "no" and, if necessary, slapping the child on the hand contingent upon self-stimulation. When these interfering behaviors were suppressed the children rapidly learned the correct discrimination.

In a related study, Koegel, Firestone, Kramme, and Dunlap (1974) reported a dramatic increase in spontaneous, appropriate toy play when the self-stimulation of two autistic children was suppressed. In this study spontaneous toy play was never explicitly reinforced. Prior to and following the removal of the suppression contingency, appropriate toy play occurred at near zero levels, while self-stimulation occurred nearly 100% of the time. Conversely, when self-stimulation was punished, its rate fell to zero, and appropriate toy play rose to very high levels.

At the physiological level, several studies seem to support and clarify these findings. Stone (1964) found sleep-like EEG activity following self-stimulation in blind children. Stone speculated that the stimulation involved in some self-stimulatory behaviors is sleep-inducing. Under conditions of continuous auditory stimulation, Brackbill, Adams, Crowell, and Gray (1966) reported decreased arousal levels and more rapid onset of sleep in normal children. They suggested that almost any continuous, monotonous stimulation, including tactile and kinesthetic, could probably produce a similarly decreased arousal level. Sroufe, Stuecher, and Stutzer (1973) interpreted their finding that finger-flicking in an autistic boy was associated with heart rate acceleration as being consistent with Lacey's (1967) conclusion that heart rate acceleration correlates with the withdrawal of attention from the external environment.

At the overt behavioral level, our attempt to understand the relationship between self-stimulation and decreased responsivity to external stimulation has led us to consider the possibility that the stimulation arising from self-stimulatory behavior is strongly reinforcing. Our data (Lovaas et al., 1971; Koegel & Covert, 1972; Koegel et al., 1974) suggest that the child is confronted with the choice between two kinds of reinforcers: self-stimulatory (sensory) reinforcers as opposed to food and social reinforcers. The relative potencies of these two kinds of reinforcers is reflected in the extent to which a child either self-stimulates or behaves appropriately in a situation in which he has learned some appropriate behavior. If a child is hungry and has learned a response which produces food, he will respond for the strong reinforcer and is more likely to not self-stimulate. On the other hand, if the child is not hungry and food would be considered a weak reinforcer, then one is likely to observe self-stimulatory behaviors. Thus, we can often predict the direction of a child's behavior and attention in a given situation if we know the relative strength of the reinforcers which are functional for that child. Since autistic children apparently have a deficiency in socially oriented, appropriate reinforcers, we would expect a high rate of self-stimulatory behaviors. In our earlier study (Lovaas et al., 1971), we suggested that sensory reinforcers may be incompatible with other, more socially appropriate reinforcers, such that a child cannot "enjoy" both at the same time. To allow the relatively weak social reinforcers to become functional (i.e., effectively to compete with strong sensory reinforcement), we have found it necessary to first suppress self-stimulation. Self-stimulatory behavior is thus made aversive instead of reinforcing, at least within the therapy setting, in order to increase the probability that the child will attend to those environmental events which will teach him to function more adequately. Note that extinction procedures alone typically have very little effect on reducing self-stimulation, since such behavior is not maintained by externally manipulable reinforcers. Therefore, punishment procedures, paired with the teaching of more appropriate alternative patterns of responding, appear at present to be necessary for maximal therapeutic effectiveness.

Our analysis of self-stimulation and its relevance to therapeutic efforts with psychotic children can be summarized as follows:

1. Self-stimulatory behavior in psychotic children appears to be incompatible with the acquisition of socially appropriate behaviors, and the child's teacher or therapist may find it necessary to actively suppress self-stimulation in order to facilitate learning. A number of studies have been reviewed by Baumeister and Forehand (1973) indicating that self-stimulatory behaviors may be reduced or eliminated by the use of contingent punishment and by shaping incompatible responses. "Positive practice overcorrection," a recently reported technique, requires the child to practice correct, appropriate behaviors for several minutes each time he engages in self-stimulation (Azrin, Kaplan, & Foxx, 1973; Epstein, Doke, Sajwaj, Sorrell, & Rimmer, 1974; Foxx & Azrin, 1973). Such procedures merit further investigation.

2. The high degree to which psychotic children engage in self-stimulatory behaviors is apparently a function of the limited power social events have to shape and maintain more appropriate behaviors.

3. It may be useful to consider self-stimulation as operant behavior which is maintained by the sensory consequences (Kish, 1966) generated by the behavior itself. Thus self-stimulatory operant behavior may be distinguished from extrinsic or socially controlled operant behavior. In the case of self-stimulatory operants, the person himself controls the reinforcers which maintain the behavior. In the case of extrinsic or social operants, others control the reinforcers and thus the acquisition and maintenance of certain behaviors. Such a distinction poses a number of interesting problems for future research. First, it invites a more detailed analysis of the nature of self-stimulatory reinforcement. Second, it implores us to find techniques which will enable social stimuli to compete more effectively with self-produced sensory reinforcers in these children. These are more properly questions of motiva-

tion, and we will return to them in a later section of this chapter.

Self-mutilation and self-stimulation typically make up the larger part of the behavioral repertoires of severely psychotic children. Other, less pronounced behaviors have not yet been investigated, or we have investigated them without arriving at a satisfactory understanding of their controlling variables. For example, behaviors assumed to indicate a "preference for order" (e.g., resisting changes in furniture arrangement, lining up toys in neat rows), a strong liking for music, and an extensive rote memory remain to be analyzed experimentally. Some of these may be extensions of self-stimulation, and the potential reinforcers which back up these behaviors should be important stimuli to analyze.

Echolalic speech is a phenomenon about which we know very little despite years of effort. Recently, however, Carr, Schreibman, and Lovaas (1975) have presented data suggesting that one of the factors governing immediate echolalia is the incomprehensibility of speech stimuli. Echolalic autistics selectively echoed questions and commands to which no appropriate responses were possible, but did not echo questions and commands to which they could make appropriate responses. Similarly, Baltaxe and Simmons (1975) believe that echolalia reflects "the autistic child's inability to recognize and operate in terms of functional relationships" (p. 453). In another study, Lovaas, Varni, Koegel, and Lorsch (1976) presented data which showed that delayed echolalia did not extinguish over a large number of sessions in controlled situations where no nutritive or social reinforcement was available. In this respect, delayed echolalia resembles the "verbal play" exhibited by young normal children when they are alone and may constitute a more sophisticated form of self-stimulation.

We will now look at programs which have been designed to help these children acquire normal, socially adaptive behaviors. Our focus will be on the programs devised to teach language to psychotic children. Language is the most complex phenomenon we have attempted to teach these children, and our language-training procedures subsume many of the techniques for establishing more "elementary" behaviors.

TEACHING LANGUAGE

Most children acquire language as a matter of course, without anyone quite knowing how or why they do so. However, autistic children are usually without functional language, being either mute or echolalic. In order to help such children talk, we need to know how language comes about. Traditional attempts to help autistic children learn language have apparently been neither systematic nor very successful. Such attempts have been concerned with viewing the child's language problems as symptomatic of an underlying psychodynamic aberration or expressive of some cognitive dysfunction, with emphasis on providing some relatively nonspecific remedial experiences. However, rather than focus our attention on the emotional or cognitive aspects of language, we chose to view it functionally by attempting to manipulate specific learning variables as precisely as possible in order to produce predictable language acquisition. While our approach may not delineate the etiology of the child's language problem, it may bring about important changes now. Furthermore, what we learn about teaching language to psychotic children can prove useful to many—to parents, teachers, and clinicians engaged in remedial language training with many kinds of language problems.

It is possible to consider language acquisition as the learning of at least two events. First, the child must acquire verbal responses which differ in levels of complexity. One level includes phonemic acquisition (i.e., the basic speech sounds of the consonants and vowels); another level concerns morphemic behavior (words and parts of words); still another involves grammatical response patterns (arrangement of words in sentences). A large repertoire of verbalizations does not by itself constitute what we call language; utterances can easily exist without meaning. Verbalizations are meaningful only insofar as they are appropriate to the context in which they occur. That is, certain aspects of the child's environment must acquire stimulus functions which serve to regulate the occurrence of his vocal output. To achieve this, a child must learn which stimuli or cuing conditions, be they external or internal, give rise to which utterances. The child must also learn what stimulus functions the utterance itself should possess, that is, what further verbal or nonverbal behavior, in himself or others, may be evoked by that verbalization. Thus the second requisite for language is the acquisition of stimulus functions, or in linguistic terminology, *semantics*.

In working with nonlinguistic children, one soon realizes how handicapped they are without language. They appear to have little or no comprehension of what is said to them; similarly, they have no easy way to express how they feel or what they want. Our goal is for language to become a means for facilitating social interactions and to help the child recognize, express, and cope with his feelings. Early in our work, we had in the back of our minds a notion that if the child learned to talk, somehow a "conception of himself" would emerge, that he might become "more defined as a person," that he might show more self-control.

Before we begin trying to teach language per se, we must "prepare" the child for the teaching situation. If the child is self-mutilative, we attempt to suppress that behavior. Also, as has previously been mentioned, a special effort is made to suppress self-stimulation in order to maximize the probability that the child will attend to the therapist. Simultaneous with the suppression of inappropriate behaviors, the therapist attempts to establish some early forms of stimulus control. For example, the child is required to comply with some very simple demands, such as sitting quietly in a chair for half-a-minute. Since even such a minimal request often evokes tantrums, self-destruction, or self-stimulatory behavior, the establishment of this basic stimulus control and the reduction of aggression and self-stimulation proceed together. It is generally impossible to work on the acquisition of appropriate behaviors until one has achieved some reduction of pathological behaviors. A more complete intervention program for building language within a behavioral framework has been presented in a book (Lovaas, 1977) and on film (Lovaas, 1969), but the basic outline will be presented here. Additional sources for procedures very similar to ours are Kent (1974) and Kozloff (1974).

BUILDING A VERBAL TOPOGRAPHY.

With the therapist and child sitting closely facing each other and the child attending to the therapist's face, one can begin teaching verbal behaviors through imitation. The basic paradigm involves building various discriminations. This is done by reinforcing a response that occurs when a stimulus is presented and attended to, and withholding reinforcement if the response occurs to another stimulus. Reinforcement is also withheld if another, incorrect response, occurs to the training stimulus. With consistency, a particular stimulus becomes discriminative for the appropriate response; we say that the stimulus "occasions" the response because it signals that the response will be reinforced in its presence. An imitative response is one which has the same topography as its controlling discriminative stimulus. That is, the response "resembles" its stimulus such that when the therapist says "ah," the child says "ah." Verbal imitation training usually progresses along the following steps. In Step 1, the therapist attempts to increase the child's vocalizations by rewarding him with praise and perhaps bites of food contingent upon any vocalizations. The child is fondled, tickled, etc., in order to make the situation more conducive to emitting sounds. We do this with mute children in order to obtain some vocalizations with which to work. Step 2 involves teaching the child to make a temporal discrimination: His vocalizations are reinforced only if they occur within about 3 seconds after the therapist's vocalizations. In Step 3 closer approximations of the therapist's vocalizations are reinforced. Successively closer approximations to the therapist's speech sound are reinforced until the child matches the particular sound given by the therapist (e.g., emits "ah" soon after the therapist says "ah"). The sounds to be imitated are selected according to several criteria. Usually they are those sounds most frequently emitted while the frequency of vocalizations was being increased (Step 1). Second, sounds are chosen that have concomitant visual components which can be exaggerated by the therapist. Finally, some sounds are particularly easy to prompt manually; that is, the child's mouth can be held in the appropriate shape while he vocalizes. For example, the sound "mm" is prompted by holding the child's lips together when he vocalizes. In Step 4, the therapist repeats Step 3 with a second sound very different from the first one. For example, if "ah" was the first sound, "mm," "be," or "t" would be an appropriate second sound. Once the child can reliably imitate the second sound, the therapist intersperses the two sounds and reinforces the child only for correct productions. Increasingly finer discriminations are required as new sounds are added, then syllables, words, and sentences are taught as the child becomes able to master them.

The course of acquisition of verbal imitation for Billy and Chuck, the first two mute psychotic children we taught to imitate, is presented in Figure 22-4. Phonemes and words are presented in lower case letters on the days they were introduced

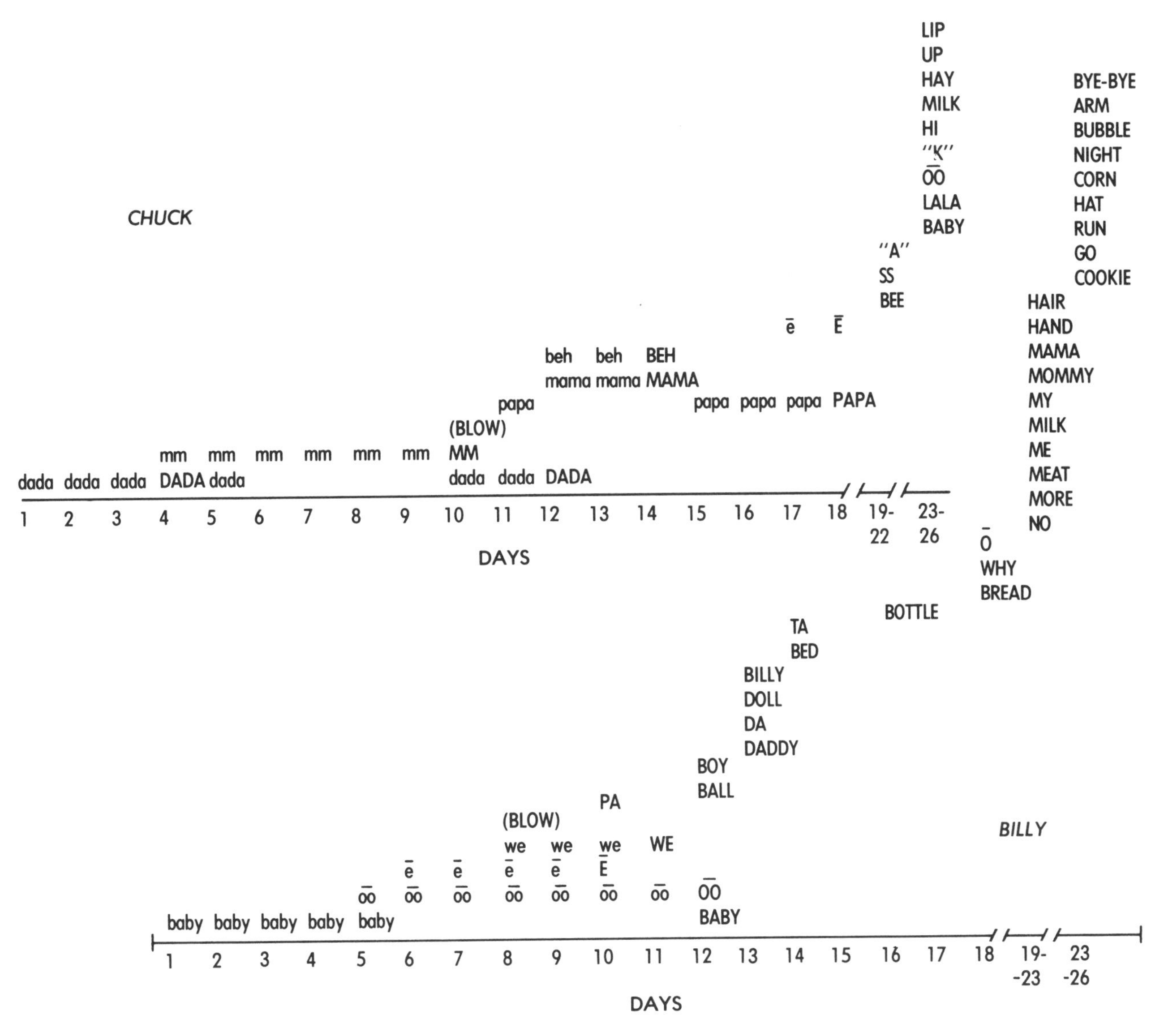

Figure 22-4 The first 26 days of verbal imitation training for Billy and Chuck, psychotic boys who were mute before training. The sounds and words are printed in lower case letters on the days they were introduced and in capitals on the days they were mastered.

and practiced, and in capital letters on the days they were mastered. Notice that each cumulative curve is positively accelerated, indicating that each child learned new verbal discriminations more and more easily and rapidly as imitation training progressed. Obviously, if the child exhibits echolalia, verbal imitation training can proceed more quickly than if the child is mute.

TEACHING MEANING (STIMULUS FUNCTIONS).

While a child may come to imitate the vocalizations of others, he will not automatically know the meanings of the words he utters. The acquisition of meaningful speech involves establishing a *context* for speech, which we view as learning two basic discriminations. An expressive discrimination involves a nonverbal stimulus and a verbal response (e.g., labeling and describing). The second, termed a receptive discrimination, consists of a verbal stimulus and a nonverbal response. This refers to speech comprehension where the child and his behavior come under the verbal control of others. It is true, of course, that most language situations are neither strictly "expressive" nor "receptive" but involve components of both discriminations.

The speech program based on teaching these two discriminations begins with labeling of objects and events and is made functional as soon as possible. Once the child can label objects and events in his environment, we demand that he use these labels to receive access to what they denote. In this way, talking becomes rewarding for the child, and we try to make speaking intrinsically rewarding in and of itself without any external prompts or reinforcers. The program gradually moves on to helping the child become increasingly proficient in language, including teaching more abstract terms such as pronouns and adjectives, verb tenses, and the use of language to please others in such activities as recall or story telling.

Throughout language training, we place particular emphasis on requiring the child to use the words, phrases, and sentences that he knows. That is, once a particular level of competence has been reached, anything below that level becomes unacceptable, so that the child is required to use his "best" or most complex language forms at any given time. For example, if the child has previously and reliably (on several occasions) demonstrated that he can say "I want a piece of gum," we would not accept "piece of gum" or "gum."

Figure 22-5 presents data on the acquisition of verbal labels for some body parts and common objects by two previously mute psychotic children. The similarity between Figures 22-4 and 22-5 is most probably attributable to the communality and lawfulness of the process we believe underlies verbal imitation and acquisition of meaning, namely discrimination learning. The high degree of behavioral complexity we have achieved with some of these children is amply illustrated by our procedures and data on teaching abstract concepts, such as prepositional and time relationships, and on grammar (Lovaas, 1977). In these programs, the children have learned to generate their own sentences and to respond to stimuli they had not previously encountered.

It may be useful to review our work and that of others as it relates to the more traditional ways in which language has been considered to develop. We will discuss how the phonetic, semantic, and syntactic aspects of language can be viewed within a learning theory framework. In doing so, it will be apparent that there are some significant gaps in our knowledge; these serve as impetuses for further research because the strengths of our approach are clearly reflected in the children with whom we have spent any large amount of time.

SEMANTICS.

A major question in language development concerns the acquisition of meaning, or how verbalizations become associated with the appropriate context. There are at least two dimensions that characterize this "context": the environmental stimuli that trigger the vocalizations and the verbal behavior itself, which cues further responding in either the speaker or the listener.

In our own therapeutic efforts, we have repeatedly found that the verbalizations of autistic children can be brought under the control of a large range of environmental stimuli, both external and internal (Lovaas, 1977). Through differential rein-

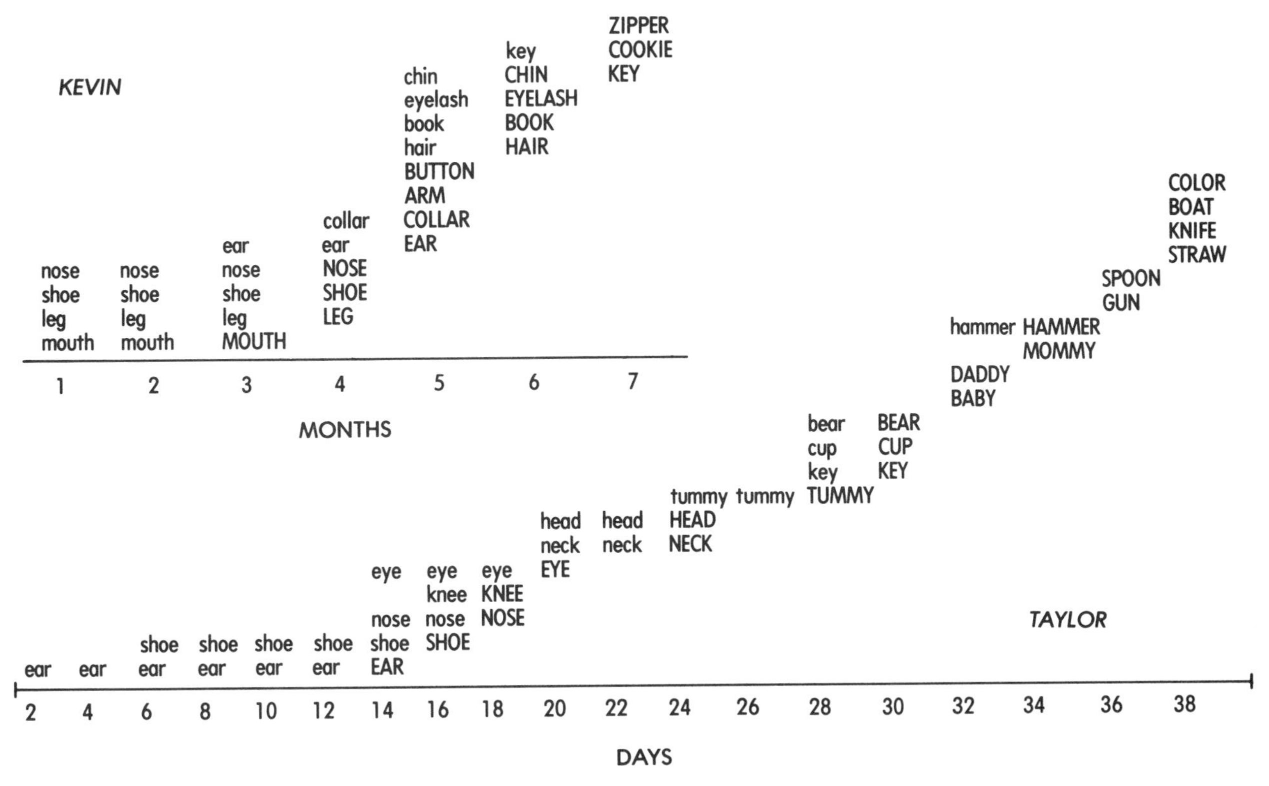

Figure 22-5 Acquisition of expressive labels by two previously mute psychotic boys. Introduction and mastery of labels are differentially indicated by lower case and capital letters as in Figure 22-4. The different scales of the abscissae indicate the range of acquisition rates for these psychotic children.

forcement, we have taught discriminations between purely internal events such as various feeling states (e.g., anxious, relaxed, happy, hungry), and among such structurally similar statements as "Ricky is a bad boy," "Is Ricky a bad boy?" and "Ricky is a big boy." Our data on the acquisition of meaning (semantics) is perhaps our strongest point and relates to a small body of similar investigations that have been published in the last few years.

A group of researchers at the University of Kansas has provided one of the more detailed accounts of operant procedures for language acquisition, including semantics. These studies describe prompting, prompt fading, stimulus rotation, timing of reinforcement, and a number of additional procedures similar to those we employ. Their first study (Wolf et al., 1964) described the establishment of a 10-word labeling vocabulary in a $3\frac{1}{2}$-year-old psychotic echolalic boy. Risley and Wolf (1967) presented data on the acquisition of broader classes of functional speech (i.e., beyond simple labeling) in four psychotic children.

Although the two programs were developed independently, the techniques employed by the Kansas group are strikingly similar to those we have outlined. In addition to demonstrating the positive acceleration in learning (savings over tasks) that characterizes our results, these researchers comment on many of the same learning difficulties we have enountered, such as the loss of previously mastered material as new stimuli are introduced and the difficulty in shifting correct responding from prompt to training stimuli. Accounts of similar programs designed to establish labeling vocabularies are reported by Cook and Adams (1966), Hewett (1965), Risley and Wolf (1966), Salzinger, Feldman, Cowan, and Salzinger (1965), and Sloane, Johnston, and Harris (1968).

Another aspect of semantics is concerned with

teaching verbal comprehension, that is, appropriate nonverbal responses to verbal instructions, questions, and commands. Studies by Davison (1964), Hartung (1970), Schell, Stark, and Giddan (1967), and Stark, Giddan, and Meisel (1968) are representative of this area. Their data again show positive acceleration in that the child acquires mastery over each successive task in a lesser number of trials.

The literature pertaining to the acquisition of abstractions (pronouns, prepositions, etc.) is scarce compared to that for simple labeling. Sailor and Taman (1972), for example, evaluated the effects of using the same stimulus objects to train both "on" and "in" as opposed to using a different pair of objects with each word. As one might expect, they found that correct usage of the prepositions was much more likely to occur when each word was trained with a separate set of objects.

Historically, the importance of learning or experience in the development of meaning has not been debated by most writers. Perhaps this accounts for the relative paucity of research into this area. Yet there are many issues related to the acquisition of semantics that have not been adequately resolved. For example, it seems that we need to know what actually constitutes a stimulus, which apparently is the critical issue in teaching semantics. We need to know what the child is learning about his environment, how subtle a difference between stimuli he can be taught to respond to and at what ages, how broad a range of events may constitute a stimulus, and so on.

SYNTAX

Many investigators feel that the structure of language (grammar) is too complex to be acquired through learning processes as we now know them. This problem derives in part from early attempts to define stimuli and responses solely in topographical rather than in functional terms, and to consider stimulus and response generalization in terms of physical structure rather than functional relatedness. Such definitional attempts placed severe limitations on the flexibility of learning theory formulations and virtually excluded syntax as learned behavior. The classic argument used to support the nativistic position is that people will speak grammatically correct sentences even though those particular sequences of words may have never been uttered in the past. Brown and Bellugi (1964) state the argument in this way: "Children are able to understand and construct sentences (and grammatical forms) they have never heard but which are, nonetheless, well formed, i.e., well formed in terms of the general rules that are implicit in the sentences the child has heard" (p. 151). This observation led many linguists to postulate certain theoretical concepts such as "generative" grammar and "rule-generated" language. Further, these concepts were endowed with many neurologically based innate determinants.

This argument that language is primarily innately determined is, of course, not new. For centuries, those who have wondered how such a complex phenomenon as human language comes about have emphasized either the view that language is determined by innate capacities or the position that it is learned or determined by environmental or experiential variables. Chomsky (1965) and Lenneberg (1964) are currently most closely associated with the nativistic position. The environmentalist view has been most closely associated with Skinner (1957), Mowrer (1960), and to some extent Berko (1958), Brown and Fraser (1964), and Ervin (1964). Hopefully, our research and therapy will lend more credence to one of these positions than the other, or at least point to a strong interaction between the two.

How can the flexibility reflected in correctly understanding and expressing novel and grammatically correct sentences be conceptualized within learning theory? In this regard, the concept of *response class* becomes directly useful. This concept allows for the occurrence of behavior which has not been specifically practiced or reinforced in the past, provided other responses within the same class have been executed or reinforced. Most critics of learning approaches to syntax appear not to be fully aware of the response class concept. The members of a response class are related in that an operation that changes the strength of one response indirectly alters the strength of the other responses

(Bijou & Baer, 1967, p. 78; Segal, 1972). For example, let us suppose that an infant emits the phoneme "da" and receives the attention and praise of his parents. One may well observe an increase in a large range of other phonemes, such as "ee," "ah," "ba," "oh," and "ma" and in facial movements, even though these additional responses have never been emitted or reinforced before.

One of the earliest reports relating the concept of a response class to the acquisition of grammatical forms came from the study by Salzinger and his colleagues (1965). They observed language development in one child who was reinforced for the response "gimme candy." They subsequently observed an increase in the use of the "gimme ———" response with a whole series of new words and strings of words *without* the additional "specific reinforcement of these combinations." Examples include "gimme tape," "gimme office," "gimme no more cloudy again," and a perfectly logical, although ungrammatical, request for assistance, "gimme pick it up." In this study, the concurrent appearance of these functionally similar responses illustrates the response class concept. Data consistent with the response class concept are reported by Guess, Sailor, Rutherford, and Baer (1968) and by Sailor (1971) for the acquisition of plurals and by Schumaker and Sherman (1970) in teaching past and present verb tenses.

Evidence that word classes function as response classes provides the basis for an argument that psychotic children can also learn what position different word classes may occupy in a given sentence. This hypothesis is, however, complicated by the fact that a particular word class may occupy a number of positions depending upon many diverse environmental and motivational variables. This complexity, which is at the heart of the argument that syntax cannot be learned, has led some investigators to propose that a speaker must know the rules of sentence structure in order to properly combine word classes. We suggest that such rules can be considered to be the definitions of higher order verbal response classes, and that practice and reinforcement of the grammatically permissible orders of words and classes (and non-reinforcement of nonpermissible orders) can create response classes of sentence length. Salzinger (1968) states that "a second kind of complexity is introduced by response classes of a somewhat larger size than, say, word classes. To the outside observer these response classes appear to be quite obviously based on rules. Thus the 'rule' for sentence type is a grammatical one or a series of these having to do with the arrangement of words and phrases" (p. 123). It is therefore possible to conceptualize sentences as forming the response unit of interest when considering the acquisition of sentence structures, just as it was possible to speak of words as forming the unit of interest in the acquisition of word classes.

Our efforts, as well as those of others (Salzinger, 1968; Garcia, Guess, & Byrnes, 1973), have demonstrated that it is possible to prompt and differentially reinforce a child for arranging words into phrases and sentences, and that as a function of this intervention, the child will then combine new words into novel and grammatically correct sentences. All our echolalic children, and some of the previously mute ones, have been able to acquire such verbal behavior. An illustration is provided by Wheeler and Sulzer (1970) who worked with an 8-year-old boy, variously diagnosed as autistic, brain damaged, and retarded. The child was taught to use a particular kind of sentence structure to describe a standardized set of pictures through the use of differential reinforcement, chaining, and imitative prompting techniques. The sentences used the form, "The (noun) is (present participle of the verb) the (noun)," e.g., "The girl is feeding the cat." The authors argued that a functional response class had been established since the use of this form generalized to sets of untaught and novel stimuli.

Working with a culturally disadvantaged, linguistically impoverished, nonpsychotic population, Risley, Reynolds, and Hart (1970) have also presented evidence supporting the feasibility of using prompting and differential reinforcement to build elaborate sentence structure. They give the following account of their method, which they refer to as "narration training" and which is very similar to our program for psychotic children entitled "spontaneity training."

> If the child had responded to the question, "What did you see on the way to school?" with, "A doggie," the teacher nodded and said, "What kind of doggie?" The child answered, "A German shepherd." The teacher praised the child and then asked again, "What did you see on the way to school?" He answered, "A doggie;" the teacher looked expectantly, raised her eyebrows and waited. The child then said, "A German shepherd doggie," and was again praised by the teacher. The next time the child responded to the question with, "A German shepherd doggie," the teacher nodded, smiled and asked what the doggie was doing; to which the child responded, "Fighting." This was reinforced and the child again was asked, "What did you see on the way to school?" The child responded, "A German shepherd doggie," and the teacher raised her eyebrows and waited and the child said, "A German shepherd doggie was fighting." (1970, p. 251)

Risley and co-workers (1970) present data demonstrating generalization of this elaboration of grammatical output to new situations that had not specifically been taught.

Stevens-Long and Rasmussen (1974) report similar success at building sentences. Using imitative prompts and reinforcement, they taught both simple and compound sentences to an autistic boy. Furthermore, they showed how this behavior generalized to new stimulus situations in which the child had received no direct training.

Finally, let us briefly consider Premack's (1970, 1971) work on training a chimpanzee in the acquisition of prepositions. He reports on (1) choosing and rotating stimuli in such a fashion as to allow Sarah to discriminate the correct dimensions of the training stimulus ("... to assure that our subject uses syntactic definitions from the beginning ..."); (2) using prompts to facilitate the desired response ("... to bring about the desired behavior by limiting the probability of other kinds of behavior..."); and (3) testing for generalization to new (untrained) stimuli. Premack as well as Gardner and Gardner (1971) note positive acceleration as a characteristic feature of the acquisition of language-like behaviors in chimpanzees. Both studies also report a substantial amount of stimulus generalization and interchangeability of responses within a given class. Thus, these researchers provide additional support for the utility of the response class concept and the power of discrimination training in teaching sentence structure. Other excellent discussions of the response-class model and its relationship to the acquisition of complex behavior are presented by Baer, Guess, and Sherman (1972), MacCorquodale (1969, 1970), Segal (1972), Sherman (1971), and Wiest (1967).

Phonetics

Since we already have some knowledge of how to teach a young psychotic child semantics and grammar, it would seem a relatively simple matter to engineer phonological development. But in practice this is not always the case. Although the use of discrimination training procedures to teach verbal imitation clearly assures some progress in phonological development for the mute child, clinical observations often reveal large differences between the "imitation trained," previously mute child and the echolalic child. Echolalic children clearly and effortlessly imitate an adult's speech; they talk frequently and "play" with their speech. On the other hand, the verbalizations of previously mute children often stay closely dependent on the experimental reinforcers, frequently deteriorate ("drift" away from the criterion), sound stilted, etc. Our language program has, in general, been more successful for the echolalic children than for the mute ones. Although the echolalic child often does not know the meaning of his verbalizations or how to arrange them into appropriate sentences, we find that language remediation is relatively easy. That is, we are usually very successful in rearranging the echolalic child's verbal output (syntax) and bringing it under appropriate stimulus control (semantics). However, we are often less successful in creating and maintaining new verbal topographies.

There are some important and interesting exceptions to our failure at teaching phonetics. As a result of intensive verbal imitation training, many mute children become echolalic. That is, their word production becomes extensive and takes on the qualities of the echolalic child's imitations, a phenomenon that is particularly true when treatment is begun before the child is 3 or 4 years of age. These same findings have been described by Hewett

(1965) and Hartung (1970). When working with a child who remains essentially mute after intensive, repeated attempts to teach words, it may prove useful to try to teach manual signs like those used with deaf children (Creedon, 1973; Webster, McPherson, Sloman, Evans, & Kuchar, 1973).

The building of language has been considered by many to be a most difficult and challenging task. Despite some apparent limitations on phonological development, behavioral approaches to teaching complex language have met with considerable success.

TYPICAL COURSE OF TREATMENT

This chapter has delineated certain aspects of a behavioral approach to the treatment of psychotic children. We will now present a more concise summary of the typical treatment program. When the parents first bring their child to the clinic, he is typically either completely indifferent to our first intervention attempts or reacts with severe tantrums, aggression, and self-mutilation. Occasionally, a child is alternatively indifferent and aggressively negativistic. The parents are completely befuddled. Since tantrums, aggression, self-destruction, and self-stimulation interfere with and often preclude the acquisition of more appropriate and adaptive behaviors, we attempt to suppress these pathological behaviors from the beginning. The first three appear social and may be dealt with by any of three techniques: extinction, time-out, and punishment. The last, self-stimulation, can typically be reduced only through punishment procedures combined with the establishment of incompatible, appropriate responses.

Extinction, since it is the least aversive technique, is nearly always tried first, except in cases of more severe self-destruction. Extinction requires the therapist to completely remove his attention from the child contingent upon crying, whining, aggressiveness, or mild self-injurious responses. The therapist must not look at the child, speak to him, or in any way show an awareness of what the child is doing; others in the environment must also follow the same procedure. One should be prepared for an initial increase in these behaviors; however, persistence in the correct application of extinction procedures usually results in a decrease and finally a cessation of such negativistic behaviors.

If extinction does not work in reducing the frequency of these disruptive behaviors, the therapist may then implement time-out procedures, i.e., placement of the child in a "time-out" area where there is no opportunity to obtain reinforcement. The area should be devoid of other people, toys, or objects that the child could use to entertain himself. It is important that the child remain in the time-out area for at least several minutes after the disruptive behavior has ceased *and* that the act of placing the child in time-out is not in itself reinforcing. Thus, the therapist must not spend time arguing with or elaborately explaining to the child why he is being placed in the time-out area. One must act quickly and decisively.

Punishment procedures remain the final alternative if these behaviors continue to be extreme or severe. They are indicated especially if it is felt that a self-destructive child could severely hurt himself during extinction, or if the child is using the disruptive behaviors to escape working and is thus rewarded by extinction or time-out. It should again be mentioned that self-simulatory activities, particularly if they are intense in nature, respond little, if at all, to extinction and time-out procedures. Therefore, various forms of contingent punishment are usually the most effective methods of dealing with this type of pathological behavior. As we have mentioned previously, punishment must be presented contingent upon, and immediately following, each inappropriate act. Contingent aversives can take the form of a loud "No," or if that is ineffective, one can progress to slaps on the hands, arms, or legs. We have found it necessary to use contingent shock only with children who are so severely self-destructive that they endanger their own lives. It is important to try the least aversive form of punishment first, progressing to more extreme forms only if necessary. The therapist should pair the command "No" with the delivery of the physical punishment so that the child will learn that "No" means to stop. Finally, it is most important that different therapists apply the punishment in different settings when and if the behaviors in question occur in order to promote generalization of treatment effects. The cold tone and technical language of the previous paragraphs represent a deliberate attempt on our part to state the procedures objectively in order to help the clinician avoid mistakes. Mistakes are ultimately very costly to the child. Pleasant, folksy, and "humanistic" presentations of therapeutic technique seem to benefit the therapist who cares more about discussing his work than his patients. Note that if all goes well, little or no disciplinary measures should be necessary beyond the first few weeks or months of treatment.

Concurrent with the reduction of disruptive, pathological behaviors, the therapist begins to teach more appropriate patterns of responding. It is important that these two endeavors occur simultaneously because if one were to concentrate solely on the reduction of disruptive behaviors, there would be little chance for the child to be rewarded for appropriate and incompatible behavior. Thus, one may begin treatment by teaching the child to sit in a chair properly and to visually attend to the therapist's face. Typically, the autistic child will react to these early attempts to control his behavior with tantrums, aggression, self-destruction, or self-stimulation. Proper sitting and looking are lavishly rewarded with bites of food, kisses, stroking, and whatever else may be functional reinforcers for that child.

Let us briefly summarize the teaching steps thus far. Up to this point the child has been taught to sit in a chair, to look at the therapist when the latter says "look at me," and to suppress tantrum, self-destructive, and self-stimulatory activities. We will now describe the acquisition of three major categories of behavior: (1) nonverbal imitative behavior, (2) following commands, and (3) verbal imitative behavior.

Casual observation suggests that children normally acquire a large proportion of their social and intellectual skills by imitating the actions of others. We have reasoned that the extent to which autistic children have failed in their affective, social, and intellectual development may be reflected in their lack of imitative behaviors. As such, we have found that by first requiring the child to imitate simple responses, it is possible to teach the more complex behaviors involved in early intellectual, social, and self-help skills (Lovaas, Berberich, Perloff, & Schaeffer, 1966; Lovaas et al., 1967). Therefore we spend considerable time (from weeks to months, depending on the child) teaching imitation of nonverbal behavior, such as arm-raising, hand-clapping, gestures, facial expressions, touching various body parts, etc. If the child is mute, we also concentrate heavily on imitation of simple sounds (e.g., "ma," "de") and progress to imitation of words. Throughout this period we demand the child's "best performance." That is, if he has demonstrated he can work at a certain level, we do not reinforce him for performing below his best level.

Soon after the child has acquired several imitative responses, we shift the stimulus cuing these responses from a physical to a verbal one. Thus, the child is taught to execute nonverbal behaviors when the therapist verbally requests him to do so, and such "following commands" comes to form the beginning of receptive language. Along with the acquisition of these kinds of receptive language abilities, we also begin a receptive labeling program in which the child is taught to discriminate various objects from one another. For example, a block and a spoon are placed in front of the child, who is then required to give one of the objects, upon request, to the therapist. In this way we teach the names of objects. Soon after such training in receptive labeling, the child is taught to use the names of these objects expressively.

Following the reduction of disruptive, inappropriate and bizarre behaviors and the acquisition of a relatively generalized verbal and nonverbal imitative repertoire, the remainder of our therapeutic efforts focus largely on the development of cognitive, social, and intellectual abilities. This invariably requires us to expand and enhance the child's receptive and expressive language abilities. We have previously discussed our language program at some length; however, suffice it to say that with any given child, the major part of our time and effort is spent in this language acquisition process. In addition, we try to teach all those behaviors which these children do not typically display. These include peer-play, appropriate play with toys, how to behave in public, how to express proper affect, and self-help skills such as proper eating, dressing, toileting, etc. This may seem like an enormous task, and it is, but the basic teaching steps (learning procedures) are similar for each behavior.

An important variable, especially in the early stages of treatment, concerns the exaggeration of the therapist's approval and disapproval for correct and incorrect responding, respectively. If the child does respond appropriately, the therapist lavishes him with affection and praise so that his correct responses are reinforced with as much emotionally laden and vivid social approval as the therapist can muster. On the other hand, if the child engages in pathological behaviors he engenders the therapist's immediate, harsh, and very loud disapproval. This overemphasis on the affective component of the therapist's approval and disapproval seems critical for the child's progress. Furthermore, we have found that if a child receives deserved approval for correct responses, and no disapproval for responding incorrectly, the positive reinforcement often rapidly loses its power to control any behavior at all. Our praise, love, and affection, no matter how intense and genuine, simply seem to lose any reinforcing function if they are not combined with appropriate feedback for inappropriate or incorrect responses. It should be apparent that this exaggeration of approval and disapproval far beyond that which is typically necessary to teach less severely disturbed children is indeed a very difficult thing for a therapist to learn. It often requires the therapist to be contingently harsh, punitive, and disapproving with the child and then to do an about-face and be contingently loving, reassuring, warm, and approving. Not everyone is able to do this.

It also appears that antecedent stimuli can play a very important motivating role. The affective tone of stimuli that set the occasion for a response to be reinforced clearly influences the probability of occurrence of that behavior. Thus, we place much importance on presenting our discriminative stimuli, especially verbal ones, in a lively, animated manner, and they have to be presented discretely. Monotonous, emotionally flat antecedents from the therapist typically result in either no response from the child or behavior that is itself affectively shallow and monotonic. Therefore, the therapist must not only present response consequences that are affectively heightened, but also antecedents that are animated and lively, in an effort to increase the probability that the child will respond to such discriminative stimuli.

In the initial stages of treatment we require the child's parent, typically the mother, to devote most of her day to the child, and we train the parents to become the child's primary therapists. The majority of this training is done in the child's home. As a result, the child's environment becomes totally restructured and one in which he receives treatment throughout his daily life. Simply stated, if the child is awake, he receives treatment. We also try to teach the child's siblings and neighborhood friends to function as peer-therapists. After about 6 to 8 months of treatment, we try to place the young autistic child in a *normal* preschool where we slowly fade the child into the group, train his new teacher how to cope with him, initially provide her with a teacher-aide, and so on. We rely heavily on volunteers from college classes in behavior modification to implement the program. These undergraduates are under the direct supervision of senior therapists. In short, our therapeutic efforts are *massive* and they occur in the child's normal environment.

GENERALIZATION AND FOLLOW-UP RESULTS

Let us illustrate the kinds of treatment changes and follow-up measures we have obtained from the first group of children we treated. This is included here because it demonstrates certain problems in our initial treatment efforts, and our attempts to remedy the weaknesses. Lovaas, Koegel, Simmons, and Long (1973) examined three measures of the generality of treatment effects: (1) stimulus generalization, or the degree to which behavioral changes that occurred in the treatment setting transferred to other situations; (2) response generalization, or the extent to which changes in a specific, limited set of behaviors effected changes in other broader areas of functioning; and (3) durability, or the maintenance over time of the therapeutic effects.

Five categories of behaviors were recorded in a free-play situation. The setting was different from the treatment environment and people were present who had not treated the child. Two of the behavioral categories, *echolalia* and *self-stimulation* were inappropriate. Three were appropriate: *appropriate verbal*, which was understandable and grammatically correct speech related to an appropriate context; *social nonverbal*, which referred to appropriate nonverbal interaction with another person; and *appropriate play*, which referred to the use of toys and objects in an age-related, appropriate manner. These measures were taken before treatment started, at the end of 12 to 14 months of therapy, and in a follow-up evaluation conducted from 1 to 4 years after treatment was terminated. These data are presented in Figure 22-6, which show measures before treatment (B), after about 14 months of treatment (A), and at follow-up, 2 to 4 years later (F). The children were divided into two groups—those who were later discharged to a state hospital (I) and those who remained with their parents (P).

Figure 22-6 reveals that all the children improved with treatment. After 12 to 14 months of treatment there was a substantial reduction in inappropriate behaviors and a corresponding increase in appropriate ones. The follow-up data also pose a warning: The children who were institutionalized lost most of what they had gained. Their psychotic behavior (self-stimulation and echolalia) increased and they regressed in terms of appropriate social, verbal, and play behaviors. On the other hand, the children who stayed with their parents either maintained their gains or improved further. We have data to show that a brief reinstatement of behavior therapy could temporarily reestablish the original therapeutic gains for the children who had regressed during hospitalization.

The follow-up data clearly emphasize certain important points concerning the use of behavior

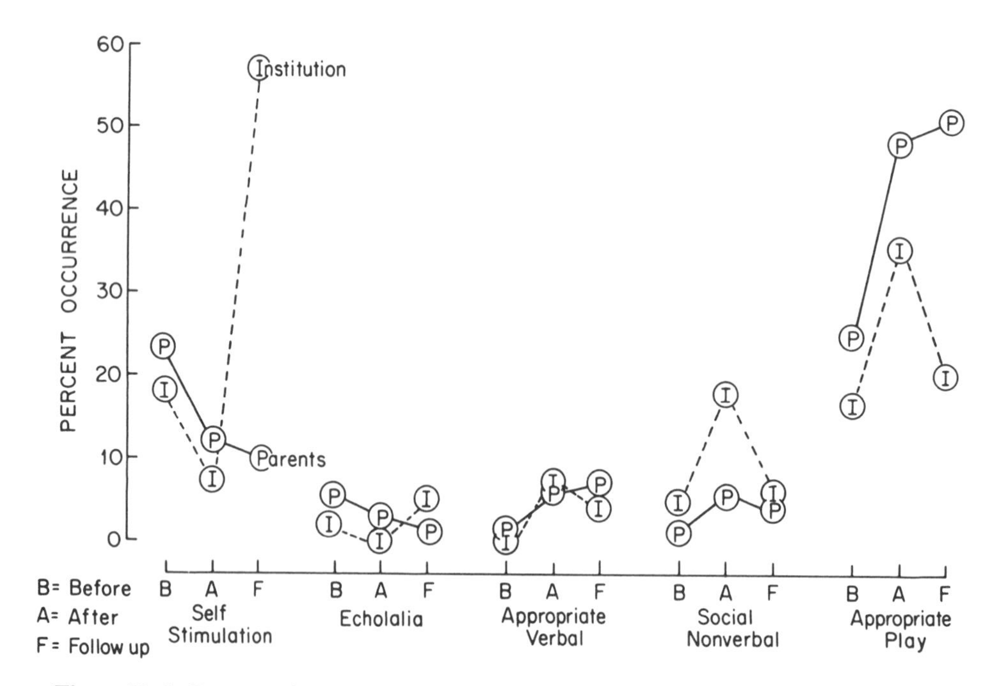

Figure 22-6 Percent of time psychotic children engaged in five classes of behaviors during sessions conducted before treatment (B), after treatment (A), and at follow-up (F). "I" refers to the average results for four children who were institutionalized after treatment; "P" refers to the average results for the nine children who lived with parents after treatment.

therapy with these children. It is simply not enough to help the child acquire appropriate behaviors and overcome the inappropriate ones; it is also necessary to provide maintaining conditions that ensure the improvements will last. Training the parents to treat their child in his home in order to promote generalization and maintenance of the treatment effects became essential. The parents are trained in an apprenticeship fashion, largely through modeling of senior therapists.

RESEARCH PROBLEMS IN MOTIVATION

Both the acquisition of new learning as well as the maintenance of that which has been learned are affected by motivational variables. In a behavioristic system such as the one we have followed, the question of motivation is essentially a question about the effectiveness of reinforcers. In our first treatment efforts with autistic children, we explored the possibility of enriching and normalizing reinforcing stimuli. For example, we were able to establish certain social stimuli as reinforcing for the autistic child by delivering smiles and verbal approval at the same time as the child was fed (Lovaas, Freitag, Kinder, Rubenstein, Schaeffer, & Simmons, 1966). We further reasoned that parents also normally acquire reinforcing functions because they help their children escape from frightening situations. Therefore we devised a "dangerous" environment for the child and proceeded to rescue him from that danger (Lovaas, Schaeffer, & Simmons, 1965). We delivered a painful but physically harmless electric shock through the floor, which was turned off as soon as the child sought us out. Ideally, we would have preferred to help the child overcome fear of a more "natural" aversive situation than shock; however, autistic children typically appear devoid of natural fears. Although we were thus able to establish ourselves as durable reinforcers, our reinforcing function was ultimately limited to the treatment room, and the procedures were too cumbersome to be of much practical significance. The children showed great affection for us when in the treatment environment but returned more and more to their previous autistic behaviors outside it, since strong consequences were not present to ensure the maintenance of socially appropriate responding.

Throughout most of our treatment we have attempted to sidestep the child's motivational deficiency by selecting powerful primary reinforcers such as food and pain, or other "artificial" reinforcers, like exaggerated social praise. There are, however, some very serious problems inherent in the use of such artificial reinforcers because they exist only in specially constructed environments—e.g., our treatment setting—and, rather logically, they generalize on a limited scale to new environments. For the same reasons, behaviors built by the use of such reinforcers probably do not maintain over time. Our use of artificial reinforcers is part of the reason why those children institutionalized after discharge from us showed behavioral regression. The institutional setting, like most environments, did not prescribe contingent primary reinforcers for the children, hence the behaviors we had built were extinguished while pathological, bizarre patterns of responding returned. Clearly, the ideal treatment setting would normalize the child's motivational structure and develop "natural" reinforcers available in his everyday environment.

The importance of learning more about motivational variables has led to a systematic inquiry into the reinforcing effects of certain sensory stimuli for psychotic children (Rincover, Newsom, & Carr, 1974). This study demonstrated that sensory events, such as music, for example, can be very powerful, long-lasting reinforcers that compare favorably to the appetitive reinforcers usually employed in behavior therapy with psychotic children. It is important to note that the ability of a specific sensory event to function as a reinforcer for a particular child can only be determined empirically. One should observe the child in his natural environment or talk with someone who has already done so, such as a parent or teacher, to narrow down the range of alternatives to be tried in therapeutic work. If the child spends a considerable amount of time self-stimulating with a particular object, an attempt could be made to exploit the reinforcement properties of that object by making access to it for brief periods contingent on appropriate behavior. Making the opportunity to engage in the more rewarding and higher probability activity conditional upon the prior performance of lower probability behaviors results in an increase in the frequency of the latter responses (Premack, 1965). Further investigation of the possibility of letting the child's self-stimulation serve as his reinforcer for engaging in appropriate behavior may contribute much to a solution of the motivational problems that exist in work with psychotic children.

RESEARCH PROBLEMS IN PERCEPTION

The unpredictable responsivity of autistic children to external stimuli, and the difficulty with which they acquire even rudimentary social and academic skills, suggests the presence of serious perceptual anomalies. Attentional processes, in particular, have been implicated. For example, several clinical studies have indicated that these children may selectively attend to only part of the stimulation provided by a therapist, such as gestural or facial cues rather than verbalizations (Lovaas, Schreibman, Koegel, & Rehm, 1971; Pronovost, Wakstein, & Wakstein, 1966; Ruttenberg & Gordon, 1967). Clinical data presented by Lovaas and his collaborators (1971) provide a striking illustration of this problem. An autistic boy was trained to imitate certain simple sounds modeled by his therapist. However, when the therapist presented the sounds while the child was looking away or while she covered her mouth, the child was unable to give the correct response. It appeared that the child had never listened to her voice during the more than 1700 trials of training.

Such observations have led us to conduct a series of laboratory investigations of the autistic child's attention to multiple cues. We were especially interested in situations in which several cues impinge simultaneously on the child and in which he is expected to learn an overt discriminative response. Such situations relate quite naturally to conditions in classrooms and language training sessions. Findings in a number of experiments indicate that autistic children typically respond to a very limited number of the relevant cues in learning tasks. Evidence for this *stimulus overselectivity* was first obtained by the Lovaas group (1971), who found that autistic children presented with a stimulus complex consisting of a light, white noise, and tactile pressure learned to respond to only one of the stimuli. Normal children responded to all three cues, while retarded children fell between these extremes, generally responding to two cues. When the autistic children were trained with one of the previously nonfunctional cues in isolation, they were able to learn to respond to it reliably. This evidence established the problem as stemming from breadth of attention rather than from a specific sensory deficit. Subsequent studies showed that autistic children mainfested the same stimulus overselectivity when they were presented with multiple cues entirely within the visual modality (Koegel & Wilhelm, 1973) or the auditory modality (Reynolds, Newsom, & Lovaas, 1974). Other experiments indicated that these children often attend to social stimuli overselectively. Schreibman and Lovaas (1973) found that autistic children distinguished between people on the basis of an unreliable and idiosyncratic cue, such as an article of clothing. Analyzing one-to-one teaching interactions, Rincover and Koegel (1975) discovered that some autistic children learned to associate the correctness of their responses with irrelevant movements of the teacher and therefore showed no generalization of those responses to a different adult.

At present we do not know the extent to which stimulus overselectivity contributes to the autistic child's severe emotional, language, and social problems, although we have speculated on ways in which it may have profound effects in these areas (Lovaas et al., 1971). Since we also know that stimulus overselectivity occurs in severely retarded and very young children (Kovattana & Kraemer, 1974; Schover & Newsom, 1976; Wilhelm & Lovaas, 1976), it is probably inappropriate to view overselectivity as causative in producing the autistic syndrome. However, the research on overselectivity has made it clear that the perceptual functioning of autistic children can be conceptualized as being at a very early developmental stage, and this consideration must enter into treatment and educational planning.

THE CHILD'S AGE AT ONSET OF TREATMENT

The primary weaknesses of behavior therapy with psychotic children concern the slow rate of change and the reversibility of the therapeutic gains. We have tried to tackle these problems in three ways.

1. We are attempting to acquire a better understanding of the psychotic child per se by investigating his perceptual and motivational deviations as we reviewed above.
2. We are attempting to generalize and extend the treatment environment by means of teacher- and parent-training programs (Koegel & Rincover, 1974; Rincover & Koegel, 1975; Koegel, Russo, Rincover, 1976). Attempts are also being made to seek treatment models which avoid reliance on large, impersonal, and nontherapeutic institutional environments, and instead emphasize the concept of professional foster or "teaching" homes (Russo, Glahn, & Lovaas, 1974). This involves an effort to extend Montrose Wolf's Kansas Achievement Place model for delinquents (Phillips, 1968) to psychotic children.
3. We are attempting to maximize treatment effects by selecting young children for treatment. Psychotic children have shown great variability in their responses to our efforts; occasionally a child has even attained normal functioning. It is becoming increasingly clear that the child's age at the onset of treatment is highly correlated with rapid, irreversible changes such that the younger the child, the better his prognosis.

In an effort to identify cases of infantile autism at an earlier age than has usually been possible, Young and Lovaas (1977) have developed a relatively comprehensive behavioral checklist, consisting of some 300 items. This scale has proven rather effective in discriminating very young autistic children (ages 2 to 3 years and younger) from normals and from other pathological situations of infancy such as mental retardation.

The observation that younger children do better under our type of treatment regime than older ones led to the young-autism (under 40 months of age) treatment project (Lovaas, Koegel, & Schreibman, 1973), whose results are most encouraging. Changes in the child's behavior usually occur quite rapidly (within the first year of treatment), large classes of behavior are involved, including the full range of social, affective, and intellectual behaviors, and the therapeutic effects appear to be quite permanent.

Several hypotheses may be suggested as to why younger autistic children do better than older ones. It is apparent that the younger children have acquired fewer and less intense behaviors, such as tantrums and self-stimulation, which interfere with treatment. Also, their behavior may be easier to bring under the control of generalized conditioned reinforcers which we see as essential to support necessary social and intellectual functioning. In other words, the older and more experienced the child, the less likely it will be that social stimuli, such as smiles, affection and other forms of attention, will achieve generalized control over his behavior. The type of exclusive control such events must possess for normal development to take place is probably acquired during infancy, because such stimuli are thereafter rarely associated with basic reinforcers (i.e., food, warmth, pain reduction, and so on). Similarly, the young child does not have a history of discrimination training which might render these reinforcers effective only in certain situations. We have described several studies involving primarily older autistic children, which showed that they can discriminate between situations in which social stimuli are reliably backed up by food or shock and situations in which they are not. On the other hand, younger children have a relatively limited practice in forming discriminations and can therefore be expected to generalize appropriate behaviors more readily and extensively across people and situations. In other words, to be maximally "hooked" on social stimuli, one has to be "hooked" early. Finally, there probably exists an "optimal age" for the acquisition of certain kinds of behaviors, such as language, so that a child at the age of one, two, or three can learn these behaviors much easier than a child of ten or eleven. In any case, our work with young autistic children looks most promising at the present time.

SUMMARY

We will conclude by briefly discussing some of the more significant contributions of a behavioral approach to the understanding and treatment of psychotic children.

1. The *methodology* used in working with psychotic children, or persons from any other clinical population, must be considered as the primary innovation (Baer, Wolf, & Risley, 1968; Leitenberg, 1973). *Measurement*, where the therapeutic interventions used and the behavioral changes are precisely specified, and *experimentation*, in which the causal status and the replicability of the effects of treatment variables are directly assessed, constitute the key components of this methodology. The use of these methodological principles offers an enormous advantage over more traditional psychotherapies since it forces us to center our inquiry on hypotheses that are capable of being disproven relatively quickly. Thus, effective interventions can be readily distinguished from merely plausible ones.

2. Extinction, time-out, and punishment procedures have led to the surprisingly rapid elimination of the more grossly pathological behaviors of the psychotic child, especially when incompatible, more appropriate responses are taught simultaneously. The effective management of self-mutilation, tantrums, and the more overt forms of self-stimulation can be undertaken by anyone knowledgeable with the existing technology.

3. The use of prompting, shaping, imitation, differential reinforcement, and other operations has made it feasible to teach the most complex of behaviors, such as receptive and expressive language. The successes which have been achieved by therapies incorporating these techniques constitute a major basis for optimism in treatment endeavors.

4. Age at onset of treatment appears highly predictive of treatment outcome. In general, the older autistic child makes relatively smaller gains in treatment, and these gains may be reversible. The younger child (before 40 months of age) apparently makes larger and irreversible gains.

5. Our ignorance of motivational factors is probably the major deterrent to the development of more optimal treatment programs. Reliance on treatment-specific, "artificial" reinforcers, such as food and physical pain, probably accounts for much of the situational and response-specificity associated with a majority of our therapeutic accomplishments to date. Our investigations into the use of affectively exaggerated response consequences and antecedents, our attempts to identify intrinsically rewarding behaviors and sensory based reinforcement, and our increased understanding of very young psychotic children all offer hope for the establishment of more normal motivation structures.

There are a number of other interesting and important aspects of research, treatment, and theory which we have been unable to broach here. Recent reviews of a variety of topics relating to psychotic children are provided by Baltaxe and Simmons (1975), Churchill, Alpern, and DeMyer (1971), Hermelin and O'Connor (1970), Hingtgen and Bryson (1972), Leff (1968), Ornitz (1973), Ross (1974), Rutter (1971), and Yates (1970).

REFERENCES

AZRIN, N. H., and HOLZ, W. C. Punishment. In W. K. Honig (Ed.), *Operant behavior: Areas of research and application.* New York: Appleton-Century-Crofts, 1966.

AZRIN, N. H., KAPLAN, S. J., and FOXX, R. M. Autism reversal: Eliminating stereotyped self-stimulation of retarded individuals. *American Journal of Mental Deficiency*, 1973, *78*, 241–248.

BACHMAN, J. A. Self-injurious behavior: A behavioral analysis. *Journal of Abnormal Psychology*, 1972, *80*, 211–224.

BAER, D. M., GUESS, D., and SHERMAN, J. Adventures in simplistic grammar. In R. L. Schiefelbusch (Ed.), *Language of the mentally retarded.* Baltimore: University Park Press, 1972.

BAER, D. M., and SHERMAN, J. Reinforcement control of generalized imitation in young children. *Journal of Experimental Child Psychology*, 1964, *1*, 37–49.

BAER, D. J., WOLF, M. M., and RISLEY, T. R. Some current dimensions of applied behavior analysis. *Journal of Applied Behavior Analysis*, 1968, *1*, 91–97.

BALTAXE, C. A. M., and SIMMONS, J. Q. Language in childhood psychosis: A review. *Journal of Speech and Hearing Disorders*, 1975, *40*, 439–458.

BANDURA, A. *Principles of behavior modification*. New York: Holt, Rinehart, & Winston, 1969.

BAUMEISTER, A. A., and FOREHAND, R. Stereotyped acts. In N. R. Ellis (Ed.), *International review of research in mental retardation* (Vol. 6). New York: Academic Press, 1973.

BERKO, J. The child's learning of English morphology. *Word*, 1958, *14*, 150–177.

BETTELHEIM, B. *The empty fortress*. New York: Free Press, 1967.

BIJOU, S. W., and BAER, D. M. *Child development: Readings in experimental analysis*. New York: Appleton-Century-Crofts, 1967.

BRACKBILL, Y., ADAMS, G., CROWELL, D. H., and GRAY, M. L. Arousal level in neonates and preschool children under continuous auditory stimulation. *Journal of Experimental Child Psychology*, 1966, *4*, 178–188.

BROWN, J. L. Prognosis from presenting symptoms of preschool children with atypical behavior. *American Journal of Orthopsychiatry*, 1960, *30*, 382–390.

BROWN, R., and BELLUGI, U. (Eds.). *The acquisition of language*. Yellow Springs, Ohio: Antioch Press, 1964.

BROWN, R., and FRASER, C. The acquisition of syntax. *Child Development Monographs*, 1964, *29*, 43–79.

BUCHER, B., and LOVAAS, O. I. Use of aversive stimulation in behavior modification. In M. R. Jones (Ed.), *Miami symposium on the prediction of behavior, 1967: Aversive stimulation*. Coral Gables, Florida: University of Miami Press, 1968.

CARR, E. G., NEWSOM, C. D., and BINKOFF, J. Stimulus control of self-destructive behavior in a psychotic child. *Journal of Abnormal Child Psychology*, 1976, *4*, 139–153.

CARR, E. G., SCHREIBMAN, L., and LOVAAS, O. I. Control of echolalic speech in psychotic children. *Journal of Abnormal Child Psychology*, 1975, *3*, 331–351.

CHOMSKY, N. *Aspects of the theory of syntax*. Cambridge, Mass.: MIT Press, 1965.

CHURCHILL, D. W., ALPERN, G. D., and DEMYER, M. K. (Eds.). *Infantile autism: Proceedings of the Indiana University colloquium*. Springfield, Ill.: Charles C. Thomas Publisher, 1971.

COOK, C., and ADAMS, H. E. Modification of verbal behavior in speech deficient children. *Behavior Research and Therapy*, 1966, *4*, 265–271.

CORTE, H. E., WOLF, M. M., and LOCKE, B. J. A comparison of procedures for eliminating self-injurious behavior of retarded adolescents. *Journal of Applied Behavior Analysis*, 1971, *4*, 201–213.

CREAK, M. Juvenile psychosis and mental deficiency. In B. W. Richards (Ed.), *Proceedings of the London Conference for the Scientific Study of Mental Deficiency 2*. Deganham: May and Baker, 1962.

CREAK, M., and INI, S. Families of psychotic children. *Journal of Child Psychology and Psychiatry*, 1960, *1*, 156–175.

CREEDON, M. P. *A simultaneous communication learning program: Rationale and results*. Paper presented at the meeting of the American Psychological Association, Montreal, August 1973.

DAVISON, G. C. A social learning therapy programme with an autistic child. *Behaviour Research and Therapy*, 1964, *2*, 149–159.

EPSTEIN, L. H., DOKE, L. A., SAJWAJ, T. E., SORRELL, S., and RIMMER, B. Generality and side effects of overcorrection. *Journal of Applied Behavior Analysis*, 1974, *7*, 385–390.

ERVIN, S. M. Imitation and structural change in children's language. In E. H. Lenneberg

(Ed.), *New directions in the study of language.* Cambridge, Mass.: MIT Press, 1964.

FERSTER, C. B. Positive reinforcement and behavioral deficits of autistic children. *Child Development*, 1961, *32*, 437–456.

FERSTER, C. B., and DEMYER, M. K. The development of performances in autistic children in an automatically controlled environment. *Journal of Chronic Diseases*, 1961, *13*, 312–345.

FERSTER, C. B., and DEMYER, M. K. A method for the experimental analysis of the behavior of autistic children. *The American Journal of Orthopsychiatry*, 1962, *32*, 89–98.

FOXX, R. M., and AZRIN, N. H. The elimination of autistic self-stimulatory behavior by overcorrection. *Journal of Applied Behavior Analysis*, 1973, *6*, 1–14.

GARCIA, E., GUESS, D., and BYRNES, J. Development of syntax in a retarded girl using imitation, reinforcement, and modeling. *Journal of Applied Behavior Analysis*, 1973, *6*, 299–310.

GARDNER, B. T., and GARDNER, R. A. Two-way communication with an infant chimpanzee. In A. Schrier and F. Stollnitz (Eds.), *Behavior of nonhuman primates* (Vol. 4). New York: Academic Press, 1971.

GUESS, D., SAILOR, W., RUTHERFORD, G., and BAER, D. An experimental analysis of linguistic development: The productive use of the plural morpheme. *Journal of Applied Behavior Analysis*, 1968, *1*, 292–307.

HAMILTON, J., STEPHENS, L., and ALLEN, P. Controlling aggressive and destructive behavior in severely retarded institutionalized residents. *American Journal of Mental Deficiency*, 1967, *71*, 852–856.

HARTUNG, J. R. A review of procedures to increase verbal imitation skills and functional speech in autistic children. *Journal of Speech and Hearing Disorders*, 1970, *35*, 203–217.

HERMELIN, B., and O'CONNOR, N. *Psychological experiments with autistic children.* London: Pergamon, 1970.

HEWETT, F. M. Teaching speech to an autistic child through operant conditioning. *American Journal of Orthopsychiatry*, 1965, *35*, 927–936.

HINGTGEN, J. N., and BRYSON, C. Q. Recent developments in the study of early childhood psychoses: Infantile autism, childhood schizophrenia, and related disorders. *Schizophrenia Bulletin*, 1972, *5*, 8–54.

KANNER, L. Autistic disturbances of affective contact. *Nervous Child*, 1943, *2*, 181–197.

KANNER, L., and EISENBERG, L. Notes on the follow-up studies of autistic children. In P. H. Hoch and J. Zubin (Eds.), *Psychopathology of childhood.* New York: Grune & Stratton, 1955.

KENT, L. R. *Language acquisition program for the severely retarded.* Champaign, Ill.: Research Press, 1974.

KISH, G. B. Studies of sensory reinforcement. In W. K. Honig (Ed.), *Operant behavior: Areas of research and application.* New York: Appleton-Century-Crofts, 1966.

KOEGEL, R. L., and COVERT, A. The relationship of self-stimulation to learning in autistic children. *Journal of Applied Behavior Analysis*, 1972, *5*, 381–387.

KOEGEL, R. L., Firestone, P. B., KRAMME, K. W., and DUNLAP, G. Increasing spontaneous play by suppressing self-stimulation in autistic children. *Journal of Applied Behavior Analysis*, 1974, *7*, 521–528.

KOEGEL, R. L., and RINCOVER, A. Treatment of psychotic children in a classroom environment. I. Learning in a large group. *Journal of Applied Behavior Analysis*, 1974, *7*, 45–59.

KOEGEL, R. L., RUSSO, D. C., and RINCOVER, A. Assessing and training the generalized use of behavior modification with autistic children. *Journal of Applied Behavior Analysis*, 1977, in press.

KOEGEL, R. L., and WILHELM, H. Selective responding to the components of multiple visual cues by autistic children. *Journal of Experimental Child Psychology*, 1973, *15*, 442–453.

KOVATTANA, P. M., and KRAEMER, H. C. Response

to multiple visual cues of color, size, and form by autistic children. *Journal of Autism and Childhood Schizophrenia*, 1974, *4*, 251–261.

KOZLOFF, M. A. *Educating children with learning and behavior problems.* New York: John Wiley, 1974.

KUSHNER, M. Faradic aversive controls in clinical practice. In C. Neuringer and J. L. Michael (Eds.), *Behavior modification in clinical psychology*. New York: Appleton-Century-Crofts, 1970.

LACEY, J. I. Somatic response patterning and stress: Some revisions of activation theory. In M. H. Appley and R. Trumbull (Eds.), *Psychological stress: Issues in research.* New York: Appleton-Century-Crofts, 1967.

LEFF, R. Behavior modification and the psychoses of childhood: A review. *Psychological Bulletin*, 1968, *69*, 396–409.

LEITENBERG, H. The use of single-case methodology in psychotherapy research. *Journal of Abnormal Psychology*, 1973, *82*, 87–101.

LENNEBERG, E. H. Language disorders in childhood. *Harvard Educational Review*, 1964, *34*, 152–177.

LEUBA, C. Toward some integration of learning theories: The concept of optimal stimulation. *Psychological Reports*, 1955, *1*, 27–33.

LOVAAS, O. I. *Behavior modification: Teaching language to psychotic children.* New York: Appleton-Century-Crofts, 1969. (Instructional film, 45 min., 16 mm-sound.)

LOVAAS, O. I. *The autistic child: Language development through behavior modification.* New York: Irvington Publishers, 1977.

LOVAAS, O. I., BERBERICH, J. P., PERLOFF, B. F., and SCHAEFFER, B. Acquisition of imitative speech by schizophrenic children. *Science*, 1966, *151*, 705–707.

LOVAAS, O. I., FREITAG, G., GOLD, V. J., and KASSORLA, I. C. Experimental studies in childhood schizophrenia: Analysis of self-destructive behavior. *Journal of Experimental Child Psychology*, 1965, *2*, 67–84.

LOVAAS, O. I., FREITAG, G., KINDER, M. I., RUBENSTEIN, B. D., SCHAEFFER, B., and SIMMONS, J. Q. Establishment of social reinforcers in two schizophrenic children on the basis of food. *Journal of Experimental Child Psychology*, 1966, *4*, 109–125.

LOVAAS, O. I., FREITAS, L., NELSON, K., and WHALEN, C. The establishment of imitation and its use for the development of complex behavior in schizophrenic children. *Behaviour Research and Therapy*, 1967, *5*, 171–181.

LOVAAS, O. I., KOEGEL, R. L., and SCHREIBMAN, L. *Experimental studies in child schizophrenia* (Research Project MH-11440-07). National Institute of Mental Health, 1973.

LOVAAS, O. I., KOEGEL, R. L., SIMMONS, J. Q., and LONG, J. S. Some generalization and follow-up measures on autistic children in behavior therapy. *Journal of Applied Behavior Analysis*, 1973, *6*, 131–165.

LOVAAS, O. I., LITROWNIK, A., and MANN, R. Response latencies to auditory stimuli in autistic children engaged in self-stimulatory behavior. *Behaviour Research and Therapy*, 1971, *9*, 39–49.

LOVAAS, O. I., SCHAEFFER, B., and SIMMONS, J. Q. Experimental studies in childhood schizophrenia: Building social behavior in autistic children by use of electric shock. *Journal of Experimental Research in Personality*, 1965, *1*, 99–109.

LOVAAS, O. I., SCHREIBMAN, L., KOEGEL, R. L., and REHM, R. Selective responding by autistic children to multiple sensory input. *Journal of Abnormal Psychology*, 1971, *77*, 211–222.

LOVAAS, O. I., and SIMMONS, J. Q. Manipulation of self-destruction in three retarded children. *Journal of Applied Behavior Analysis*, 1969, *2*, 143–157.

LOVAAS, O. I., VARNI, J. W., KOEGEL, R. L., and LORSCH, N. Some observations on the non-extinguishability of children's speech. *Child Development*, in press.

MACCORQUODALE, K. B. F. Skinner's "Verbal behavior:" A retrospective appreciation.

Journal of the Experimental Analysis of Behavior, 1969, *12*, 831–841.

MacCorquodale, K. On Chomsky's review of Skinner's "Verbal behavior." *Journal of the Experimental Analysis of Behavior*, 1970, *13*, 83–99.

Masserman, J. H. *Principles of dynamic psychiatry*. Philadelphia: Saunders, 1946.

May, J. G., McAllister, J., Risley, T., Twardosz, S., Cox, C. H., et al. Florida Guidelines for the Use of Behavioral Procedures in State Programs for the Retarded. Joint Task Force assembled by the Florida Division of Retardation and the Department of Psychology of the Florida State University, June, 1974.

Merbaum, M. The modification of self-destructive behavior by a mother-therapist using aversive stimulation. *Behavior Therapy*, 1973, *4*, 442–447.

Metz, J. R. Conditioning generalized imitation in autistic children. *Journal of Experimental Child Psychology*, 1965, *2*, 389–399.

Miller, N. E. Learning resistance to pain and fear: Effects of overlearning, exposure, and rewarded exposure in context. *Journal of Experimental Psychology*, 1960, *60*, 137–145.

Mowrer, O. H. *Learning theory and the symbolic processes*. New York: John Wiley, 1960.

Ornitz, E. M. Childhood autism: A review of the clinical and experimental literature. *California Medicine*, 1973, *118*, 21–47.

Phillips, E. L. Achievement place: Token reinforcement procedures in a home-style rehabilitation setting for "pre-delinquent" boys. *Journal of Applied Behavior Analysis*, 1968, *1*, 213–223.

Pitfield, M., and Oppenheim, A. N. Child rearing attitudes of mothers of psychotic children. *Journal of Child Psychiatry*, 1964, *5*, 51–57.

Premack, D. Reinforcement theory. In D. Levine (Ed.), *Nebraska symposium on motivation: 1965*. Lincoln: University of Nebraska Press, 1965.

Premack, D. A functional analysis of language. *Journal of the Experimental Analysis of Behavior*, 1970, *14*, 1–19.

Premack, D. Language in chimpanzee? *Science*, 1971, *172*, 808–822.

Pronovost, W., Wakstein, P., and Wakstein, P. A longitudinal study of the speech behavior of fourteen children diagnosed as atypical or autistic. *Exceptional Children*, 1966, *33*, 19–26.

Reynolds, B. S., Newsom, C. D., and Lovaas, O. I. Auditory overselectivity in autistic children. *Journal of Abnormal Child Psychology*, 1974, *2*, 253–263.

Rimland, B. *Infantile autism: The syndrome and its implications for a neural theory of behavior*. New York: Appleton-Century-Crofts, 1964.

Rincover, A., and Koegel, R. L. Setting generality and stimulus control in autistic children. *Journal of Applied Behavior Analysis*, 1975, *8*, 235–246.

Rincover, A., Newsom, C. D., and Carr, E. G. *Identifying and using sensory reinforcers with autistic children*. Paper presented at the Western Psychological Association convention, San Francisco, April 1974.

Risley, T. The effects and side effects of the use of punishment with an autistic child. *Journal of Applied Behavior Analysis*, 1968, *1*, 21–34.

Risley, T., Reynolds, N., and Hart, B. Behavior modification with disadvantaged preschool children. In R. H. Bradfield (Ed.), *Behavior modification: The human effort*. San Rafael, Calif.: Dimensions Publishing Co., 1970.

Risley, T., and Wolf, M. M. Experimental manipulation of autistic behaviors and generalization into the home. In R. Ulrich, T. Stachnik, and J. Mabry (Eds.), *Control of human behavior*. Glenview, Ill.: Scott, Foresman & Co., 1966.

Risley, T., and Wolf, M. M. Establishing functional speech in echolalic children. *Behaviour Research and Therapy*, 1967, *5*, 73–88.

Ross, A. O. *Psychological disorders of children: A behavioral approach to theory, research, and therapy*. New York: McGraw-Hill, 1974.

Russo, D. C., Glahn, T. J., and Lovaas, O. I. *Use of teaching homes for the treatment of psychotic children*. Paper presented at the meeting of the American Psychological Association, New Orleans, September 1974.

RUTTENBERG, B. A., and GORDON, E. G. Evaluating the communication of the autistic child. *Journal of Speech and Hearing Disorders*, 1967, *32*, 314–324.

RUTTER, M. Prognosis: Psychotic children in adolescence and early adult life. In J. K. Wing (Ed.), *Early childhood autism: Clinical, educational, and social aspects*. London: Pergamon, 1966.

RUTTER, M. (Ed.) *Infantile autism: Concepts, characteristics, and treatment*. London: Churchill Livingstone, 1971.

SAILOR, W. Reinforcement and generalization of productive plural allomorphs in two retarded children. *Journal of Applied Behavior Analysis*, 1971, *4*, 305–310.

SAILOR, W., and TAMAN, T. Stimulus factors in the training of prepositional usage in three autistic children. *Journal of Applied Behavior Analysis*, 1972, *5*, 183–190.

SALZINGER, K. On the operant conditioning of complex behavior. In J. K. Shlien (Ed.), *Research in psychotherapy* (Vol. 3). Washington, D. C.: American Psychological Association, 1968.

SALZINGER, K., FELDMAN, R., COWAN, J., and SALZINGER, S. Operant conditioning of verbal behavior of two young speech-deficient boys. In L. Krasner and L. Ullmann (Eds.), *Research in behavior modification*. New York: Holt, Rinehart, & Winston, 1965.

SCHELL, R. E., STARK, J., and GIDDAN, J. G. Development of language behavior in an autistic child. *Journal of Speech and Hearing Disorders*, 1967, *32*, 51–64.

SCHOPLER, E., and REICHLER, R. J. How well do parents understand their own psychotic children? *Journal of Autism and Childhood Schizophrenia*, 1972, *2*, 387–400.

SCHOVER, L. E., and NEWSOM, C. D. Overselectivity, developmental level, and overtraining in autistic and normal children. *Journal of Abnormal Child Psychology*, 1976, *4*, 289–298.

SCHREIBMAN, L., and LOVAAS, O. I. Overselective response to social stimuli by autistic children. *Journal of Abnormal Child Psychology*, 1973, *1*, 152–168.

SCHUMAKER, J., and SHERMAN, J. A. Training generative verb usage by imitation and reinforcement procedures. *Journal of Applied Behavior Analysis*, 1970, *3*, 273–287.

SEGAL, E. F. Induction and the provenance of operants. In R. M. Gilbert and J. R. Millenson (Eds.), *Reinforcement: Behavioral analyses*. New York: Academic Press, 1972.

SHERMAN, J. A. Imitation and language development. In H. W. Reese (Ed.), *Advances in child development and behavior* (Vol. 6). New York: Academic Press, 1971.

SKINNER, B. F. *Verbal behavior*. New York: Appleton-Century-Crofts, 1957.

SLOANE, H. N., JOHNSTON, M. K., and HARRIS, F. R. Remedial procedures for teaching verbal behavior to speech deficient or defective young children. In H. N. Sloane and B. MacAuley (Eds.), *Operant procedures in remedial speech and language training*. Boston: Houghton Mifflin, 1968.

SROUFE, L. A., STUECHER, H. U., and STUTZER, W. The functional significance of autistic behavior for the psychotic child. *Journal of Abnormal Child Psychology*, 1973, *1*, 225–240.

STARK, J., GIDDAN, J. J., and MEISEL, J. Increasing verbal behavior in an autistic child. *Journal of Speech and Hearing Disorders*, 1968, *33*, 42–48.

STEVENS-LONG, J., and RASMUSSEN, M. The acquisition of simple and compound sentence structure in an autistic child. *Journal of Applied Behavior Analysis*, 1974, *7*, 473–479.

STONE, A. A. Consciousness: Altered levels in blind retarded children. *Psychosomatic Medicine*, 1964, *26*, 14–19.

TATE, B. G. Case study: Control of chronic self-injurious behavior by conditioning procedures. *Behavior Therapy*, 1972, *3*, 72–83.

TATE, B. G., and BAROFF, G. S. Aversive control of self-injurious behavior in a psychotic boy.

Behaviour Research and Therapy, 1966, *4*, 281–287.

Terrace, H. S. Discrimination learning with and without "errors." *Journal of the Experimental Analysis of Behavior*, 1963, *6*, 1–27.

Webster, C. D., McPherson, H., Sloman, L., Evans, M. A., and Kuchar, E. Communicating with an autistic boy by gestures. *Journal of Autism and Childhood Schizophrenia*, 1973, *3*, 337–346.

Wheeler, A. J., and Sulzer, B. Operant training and generalization of a verbal response form in a speech deficient child. *Journal of Applied Behavior Analysis*, 1970, *3*, 139–147.

White, J. C., and Taylor, D. Noxious conditioning as a treatment for rumination. *Mental Retardation*, 1967, *6*, 30–33.

Wiest, W. Some recent criticisms of behaviorism and learning theory. *Psychological Bulletin*, 1967, *67*, 214–225.

Wilhelm, H., and Lovaas, O. I. Stimulus overselectivity: A common feature in autism and mental retardation. *American Journal of Mental Deficiency*, 1976, *81*, 227–241.

Wolf, M. M., Risley, T., Johnston, M., Harris, F., and Allen, E. Application of operant conditioning procedures to the behavior problems of an autistic child: A follow-up and extension. *Behaviour Research and Therapy*, 1967, *5*, 103–112.

Wolf, M. M., Risley, T., and Mees, H. Application of operant conditioning procedures to the behavior problems of an autistic child. *Behaviour Research and Therapy*, 1964, *1*, 305–312.

Wolff, W. M., and Morris, L. A. Intellectual and personality characteristics of parents of autistic children. *Journal of Abnormal Psychology*, 1971, *77*, 155–161.

Yates, A. J. *Behavior therapy*. New York: John Wiley, 1970.

Young, D. B., and Lovaas, O. I. *Behavior checklist: A scale for differentiating infantile autism from other disorders of infancy*. Manuscript submitted for publication, 1977.

Zubek, J. P. (Ed.) *Sensory deprivation: Fifteen years of research*. New York: Appleton-Century-Crofts, 1969.

23

CHILDHOOD PSYCHOSIS: RESIDENTIAL TREATMENT AND ITS ALTERNATIVES

Mary B. Hagamen

Although the incidence of psychoses is relatively rare compared to other psychiatric disorders of childhood, the small number of youngsters affected can create for the clinician the greatest challenge to his skill in treatment planning. In this situation there are a broad range of variables that intertwine in a perplexing way:

> The variables that pertain to the child are the level of intellect and degree of overactivity. Those that pertain to the family are the strength of their personal support systems. A third and very critical factor is the resources available for the child in the community, such as early childhood education, professional guidance, etc.

Thus, the informed professional must understand something about the natural history of the disorder, the dynamics of the effect of a handicapped child on the life of a particular family, and most of all how the resources available can best be used to create a long-term treatment plan that will allow for optimum development of the child and his family.

Perhaps the most important part of the clinician's task is to clarify all of the above factors to the parents so they are helped to participate in an informed way when making a lifetime plan for their child.

Chess (1959) pointed out that whatever the situation with the child, the plan for residential treatment should be seen as a specialized and relatively temporary service, a specific device aimed at returning the child to his place in the community equipped to make a better adjustment. Hopefully the child will be able to return to his own home, but if this is not feasible community placement in the least restrictive and most normalized environment should be the goal. Institutional care, whether in a hospital psychiatric unit for children or a residential treatment center, should be part of a total long-range plan in which 24-hour care is seen as the treatment of choice rather than as a last resort.

Although we know that many psychotic children will remain dependent throughout their lifetime and as adults will require a sheltered life existence, if not total institutional care, the point to be made is that (with the exception of those psychotic children functioning in the severe and profound range of mental retardation) during childhood every effort should be made to keep the psychotic youngster as close as possible to the mainstream of life so that he or she has an optimum chance to develop his potential.

NATURAL HISTORY OF CHILDHOOD PSYCHOSES

Much of the treatment planning done for this type of child will depend on the severity of the disorder and the course of development demonstrated by the child in question. Psychoses of childhood can be divided into two major groups according to the age of onset. Rutter (1974) has pooled the data of Kolvin (1971) and Makita (1966) to demonstrate this distribution by age of onset.

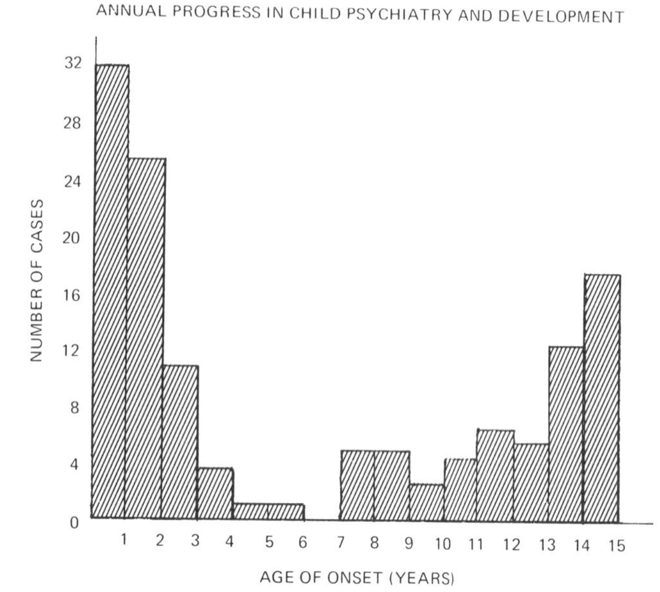

Figure 23-1 Distribution of cases of child psychosis by age of onset. Data from Makita (1966) and Kolvin (1971). From, Michael Rutter, "The Development of Infantile Autism," *Psychological Medicine,* 4 (1974), 147–63. Reprinted by permission of Cambridge University Press, New York.

The first group is the larger of the two and represents the psychoses of early childhood, that is, those children with an onset prior to age three. This is the group that is most frequently referred for residential treatment.

The incidence of psychoses with an onset between ages three and ten is remarkably low. This small number of children with later onset present initially as severe neurotics. The diagnosis is often equivocal, however, since the intensity of the child's symptoms and their permeation through every facet of his being often creates a difficult treatment problem. Most often such children are seen initially in the in-patient psychiatric service of a hospital. The outlook for their recovery is far superior to the outlook for children with developmental psychoses. Whether they are referred for continued residential treatment usually depends on the resources of the family and the community. These patients respond well to residential treatment where they have a chance to sort out their lives away from the stresses of their natural family and school environment. They can usually be titrated back to a community living plan over a summer vacation and given a chance to utilize their strengthened ability for adjustment with the onset of a new school year.

The second peak of incidence occurs in late childhood and early adolescence. Because these illnesses resemble adult schizophrenia and are frequently treated on adolescent or adult services, they are underrepresented in Figure 23-1. Pioneers in descriptive psychiatry such as Kraeplin and Bleuler have pointed out that a small percentage of their adult psychotic patients demonstrated onset prior to age ten. However, in the world of the 19th century childhood was short, and children had a very different place in society so that it is hard to evaluate the relevance of their findings. This type of late onset psychoses are actually a phenomenon of adolescence and as such fall outside the focus of our discussion.

Since by far the largest number of childhood psychoses are those that develop in early childhood, the thrust of this chapter will be devoted to a discussion of their treatment.

PROGNOSIS

The treatment of any disorder is closely related to our prognosis of its course. With childhood psychoses we face a dilemma since we can predict very little on an individual basis despite our knowledge from long-term follow-ups of groups.

In the more recent follow-up studies, approximately a quarter of the children seem to do well compared to less than 10% of those studied in the 1930s. Eisenberg attributes this to a better understanding of the parameters of the functional psychoses among later investigators. Hopefully when the results are in for the children of the 1960s who have had early intervention, there will be another increase in the percentage of children who do well.

The follow-up studies of Kanner and Eisenberg (1956) conclude that the outlook is best for those children who have useful speech by age five. This is undoubtedly true; yet Rutter has pointed out that despite the difficulty and unreliablity of IQ testing with such children, there is a close correlation between measured level of intelligence and recovery. In reviewing all the factors, Eisenberg (1967) concludes that the presence or absence of useful speech by age five as a predictor may be largely due to the high correlation between the absence of speech and low intelligence. Thus it appears that outcome is directly related to level of intelligence. Because intelligence testing in the preschool years is difficult and unreliable, it is unwise to prognosticate before age five. Even then the erratic developmental lags characteristic of the developmental psychoses continue to confuse the issues.

In considering the natural history of the disorder there are many unanswered questions. Will the new techniques of early intervention result in better outcome? How will this change long-range planning and particularly the role of institutionalization? If institutional care is necessary for those youngsters with low levels of intelligence, must it be total or is there a place for partial institutional care during the years of childhood?

From information presently available (Rutter, 1974), we know that three-fourths of the children with psychoses of early childhood are retarded. Experience to date involving the treatment of these children with the newest educational methods combined with a strong parent-professional partnership suggests that in most cases of psychoses in which the child is retarded, the youngster's level of functioning can be raised a step or two—i.e., from the severe to the moderate level of retardation. To those who have not been intimately involved with such children, this may seem like a small reward for a very large investment, yet when we look at the status of adult care for the severely retarded compared to the options available to those who can function in the moderate range, the benefits appear worthwhile to all involved—parent, professional, and taxpayer.

THE FAMILY AND THE PSYCHOTIC CHILD

It is hard to consider any area in the life of a psychotic child without thinking of his family. This is particularly true when we discuss treatment, since no matter what the treatment plan advises, the family is the party responsible to a large degree for its coordination and implementation.

When viewed as a group, the families of psychotic children show some interesting characteristics. A far larger proportion of those children with psychoses come from intact families than do the general population of children with psychiatric disorders. Also, it has been repeatedly observed both in this country (Kanner, 1943; Goldfarb, 1962; Rimland, 1964) and abroad (Rutter, 1974) that while individual cases can be found on all socioeconomic levels, a proportionately greater number of psychotic children are the offspring of better educated individuals at the middle and upper socioeconomic levels (Wolman, 1970).

As stated earlier, no characteristic of the child is more significant than his level of intellectual functioning. When, in addition to deficits in the areas of affect and language development, a child also functions in the severely retarded range, he or she will require lifelong supervision of the type given to a preschooler. Such a child puts a tremendous strain on his caretakers. Unless arrangements can be made to spread this exhausting 24-hour responsibility to other than the mother, such a child is a prime candidate for early institutionalization. Despite the lack of feedback characteristic of psychotic children, they do tend to evoke a good amount of heroic zeal in those who care for them, particularly parents. This can generate an unfounded hope for future progress. Occasionally, however, a very slow child does learn to communicate between his fifth and tenth year and the hope has been warranted inasmuch as progress continues once some mode of communication has been established. On the other hand, with those children who are profoundly retarded, hope may slowly fade when some signs of development do not become evident. Frequently during the first ten years of life we are not sure whether this level of retardation represents a permanent plateau or whether there will be a continued, if slow, growth to follow.

THE NEEDS OF THE CHILD

In planning for any child, it is wise to take a look at what is needed to promote growth. A primary need of every youngster, whether handicapped or not, is a home setting where he or she is loved and cared for. This means that there must be shelter, food, clothing, and most important, the sense of belonging that exists in a warm, accepting environment. There must be an opportunity for education and also for socializing and having fun with peers. In addition, every child must have access to specialized care when needed. With normal children the pediatrician and the dentist usually suffice. However, when there is a psychotic process it is necessary to have available the services of a psychiatrist, a psychologist, and a social worker, all with the special skills needed to help families care for their child.

In most situations the psychotic child is accepted and protected in his own home, particularly during early childhood. As has been mentioned, there is an increasing number of publicly funded educational programs that can provide well for his training. So far as socialization is concerned, this may be a problem since psychotic children do not relate well to other children and tend to be viewed as odd by their peers.

The need for psychiatric services varies greatly with the age and stage of the child. Certainly it is important that the youngster be subjected to thorough assessment by experienced professionals as soon as psychosis is suspected. Continued monitoring by a seasoned child psychiatrist or psychologist who can educate and advise the family with some confidence as to what they must do to plan for their child is a must. Such a person should be available for crisis consultations which can be done over the phone. It is important to be available to parents and to be able to support them in their decision making.

Taking only the child into account, we rarely see an advantage in residential care if the child's needs can be provided by his home, school, and community.

THE NEEDS OF THE FAMILY

The needs of the other members of the family must also be considered when making a long-range treatment plan. As do parents of non-handicapped children, mothers and fathers of children with early childhood psychoses should have a chance for rest and recreation in order to maintain an adequate energy level for coping. They also need an opportunity for social interaction in family and community affairs. In addition, they need the professional services of specialists able to serve them in educational and health matters related to raising a family. The needs of the normal children in the family must also be taken into consideration. In these families so much depends on the relative ages of the children involved; because of the prolonged period of dependency characteristic of youngsters with the developmental psychoses, the needs of both younger and older siblings may be impinged upon. When there are younger siblings the mother may become exhausted if she tries to cope with the demands of the psychotic child as well as the needs of the younger offspring. Psychotic children are so forceful in their demands that they may usurp maternal energy that should be devoted to the younger child. If the siblings are older than the affected child, their social life may be limited by the extra responsibility they have for sharing in the care of their psychotic sibling.

Families vary dramatically in their ability to

cope successfully with the problems presented. Children in affected families model after their parents and tend to accept the disorder in a matter-of-fact, constructive way if their parents allow them to do so. For this reason it is important that parents be educated and supported in understanding the family dynamics related to having a handicapped youngster in their midst.

The incidence of psychoses is greater among males and particularly first born males. This is a cause for deep grief and profoundly affects the dynamics of all family interaction. That parents need support in working out their reactions to the realities of their situation is a vital factor that must be recognized by the professional who works with the family.

There is an equation that inevitably evolves in discussing planning for the very disturbed youngster at home. On one side of the equation we have the strain that such a child puts on the family and on the other side we can put the resources the family has to support such a strain. When the strain exerted by the child is greater than the resources the family has available for coping, then something must be done to change the equation. We can either work to change the child's behavior and thus reduce the strain, or we can develop ways to support the family and increase their coping resources.

In our experience at Sagamore Children's Center, we have found that the greater the component of functional retardation in the child's psychosis the less likely it is that we will be able to reduce the strain by treating the child. In these cases, we have looked to ways of increasing resources available to the family, such as providing homemakers, family aides, and programs of rotating respite.

Families must be assessed just as the children are if we are to understand what additional resources are most needed to help them comfortably manage their child at home.

COMMUNITY RESOURCES

As discussed earlier, in addition to a supportive home situation, the child must have an appropriate educational program. Such programs, although unknown prior to the 1950s, have gradually developed throughout the country. The pioneer work of Carl Fenichel at the League School in Brooklyn created the model that has been followed by public and private agencies. A strong educational program is the backbone of any treatment plan.

Such programs have become increasingly available at the community level since 1970. Special education in this country has been developmentally delayed compared to educational programs for normal children. Although special schools for the deaf were begun as early as 1817 in Connecticut, and these were closely followed by schools for the more severe handicaps such as blindness and severe retardation, schools for children with emotional problems have been the last to develop. With the enforcement of compulsory education laws, school boards have begun to accept responsibility for the education of all handicapped children including the emotionally disturbed. The civil rights movement of the 'sixties has rippled through the lives of all minority groups, including the handicapped, so that in the 'seventies special education has become a civil right. Another factor that has led to increased availability of community schools for children with psychoses has been the present decrease in the overall child population, which has released available space in special education programs for the more severely handicapped. A corollary of all the above facts has been the national trend toward mainstreaming. Thus, the outlook throughout the country for appropriate community schools for psychotic children is improving.

When schools are available in the community, families are much better able to cope with their children. Because of the psychotic child's tendency to intellectualize, he or she often does very well once engaged in a good educational program. This is also true for the severely handicapped youngster of the autistic type who needs special training in order to communicate. Schools provide parents with daily respite from the 24-hour care of their child. They also provide tremendous emotional support via contact with parents who have children with similar problems.

Recreational programs are also increasingly

available for handicapped children who live in suburban areas. These take the form of Saturday groups or day camp programs in the summer. Many communities provide publicly supported recreational programs, and there are a variety of recreational day camps for the handicapped available in heavily populated communities.

Another resource increasingly available in the community is the well-trained psychologist or child psychiatrist who is able to support and guide parents through the difficult years as well as to provide appropriate psychiatric treatment for the child. All of this points toward more services at the community level to meet the major needs of psychotic children and their parents.

RESIDENTIAL TREATMENT CENTERS

In the broadest sense, residential treatment centers can be defined as any 24-hour care facility that devotes itself exclusively to the treatment of emotionally disturbed children. There are three basic models. (1) the hospital—the medical model; (2) the school—the educational model; and (3) the child-care institution—the social service model. Such models seldom exist in pure form. Although the medical model is usually seen in a hospital setting, such units have extensive educational and social service facilities. The same blend is also seen among educational and social service models. Each is designed to meet all the needs of children but each has a particular focus. In the medical model the primary thrust is toward diagnosis, evaluation, and psychiatric treatment, whereas in the educational model the thrust is primarily toward school needs. The social service model was developed to provide the supportive home environment so often needed by children who do not have families. We might say that the more serious the psychosis, the more one might refer the child to a hospital. The greater the degree of retardation, the more one would expect to see a child referred to a school program. Or, focusing on joint child-family problems, the more social service needs are apparent, the more the child might be referred to a child-care institution.

As with the treatment of psychoses in adults, there has been a trend away from institutionalization of psychotic children. The reasons are multiple. Perhaps the most important factor in this regard has been the awareness that day treatment programs for children developed on an educational model provide the same results as residential treatment (Goldfarb, 1969). Another factor that plays a prominent but little discussed role in the trend away from residential care is the difficulty inherent in creating good residential treatment programs. The expenditure involved not only in money but also in human energy is enormous. In publicly operated facilities such as children's units of state hospitals, the complexity of size, funding, and personnel practice within the bureaucratic framework limit ideal utilization of resources. Although voluntary nonprofit agencies have a good bit of freedom of operation, they must devote time and energy to fund raising which often offsets the advantages of operating outside the bureaucracy. Thus, good residential programs for psychotic children are very scarce and of a cost that is prohibitive to parents who are not independently wealthy or eligible for aid from public resources. It should be remembered that the long-range goal of treatment planning is to help the child develop into an adult who can cope in the least restrictive environment possible. For bright psychotic children, solutions may evolve almost naturally, just as normal children seem to outgrow their problems. However, for the vast majority who exhibit some form of retardation, parents must be helped to create a lifetime plan for their child.

Efforts should be made to keep the child in a family environment during the developmental years. This time span may be grossly extended compared to that of normal children. If the natural family is unable to care for the psychotic child, a foster family should be recruited. Except for extremely short-term care, residential treatment should be avoided in the preschool years.

There are several guidelines that aid the clinician in referring the child for residential care: The more severe the level of retardation, the earlier the need for residential care in a long-term facility. The greater the degree of hyperactive destructive behavior, the greater the need for a residential program during middle childhood.

The more the psychotic child impinges on the needs of others in the family, the greater is the need for a period of residential care. As other family members become more independent and their needs change, it is then possible to reintegrate the child back into the home or at least the community.

If the educational needs of the child cannot be met at the community level because of physical isolation, as occurs in farm families, there will be a need for a residential school program. Residential placement also is necessitated when the emotional needs of the child cannot be met at home, because of other family stresses. If the professional needs of the child and his family cannot be met at a community level, there may be a need for residential care in the form of an inpatient evaluation with follow-up guidance.

INDICATIONS FOR RESIDENTIAL TREATMENT

MEDICAL MODEL—CHILDREN'S PSYCHIATRIC HOSPITAL

In the past, psychotic children have been hospitalized for life at an early age because their needs could not be met at a community level. The results of such treatment have been poor. Kanner (1971) found those children who had been in total institutional care had the worst outcome. Whether they were institutionalized because of the severity of their disease or whether they became worse from institutional care is not clear. The best use of hospitals is for evaluation and short-term inpatient care to provide for a specific phase of treatment. Potter in 1934 provided some criteria for admission to the New York State Psychiatric Institute, New York City. His guidelines are as relevant today as they were when originally written:

Potter states that admission for *diagnosis* may be needed in three main situations:

1. for the investigation of a suspected underlying physical condition;
2. to assess the ability level, chiefly of children under five or six years of age, in cases where emotional disorder is, or may be, adversely affecting intellectual function and assessment;
3. where there is an organic element to a child's condition but it is unclear how far the disability is due to resulting oversolicitude or spoiling by the parents.

The Institute admitted children for *treatment* of four main types of problems:

1. children so disturbed in their conduct that care at home and outpatient treatment was impracticable;
2. where severe neurotic or psychotic reactions rendered children incapable of adjusting at home or at school, and where intensive and extensive psychotherapy was necessary;
3. where the home situation was so difficult that admission to the hospital was required to relieve the tension in the family;
4. where children needing residential child-care treatment showed behavioral or neurotic symptoms so severe that a period of in-patient treatment was needed before they were placed in a children's home or foster home.

EDUCATIONAL MODEL

Since psychotic children respond best to a firmly structured educational program, the residential school that can devote itself to an individualized educational program is often the treatment of choice during the child's later school years. Such programs allow the child to maintain contact with his family on holidays much the same as a normal child would if he were being educated in a boarding school. Family contacts should most always be nurtured and the educational model provides nicely for this.

If the family cannot meet the child's needs, or if the child drains the resources of the family, residential school may provide the best plan. When the child's level of development is very low, i.e., in the severe or profound range, a state facility for the retarded (often called a school) can be used in the same manner. Again, efforts should be made to help families maintain contact with their youngster in order to help alleviate the inevitable guilt that results from such a placement.

CHILD-CARE AGENCY

Residential facilities run by social agencies tend to overlap to a great extent with facilities run on an educational model since some child-care agencies have their own school programs. However, this is becoming less true as more children from all aspects of life are mainstreamed into the community. Thus, many residential facilities send their children into the community for school. Placement in such centers must be fitted to the needs of the individual child. For certain psychotic children whose families are unable to care for them, this may be the treatment of choice.

AVAILABILITY OF RESIDENTIAL TREATMENT CENTERS

Residential treatment is frequently recommended and infrequently available. As has been noted, 24-hour care is very expensive no matter what the model. Most families will require some type of public support if they are to utilize the facilities of residential placement. In the medical model, health plans frequently provide for such care. Funds from State departments of education have become increasingly available to supplement family resources in providing for a residential school. Members of such parent groups as the National Society for Autistic Children often have become expert in advising parents how to apply for public funds to help them support their child in a residential facility. Such information should also be available through local social service agencies.

ALTERNATIVES TO RESIDENTIAL CARE

Because residential care is difficult to find and hard to fund, alternatives to 24-hour care have been sought. As discussed earlier, the goal of the professional should be to work out a plan with the family that would best meet the needs of *all* family members. It has been pointed out (Hagamen, 1976) that requests for residential care are seldom due to a change in the child's behavior. The conditions that precipitate requests for institutionalization are usually some kind of family stress such as the birth of a baby, the exhaustion of a mother, the illness of a family member, marital discord, or any of a variety of other stresses. Thus it appears that efforts to help the family and work out ways to reduce the strain involved in caring for the psychotic child may provide growth opportunities for all involved.

At Sagamore Children's Center, a facility of the New York State Department of Mental Hygiene, programs were developed to provide home support and, in addition, parent-training programs were designed to educate interested family members in behavior modification skills that would aid them in the management of their psychotic child. The home support services included a Family Aide Program that involved the training of high-school and college students in behavior management techniques so that they could relieve families that were caring for psychotic children. Family Aides provided individual attention to the child and were used in a variety of ways from baby-sitters to communication tutors. The goal of this program was to help families avoid the social isolation that is often the result of their being "on duty" 24 hours a day. This Center also provided professional homemakers to help families through the crises of birth, death, family illness, etc. that previously had resulted in requests for total institutional care. Another aspect of the home support system was a "rotating respite," in which psychotic children were admitted to the hospital on Friday afternoon and remained for the weekend, rejoining their families on Sunday night so that they could attend the community school. In addition to providing the child with a socializing experience, this program gave the parents the opportunity for weekend respite, a chance to spend time with their other children and to enjoy social activities without the stress of having their disturbed youngster in the house. Such a program is replicable in almost any setting, e.g., in a foster care model, and need not involve a hospital. Such alternatives to total institutional care—because they are available, less costly, and promote better development of the child and his family—can be seen as treatment of choice in most instances for children under the age of twelve.

SUMMARY

The recommendation by the professional for residential care of the psychotic child should be based on a careful evaluation of the needs of the child, the needs of the family and the availability of appropriate residential programs.

Except in the case of the severely retarded child efforts should be made to keep the child in a family setting during the developmental years. However, when the psychotic child remains at home it is imperative to provide a family support system that will minimize any negative effect such a child may have on other family members.

REFERENCES

CHESS, S. *An introduction to child psychiatry*. New York: Grune and Stratton, 1959.

EISENBERG, L. Psychiatric disorders of childhood. In A. FRIEDMAN and H. KAPLAN. (Eds.), *Handbook of psychiatry*. Place: Php., 1967.

EISENBERG, L., and KANNER, L. Early infantile autism. *Am. J. Orthopsychiatry*, 1956, *26*, 556.

FENICHEL, C. Psychoeducational approaches for seriously disturbed children in the classroom. Intervention approach in educating emotionally disturbed children. New York: Syracuse University, Division of Special Education and Rehabilitation, 1966.

GOLDFARB, W. Childhood schizophrenia. Cambridge, Mass.: Harvard University Press, 1961.

GOLDFARB, W., MINTZ, W., and STROOK, K.W. *A time to heal—Corrective socialization—A treatment approach to childhood Schizophrenia*. New York: New York International Press, Inc., 1969.

HAGAMEN, M.B. and VAN WITSEN, B. Early intervention in childhood schizophrenia; The role of special education. *Strategic Intervention in Psychiatry*. Cancro/Fox/Shapiro, 1974.

HAGAMEN, M. B. Family-Support Systems. Their effect on long-term psychiatric hospitalization in children. *Journal of the American Academy of Child Psychiatry*. Winter 1977, *16*, 1, 53–66.

KANNER, L. Autistic disturbances of affective contact. *Nervous child*, 1943, *2*, 217–250.

KANNER, L. Follow-up study of eleven autistic children originally reported in 1943. *J. of Autism & Childhood Schizophrenia*. 1971, *1*, 119–145.

KAUFMAN, K. Behavioral approaches to autism: Home and school. Paper presented at the panel "A Plan for Autistics-Long Island, 1974" at the annual convention of the American Psychiatric Association, Detroit, Michigan, Apr. 1974.

KOLVIN, I. Psychoses in childhood—a comparative study. In M. Rutter (Ed.), *Infantile Autism: Concepts, Characteristics and Treatment*. London: Churchill Livingstone, 1971.

MAKITA, K. The age of onset of childhood schizophrenia. *Folia Psychiatrica Neurologica Japonica*, 1966, *20*, 111–121.

POTTER, H. W. The treatment of problem children in a Psychiatric hospital. *Am. J. of Psychiatry*, Jan. 1935, *91*, pp. 869–880.

RIMLAND, B. *Infantile autism*. Englewood Cliffs, N.J.: Prentice-Hall, 1964.

RUTTER, M. Goulstonian Lecture given at Royal College of Physicians on 17 April 1973. *Psychological medicine*, 1974, *4*, 147–163.

WOLMAN, B. B. (Ed). *Children Without Childhood; a study of childhood schizophrenia*. New York: Grune and Strattor, 1970.

24

CHILD ABUSE

Arthur H. Green

The main objective of this chapter is to provide the reader with a dynamic understanding of the many facets of the child-abuse syndrome so that appropriate strategies for its treatment and prevention may be presented in detail. Child abuse will be defined and demographic data will be presented to illustrate the scope of the problem. An overview of the legal aspects of child abuse consisting of mandatory reporting, investigation, and supervision of child-abusing families in New York State will be included. The major etiological factors in child abuse will be described: the characteristics of abusing parents which impede their capacity for child rearing, the contributions of the child to his scapegoating and abuse, and the environmental factors which exacerbate and perpetuate the child abuse syndrome. Crucial psychodynamic issues underlying this type of pathological family interaction will be explored, as well as the impact of abuse on the behavior and psychological functioning of the children. The elaboration of a conceptual model for the child abuse syndrome based on an understanding of its basic components will offer a rationale for the comprehensive treatment of the abused children and their families.

The material in this chapter is based on the recent literature on child abuse and the author's extensive clinical and research experience with abused children and their families at the Downstate Medical Center.

SCOPE OF THE PROBLEM

The age-old phenomenon of child maltreatment has only recently attracted the attention of mental health professionals. Psychiatric and psychological exploration of child battering has lagged two decades behind the pioneering efforts of pediatricians and radiologists in establishing medical diagnostic criteria for physical abuse in children. Kempe's (Kempe, Silverman, Steele, Droegemueller, and Silver, 1962) classic description of "The Battered Child Syndrome" stimulated widespread interest in child abuse, which soon became recognized as a major pediatric problem. Between 1963 and 1965, the passage of laws by all 50 states requiring medical reporting of child abuse ultimately subjected the abusing parents to legal process and catalyzed the formation of child protective services throughout the nation. The first psychological studies of abusing parents were carried out during this period.

Because of improved reporting procedures and legal pressure to investigate all possible incidents of child abuse and neglect, the true magnitude of the problem in the United States has finally become apparent. The child abuse law in New York State became effective on July 1, 1964. During the first 12-month period, 313 cases of child abuse were reported in New York City with 16 deaths.[1] The latest New York City statistics (1975) indicate that 4,285 cases were reported with 100 deaths. An additional 22,227 children were reported to be neglected. The ten-fold increase in reported abuse over a 9-year period undoubtedly reflects an improvement in reporting procedures as well as an absolute increase in the incidence of child abuse. This impression is supported by similar increases in reported child abuse throughout the country. One author (Light, 1973) has utilized Gil's 1965 survey and 1970 U.S. Census statistics to project an estimated 200,000 to 500,000 abuse cases nationally. This projection refers to cases of physical abuse exclusively and does not include sexual abuse or neglect.

A New York State Department of Social Services estimate of the percentage of severe neglect or sexual abuse cases enables Light to project 465,000 to 1,175,000 such incidents across the nation annually. Combining all types of maltreatment leads to an upper projection of over 1,500,000 cases per year. This figure is approximately equivalent to an estimate by Mr. Douglas Besharov, Director of The National Center on Child Abuse and Neglect. Mr. Besharov indicated that 1.6 million cases of child abuse or neglect are reported each year with 2,000–4,000 deaths (1975). These estimates were based on a recent statistical survey carried out by the Center.

Child maltreatment is currently regarded as the leading cause of death in children and a major public health problem. The proliferation of child abuse and neglect might bear some relationship to the alarming general increase of violence in our society demonstrated by the rising incidence of violent crimes, delinquency, suicide, and lethal accidents. In the last 10 years, child abuse has become a major focus of research and clinical study. A concerted effort is being made by the Federal, State, and local governments to develop programs for the study, prevention, and treatment of child abuse.

[1]New York Central Registry for Child Abuse and Neglect, 1975.

Owing to its complexity and far reaching consequences, the problem of child abuse has attracted the attention of professionals from widely divergent backgrounds. Contributions to this area have come from the fields of pediatrics, psychiatry, psychology, social work, sociology, nursing, education, law, and law enforcement. Such multidisciplinary involvement has been essential in tracking down cases, locating medical treatment, and arranging for protective intervention and long-term planning with the families. At the same time it has become a source of confusion as a result of the differing roles, frames of reference, and terminology of each specialty. Exclusively cultural, socioeconomic, psychodynamic, and behavioral interpretations of the child abuse syndrome have failed to present the full picture. It is the purpose of this chapter to present a comprehensive understanding of the child abuse syndrome by examining its background and the roles of each participant in this tragic process. With this accomplished, one may proceed to develop a logical plan for the prevention, intervention, and treatment of this syndrome.

DEFINITION OF CHILD ABUSE

The definition of child abuse has been continually expanding in recent years. In a classic paper, "The Battered Child Syndrome", Kempe and his collaborators (1962) described child abuse as the infliction of serious injury upon young children by parents and caretakers. The injuries, which included fractures, subdural hematoma, and multiple soft tissue injuries, often resulted in permanent disability and death. Fontana's concept of the "Maltreatment Syndrome" (1964) viewed child abuse as one end of a spectrum of maltreatment which also included emotional deprivation, neglect, and malnutrition. Helfer (1975) recognized the prevalence of minor injuries resulting from abuse and suspected that abuse might be implicated in 10% of all childhood accidents treated in emergency rooms. Gil (1974) extended the concept of child abuse to include any action which prevents a child from achieving his physical and psychological potential.

In this chapter, child abuse will refer to the nonaccidental physical injury inflicted on a child by a parent or guardian, and will encompass the total range of physical injury. Child abuse will be differentiated from child neglect, and the term "maltreatment" will be used as a general reference to both abuse and neglect. The terms *child abuse* and *neglect*, based on the legal definitions stated in the New York State Child Protective Services Act of 1973, will be used as follows:

> *Definition of Child Abuse.* An "abused child" is a child less than 16 years of age whose parent or other person legally responsible for his care:
> 1) inflicts or allows to be inflicted upon the child serious physical injury, or
> 2) creates or allows to be created a substantial risk of serious injury, or
> 3) commits or allows to be committed against the child an act of sexual abuse as defined in the penal law.
>
> *Definition of Child Maltreatment.*[2] A "maltreated child" is a child under 18 years of age who has had serious physical injury inflicted upon him by other than accidental means.
>
> A "maltreated child" is a child under 18 years of age impaired as a result of the failure of his parent or other person legally responsible for his care to exercise a minimum degree of care:
> 1) in supplying the child with adequate food, clothing, shelter, education, medical or surgical care, though financially able to do so or offered financial or other reasonable means to do so; or
> 2) in providing the child with proper supervision or guardianship; or
> 3) by unreasonably inflicting or allowing to be inflicted harm or a substantial risk thereof, including the infliction of excessive corporal punishment; or
> 4) by using a drug or drugs; or
> 5) by using alcoholic beverages to the extent that he loses self-control of his actions; or
> 6) by any other acts of a similarly serious nature requiring the aid of the family court.
>
> A "maltreated child" is also a child under 18 years of age who has been abandoned by his parents or other person legally responsible for his care.

[2]In this legal definition, "maltreatment" refers to neglect.

Child Protective Services

Child protective services are specialized agencies existing under public welfare auspices which are responsible for receiving and investigating all reports of child abuse or maltreatment for the purpose of preventing further abuse and providing services necessary to safeguard the child's well-being and to strengthen the family unit. These agencies are responsible for maintaining service until the conditions of maltreatment are remedied. They also have the mandate to invoke the authority of the juvenile or family court to secure protection and treatment of children whose parents are unable or unwilling to utilize their services.

In New York State, the Child Protective Services Act of 1973 requires every local Department of Social Services to establish a child protective service, which is the sole public agency responsible for receiving and investigating all reports of child abuse or maltreatment on a 24-hour, seven-day-a-week basis. The investigation must commence within 24 hours of the receipt of the report, and must determine within 90 days whether the report is "indicated" or "unfounded." The child protective service is also obligated to send a preliminary written report of the initial investigation to the state central registry of child abuse and maltreatment. Child protective services arrange for and monitor rehabilitative services for children and their families on a voluntary basis or under an order of the Family Court.

The following three sections will be devoted to an exploration of the major components of the child abuse syndrome—the characteristics of the abusing parents, the children who become their victims, and the environmental context in which the abuse takes place.

CHARACTERISTICS OF ABUSING PARENTS

A multitude of behavioral characteristics and psychopathology has been attributed to parents and other adults who engage in child abuse. They have been described as impulsive (Elmer, 1963), immature (Cohen, Raphling, & Green, 1966), rigid and domineering (Merrill, 1962), dependent and narcissistic (Pollock & Steele, 1972), chronically aggressive (Merrill, 1962), isolated from family and friends (Steele & Pollock, 1968), and experiencing marital difficulties (Kempe et al., 1962). One observer noted that abusive mothers were "masculine while their husbands were passive" (Galdston, 1965).

More insightful impressions of the personalities and underlying psychopathology of abusing parents have been gained by observing them during their psychiatric treatment and while interacting with their children. Steele (1970) described specific key psychodynamics contributing to the parental dysfunction encountered in child abuse. He stressed the importance of the parent's closely linked identifications with a harsh, rejecting mother and with a "bad" childhood self-image, both of which are perpetuated in the current relationship with the abused child. The abusive parents submit their children to traumatic experiences similar to those they endured during childhood. Steele observed the use of such defense mechanisms as denial, projection, identification with the aggressor, and role reversal. The last, a maneuver by which the abusing parent turns toward the child for an inordinate amount of dependency gratification, has been noted by other investigators (Morris & Gould, 1963; Simons, Downs, Hurster, & Archer, 1966) as well. Galdston (1971) studied the parents of abused preschool children who attended a therapeutic day care center. He emphasized the importance of unresolved sexual guilt surrounding the conception of the child, who is subsequently abused. Feinstein and his associates (1964) explored the behavior of women with infanticidal impulses in group therapy. These women displayed deep resentment toward their parents for failing to satisfy their dependency needs. They frequently demonstrated a hatred of men which could be traced to intense sibling rivalry with their brothers. Many of these women had witnessed or been subjected to excessive parental violence. They manifested phobic and depressive symptoms in addition to their fears about harming their children.

The wide variety of behavior and personality traits observed in abusing parents suggests that a specific "abusive" personality does not exist. Rather, individuals with a certain psychological makeup operating in combination with the burden of a painfully perceived childhood and immediate environmental stress might be likely to abuse the offspring who most readily elicits the unhappy childhood imagery of the past.

The greatest area of agreement in the field of child abuse has pertained to the history and background of the abusive parents themselves. These individuals have usually experienced abuse, deprivation, rejection, and inadequate mothering during childhood. As children they were subjected to unrealistic expectations and premature demands by their parents.

A study of 60 abused children and their families carried out at The Downstate Medical Center by Green, Gaines, and Sandgrund (1974) demonstrated the following personality characteristics of abuse-prone parents:

1. The parents rely on the child to gratify dependency needs that are unsatisfied in their relationships with their spouses and families. This constitutes role reversal.

2. They manifest impaired impulse control based on childhood experience with harsh punishment and identification with violent adult models.

3. They are handicapped by a poor self-concept. They feel worthless and devalued, which reflects the rejection and criticism accorded them by adults during their own childhood.

4. They display disturbances in identity formation. Identifications are shifting and unstable and are dominated by hostile introjects derived from the internalization of "bad" self and object representations of early childhood.

5. They respond to assaults on their fragile self-esteem with a compensatory adaptation. Because of their need to maintain a positive facade they must desperately defend themselves against the awareness of underlying feelings of worthlessness by the frequent use of projection and externalization as defense mechanisms.

6. The projection of negative parental attributes onto the child causes him to be misperceived and used

as a scapegoat in order to bear the brunt of the parent's aggression.

Psychodynamics

The psychodynamics in a given case of child abuse are largely determined by the "abuse-prone" personality traits of the parent. The relationship between the abusing parent and his child is distorted by the cumulative impact of the parent's own traumatic experiences as a child reared in a punitive, unloving environment. Individuals who abuse their children cannot envision any parent-child relationship as a mutually gratifying experience. The task of parenting mobilizes identifications with the parent-aggressor, child-victim dyad of the past. The key psychodynamic elements in child abuse are role reversal, excessive use of denial and projection as defenses, rapidly shifting identifications, and displacement of aggression from frustrating objects onto the child.

Role reversal occurs when the unfulfilled abusing parent seeks dependency gratification, which is unavailable from his spouse and family, from his "parentified" child. It is based on an identification with the "child-victim." The child's inability to gratify the parent causes him to be unconsciously perceived as the rejecting mother. This intensifies the parent's feelings of rejection and worthlessness which threaten his narcissistic equilibrium. These painful feelings are denied and projected onto the child, who then becomes the recipient of the parent's self-directed aggression.

This is accomplished by a shift toward identification with the aggressive parent, terminating the role reversal. By beating the child, the abuser assuages his punitive superego and attempts actively to master the traumatic experiences passively endured as a child. The scapegoating process continues as the child becomes the target for additional aggression displaced from various despised and frustrating objects in the parent's current and past life, such as a rejecting mate or lover, a hated sibling rival, or a depriving parent substitute. These objects are unconsciously linked to the original "parent-aggressor."

The choice of particular child for scapegoating might depend upon accidental factors such as time of birth, physical appearance, temperament, and/or sex, in addition to actual physical or psychological deviancy.

Differences Between Abusing Fathers and Mothers

While abusing fathers and mothers share some specific personality traits and psychodynamics, differences in sex, family role, and environmental influences create typical contrasts in maternal and paternal child abuse patterns (Green, 1976b). The mother's greater responsibility for child care and homemaking and the father's more peripheral involvement with the family are a major cause of divergent parental behavior in child rearing.

The abusing father regards his spouse as his major source of dependency gratification and expects her to compensate for his earlier parental deprivation. He cannot tolerate the nurturing interaction between his spouse and children, who are unconsciously perceived as rejecting mother and sibling rivals. The abusing father typically abuses his wife and child simultaneously. These fathers are unable to acknowledge and verbalize their feelings of deprivation and dependent longings for their spouse. Expression of these feelings is further discouraged by society's intolerance of male "weakness and passivity." The father's wishes for nurturance are more easily satisfied in the socially acceptable ritual of drinking. Excessive alcohol intake permits the fulfillment of regressive oral fantasies while absolving the father from any responsibility for the act. Thus, drinking, denial of dependency, and spouse abuse are typical characteristics of abusing fathers. These characteristics are, however, often absent in abusing mothers.

Since her spouse and family are incapable of providing nurturance and satisfaction, the abusing mother seeks gratification primarily from her children. These mothers can express their dependency yearnings more easily than the fathers yet they remain essentially unfulfilled. Their more intense involvement and identification with their children make them less dependent on alcohol for gratification. They are unable to express their frustration and rage directly toward their mates. These, then, are conveyed indirectly through abuse of the children and refusal to perform domestic responsibilities, which are then delegated to the spouse.

Another contrast between abusing mothers and fathers is observed in their reactions to their spouse's participation in child rearing activities. Abusing fathers react with jealousy and resentment to their spouse's contact with the children. Abusing mothers, on the other hand, welcome their spouse's all too infrequent involvement with the children. Abusing mothers exhibit envy of their children's attachment to the father only after the husband-wife relationship has terminated, and he is no longer living at home.

One may also observe differences in the quality of role reversal as perceived by abusing mothers and fathers. The abusing mother cherishes the child's premature independence as a source of physical and emotional support which is not forthcoming from spouse or family. The abusing father expects premature performances from his children so they will be able to relinquish their claims on his spouse. These fathers often expect their sons to be aggressive and violent as a means of confirming the parents' own masculinity. Abusing mothers, however, do not easily tolerate aggressive behavior in their sons because it often evokes the image of a despised husband or spouse.

Thus, different patterns of parental identification with the child, based on sex, influence the quality of abuse. The greater ease of parental identification with a child of the same sex makes this child a convenient scapegoat for the projection of the parent's own shortcomings. Parental abuse of the opposite sex child is more likely to be based upon this child's link to the despised spouse.

Nonabusive mothers whose children have been battered by husbands or boyfriends exhibit a slight variation in the psychodynamic pattern. The interaction between mother and child begins in a similar fashion as the mother endows the child with the attributes of her own rejecting parents. However, the resulting "bad" childhood self-image derived from her parents is partly maintained and partly transferred to the child, while the internalized "parent-aggressor" is projected onto the abusive mate. The mother retains her identification with the "child-victim" rather than with the "parent-aggressor."

These women submit to the physical cruelty of their mates as a masochistic repetition of their childhood victimization by rejecting, aggressive parents. The pain-dependent attachment to the spouse serves as a defense against their hostility toward the child. This is confirmed by the tenacity with which these women cling to brutal and humiliating relationships, and by their tendency to assume the abusive role if the spouse leaves.

CHARACTERISTICS OF ABUSED CHILDREN

Recent efforts to document the psychological damage sustained by abused children have uncovered a variety of cognitive and emotional difficulties, but these have yet to be integrated into a comprehensive psychodynamic understanding of the abused child in the context of his traumatic family environment. Elmer (1965) studied the effects of abuse by comparing abused and non-abused children who had been hospitalized for multiple bone injuries. The abused children showed a higher incidence of mental retardation and speech difficulties. Martin (1972) reported a study in which one-third of a sample of abused children was mentally retarded, 43% were neurologically damaged, and 38% exhibited delayed language development. Morse, Sahler, and Friedman (1970) discovered mental deficiency in 70% of a group of children whose injuries resulted from abuse or neglect.

Behavioral observations of abused children have found them to be stubborn, unresponsive, negativistic and depressed (Johnson & Morse, 1968), fearful, apathetic, and unappealing with a blunting of their appetite for food and human contact (Galdston, 1965) and likely to provoke physical attack from others. Green (1968) documented a link between physical abuse and subsequent self-mutilation in schizophrenic children.

The severity and wide range of psychological impairment attributed to abused children clearly warranted further clinical investigation and research. This stimulated the author's interest in exploring the psychological sequelae of abuse in 60 schoolage battered children at the Downstate Medical Center (Green, Sandgrund, Gaines, & Haberfeld, 1974). Psychiatric evaluation and psychological testing of these children documented the cognitive impairment described by others. The abused children exhibited significantly lower mean IQ scores than matched normal controls. Twenty-five percent of the abused children were found to be mentally retarded with IQ's of less than 70. These children also demonstrated severe deficits in a wide variety of ego functions, such as impulse control, defensive functioning, reality testing, object relations, thought processes, body image, and overall ego competency. The abused children also exhibited a rather typical pattern of depressive affect with low self-esteem, which was often accompanied by self-destructive behavior. These abnormalities were attributed to the disruptive impact of physical and emotional trauma on the normal development of the child's cognitive and adaptive ego functions as a consequence of deviant parenting. In some cases, however, the defects of the child preceded and precipitated the maltreatment (Sandgrund, Gaines, & Green, 1974).

Most of the abused children required intensive psychotherapeutic and psychoeducational intervention in order to overcome severe behavioral and educational difficulties. This led to the development of a pilot treatment program for abused children and their families under the auspices of the Division of Child and Adolescent Psychiatry. Approximately 20 abused children were involved in out-patient individual psychotherapy from 1972 through 1975. The treatment of the children was complemented by various modes of therapeutic involvement with the parents, such as counseling, crisis intervention, and home contact by visiting nurses. The children ranged in age from 5 to 12, and most of them were seen twice weekly for at least one year. A major purpose of the treatment program was the in-depth exploration of the psychopathology and psychodynamics typical of abused children, and their genetic relationship to a hostile environment. Another aim was the development of specialized therapeutic techniques designed to reverse the psychopathology of the child and to prevent further maltreatment. To the author's knowledge, this is the only specialized program involved in the intensive study and treatment of abused children.

Psychopathology of Abused Children

A more profound understanding of the psychological functioning of abused children was obtained from material derived from these psychotherapeutic interventions. This study permitted the exploration of the abusive interaction between each child and his family within the context of their physical and psychological environment. Child abuse was regarded as a complex experience consisting of several components rather than as a single variable. The following elements were identified:

1. An acute physical and psychological assault conveying parental rage and hostility which confronted the child with the threat of annihilation and/or abandonment.
2. The abuse occurred within a background of poverty, family disorganization, and the interruption of maternal care, resulting in early experiences of object loss and emotional deprivation. The precipitating cause was often a step-wise family migration from rural areas to the urban ghetto. The children were frequently left with grandparents while the mothers attempted to secure housing and employment in the new surroundings.
3. Deviant psychological and constitutional endowment of the child often complemented the pathological environment as a crucial variable associated with abuse.
4. The abused child was usually a scapegoat and was perceived as the major source of the family's frustrations. The scapegoating process, which consists of the projection of negative parental attributes onto the child, was also influenced by the latter's inherited or acquired behavioral deviancy.

These immediate and long-term adverse experiences left a characteristic impact on the cognitive apparatus, ego functions, object relationships, identifications, and libidinal organization of the abused children. Specific disturbances in ego functions, behavior, and character structure with their pathological sequelae may be outlined in the following manner.

Overall Impairment in Ego Functioning. When viewed globally, the abused children exhibited an overall impairment in ego functioning associated with intellectual and cognitive deficits. They displayed a higher incidence of delayed development and CNS dysfunction than their nonabused peers. Many were mentally retarded. They were often found to be hyperactive and impulsive, with minimal frustration tolerance. Motor activity, rather than verbalization, was the preferred mode of expression. Many abused children manifested aberrant speech and language development. Although these children were of latency age, they failed to demonstrate the progressive ego growth and reorganization characteristic of this stage. There was an absence of those typical latency defenses that enable the normal child to bind anxiety from internal and external sources and cope with phase specific stresses and conflicts. The abused children's preoccupation with external danger and overstimulated drive activity deprived them of the energy necessary for learning and mastery.

"Traumatic" Reaction with Acute Anxiety State. The frightening physical and psychological assault experienced by these children during an abusive episode exposed them to the threat of annihilation and/or abandonment. Many of the children were overwhelmed by both the quality and quantity of the noxious stimulation, which paralyzed ego functioning and resulted in severe panic. This situation resembled Freud's concept of traumatic neurosis and the breaching of the stimulus barrier (1920). The anxiety states the children manifested occurred prior to or during a beating, or in anticipation of an attack. Under these conditions they frequently displayed psychotic behavior, attributable to severe ego regression with the temporary suspension of reality testing.

These children also exhibited a striking tendency continually to reenact the traumatic situation. Repetition of the trauma was observed in overt behavior and in symbolic activities such as fantasy, play, and artistic productions. It was also encountered in the therapeutic relationship when the abused child acted out the role of the "bad child" and sought punishment from the therapist. This "fixation to the trauma" may be considered as a defensive reaction which permits the abused child actively to recreate, master, and control the painful affects and anxiety which otherwise might be instigated by the environment. The maladaptive aspects of this pattern are quite obvious. It may lead to further maltreatment and punishment and ultimately result in a pain-dependent orientation.

Khan's concept of "cumulative trauma" (1963) might explain the long-term interference with the abused child's development caused by the mother's failure to function as a protective shield.

Pathological Object Relationships. Early and pervasive exposure to parental rejection, assault, and deprivation has an adverse effect on the development of subsequent object relationships. Potential new objects are regarded with fear and apprehension, and Erikson's stage of basic trust (1950) is apparently beyond their reach. These children learn to expect frustration and maltreatment from all adults and to view human encounters as basically violent and rejecting. They are involved in a perpetual search for "good" objects to protect them from the "bad" ones.

Psychotherapeutic involvement with abused children has provided us with a good opportunity to study the vicissitudes of their object relationships in *statu nascendi.* The typical abused child initially appeared detached and guarded, and was ingratiating in order to please the therapist and avoid punishment. Once he felt safe, he displayed an enormous object hunger. The therapist was overidealized, and the child attempted to capture and incorporate this "good parent" as a source of dependency gratification and as a means of protection against his "bad" parental objects. However, the inevitable frustrations and limitations in the therapeutic relationship incited the child's rage and disillusionment.

The child's increasing anger and provocative behavior led to his anticipation of punishment by the therapist, who was rapidly transformed into the "bad parent." Projecting his own rage onto the therapist, the child only succeeded in compounding this negative image and increasing his fear of retaliation. At this point he adopted the negative self-image of the "bad child" which represented an "identification with the aggressor" (his own bad parent) in the face of increasing anxiety and helplessness in the treatment situation. The child then proceeded to reenact his relationship with the abusing parent with the therapist. He sought to achieve mastery and control over anticipated punishment through provocative and testing behavior. The rapidly fluctuating self and object identifications of the child were facilitated by the utilization of primitive defense mechanisms which will now be described.

Primitive Defense Mechanisms. The abused children relied on an excessive use of primitive defenses such as denial, projection, introjection, and splitting in order to cope with threatening external and internalized parental images. They were unable to integrate the loving and hostile aspects of their parents and others. This accounted for the baffling tendency of some of these children completely to support their parent's transparent denials and rationalizations concerning inflicted injuries.

While this need to suppress knowledge of parental wrongdoing was occasionally motivated by fear of additional punishment, it also represented the child's need to protect himself from the awareness of the actual and internalized destructive parent and to safeguard the parent from his own murderous rage. The image of the "bad parent" was subjected to denial and was projected onto some other person, allowing the child to maintain the fantasy of having a "good parent." At times the child assumed this negative identification in compliance with parental wishes for a scapegoat. In this situation, the child acted as a willing prop for the projection of the parent's bad, unacceptable self-image. Splitting mechanisms were more frequently observed in those children who were abused by the parent who provided most of their nurturing. Their acknowledgement of the destructiveness and malevolence of the primary caretaker, usually the mother, would have placed their tenuous dependent relationship in jeopardy.

Impaired Impulse Control. The abused children were often cited for aggressive and destructive behavior at home and in school. Bullying, fighting, and assaultive behavior were observed in their contact with peers and siblings. The younger children were frequently restless and hyperactive, while the older children and adolescents were commonly involved in antisocial and delinquent behavior. The origin of this problem was overdetermined. The abused children formed a basic identification with their violent parents, which facilitated the use of "identification with the aggressor" as a major defense against feelings of anxiety and helplessness. Hyperaggressive behavior typically followed incidents of physical abuse. Loss of impulse control was further enhanced by the presence of CNS dysfunction. These children also lacked the usual superego restraints found in normal children during latency due to inadequate superego models and faulty internalization. Impulse control was precarious and inconsistent, achieved largely through externalization and fear of punishment.

Impaired Self-Concept. The abused children were frequently sad, dejected, and self-deprecatory. Their poor self-concept was an end result of chronic physical and emotional scarring, humiliation, and scapegoating compounded and reinforced by each new episode of physical abuse. One may hypothesize that the preverbal infant who is repeatedly assaulted acquires an unpleasurable awareness of "self" consisting of painful sensations and painful affects linked to primary objects. With the development of cognition and language, this painful self-awareness becomes transformed into a devalued self-concept. These children ultimately regard themselves with the same displeasure and contempt that their parents directed toward them. Young children who are repeatedly punished, beaten, and threatened with abandonment assume that it is a consequence of their own behavior, regardless of their actual innocence. Our subjects' loathsome self-image often created such anxiety and discomfort that it was projected or displaced onto others. These negative self representations were often attributed to a specific doll or puppet in the playroom. At times the poor self-concept was disguised by compensatory fantasies of grandiosity and omnipotence.

Masochistic and Self-Destructive Behavior. Abused children commonly exhibit overt types of self-destructive behavior such as suicide attempts, gestures, threats, and various forms of self-mutilation. These are often accompanied by more subtle forms of pain-dependent activity in the form of provocative, belligerent, and limit-testing behavior which easily elicit beatings and punishment from parents, adults, and peers. Accident proneness is another form of self-destructive activity frequently observed in this population. Forty percent of our research population of abused children manifested direct forms of self-destructive behavior, a significantly higher incidence than in the neglected and normal controls (Green, 1976c). In the majority of cases, the self-destructive behavior was precipitated by parental beatings or occurred in response to actual or threatened separation from parental figures. This finding is of special importance since self-destructive behavior is seldom observed among latency and pre-adolescent children in the general population. Thus, certain events that occur in normal latency and seem to have self-preservative functions are interfered with in the abused child.

The overall impairment of ego functions and impulse control in these children facilitated their reenactment of parental hostility and rejection. Self-destructive behavior represented the child's compliance with parental wishes for his destruction and/or disappearance. The child's acting out of parental hostility directed toward him has been described as an important factor in the etiology of adolescent suicidal behavior (Sabbeth, 1969). The self-destructive behavior of the abused child may also be conceived as the end result of the transformation of feelings of low self-esteem and self-hatred into action.

Difficulties with Separation. The abused children often reacted to actual or threatened separation and object loss with intense anxiety. This was frequently traced to numerous experiences of separation and abandonment with parental figures during infancy and early childhood. Hypothetically, chronic physical abuse might have increased the vulnerability of these children to separation because each beating implies the parent's withdrawal of love and wish to be rid of the child. The abused child's frequent lack of object constancy resulting from cognitive impairment and/or cerebral dysfunction was another contributing factor to the separation problem. This interfered with the construction and internalization of the mental representation of the absent object. Acute separation anxiety in the clinical situation was often observed in response to the therapist's vacations or departure from the hospital. Abused children were commonly unable to leave the playroom unless they were given a tangible object which they could utilize to represent the absent therapist.

Difficulties in School Adjustment. Most of the abused children exhibited major problems in school adjustment. Their limited attention span, frequent hyperactivity, and cognitive impairment led to deficient academic performance. At times they demonstrated specific learning disabilities such as dyslexia, expressive and receptive language disorders, and perceptual-motor dysfunction contingent on minimal brain dysfunction or maturational lag. Their aggressivity and poor impulse control contributed to behavior problems with peers and teachers. Their parents were frequently called to school because of their disruptive behavior and learning difficulties, which often led to further abuse. A vicious cycle often ensued, consisting of academic and behavioral problems, parental beatings, and increased disruptiveness in the classroom due to the displacement of anger at the parents onto the teachers. Chronic school difficulties leading to disciplinary action and placement in special classes for the emotionally or intellectually handicapped produced further adverse effects on the abused child's previously damaged self-esteem.

ENVIRONMENTAL FACTORS ASSOCIATED WITH CHILD ABUSE

While environmental stress has often been suggested as a prominent etiological factor in child abuse, the precise definition of this relationship has eluded most investigators. One author has attributed child abuse almost exclusively to socioeconomic determinants (Gil, 1968, 1970), but most researchers agree that environmental stress is basically only the catalyst, in many instances, for an abuse-prone personality.

In addition to Gil's studies, economic pressures were important findings in studies by Elmer (1967), Kempe et al. (1962), Young (1964), Johnson and Morse (1968), and Bennie and Sclare (1969). Contrary evidence can be obtained in Paulson and Blake (1969) and Steele and Pollock (1968), who observed child abuse in economically advantaged populations. These and other authors (Adelson, 1961; Allen, Ten Bensel, & Raile, 1969; Holter & Friedman, 1968; Kempe et al., 1962; Simons et al., 1966; Green, 1976a; Green et al., 1974) place far greater emphasis upon personality factors and intrafamily dynamics.

The stress argument has at least in part been predicated on the high percentage of low socioeconomic status, multiple problem families in child abuse registers throughout the country. It is probable that reporting procedures themselves have led to the greater emphasis on socioeconomic determinants. Any controlled study which matches for SES (Socioeconomic Status) is compelled to look beyond such variables as family income for the origin of child abuse. The conclusion that Spinetta and Rigler (1972) reach in their review of the literature is far more likely—that environmental stress is neither necessary nor sufficient for child abuse but that it does, in some instances, interact with other factors, such as parent personality variables and child behaviors, to potentiate child battering.

Environmental stress includes current events that widen the discrepancy between the limited capacity of the parents and increased child-rearing pressures. The stress may consist of a diminution of child rearing resources owing to a spouse's illness or desertion, or to the unavailability of an earlier caretaker, such as a neighbor or some other family member.

Another environmental stress is the actual or threatened loss of a key relationship that provides the parent with emotional security and dependency gratification. This may occur when the spouse becomes physically or emotionally unavailable or when ties with parents or important relatives are severed due to estrangement, illness, or death. Additional child-rearing pressures, such as the birth or illness of another child, or the assumption of temporary care of other children, create environmental stress that may also lead to child abuse.

Justice and Duncan (1975) described the contribution of work-related pressures to environmental stress in situations of child abuse. They cited four types of work-related situations: unemployed fathers caring for children at home, working mothers with domestic obligations, overworked husbands who neglect their wives, and traumatic job experiences resulting in undischarged tension. Justice and Justice (1975) were able to document the importance of stress in terms of excessive life changes in child-abusing families by means of the Social Readjustment Rating Scale developed by Holmes and Rahe (1967).

Conceptualization of the Child Abuse Syndrome

Reviewing the characteristics, motivation, and pathological interaction of the abused children and their parents in the context of their surroundings leads this writer to regard child abuse as a dysfunction of parenting in which the parent misperceives the child because of his own frustrating childhood experiences. In beating the child, the parent attempts actively to master the trauma he passively endured during his early life. The etiology of child abuse is based upon an interaction among three factors: the personality traits of the parents that contribute to "abuse proneness"; the child's characteristics that enhance his scapegoating; and environmental stress which widens the discrepancy between the limited child-rearing capacity of the parents and increased child-rearing pressures. This viewpoint coincides with that of Kempe and Helfer (1972) who described the parent with abusive potential, the special child, and a precipitating crisis as the combination of factors which lead to abuse.

The next section will deal with the treatment and prevention of child abuse. Our society's urgent need for programs providing treatment and rehabilitation for the increasing numbers of abusing families will be considered along with some recent progress made in this direction. The heightened interest in treatment reflects a shift away from the previous emphasis on placement of abused children in foster homes and institutions.

The major techniques of crisis intervention and treatment designed to modify the etiological components of the child abuse syndrome and preserve the integrity of the family will be discussed. We will consider both specialized therapeutic methods tailored to the specific needs and problems of the abusing parents and the outpatient psychotherapy of abused children, including the delivery of vital social and health services to reduce the environmental stress impinging on these families.

We will propose a comprehensive treatment program in the setting of a medical center with its numerous therapeutic and rehabilitative components as the most effective vehicle for improving the parental functioning of abusing families and maintaining the physical and psychological development of the abused children. The composition of such a multidisciplinary staff and the specific functions of each member will be described. Finally, we will discuss the prevention of child abuse with a two-fold focus on educational programs for the general public and primary intervention with those families considered to be at risk for abuse.

TREATMENT OF CHILD ABUSE

GENERAL CONSIDERATIONS

Unfortunately, efforts toward the rehabilitation of abusing families have not kept pace with the recent nationwide increase in the reporting and public awareness of child abuse. Social scientists have deplored the inability of states and cities to supply services and treatment for the great influx of maltreating families (DeFrancis, 1972; Oviatt, 1972; Nagi, 1975). The impact of punitive societal attitudes toward abusing parents is still reflected in the investigation and management of newly reported cases. In many states, cases of abuse are reported to law enforcement officials rather than to protective service agencies. The initial contact with abusing families emphasizes investigation and confirmation of the alleged incident, a practice that is usually incompatible with the development of a therapeutic strategy. Placement of the children in foster homes and institutions has become the major mode of intervention owing to the relative scarcity of social and psychiatric services for abusing families and the difficulties experienced in involving abusing parents in traditional counseling and psychotherapy. Abusing parents are still too frequently presumed to be unmotivated for help and therefore beyond rehabilitation.

Some progress has recently been made toward the development of child-abuse treatment programs through the pioneering efforts of a group of pediatricians, psychiatrists, and social workers at the University of Colorado Medical Center at Denver, Colorado. The Denver group was the first systematically to describe the clinical dimensions and psychology of child abuse and to base innovative treatment techniques on this body of knowledge. This group collaborated in the publication of two basic texts on child abuse edited by Helfer and Kempe (1968, 1972), which stimulated the initiation of child-abuse treatment facilities in other parts of the country. In January 1974, the Child Abuse Prevention and Treatment Act (P.L. 93–247) established a National Center on Child Abuse and Neglect in Washington, D.C., under the direction of the U.S. Department of Health, Education and Welfare, Office of Child Development. The role of the National Center is to conduct research, provide grants for the improvement of state protective services, establish training programs for professionals, and to fund demonstration treatment programs in the area of child abuse and neglect. Helfer (1975) estimated that 70 to 75% of families involved in child abuse or neglect can be expected to show significant improvement within 6 to 9 months after the beginning of treatment. Pollack and Steele (1972) reported that, under optimal conditions, 80% of these parents can be treated satisfactorily. Multidisciplinary child-abuse consultation teams are now being established in various parts of the country to improve the diagnosis and management of cases of abuse and maltreatment. Child-abuse treatment centers have been initiated in certain hospital and community settings with the aim of providing rehabilitation and social services to strengthen abusing and neglecting families in crisis. However, these direly needed facilities are so few in number that the vast majority of maltreating families receive no therapeutic intervention during or after the initial investigation by protective service personnel. In New York City, 26,512 cases of child abuse and maltreatment were reported in 1975,[3] yet only three relatively small comprehensive treatment programs are in existence, only one of which is partially supported by the city.

An intensification of this trend toward treatment and rehabilitation with an emphasis on crisis-oriented intervention in the home can be expected in the future. The greater availability of treatment facilities designed to strengthen and maintain the integrity of the family will significantly reduce the number of children requiring costly placement in foster homes and institutions, and hopefully result in substantial savings, both in terms of finances and human resources, to communities and municipalities.

Any plan for the prevention or treatment of child abuse must be designed to create a safe environment for the child and to modify the potentiating factors underlying abuse. Therefore, an effective treatment program must deal specifically with the parental abuse proneness, those characteristics of the child which make him vulnerable for scapegoating, and the environmental stresses that trigger the abusive interaction.

Goals and Objectives of a Comprehensive Treatment Program for Child-Abusing Families

The major objective of an ideal treatment program is to provide both parent and child with a broad, comprehensive, and relevant spectrum of services in order to strengthen and maintain the family constellation when possible. The program elements should be designed to modify the three important etiological factors underlying the maltreatment process.

A. *Abuse Proneness of the Parents*

1. Helping the parent establish a trusting, supportive, and gratifying relationship with the therapist and with other adults.

2. Helping the parent improve his chronically devalued self-image.

3. Enabling the parent to receive satisfaction from his own accomplishments and from contacts with others so that he will no longer depend on his children to bolster his self-esteem.

4. Providing the parent with a positive child-rearing model for identification.

5. Enabling the parent to derive pleasure from the child, and increasing the parent's capacity to "give" (love, warmth, attention, etc.) to the child so that the role reversal will be eliminated.

6. Providing the parent with basic information about child rearing and child development. Special counseling will be made available to parents of vulnerable children with physical, emotional, and intellectual impairment.

7. Helping the parent to understand the relationship between the painful experiences of his own childhood and his current misperception of the child.

B. *The Children*

1. Safeguarding the children from further abuse and maltreatment.

2. Reversing the physical, psychological, and cognitive damage already inflicted on the child.

3. Preventing future social, educational, and psychiatric maladaptation.

C. *Environmental Stress*

1. Eliminating the discrepancy between the limited parental capacity of the family and the increased child-rearing pressures by providing help with direct child care (baby-sitting, day care facilities). Homemaking assistance or visiting nurses should be made available when appropriate, as well as the material resources required by each family such as food, clothing, and shelter.

[3] New York City Central Registry for Child Abuse and Neglect, 1975.

2. The treatment staff should be available for emergencies on a 24-hour basis.

SPECIAL PROBLEMS IN THE TREATMENT OF ABUSING PARENTS

The treatment of child-abusing parents poses special difficulties beyond those usually associated with a psychologically unsophisticated, primarily lower-class, multiproblem population. The following characteristics of the abusing parents must be dealt with before a therapeutic relationship can be established.

1. These parents are often unmotivated to seek help, or even overtly hostile to the suggestion that they may suffer from emotional difficulties. They typically lack insight and deny and project their problems onto other people or situations. Confronting them about these tactics would be counterproductive. It is more effective to accept their projections and empathize with their frustrations in dealing with significant persons and situations. One might initially focus on the "difficult child" or on material issues such as financial and housing problems, where intervention might be less threatening and even considered helpful.

2. Their suspiciousness and basic mistrust of authorities interferes with the formation of a therapeutic alliance. This is a result of their life-long experience of humiliation and criticism at the hands of their parents and subsequent authority figures.

3. The fragile self-esteem of these parents impairs their capacity to accept help and counseling from the therapeutic team. Constructive suggestions concerning child rearing and home management might be rebuffed if construed as criticisms. The parents require continual reassurance and support, especially during the initial stages of treatment. Their basic dependency needs must be gratified before "demands" can be placed on them.

4. The abusive parents are masochistic and provocative, and they exhibit a stubborn tendency to turn the treatment situation into a repetition of their frustrating and humiliating interaction with their parents and spouses. The treatment staff must be trained to handle this provocative behavior without counter-reacting.

5. The impact of ongoing investigative and punitive procedures by protective services or the court, inhibits the establishment of a confidential and trusting relationship with the therapist. The problem of confidentiality may be eased by divorcing the investigation and court-related activities from the treatment process. Psychiatric evaluations and recommendations required by the court should be performed independently by their own personnel.

The next group of obstacles to treatment is primarily determined by personal attitudes and feelings elicited in therapists by abusive parents and the act of child abuse itself.

1. The phenomenon of negative countertransference is such an obstacle. This involves the natural tendency of the therapist instinctively to condemn and dislike a parent who would cruelly assault and humiliate a helpless infant or child. The primary therapist of the abusive parent, as well as the entire treatment staff, must learn to control feelings of anger and self-righteous indignation toward the parent. Such expressed attitudes, needless to say, preclude the development of a therapeutic alliance.

2. The therapist tends to act out the role of a "good parent" who rescues the child from his brutal family. These rescue fantasies are often accompanied by premature efforts to transform the abusing mothers and fathers into model parents. Abusing parents are unable to tolerate this competitive and patronizing attitude of the therapist, which evokes deep-seated feelings of inadequacy experienced during confrontations with their own parents.

3. The marked degree of parental ambivalence toward therapeutic involvement characterized by rapidly alternating periods of infantile demands for dependency gratification and hostile withdrawal typically engenders a great deal of frustration in the therapist. Child-abusing parents also frequently arrive late or miss their appointments and seem unappreciative of the therapist's investment of time and energy. Their apparent lack of cooperation and commitment to the treatment process is a threat to the narcissistic gratification of the therapist.

These formidable obstacles to the development of a viable therapeutic relationship with abusing parents initially discouraged many workers in the field about the value of therapeutic intervention in modifying their behavior. For many, placement of abused children in foster homes and institutions seemed to be the safer and more expedient solution, despite its great expense and obvious limitations. However, many of those who continued to work with abusing parents realized that their failure to adapt to the traditional out-patient model of psychiatric and social service intervention could be remedied by major modifications of these techniques. A multidisciplinary "team" approach with a shift in focus from the out-patient clinical setting to the home was found to be effective. The delivery of comprehensive services such as crisis-oriented home visits, telephone hot-lines, parent groups, homemaking assistance, visiting nurse intervention, and day care facilities for infants and small children in the abusing families reduced adverse environmental pressures and fostered a strengthening and stabilization of crisis-ridden families. This comprehensive intervention has helped overcome the above-mentioned obstacles to therapeutic involvement and has facilitated positive changes in the child-rearing patterns of abusing parents. The crucial ingredient of any treatment program for abusing parents is still found in the parent's involvement in a therapeutic relationship with an accepting, gratifying, and uncritical adult. The helping person need not be a psychiatrist, physician, psychologist, or social worker. Nurses, nursing students, graduate students in the behavioral sciences, and mature volunteers who have mothered successfully may be trained to help abusing parents.

Treatment of Abused Children

The initial goal of intervention with abused children is to protect them from further maltreatment. This may be accomplished by strengthening parental functioning where possible or by temporary removal from the home. Once these children are in a safe environment, every effort should be made to reverse the serious emotional and cognitive impairment associated with their traumatic life experience and frequent constitutional vulnerability. Since most of the abusive parents were subjected to abuse during their own childhood, the abused children might become the violent child-abusing adults of the next generation if they are not helped.

A wide range of psychotherapeutic and educational techniques have proven successful in reducing the symptoms and problems of abused children. Psychoanalytically oriented play therapy and psychotherapy have been used effectively at the Downstate Medical Center's treatment program for abused children. However, certain modifications of therapeutic technique were necessary to deal with the high incidence of developmental deviation and psychopathology. In general, these children presented with ego deficits and cognitive impairment to such a degree that an emphasis on ego integration, reality testing, containment of drives and impulses, and the strengthening of higher level defenses (similar to those techniques applied to borderline and psychotic children) proved necessary.

Strengthening of ego functions is achieved by a supportive approach in which the therapist allows himself to be used as a primary object by the child. The therapist encourages verbalization and containment of impulse and action, and helps the child gradually increase his tolerance for frustration. The child is permitted to reenact the traumatic beatings in play and fantasy as a means of achieving ego mastery. In contrast to the hostile parents, the therapist offers himself as a benign object for incorporation of ego and superego functions sorely needed by the abused child. This facilitates a strengthening of psychic structure and a gradual internalization of the therapist's attitudes and controls. With the emergence of more effective defenses such as repression, sublimation, and reaction formation, the child will begin to experience internal conflict and neurotic symptom formation. The therapist also helps the child with reality testing and encourages him to participate in the typical structured "games" of latency. One major goal of treatment is to foster more adaptive controls and defenses so that the child can finally experience a "latency" period relatively free from excessive external and internal stimulation.

Strengthening of impulse control is another crucial task of therapeutic intervention, since the abused child's aggressive, assaultive, and destructive behavior is the major source of his difficulty at home and in school and the cause of his referral for psychiatric treatment. The therapist can foster impulse control by careful structuring of the therapy sessions. Direct manifestations of aggression such as hitting, or destroying toys and playroom materials should not be permitted. Instead, the child is encouraged to verbalize anger or express it through play. Limit setting must be clearly defined with respect to entering and leaving the playroom, removing toys and materials, and the length of the sessions. By gradually identifying with the therapist and internalizing his warm and accepting attitudes, the child will be able to counteract his tendency to use "identification with the aggressor" as a primary mode of communication. The abused child's capacity to "neutralize" aggression will increase with the consolidation of his libidinal and affective bonds with the therapist. If impulsivity is associated with hyperactivity and minimal cerebral dysfunction, psychotherapeutic techniques should be complemented with the use of amphetamines or Ritalin.

Improvement of object relationships is another treatment objective. The therapist helps the child gradually overcome his basic mistrust of significant objects by establishing a gratifying, consistent, and dependable relationship. Initially, the therapist is indulgent and allows the child some measure of regression and gratification of unfulfilled dependency yearnings. He might provide the child with food, candy, and gifts on appropriate occasions, etc. As the therapist rapidly evolves into an overidealized "good" parent for the child, he makes use of the child's positive attachment to strengthen the therapeutic alliance. This is necessary to protect the relationship when the therapist is ultimately regarded as the "bad parent."

During this phase of treatment, the child's attempts to provoke the therapist into punishing him and recreating the original "bad parent"/"bad child" relationship can be interpreted. The therapist can also indicate the child's projection of his own anger onto the therapist with the resulting fear of retaliation. Although the child's proneness for using primitive defenses (denial, projection, and splitting) may initially be refractory to interpretation, this tendency should gradually fade as ego functioning is strengthened during the course of treatment. Once the child is able to integrate the "good" and "bad" aspects of himself and others, he will be able to resist the tendency to assume the role of the "scapegoat," thus reducing his motivation for acting out.

Improvement of self-esteem occurs during the ongoing climate of warmth and acceptance by the therapist. The abused child will gradually readjust his self-esteem to coincide with the therapist's positive view of him. The child needs to be told that his frequent beatings usually resulted from parental problems rather than as a result of his "badness." Improvement in the child's overall ego functioning and behavior should boost his self-esteem, as he evidences greater mastery in daily experience and improved capacity to form gratifying object ties.

Improved parental functioning and cessation of abuse as a consequence of therapeutic intervention with the family will also contribute to the enhancement of the child's self-regard.

The child's tendency toward self-destructive and masochistic behavior can ultimately be interpreted as a repetition of parental hostility directed toward him. This "turning inward" of aggression originally directed externally is often observed in the playroom as an expression of anger with the therapist. The child's internal displacement of aggression can be effectively interpreted in this situation.

Strengthening Object Constancy and the Ability to Tolerate Separation. Since the abused child soon realizes that he is safe from physical attack by the therapist, his major anxieties center around fears of rejection and abandonment. These anxieties are frequently increased following provocative "acting out" behavior. Cancelled sessions, lateness, and longer interruptions in treatment by the therapist are inevitably interpreted as punitive types of rejection. The abused child often displays "hide-and-seek" behavior at this time in an attempt to master and reverse the fear of abandonment. He is intolerant of the therapist's involvement with other children and frequently manifests difficulty in leaving the playroom at the end of the session, often requesting to take home play materials. At this point, the child requires active assurance by the therapist concerning his ongoing interest despite interruptions in contact. Children at this stage of treatment may be allowed to take home token "symbols" of the therapist (drawings, pencils, candy, etc.) to promote internalization of his mental representation during his absence.

Improvement of School Performance. Most abused children of school age require psychological testing and language assessment to document specific learning disabilities. Special remedial intervention or placement in a special class might be necessary. The therapist should maintain contact with the child's teacher or guidance counselor and act as an intermediary between the child's parents and the school. The child's adjustment at school should become a major focus of the treatment. One may interpret the child's tendency to utilize classmates and teachers as targets of aggression originally directed toward the family. The parents need counseling about the child's learning disabilities, as they are prone to regard any academic difficulty as a sign of willful disobedience which requires punishment. The vicious cycle of academic failure, physical abuse, and increased disruptiveness in school must be interrupted. Better functioning in school can be an important factor in the improvement of the child's self-esteem.

REQUIREMENTS FOR A COMPREHENSIVE TREATMENT CENTER FOR ABUSED CHILDREN AND THEIR FAMILIES

The following design for a comprehensive treatment center for abused children and their families is based on the combined clinical experience of numerous child abuse treatment programs that have been recently developed in various parts of the country. The treatment modalities which have proven successful will be discussed in turn as components of the ideal treatment center. This concept has also been influenced by the author's experience in developing a comprehensive pilot treatment program for abused children and their families at the Kings County Hospital/Downstate Medical Center complex, a project that required the coordination of a great many clinical services of the medical center. This pilot program is gradually being expanded to encompass the structure and functions of the larger center.

The ideal center should offer comprehensive long-term and crisis-oriented treatment services carefully adapted to the needs of maltreated children and their families. The logical location for such a treatment facility is in a medical center. The treatment center should have a director who would coordinate component services from the departments of pediatrics, psychiatry, social service, and nursing. The treatment center would operate in liaison with the local protective service unit and the courts, and would receive referrals from these agencies.

A multidisciplinary child abuse consultation team discusses referrals and decides on an appropriate treatment intervention for each case. The consultation team makes recommendations concerning the feasibility and timing of the child's discharge, the need for home-based crisis intervention, and the suitability of the family for long-term treatment on an out-patient basis. The out-patient treatment program would consist of psychotherapy and/or counseling for the parents and children, parent group psychotherapy, family therapy, social service intervention, homemaking services, and visiting nurses. Each center operates or affiliates with a satellite day care program for infants and preschool children in maltreating families. Specialized services of the medical center especially relevant to the specific needs of the child-abuse population—such as addictive disease facilities, family medicine programs, and developmental evaluation and learning disability clinics for the abused children—are made available. Preventive intervention in high-risk families detected in prenatal and pediatric care is also provided by the treatment center. The center offers training and education to the community in the area of child abuse and neglect, a service that may be utilized by physicians, nurses, community service organizations, personnel from protective services, the courts, and the local school system.

COMPONENTS OF THE COMPREHENSIVE TREATMENT PROGRAM

Child Abuse Consultation Team (CACT)

The child abuse consultation team acts as the primary screening and evaluation unit for the referrals from the Department of Pediatrics. All suspected cases of maltreatment seen in the pediatric in-patient service, OPD, and emergency room are directed to the child-abuse consultation team, developed along the lines of the Denver model (Kempe & Helfer, 1972). It includes professionals from the several departments in the hospital concerned with the diagnosis, treatment, and long-term rehabilitation of abused and neglected children and their families. The child abuse consultation team (CACT) should consist of an attending pediatrician, a radiologist, a pediatric social worker, a pediatric nurse, and a full-time team coordinator and legal consultant.

The *pediatrician* acts as a consultant to the emergency room and to staff physicians and nurses. He collects historical data, interprets physical findings and laboratory results, and maintains communication with the family, protective agency personnel, and community workers. He also coordinates follow-up medical care and chairs the dispositional conference.

The *radiologist*, who has special expertise in pediatric radiology, aids in the diagnosis of child abuse. He interprets x-ray findings and acts as a consultant to the pediatric staff. He also determines the most appropriate radiological procedures for each case.

The *pediatric social worker* develops a relationship with the family and, if possible, assesses the family psychodynamics through careful observation and the subtle gathering of information. He maintains contact with the medical staff, child protective agency personnel, and various social agencies that might be involved with the family and also makes an assessment of the immediate and long-term requirements of each family with respect to medical care, child care, household management, financial assistance, counseling and psychiatric treatment, etc.

The *pediatric nurse* develops a relationship with the hospitalized children and their families. She observes the contact between child and family during hospital visits and notes the interactions of child and family with the hospital staff and fellow patients. She discusses the social and psychological aspects of the family situation with the nursing staff and acts as a liaison between them.

The *team coordinator:*

1. Establishes an early and on-going relationship with children suspected of maltreatment and their parents in an effort to (1) provide families with information regarding the status and expected progress of legal and medical procedures undertaken in their case, and (2) communicate the parent's wishes and needs to members of the child-abuse consultation team.
2. Meets frequently and as often as is necessary with members of the CACT so that the entire team is aware of existing case-related problems and the measures formulated to solve them.
3. Promotes as speedy and thorough an evaluation and disposition of instances of child abuse and neglect as possible.
4. Consults with all appropriate outside agencies and individuals as indicated by the nature of each particular case.
5. Reports regularly to the CACT regarding the problems encountered in evaluating and arranging disposition of cases of child abuse and neglect.
6. Maintains a file of cases and suspected cases of child abuse and neglect and issues periodic reports indicating the number of families evaluated and the results of the evaluations. In providing these liaison and specific services, it is hoped that the coordinator might also increase the parent's motivation to enter the therapeutic program.

In addition to the above-mentioned CACT representatives from the Demonstration Center Treatment Staff, a *child psychiatrist* and a *psychiatric social worker* serve both as members of the team and as members of the Screening and Evaluation Unit of the Treatment Program, along with the program director. They act as the major link between the CACT and the Treatment Program. Subsequent to confirmation of abuse or neglect, the psychiatric social worker from the Treatment Program's Screening and Evaluation Team implements each referral by contacting the family and arranging for an evaluation. If a child has been hospitalized because of the severity of his injuries or his need for protection, the evaluation is conducted prior to the child's return to the home.

SCREENING AND EVALUATION UNIT OF THE TREATMENT PROGRAM

This unit, consisting of numerous clinical staff members of the treatment program (psychiatrist, psychologists, social workers), is directed by the screening committee composed of the program director, child psychiatrist, and psychiatric social worker. In addition to referrals from the Pediatric and Psychiatric in- and out-patient services, this unit will receive additional referrals from child protective services, family court, neighboring hospitals, voluntary child care agencies, and the local public schools.

Families screened by the Child Abuse Team undergo a thorough psychiatric and psychological evaluation with consultation from other departments, e.g., neurology, available when necessary. The evaluation consists of a diagnostic interview with either or both parents and the abused child, as well as a social service investigation into the family's psychosocial history. The family's current living situation is assessed through home visits by a member of the program's social work staff.

Following the evaluation, the screening committee recommends one of three plans for the abused child and his family:

1. Child and family are amenable and appropriate for the treatment program and assigned to either the out-patient schoolage component or the day-care component contingent upon the age of the abused child.
2. Child and family do not warrant or would not profit from on-going treatment at this time; however, crisis intervention in the form of parent counseling, visiting nurse, concrete social work intervention (e.g., contacting the school guidance counselor) would be useful.
3. Family is not amenable to comprehensive treatment but would be more appropriately followed by another specialized agency, e.g., the Developmental Evaluation Clinic. Referrals are followed up to ensure that they are implemented or, in cases where the parents refuse to cooperate, to enlist the assistance of the child protective service agency.

All treated, schoolage abused children are assigned to the Child Psychiatry Staff for intensive psychotherapy, while their parents receive either individual or group therapy. Parents of preschoolers similarly receive either one or both of these modalities.

Day Care Center for Preschool Abused Children

A day care program for abused infants and preschool children can serve the following objectives:

1. It relieves the mother's burden of child care for 6 to 8 hours daily, simultaneously reducing the likelihood of physical abuse when the child is at home.
2. The program serves as a focus for the parent's involvement in the adult treatment program.
3. In reducing the risk for repeated abuse, it allows vulnerable preschool children who might otherwise require institutional or foster care to remain at home.
4. This type of program provides an invaluable source of information regarding the impact of physical abuse on the earliest psychological and developmental processes. It will also permit the observation and analysis of the crucial interaction between the abusing mother and the abused child.

The value of such a day care program for preschool abused children has been documented by Galdston (1971), who organized a Parent's Center Project in Boston. The day care program is staffed by full-time paraprofessionals and mother surrogates, supervised by a child psychiatrist and a psychiatric social worker.

In addition to the structured milieu of the regular day care playrooms, staffed by a teacher and paraprofessionals, each preschool abused child is assigned to a treatment program staff member for observation of his daily activities. The therapeutic components of the day care program consist of regular supervision of mother-child interaction by a treatment staff member (psychiatrist, psychologist, social worker) and consultation to the day care teachers and paraprofessionals.

The treatment staff provides other therapeutic services such as referrals to Pediatrics, Developmental Evaluation Clinic, or Child Psychiatry. The day care center may also become the site for mothers' group therapy and family therapy.

The educational components consist of seminars on child development with special emphasis on the needs of the preschool child for the day care staff. Classes on infant care and early development are presented to the mothers. The educational input is coordinated by the psychiatrist in charge of the day care program.

Periodic development testing of all children may be performed in order to evaluate the effect of the treatment program on their psychological growth and development.

Crisis intervention is considered to be an integral part of the treatment program for both the preschool and schoolage children and their families. Home visits will be arranged on a routine basis as well as for emergencies.

The day care program facilities may be extended to abused preschool children in temporary placement. The therapeutic efforts with their mothers are designed for the strengthening of maternal functions. Arranging limited supervised contact between mother and child in the day care setting can be beneficial to the mother in enhancing the understanding of her child and her acquisition of more appropriate child-rearing techniques. This controlled reexposure of the abused preschooler to his mother will also serve as a gauge of the mother's progress toward regaining full responsibility for the care of the child.

OUT-PATIENT TREATMENT CENTER FOR SCHOOLAGE CHILDREN AND THEIR FAMILIES

This component provides schoolage children and their families with more definitive psychiatric evaluation and treatment. The child's evaluation consists of a developmental history, mental status, and psychological testing. If needed, pediatric and neurological evaluations are arranged through the Department of Pediatrics. Evaluation of the parent(s) consists of a psychiatric examination with psychological testing when deemed necessary. Evaluation of the mother includes an observation of the mother-child interaction. The children receive moderately intensive (two sessions per week) short-term (1 to 2 years) psychotherapy with child psychiatrists. Their parents are assigned to a psychiatric social worker for supportive psychotherapy and the active provision of social services in collaboration with the psychiatrist. Parents with more severe forms of psychiatric impairment are treated by a psychiatrist.

EVALUATION AND REFERRAL SERVICE

Other abused and neglected children and their families who might be unsuitable for the treatment program may receive psychiatric evaluation and social service support, including crisis intervention. They may be referred to various services of the medical center appropriate to their needs, i.e., pediatric neurology, developmental evaluation clinic, addictive disease hospital, family planning, etc. Others might receive crisis intervention while awaiting an opening in the treatment program.

GROUP THERAPY

Group therapy is available to some mothers receiving individual psychotherapy as an additional therapeutic modality, or it may be offered as the major form of treatment to some of the mothers not involved in a one-to-one therapeutic relationship. Mothers' groups may operate in both the day care facility and in the out-patient treatment facility. Group therapy for both parents, or for fathers exclusively, might be appropriate for certain families.

Groups are led by treatment staff members who are experienced in group psychodynamics and treatment. If possible, two leaders, a male and female, are assigned to each group, in order to replicate a family constellation with two parents. Group therapy can be useful to abusing parents in the following ways: It may act as a bridge to therapeutic involvement in extremely defensive and mistrustful parents who are threatened by a one-to-one relationship. The realization that their problems are shared by others tends to diminish their guilt and low self-esteem. The permissive atmosphere of frank and open discussion facilitates the expression of long-suppressed personal feelings and reduces vulnerability to criticism. Finally, the establishment of personal ties with other group members fosters social contact with others. Group therapy is often the treatment of choice for abusing fathers, who are notoriously reluctant to seek help because of their difficulty in acknowledging passive-dependent wishes.

Self-help groups, such as Parents Anonymous, have been beneficial to individuals who are more comfortable in a peer-group milieu divorced from an organized treatment center. This type of group might also serve as an after-care facility in the community for those parents who have successfully terminated their out-patient treatment.

Homemaker Services

Homemaking assistance and home visits are provided by female homemakers who are assigned on the basis of family needs and receptivity. Mothers overburdened with the care of infants and preschool children might derive the greatest benefit from this service. The homemaking is integrated into the entire treatment program of the involved family, and the homemakers receive supervision and training from the psychiatric and social work staff. The presence of a homemaker might be pivotal in keeping a family intact during a crisis.

Parent Aide Program

The successful use of parent aides or "lay therapists" with abusing families was first described by Kempe and Helfer (1972). Parent aides are assigned to certain families in which the mother's social isolation, maternal deprivation, immaturity, and failure to develop maternal feelings are outstanding. The parent aides are usually mature women who have mothered successfully. They try to develop a noncritical, supportive relationship with the abusive mothers and act as maternal role models. Parent-aides are trained by the psychiatric and social work staff and their intervention is integrated into the overall treatment program of the involved family. If possible, parent aides and abusing parents should be matched according to socioeconomic level.

Nursing Intervention

Nursing intervention is an integral part of the treatment program for abusing and neglecting families. The nurses carry out the following functions during home visits:

1. physical assessment of the children;
2. consultation regarding physical illness of both children and adult family members, and eventually referral to medical specialists;
3. basic child care education to the parents including knowledge of the various stages of normal child development, assessment of developmental abnormality, information about feeding practices, nutrition, and home enrichment.
4. supervision of medical care in case of illness of a family member, e.g., supervising medication or help with special medical management, e.g., changing bandages, application of medical appliances.

The nurses also act as instructors in a parent education program carried out in the OPD or day care setting. This program makes use of audiovisual equipment and materials.

Family intervention as practiced by the nurses is under the overall supervision of the treatment team consisting of the psychiatrist and social worker. If the treatment program is located in a hospital or medical center affiliated with a nursing school, student nurses may participate in the program as an elective during their training. A singular advantage of utilizing students lies in their youth, enthusiasm, and capacity to provide assistance with child care without evoking the image of the "critical mother" which usually occurs when an older woman intervenes in the home.

Intervention During Placement of Children

Far too often, placement of maltreated children in foster homes or institutions has become the expedient solution for overburdened and understaffed child protective facilities in large reporting areas. The basic difficulties in adjustment facing the three major participants in the placement process have usually been ignored by the involved agencies.

The *maltreating parents* often receive no counseling or rehabilitation to help them prepare for the ultimate return of their children. Left to their own devices, these parents become depressed following their experience of humiliation and loss, and many of the mothers become pregnant within the year after removal of their children. The new infants will obviously be at-risk for future scapegoating, role reversal, and abuse.

The *maltreated children* are traumatized by the forced separation from their families, and they face formidable problems in adjusting to unfamiliar foster parents and siblings. Their severe psychopathology increases the likelihood of an unsatisfactory placement experience. These children are notoriously prone to frequent changes in foster placement.

The *foster parents*, who are equally susceptible to the "rescue fantasies" manifested by the treatment staff, are often unaware of the difficulties posed by abused children. The numerous problems these children present are often minimized by the foster care agencies.

The facilities of the treatment program are, therefore, made available to abusing families from which the children have been temporarily removed to foster care. The main goal of treatment is the reversal of the pathological child-rearing climate so the children can ultimately return home.

The abused children are provided with day care or out-patient psychiatric treatment during their placement with the emphasis on solving their problems of separation, foster care adjustment, and eventual reintroduction to their original homes.

The foster parents receive counseling regarding the specific management problems of the abused children and their relationship with the natural parents.

HOT-LINE

A "hot-line" is available for the use of all participants in the treatment program on a 24-hour basis. The hot-line is handled by one of the permanent members of the treatment staff, therefore assuring continuity of case management as well as the immediate knowledge of the patient's prior history. This leads to effective intervention in a particular crisis.

The hot-line may be considered a rehabilitative mechanism within the treatment program context only. Based upon the perceived need of the client at the time of the call and the resources available, it is immediately determined which services are required on a crisis basis.

In addition to providing any of the services available within the treatment center, the hot-line has been observed to have an anxiety-reducing effect upon the program participants, thereby facilitating both rapport and therapeutic intervention.

VOCATIONAL REHABILITATION

The social work staff assesses the vocational needs and capabilities of the parents of the abused children. Parents are encouraged to improve current vocational skills or learn new ones when appropriate. The staff may also assist the parents in seeking employment and continuing their education. Liaison is established with the local Department of Vocational Rehabilitation in order to provide job training for those parents exhibiting psychiatric or physical impairment.

SCHOOL CONSULTATION

The treatment staff consults with the teachers and guidance counselors of the schoolage abused children, and with child care personnel in cases of infants and young children attending day care centers. The treatment staff gathers detailed information about the child's school performance and behavior and provides consultation regarding classroom management and special class placement. The staff also assumes an educational role with the parents of local school districts by providing them with information about child abuse and neglect through meetings and discussion groups.

LEARNING DISABILITY CENTER

This center, part of the Department of Pediatrics or Child Psychiatry, is frequently utilized as a referral service to schoolage abused children whose overall impairment usually precludes normal academic performance. The center operates after school hours and provides psychoeducational testing, diagnosis of specific learning disabilities, and special educational rehabilitation for these impairments.

LEGAL ASSISTANCE

The legal consultant secures rights not generally accorded without legal thrust, most specifically direct services such as housing and increased welfare benefits when applicable. In this manner, the legal assistant, as a provider of direct services, is viewed by the parent as an integral member of the treatment team. He or she does not participate in court-related activities of the parents.

Training and Education

A significant function of the treatment staff is the training and education of professionals, paraprofessionals, and students in the fields of medicine, pediatrics, psychiatry, social work, nursing, education, psychology, child development, homemaking, child protection, and the law.

PREVENTION OF CHILD ABUSE

Our ideal objective in studying and treating child abuse on a nationwide scale is, as with any major public health problem, the development of a strategy for prevention. Thus far, early case finding and protective intervention in abusing families have been the primary areas of interest for workers in this field. As more basic knowledge is accumulated about the child-abuse syndrome through clinical experience and research, one can envision a logical shift in focus from treatment and rehabilitation (secondary prevention) to primary intervention. There are several types of preventive measures which may be utilized on a large scale to reduce the abusive potential of a given population.

General Educational Programs

Our society's inadequate preparation for infant and child care has been revealed by the enormous popularity of "how to" books about children and child rearing. With the demise of the extended family in this country, Spock and other child-rearing specialists have replaced grandparents among the general public as the traditional source of wisdom about raising children. Educational programs concerned with child development and parenting, therefore, might satisfy a basic need of our society. Socioeconomically and educationally deprived segments of the population might particularly benefit from such programs. The subject matter could be introduced into the high-school curriculum and might be presented to the parent population through adult education programs, community organizations, religious groups, day care centers, and obstetric and pediatric clinics. These programs would include information about community resources for child care, and provide education about child abuse and neglect.

Identification of Families at-Risk for Child Abuse

There have been recent attempts to develop predictive questionnaires for the identification of abuse-prone parents (Schneider, Pollock, & Helfer, 1972). When perfected, these instruments will be able to identify parents most likely to become abusive. Research is currently in progress at the Downstate Medical Center (Green et al., 1975) designed to develop instruments for predicting parental abuse proneness, environmental stress, and the child's vulnerability for abuse. The first two variables will be assessed by questionnaires, and the last by a rating of neonatal deviancy.

With recent advances in clinical and theoretical understanding of the child-abuse syndrome, experienced professionals are now capable of identifying high-risk parents, vulnerable children, and a stressful environment through careful interviewing, mother-child observation, and home evaluation.

Predictive questionnaires and interview techniques could be routinely deployed in prenatal clinics, obstetric wards, and pediatric clinics as a screening device to identify families at-risk for child abuse.

Preventive Intervention

Once the high-risk family has been identified, an appropriate intervention strategy can be developed according to the relative contributions of each potentiating factor. For example, if a mother exhibits a typical abuse-prone background and personality and is experiencing considerable environmental stress during visits to a prenatal clinic, a visiting nurse might be assigned to the family after the mother gives birth. The situation would entail an even greater potential for abuse if this mother gave birth to a vulnerable "high-risk" child requiring a greater amount of care or viewed as different or unsatisfying due to a physical or congenital abnormality.

This conceptual model could be especially effective in that it identifies those factors that figure most prominently in the abusive process and thus allows preventive interventions to be employed where they will have the greatest impact. For example, if parental personality variables were found to be more significant than either child deviancy or stress, psychotherapy or casework might be considered the treatment of choice. If, on the other hand, family stresses were found to have made the greatest contribution, the deployment of parent aides, homemakers, or visiting nurses in the home could present a more effective intervention. Kempe and Helfer (1972) describe the routine placement of health visitors (visiting nurses) in Aberdeen, Scotland, in all homes following the birth of a child. These nurses are trained to identify families at-risk for abuse.

REFERENCES

ADELSON, L. Slaughter of the innocents: A study of forty-six homicides in which the victims were children. *New England Journal of Medicine*, 1961 *264*, 1345–1349.

ALLEN, H., TEN BENSEL, R., and RAILE, R. The battered child syndrome. *Minnesota Medicine*, 1969, *52*, 155–156.

BENNIE, E. H., and SCLARE, A. B. The battered child syndrome. *American Journal of Psychiatry*, 1969, *125*, 975–979.

BESHAROV, D. Child Abuse Rate called "Epidemic." *The New York Times*, November 30, 1975.

COHEN, M., RAPHLING, D., and GREEN, P. Psychological aspects of the maltreatment syndrome of childhood. *Journal of Pediatrics*, 1966, *69*, 279–284.

DEFRANCIS, V. The status of child protective services. In C. H. Kempe and R. E. Helfer (Eds.), *Helping the battered child and his family*. Philadelphia: J. B. Lippincott, 1972.

ELMER, E. Identification of Abused Children, *Children* 1963 *10*, 180–184.

ELMER, E. The fifty families study: Summary of phase I, neglected and abused children and their families. Children's Hospital of Pittsburgh, Pa., 1965.

ELMER, E. *Children in jeopardy: A study of abused minors and their families*. Pittsburgh: University of Pittsburgh Press, 1967.

ERIKSON, E. H. *Childhood and society*. New York: Norton, 1950.

FEINSTEIN, H., PAUL, N. and PETTISON, E. Group therapy for mothers with infanticide impulses. *American Journal of Psychiatry*, 1964, *120*, 882–886.

FONTANA, V. *The maltreated child*. Springfield Illinois: Charles C. Thomas, 1964.

FREUD, S. *Beyond the pleasure principle* (std. ed., Vol. 18). London: Hogarth Press, 1955. (Originally published, 1920).

GALDSTON, R. Observations on children who have been physically abused and their parents. *American Journal of Psychiatry*, 1965, *122*, 440–443.

GALDSTON, R. Violence begins at home. *Journal of the American Academy of Child Psychiatry*, 1971, *10*, 336–350.

GIL, D. Incidence of child abuse and demographic characteristics of persons involved. In R.E. Helfer and C. H. Kempe (Eds.), *The battered child*. Chicago: University of Chicago Press, 1968.

GIL, D. *Violence against children*. Cambridge: Harvard University Press, 1970.

GIL, D. *A holistic perspective on child abuse and its prevention*. Paper presented at the Conference on Research on Child Abuse, National Institute of Child Health and Human Development, 1974.

GREEN, A. H. Self-destructive behavior in physically abused schizophrenic children. *Archives of General Psychiatry*, 1968, *19*, 171–179.

GREEN, A. H. A psychodynamic approach to the

study and treatment of child abusing parents. *Journal of the American Academy of Child Psychiatry*, 1976, *15*, 414–429. (a)

GREEN, A. H. *Child abusing fathers.* Unpublished manuscript, 1976. (b)

GREEN, A. H. *Self-destructive behavior in battered children.* Unpublished manuscript, 1976. (c)

GREEN, A. H., GAINES, R., and SANDGRUND, A. Child abuse: Pathological syndrome of family interaction. *American Journal of Psychiatry*, 1974, *131*, 882–886.

GREEN, A. H., GAINES, R., and SANDGRUND, A. Identification and definition of factors causally associated with child abuse and neglect. (DHEW Grant No. 90-C-421). Washington, D.C.: Office of Child Development, 1975.

GREEN, A. H., SANDGRUND, A., GAINES, R., and HABERFELD, H. *Psychological sequelae of child abuse and neglect.* Paper presented at the 127th annual meeting of the American Psychiatric Association, Detroit, May 1974.

HELFER, R. E. The diagnostic process and treatment programs. (DHEW publication No. (OHD) 75-69). Washington, D.C.: U.S. Department of Health, Education and Welfare, National Center for Child Abuse and Neglect, 1975.

HELFER, R. E., and KEMPE, C. H. (Eds.). *The battered child.* Chicago: University of Chicago Press, 1968.

HOLMES, T., and RAHE, R. The social readjustment rating scale. *Journal of Psychosomatic Medicine*, 1967, *11*, 213–218.

HOLTER, J., and FRIEDMAN, S. Principles of management in child abuse cases. *American Journal of Orthopsychiatry*, 1968, *38*, 127–136.

JOHNSON, B., and MORSE, H. Injured children and their parents. *Children*, 1968, *15*, 147–152.

JUSTICE, B., and DUNCAN, D. *Child abuse as a work-related problem.* Paper presented at American Public Health Association, Chicago, November 1975.

JUSTICE, B., and JUSTICE, R. *The abusing family.* Unpublished manuscript, 1975.

KEMPE, C. H. A practical approach to the protection of the abused child and rehabilitation of the abusing parent. *Pediatrics*, 1973, *51*(4), Part II Suppl., 804–809.

KEMPE, C. H., and HELFER, R. E. (Eds.). *Helping the battered child and his family.* Philadelphia: J. B. Lippincott, 1972.

KEMPE, C. H., SILVERMAN, F., STEELE, B., DROEGEMUELLER, W., and SILVER, H. The battered child syndrome. *Journal of the American Medical Association*, 1962 *181*, 17–24.

KHAN, M. The concept of cumulative trauma. In *The Psychoanalytic Study of the Child*, New York: International Universities Press, 1963, *18*, 286–306.

LIGHT, R. J. Abused and neglected children in America: A study of alternative policies. *Harvard Educational Review*, 1973, *43*, 556–598.

MARTIN, H. The child and his development. In C. H. Kempe and R. E. Helfer (Eds.), *Helping the battered child and his family.* Philadelphia: J. B. Lippincott, 1972.

MERRILL, E. Physical abuse of children: An agency study. In V. DeFrancis (Ed.), *Protecting the battered child.* Denver: American Humane Association, 1962.

MORRIS, M., and GOULD, R. Role reversal: A necessary concept in dealing with the battered child syndrome. *American Journal of Orthopsychiatry*, 1963, *33*, 298–299.

MORSE, W., SAHLER, O. J., and FRIEDMAN, S. B. A three-year follow-up study of abused and neglected children. *American Journal of Diseases of Children*, 1970, *120*, 439–446.

NAGI, S. Child abuse and neglect programs: A national overview (DHEW publication 75-14). *Children Today*, May-June 1975, 13–17.

New York City Central Registry for Child Abuse, 1974.

OVIATT, B. After child abuse reporting legislation—what? In C. H. Kempe and R. E. Helfer (Eds.), *Helping the battered child and his family.* Philadelphia: J. B. Lippincott, 1972.

PAULSON, M., and BLAKE, P. The physically abused child: A focus on prevention. *Child Welfare* 1969, *48*, 86–95.

POLLOCK, C., and STEELE, B. A therapeutic approach to parents. In C. H. Kempe and R. E. Helfer (Eds.), *Helping the battered child and his family*. Philadelphia: J. B. Lippincott, 1972.

SABBETH, J. The suicidal adolescent. *Journal of the American Academy of Child Psychiatry*, 1969, *8*, 272–286.

SANDGRUND, A., GAINES, R., and GREEN, A. H. Child abuse and mental retardation: A problem of cause and effect. *American Journal of Mental Deficiency*, 1974, *79*, 327–330.

SCHNEIDER, C., HELFER R., and POLLOCK, C. The predictive questionnaire; preliminary report. In C. H. Kempe and R. E. Helfer (Eds) *Helping the battered child and his family*. Philadelphia: J. B. Lippincott, 1972.

SIMONS, B., DOWNS, E., HURSTER, M., and ARCHER, M. Child abuse. *New York State Journal of Medicine*, 1966, *66*, 2783–2788.

SPINETTA, J., and RIGLER, D. The child abusing parent: A psychological review. *Psychological Bulletin*, 1972, *77*, 296–304.

STEELE, B. Parental abuse of infants and small children. In E. Anthony and T. Benedek (Eds.), *Parenthood: Its psychology and psychopathology*. Boston: Little, Brown & Co., 1970.

STEELE, B., and POLLOCK, C. A psychiatric study of parents who abuse infants and small children. In R. E. Helfer and C. H. Kempe (Eds.), *The battered child*, Chicago: University of Chicago Press, 1968.

YOUNG, L. *Wednesday's children: A study of child neglect and abuse*. New York: McGraw-Hill, 1964.

INDEX

AUTHOR INDEX

SUBJECT INDEX